CLINICAL AND DIAGNOSTIC VETERINARY TOXICOLOGY

CLINICAL AND DIAGNOSTIC VETERINARY TOXICOLOGY

SECOND EDITION

EDITED BY GARY A. VAN GELDER

William B. Buck, D.V.M., M.S.

College of Veterinary Medicine
University of Illinois
Urbana, Illinois

Gary D. Osweiler, D.V.M., M.S., Ph.D.

Gary A. Van Gelder, D.V.M., M.S., Ph.D.

Veterinary Anatomy—Physiology
University of Missouri
Columbia, Missouri

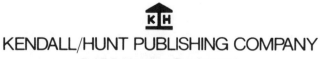

KENDALL/HUNT PUBLISHING COMPANY
2460 Kerper Boulevard,
Dubuque, Iowa 52001

ISBN 0–8403–0720–9

Fourth Printing, 1982

C   400720   07

CONTENTS

PREFACE
FIRST EDITION

In 1965, the Toxicology Section of the Veterinary Diagnostic Laboratory, Iowa State University, assumed responsibility for teaching toxicology in the professional curriculum of veterinary medicine. The authors began preparing handouts pertaining to the various toxicants as teaching aids. In 1971, these handouts were collated and copyrighted as *Veterinary Toxicology Notes*. The demand for these notes by practicing veterinarians and instructors in other colleges of veterinary medicine throughout the United States soon exhausted our supply. *Clinical and Diagnostic Veterinary Toxicology* is a product of the notes, with most of the sections having been completely rewritten.

This publication is directed primarily toward the veterinary student and the practicing veterinarian. It is not a complete textbook on veterinary toxicology nor is that its purpose, since at least two other such publications are now in existence. We have allotted considerable space to clinical and diagnostic aspects of veterinary toxicology. It is, no doubt, more complete in its discussion of chemical toxicants encountered in feed-grain, livestock-producing areas of the United States. We have not attempted to include all the toxic plants, since there are several excellent publications on this subject.

We have included actual case histories taken from our files in the discussion of many of the common toxicants in veterinary medicine. Also, we have provided perforated worksheets with problems and questions which can be used by the instructor or the student for self-evaluation. The authors encourage the reader to work the problems and answer the questions. We have purposefully not supplied the answers in order to make them of value to an instructor wishing to use them for teaching and evaluating purposes.

We wish to thank Dr. Vaughn A. Seaton, Head, Veterinary Diagnostic Laboratory, Iowa State University, for his support and cooperation in the development of the Toxicology Section. One usually thinks of a diagnostic laboratory as being only service oriented. With Doctor Seaton's support and encouragement, the research and teaching aspects of veterinary toxicology have been closely coordinated with the diagnostic service work. It is from the field cases that we have gained most of our personal knowledge in the field of veterinary toxicology. Questions and hypotheses regarding various toxicants have come through our work with field problems. These have provided excellent topics for research proposals and for training of veterinarians in the specialty of toxicology.

We especially thank Mrs. Judy Berndt and Miss Ginger Horak for typing the manuscript and editorial assistance. Special recognition is due Dr. W. E. Lloyd, Professor of Veterinary Toxicology, ISU, for writing the sections on sulfonamides and nitrofurans. We also appreciate the valuable criticism and suggestions offered by numerous colleagues.

W. B. Buck

G. D. Osweiler

G. A. Van Gelder

PREFACE
SECOND EDITION

The second edition of *Clinical and Diagnostic Veterinary Toxicology* continues the ten-year tradition of constant revision and updating. Although the three authors are currently employed in two colleges of veterinary medicine, they have pooled their expriences, knowledge and ideas in writing this second edition.

The primary emphasis remains the same, namely, to present pertinent current knowledge on chemical toxicants of significance to livestock production and the welfare of companion animals. The second edition includes information published after the manuscript for the first edition was completed. Most of the chapters have been revised and updated.

More information on the fundamental principles of toxicology has been included. The general population is becoming increasingly aware of the potential harmful effects of the many compounds encountered daily. The questions being asked are more sophisticated and probing. In many instances it is no longer sufficient to just identify the cause of disease or death but questions are raised as to how and why. Residue and contamination problems are frequently encountered that require a firm understanding of the basic concepts, toxicology, metabolism and excretion kinetics. A chapter has been added to provide background information on the types of tests used to evaluate the toxicity and safety of commercial products.

Other new chapters are: Dose-Response Relationships; Iodine; Plant Teratogens; Polybrominated Biphenyls and a chapter on Miscellaneous Rodenticides which includes alpha-chloralose, castrix, norbormide, red squill and vacor.

For the first time some photographs have been included. More graphs and tables have been used to better present data and concepts.

The presentations of the toxicology of insecticides and fungicides has been expanded and new compounds included. These are areas of rapidly changing information as new products are introduced into industry and agriculture. The section on insecticides has been divided into three chapters for easier reference. More information on the lesions and clinical signs of mercury toxicosis is included. The chapters on arsenic have been reorganized emphasizing compounds with similar biologic effects. The chapter on lead has been expanded to include more data on background residues and levels associated with toxicosis.

The second edition, like the first, is intended for use by veterinary students in toxicology, teachers of toxicology, practicing toxicologists and by practicing veterinarians who deal with both large and small animal toxicoses. Each chapter is designed for reference use through the use of headings including source, toxicity, mechanism of action, clinical signs, physiopathology, diagnosis, and treatment. Important literature citations are included at the end of each chapter.

The authors thank their colleagues who found errors in the first edition and were kind enough to write and tell us.

Special recognition is extended to Dr. W. E. Lloyd, Professor of Veterinary Toxicology, Iowa State University, for the chapters on sulfonamides and nitrofurans; and to Mr. Arden E. Shenker, Attorney at Law, Portland, Oregon, for the chapter on medical-legal toxicology. Mr. Shenker has experience with the legal aspects of veterinary toxicology problems and very graciously accepted the invitation to provide this chapter.

We appreciate the valuable criticism and suggestions offered by numerous colleagues.

G. A. Van Gelder
G. D. Osweiler
W. B. Buck

Concepts and
Basic Toxicology

INTRODUCTION

Clinical and Diagnostic Veterinary Toxicology has been written primarily for the veterinary student, veterinary toxicologist and the veterinary practitioner. It is intended to supplement the several books available on veterinary toxicology. Toxicologic problems that commonly occur in food animal production and the maintenance of companion animals are emphasized. The fact that the authors are located in the Midwest influences the types of problems encountered in their practice of veterinary toxicology and consequently, the contents of this book.

Basic information on dose-response and types of toxicology tests conducted on new compounds to determine safety and toxicity has been included so that the student has some idea of the type of information available and how it is obtained.

Terminology

Toxicology can be defined as the knowledge of poisons, including their chemical properities, identification, biologic effects and treatment of disease conditions caused by poisons. This simple definition readily points out the broad background needed by a clinical veterinary toxicologist. The *clinical veterinary toxicologist* is a veterinarian who has specialized training and experience with the various chemical substances, forms of energy and poisonous substances produced by plants and animals that may be the direct cause of disease conditions in animals under veterinary care. As such, he freely uses his knowledge of physiology and pathology to separate the normal from the abnormal. He also draws on his clinical medicine and infectious disease training to differentiate infectious diseases and metabolic conditions from those caused by poisons. Pharmacology and toxicology share many common interests including biodynamics of uptake and elimination, mechanisms of action, principles of treatment, and dose-response relationships. Some therapeutic drugs can also become poisons under certain conditions of use and both the pharmacologist and toxicologist share in-

terest in adverse drug reactions. The veterinary toxicologist, however, is also concerned with a wide variety of agricultural chemicals, feed additives, environmental contaminants, ionizing radiation, poisonous gases and poisons of plant and animal origin that may adversely affect the health of animals.

There are many specialty areas within the broad scope of toxicology, and consequently there is a wide variety of backgrounds among professional toxicologists. Some toxicologists are concerned with safety testing of new drugs and industrial and agricultural chemicals. The increased public awareness of possible deleterious effects of drugs and chemicals has resulted in greater emphasis on toxicology testing prior to release and use of new substances. Other toxicologists are involved in industrial and environmental health both in research and practice. The current emphasis on the effects of pollution has brought about a large expansion in environmental toxicology. Toxicologists are also employed by governmental agencies in supervisory, regulatory and research roles. Still another major area of toxicology is in clinical medicine. Clinical toxicologists specialize in the diagnosis and treatment of poisonings, and also frequently become involved in medicolegal aspects. The clinical veterinary toxicologist is a veterinarian and also a specialist in the cause, identification and treatment of animal poisonings. Other toxicologists may have background training in human medicine, pharmacology, physiology, pathology and chemistry. It is difficult to draw distinct lines between one academic area and another. The study and practice of toxicology is a prime example of the need for and utility of integrating traditional academic medical specialties and applying the total sum of this knowledge and experience toward the solving of practical problems.

A *poison,* as the term is used in this book, is any solid, liquid or gas that when introduced into or applied to the body can interfere with the life processes of cells of the organism by its own inherent qualities without acting mechanically and irrespective of temperature. Another term for poison is *toxicant.* Since the term poison

3

has acquired a harsh meaning as a result of its historic usage, some people prefer to talk about toxicants rather than poisons. This is particularly true when the substance being considered is intended for use as a feed additive, agricultural chemical or a therapeutic drug and only becomes a poison when used incorrectly or when used under special circumstances.

Poisons may be of biologic origin such as tetrodotoxin, nicotine, or botulism toxin; may be the result of some physical process such as carbon monoxide resulting from incomplete combustion of hydrocarbon fuels; may be a naturally occurring chemical element such as lead; or may be manufactured chemicals or drugs such as insecticides and feed additives. The term *toxin* is usually reserved to describe poisons that originate from biologic processes and are generally classified as *biotoxins*. Some examples of biotoxins are *zootoxins* (animal origin); *bacterial toxins*, which are subdivided into endotoxins and exotoxins; and *phytotoxins* (plant origin). In describing the effects of a poison on a living system the term *toxic* is used. For example, one might describe the toxic effect of warfarin in dogs as being anticoagulation. The term toxicity is often misused for toxic. It is incorrect to speak of the toxicity of parathion as being excessive salivation. The exessive salivation is a toxic effect of parathion and a dog poisoned with parathion would be described as suffering from parathion toxicosis. Thus, the term *toxicosis* is used to describe the disease state which results from exposure to a poison or toxicant. *Toxicity* refers to the amount of poison that under a specific set of conditions will cause toxic effects or stated another way, will result in detrimental biologic changes. For mammals *toxicites* are usually expressed as the mg of toxicant per kg body weight required to produce the stated biologic effect. For example, the amount of parathion required to kill 50 precent of a group of rats (i.e., the LD_{50}) is 5 mg/kg. Simply stated then, the LD_{50} toxicity of parathion in rats is 5 mg/kg. However, the literature, especially the older literature, contains numerous reports where the toxicity is expressed on the basis of "adult steers" or "young calves" without adequate reference to the weight or age of the animals. This has been unavoidable in some reports of field observations. Such data is of limited use because it is very difficult to apply to similar situations. If there is one common value of the toxicity of compounds that allows comparison with other compounds it is the acute oral LD_{50} in the laboratory rat. The LD_{50} value is usually based on the effects of a single oral exposure with the rats observed for several days after the chemical is administered. Usually the successive dosage levels are spaced at logarithmic or geometric intervals. The end point is death and the published LD_{50} value says nothing about the severity of clinical signs observed in the surviving rats. You would expect to use twenty or more animals in order to arrive at a good estimate of the LD_{50}. It is this reason that prohibits the determination of LD_{50} values in most animals of economic significance.

In other species such as birds or fish the oral toxicity is often expressed on the basis of the concentration of the substance in the feed or water. The acute oral toxicity for birds is expressed as the LC_{50}, meaning the mg of compound per kg of feed. For fish, the LC_{50} refers to the concentration of toxicant in the water.

There are other terms used in the literature to define toxicity of compounds. The *highest nontoxic dose* (HNTD) is the largest dose that does not result in hematologic, chemical, clinical or pathologic drug induced alterations. The *toxic dose-low* (TDL) is the lowest dose to produce drug induced alterations and administering twice this dose will not result in lethality. The *toxic dose-high* (TDH) is the dose which will produce drug induced alterations and administering twice this dose will result in lethality. The *lethal dose* (LD) is the lowest dose that causes drug induced deaths in any animals during the period of observation. Various percentages can be attached to the LD value to indicate doses required to kill 1 percent (LD_1), 50 percent (LD_{50}) or 100 percent (LD_{100}) of the test animals.

Another term occasionally used is MTD. Some use it to mean *maximum tolerated dose* and others use it to mean *minimal toxic dose*.

Acute toxicity is a term usually reserved to mean the effects of a single dose or multiple doses during a twenty-four-hour period. The toxic effects may become apparent over a period of several days or weeks. *Chronic toxicity* refers to effects produced by prolonged exposure with the duration of exposure being three months or longer. These definitions obviously leave a large gap between one day and ninety days. Some use the term subchronic to define this time period while others avoid the problem by stating the time, such as the fourteen-day toxicity was 5 mg/kg. The duration of exposure can greatly affect the toxicity. The single dose LD_{50} of warfarin in dogs is about 50 mg/kg while a dose of 5 mg/kg for five to fifteen days may be lethal. In rats the single dose LD_{50} of warfarin is 1.6 mg/kg while the ninety-day LD_{50} is only 0.077 mg/kg. On the other hand, compounds which are rapidly metabolized have about the same ninety-day LD_{50} as the single dose LD_{50}. For example, the single dose LD_{50} for caffeine in rats is 192 mg/kg and the ninety-day LD_{50} is slightly lower at 150 mg/kg. At the other extreme animals may develop a tolerance for a compound such that repeated exposure increases the size of the dose required to produce lethality. The single dose LD_{50} of potassium cyanide in rats is 10 mg/kg, while rats which are given potassium cyanide for ninety days are able to tolerate a dose of 250 mg/kg without lethality. This has led some toxicologists to calculate the ratio of the acute to chronic LD_{50} doses and call this the *chronicity factor*. Compounds which have pronounced cumulative effects have larger chronicity factors. In the examples used above the chronicity factors are: warfarin = 20; caffeine = 1.3; and potassium cyanide = 0.04.

Several guidelines have been developed as aids in classifying the relative toxicities of compounds. It is nearly impossible to remember the exact toxicities of the wide variety of toxicants that affect animals. It is easier to remember that some compounds are highly toxic while others are of relatively low toxicity. Table 1 shows one scheme for classifying relative toxicities.

TABLE 1
Scheme for Classifying Relative Toxicities and Equivalent Volume (Unity Density) for a Dog and Cow Based on Highest Dose of Each Level

Class	Toxicity	Volume Dose Dog-20 kg	Cow-450 kg
Extremely toxic	1 mg/kg or less	.004 teaspoon	.09 teaspoon
Highly toxic	1-50 mg/kg	0.2 teaspoon	4.5 teaspoon
Moderately toxic	50-500 mg/kg	2 teaspoon	1 cup
Slightly toxic	0.5-5 gm/kg	0.45 cup	2.5 quarts
Practically nontoxic	5-15 gm/kg	1.34 cup	2 gallons
Relatively harmless	more than 15 gm/kg	>1.34 cup	>2 gallons

For example, all compounds with either acute or chronic toxicities of 1 mg/kg or less are considered to be extremely toxic, while compounds with toxicities between 1 and 50 mg/kg are considered to be highly toxic. The use of such a system reduces the need for trying to remember that compound X has a toxicity of 13 mg/kg and compound Y has a toxicity of 20 mg/kg. For most purposes of the veterinary student and practitioner it is sufficient to recall only that both compound X and Y are highly toxic. Table 1 also shows the equivalent volume of material for a 20 kg (44 pound) dog and a 450 kg (992 pound) cow. Unity density was assumed in converting from weight to volume.

The toxicity of a compound will vary with the route of exposure. Usual routes of exposure are oral, dermal, inhalation, intravenous, intraperitoneal and subcutaneous. In clinical veterinary toxicology, oral and dermal routes of exposure are most commonly encoun-

tered. The parenteral routes of exposure are encountered when dealing with adverse drug reactions.

Another factor that can accentuate the toxic effects of a compound is concurrent organ damage due to other causes. For example, maleic acid will cause proximal tubule kidney damage resulting in elevated glucosuria for two or three days. If aspirin is given along with maleic acid then the glucosuria persists for eight days or longer. Rats with CCl_4 induced liver damage are able to maintain near normal body temperature under hypothermic conditions. However, if chlordiazepoxide is administered to these same animals then body temperature is depressed by 3° C over control animals given the same dose of chlordiazepoxide.

Concurrent infectious disease can also alter toxicity. The toxicity of digitoxin in control mice is 1.9 mg/kg while it is 1.4 mg/kg in mice with a sixty-day duration TB infection.

Brahman cattle, especially bulls, are more sensitive to Ciodrin®, an organophosphorous insecticide, than are Herefords. This is an example of a breed difference. Young sheep, goats and cattle are more sensitive to coumaphos, a systemic insecticide, than are older animals of the same species. The oral LD_{50} for dieldrin, a chlorinated hydrocarbon insecticide, in male rats is 213 mg/kg while in female rats it is 119 mg/kg. This nearly twofold difference is due to differences in rates of dieldrin metabolism by the liver in males and females. When female mice were given bedding material suitable for nesting behavior, early mortality decreased from 19 percent to 1 percent. Placing three female mice versus one mouse per cage has been shown to decrease the number of offspring produced per female by 50 percent.

There are a large number of physiologic and environmental factors, which are listed in table 2 that are known to alter the response of animals to drugs and toxicants. The list is long and there is a danger of becoming frustrated by the large number of factors that can be involved. Most of these are based on work done with small laboratory rodents and consequently, may or may not be directly germane to domestic animals. However, it is necessary to be aware of these factors. It is likely that one or more of these factors has an impact on domestic animal toxicosis and is the reason for the variety of responses observed in field situations by veterinarians. It is recognized that many of these factors cannot be measured or are simply unknown under field conditions. The research toxicologist must recognize the potential impact of these factors and carefully standardize the testing conditions and make sure that treated and control animals are handled as identically as possible.

There is not space to include discussion of every factor listed in table 2 but several examples are given. The

TABLE 2
Factors That Can Alter the Response of Animals to Toxicants

Physiological Factors

Genus
Species
Strain
Breed
Age
Sex
Maturity
Estrous cycle
Pregnancy
Lactation

Environmental Factors

Season
Temperature
Humidity
Atmospheric contaminants
Air circulation
Light intensity
Light spectrum
Light/dark cycles
Transportation

Water

Quality
Quantity
Mode of delivering

Diet

Constituents
Protein level
Quantity
Quality
Contaminants

Caging

Size
Material
Shape

Bedding

Type
Quantity

Animal Handling

Physical contact
Noise
Commotion
Temperament of handler

Health

Deficiencies
Immunity
Latent infections
Clinical illness

Dogs raised in groups are known to be more active than single raised dogs.

The point to remember is that there are many factors known to alter responses and many of these contribute to what appears to be biologic variations.

From a public health and diagnostic toxicology perspective it is also essential to know what exposure level will not cause any adverse health effect. This level is usually referred to as the *"no-effect level."* It can also be thought of as the *maximum nontoxic level.* This is the amount that can be ingested without any deaths, illness or physiopathologic alterations occurring in any of the animals fed the toxicant for the stated period of time. Usually no-effect levels in laboratory animals are based on chronic exposures ranging from ninety days to two or more years depending on the species. However, in domestic animals of economic significance the little available no-effect data is often based on much shorter exposure times, for example, one to four weeks. It is emphasized that the no-effect level is the *largest* dosage that does not result in detrimental effects.

A very important concept to understand is hazard. *Hazard* refers to the likelihood of poisoning occurring under the conditions of usage and likelihood of exposure to a particular toxicant. A clear distinction is made between toxicity and hazard. A compound may have a very high toxicity, that is only a few milligrams or micrograms need to be consumed to produce toxicosis, but if animals are never exposed to the compound, then the hazard is very low. For example, pigweed is quite toxic to pigs raised in a drylot and then allowed to graze the fresh weed. However, if the pasture containing

manyfold variation (table 3) in the LD_{50} of compound 1080 or sodium fluroacetate, a rodenticide, is a good example of species variation. The LD_{50} values range from 0.05 mg/kg in the pocket gopher to more than 500 mg/kg in the toad.

Other examples of species differences include the rodenticide ANTU. In rats the oral LD_{50} is 7 mg/kg, in dogs it is 38 mg/kg, in chickens and rhesus monkeys it is 4,200 mg/kg. Norbormide is another rodenticide with a very marked species difference in toxicity. In rats the oral LD_{50} varies with species from 0.6 to 50 mg/kg. In the cat, dog, duck, fox, ground squirrel, sheep, pig and many other animals oral doses of 1,000 mg/kg have no effect.

In an interesting study on the effect of isolation on the LD_{50} of isoproterenol it was shown that rats housed singularly were sixteen times more sensitive. The LD_{50} in the rats housed as a group was 800 mg/kg while in isolated rats the LD_{50} was less than 50 mg/kg. Returning isolated rats to groups resulted in the LD_{50} returning to 800 mg/kg after several weeks.

TABLE 3
Species Variation in the Acute Oral LD_{50} (mg/kg) of Sodium Fluroacetate

Species	LD_{50} (mg/kg)
Dog	0.1
Cat	0.2
Cow	0.4
Horse	0.4
Sheep	0.25
Rhesus monkey	4.0
Spider monkey	15.0
Opossum	60.0
Pocket gopher	< 0.05
Norway rat	2.0
House mouse	8.0
Mallard duck	9.0
Frog	54
Toad	> 500

the pigweed is well fenced and the pigs cannot gain access to the pasture, then the hazard is low. On the other hand, if the pigs are allowed into the pasture, then both the toxicity and hazard are high. Perhaps this example is a little simple, but the point to keep clearly in mind is that just because a poison has a high toxicity does not directly imply that it is dangerous to use. It is the individual conditions that prevail in a given situation that determine the hazard.

Biologic Variation

Most veterinary students gain some appreciation for biologic variation by the time they have completed their physiology courses. It does not take too long for the student to discover that animals differ in their response to sodium pentobarbital. This individualized response to a drug is said to be due to biologic variation, which is variation due to the inherent differences in biochemical and membrane properties among animals. A good example of biologic variation is the LD_{50}. In a valid LD_{50} determination the animals are of similar (but not identical) genetic makeup, have been maintained on the same diet, housed in an identical manner and handled in as nearly identical ways as possible. And yet, by definition, half the animals given the same dosage die and the remaining half survive.

If all animals were the same you would expect all of them to die or all of them to survive. The same type of biologic variation operates in clinical cases encountered by the practitioner and clinical toxicologist. It is because of this uncontrolled biologic variation that statistical procedures are used to determine the probability that the observed differences are due to the difference in treatments as opposed to being due to naturally occurring differences among animals.

Biologic Variation and Toxicity Data in Veterinary Practice

Let us examine the situation that the diagnostic veterinary toxicologist encounters on a daily basis and the toxicologic information that he needs in order to arrive at a conclusion or diagnosis. Assume you are involved in a field case in which some cattle in a herd are sick and several have died. Further assume that the clinical picture is compatible with two toxicoses and one or more infectious diseases or herd management problems. Your task is to sort out the facts and arrive at a diagnosis. In doing so you find out what the exposure level was of the one or two toxicants you suspect and you also culture for microorganisms and submit specimens for histopathology. And perhaps you determine tissue levels of the toxicant from the dead animals. At this point your job is to pull this information together.

From the toxicologic perspective you need to decide if the exposure levels you found were high enough to cause the problem under investigation. In order to do this you need to know what the toxicity of the chemical is in the species involved, cattle in this example. In fact, what you would like to know is what exposure is necessary to produce deaths, what exposure is necessary to produce clinical toxicosis without deaths, and finally what level will result in no obvious detrimental effects. If the exposure occurred over a period of days, then the informational problem is even more difficult since you need to know the *chronic toxicity*. Unfortunately, many times not all of this information is available and the practitioner or the toxicologist is forced to make best-estimate evaluations based on his experience and the experience of others.

In addition to knowing what dosage is required to cause deaths you need to know what dosage causes illness without deaths. Most of the information of this type is based on reports of field-poisoning episodes. But because animal husbandry practices vary extensively throughout the world you can expect the data, at best, to be a guideline for a particular episode.

Probably one of the most difficult situations for the toxicologist involves a case where only a few of the animals in a herd are ill and the clinical signs observed are of slight severity. Extensive case workup and chemical analyses may prove that the toxicant is present. However, the level present may not be high enough to warrant a definitive diagnosis. The dilemma then is to decide whether you should try to find another cause for the illness or conclude that the toxicant found is the cause of the problem. This perplexing problem is brought on by one or more of the following. First, for most toxicants there is insufficient information on the effects of low-level exposures. Secondly, individual animals react differently. And thirdly, individual environmental and animal husbandry conditions vary which affects the severity of response of a given set of animals to a particular level of a toxicant. The proceeding is stated not to discourage or confuse the clinical toxicologist or practitioner, but rather to acknowledge that this situation exists and, therefore, even though a thorough investigation and good laboratory work are done, you will not be able to arrive at a firm unequivocal diagnosis in every case.

Veterinary Toxicology Organizations

The American College of Veterinary Toxicologists (ACVT) was organized January 15, 1958 to foster and encourage sound education, training, and research in veterinary toxicology. The organization recognizes membership in three categories; namely, Fellow, Associate Fellow and Affiliate in Toxicology. The type of membership depends on the background of the applicant and his or her prior experience in veterinary toxicology. Detailed information can be obtained from the authors. ACVT sponsors seminars, colloquiums, training workshops and scientific meetings. The ACVT also maintains a directory of its members and their areas of expertise and also publishes a periodical called *Veterinary Toxicology* which contains reports, abstracts and notices of interest to veterinary toxicologists.

The American Board of Veterinary Toxicology (ABVT) was organized in 1967 with three charter members. The ABVT serves to recognize individuals as qualified specialists in veterinary toxicology. Membership is obtained by satisfactorily completing a qualifying examination. In 1976 there were thirty-three diplomats of the American Board of Veterinary Toxicology.

Other toxicology organizations of interest to veterinary toxicologists include the Society of Toxicology organized in 1963. This organization publishes the *Journal of Applied Pharmacology and Toxicology*. Another organization is the American Academy of Clinical Toxicology.

CALCULATIONS IN TOXICOLOGY

The ability to accurately manipulate numbers is fundamental to the practice of medicine. The practitioner is constantly calculating drug dosages based on estimates of body weight and food consumption. Similarly, the toxicologist is faced with the problem of relating the level of contamination in a feed to the clinical signs observed in a suspected poisoning. In this section several guidelines will be developed to help the toxicologist and practitioner interpret the significance of numbers resulting from laboratory analyses or estimates of probable exposure.

Terminology

In veterinary toxicology the preferred method of expressing concentrations of most toxicants in feeds, water, solvents, sprays and animal tissues is to use parts per million or related terms such as parts per billion or parts per trillion. Occasionally when high concentrations are involved, such as with insecticide concentrates, the concentration is expressed as a percentage on a weight/weight basis. A part per million, abbreviated ppm, is one part of X in 999,999 parts of Y on a weight/weight basis. Using metric units, then 1 ppm is 1 mg per 1,000,000 mg or, more simply, *1 ppm is equal to 1 mg/kg*. This relationship is fundamental and must be firmly committed to memory. If this basic relationship is understood, then the toxicologist can calculate the equivalent in any other units of weight. For example, 1 microgram (μg) per gram is also 1 ppm.

The definition of 1 part per billion, abbreviated ppb, follows in a similar manner, namely 1 part in 1,000,000,000 parts or 1 μg/1,000,000,000 μg which progressively reduces to 1 μg/1,000,000 mg = 1 μg/1,000 grams = 1 μg/kg. Again this is a basic relationship that should be firmly retained. The definition of 1 part per trillion (ppt) follows in a similar manner.

Fortunately there is a direct relationship between percentage concentration and parts per million. This relationship can be discovered by calculating the percentage equivalent of 1 ppm as given in example 1.

Example 1: Determining percentage equivalent of 1 ppm.

    a. 1 ppm = 1 mg/kg = 1 mg/1,000,000 mg.

    b. $1 \div 1,000,000 = 0.000001$.

    c. Convert to % by multiplying by 100.

    d. $0.000001 \times 100 = 0.0001\%$.

    e. Therefore, 1 ppm is the same as 0.0001%.

From this relationship a conversion table can be calculated as given in table 1.

TABLE 1
Relationship Between PPM and Percentage

PPM			Percentage
0.001	ppm =	1 ppb	0.0000001%
.01	ppm =	10 ppb	0.000001%
.1	ppm =	100 ppb	0.00001%
1	ppm		0.0001%
10	ppm		0.001%
100	ppm		0.01%
1,000	ppm		0.1%
10,000	ppm		1.0%

A rule of thumb that is most useful is: to *convert ppm to percentage, move the decimal point 4 places to the left. And, to convert percentage to ppm move the decimal point 4 places to the right.* Using this rule of thumb it is easy to see that 124 ppm is the same as 0.0124% and that 0.5% is the same as 5,000 ppm.

A commonly encountered situation in clinical veterinary toxicology is the addition of drugs to animal feeds where the concentration is expressed as grams of drug per ton of feed. Example 2 shows how this can be expressed on a ppm basis.

Example 2: Show that 1 gm/ton is equal to 1.1 ppm.

   a. Basic definition: 1 ppm = 1 mg/kg.

   b. 1 gm/ton = 1,000 mg/2,000 pounds.

   c. (1,000 mg) ÷ (2,000 pounds ÷ 2.205 pounds/kg.)

   d. = 1,000 mg/907 kg.

   e. = 1.102 mg/kg.

   f. = 1.102 ppm, therefore 1 gm/ton is equal to 1.1 ppm.

   g. And furthermore, 100 gm of drug/ton is equivalent to 110 ppm.

This provides another useful rule of thumb; namely, that *100 gm/ton gives a concentration equivalent to 110 ppm.*

Example 3 shows several ways of using the above information in solving an applied problem.

Example 3: Preparation of 2 tons of pig grower feed containing 400 ppm arsanilic acid.

Method 1—Use rule of thumb that 100 gm/ton is equal to 110 ppm.

   a. $\dfrac{400 \text{ ppm}}{110 \text{ ppm}} = \dfrac{X \text{ gms/ton}}{100 \text{ gms/ton}}$

   b. $X = \dfrac{400 \times 100}{110} = 364 \text{ gms/ton}$

   c. Therefore, you need 2 × 364 = 728 grams of arsanilic acid to prepare 2 tons of medicated feed.

Method 2—Use the rule of thumb in converting ppm to percentage.

   a. 400 ppm = 0.04%.

   b. 2 tons = 1,814 kg.

   c. 1,814 kg × 0.04% = 1,814 kg × 0.0004 = 726 grams.

(Answers differ because of rounding error)
Either method is correct and each individual needs to decide which method he personally prefers to use.

Expressing Concentrations of Substances in Body Fluids

The lack of uniform methods among toxicologists for expressing concentrations of substances in blood or other fluids can lead to appreciable confusion. Units used include ppm, mg%, mg/100 ml, milliequivalent, mg/liter, μg/100 ml, and probably others. Examples 4 shows different ways of expressing blood lead levels.

Example 4: Assume you have a report on the analysis of a whole blood sample from a dog suspected of having lead poisoning and the report comes back as 0.8 ppm. What are the other ways of expressing this residue?

  1. As mg/100 ml

     a. 0.8 ppm = 0.8 mg/kg.

     b. 0.8 ppm = .08 mg/100 ml.
       (Assuming specific gravity of blood to be 1, although we know that the specific gravity of blood of domestic animals is in the range of 1.039 to 1.061)

     c. This is also the same as 80 ug/100 ml.

  2. As μg/ml

     a. 0.8 ppm = .08 mg/100 ml.

     b. 1 mg = 1,000 micrograms.

     c. .08 mg/100 ml = 80 μg/100 ml.

     d. = .8 μg/ml.

  3. As mg%

     a. 1 mg% = 1 mg/100 ml.

     b. 0.8 ppm = .08 mg/100 ml.

     c. = 0.08 mg%.

Problems Encountered in Expressing Exposure

Frequently animal toxicology studies are done with the toxicant administered on a weight of drug per unit body weight basis (i.e., mg drug/kg body weight). However, in field cases encountered in veterinary toxicology the estimated exposure is often based on a feed analysis which results in X ppm toxicant in the feed. The problem then is to estimate how much of the suspect feed the animal consumed and to calculate an estimated dosage. Fortunately, sources of information are available for estimating the average amount of feed each of the common domestic animals consumes during various stages of its life cycle. One source is the information published by the National Academy of Sciences—National Research Council, as follows:

1. Nutrient Requirements of Beef Cattle, Fourth revised edition, 1970.
2. Nutrient Requirements of Poultry, Sixth revised edition, 1971.
3. Nutrient Requirements of Dairy Cattle, Fourth revised edition, 1971.
4. Nutrient Requirements of Sheep, Fourth revised edition, 1968.
5. Similar documents are available for horses, swine, dogs, rabbits, mink, and foxes.

Another publication of the NAS/NRC that contains extensive data on animal feeds is "United States—Canadian Table of Feed Composition," Second revision, 1969.

The general formula for converting a level of drug in feed (ppm) to the estimated equivalent on a mg/kg basis is:

$$\frac{(\text{Level in feed (ppm)}) \times (\text{kg feed eaten})}{\text{body weight in kg}} = \text{mg drug/kg body wt}$$

One additional factor to consider when making these conversion estimates is the increased toxicity that may occur when the dose is given in one, single oral exposure rather than more uniformly throughout the daily eating period. By the same token, a toxicant given in one dose may induce vomition (organic mercurials) while the same amount incorporated in the daily food may be tolerated by the stomach to the detriment of the organism.

Example 5: If the toxic level of drug XYZ in the feed is 25 ppm for a 10 pound pig, what is the estimated toxicity of drug XYZ on a mg/kg body weight basis? [Assumptions: feed is air dried, drug is evenly distributed in feed, 10 pound pig eats 0.8 pounds feed/day (8% of body weight), and the drug does not depress appetite.]

a. Formula $= \dfrac{(\text{level in feed in ppm}) \times (\text{kg feed eaten})}{\text{body weight in kg}}$

b. 25 ppm = 25 mg/kg

c. $= \dfrac{(25 \text{ mg/kg}) \times (.8 \text{ pound} \div 2.205 \text{ pounds/kg})}{(10 \text{ pounds} \div 2.205 \text{ pounds/kg})}$

d. $= \dfrac{(25 \text{ mg/kg}) \times (.3628 \text{ kg})}{(4.535 \text{ kg})}$

e. $= \dfrac{9.07 \text{ mg}}{4.535 \text{ kg}}$

f. = 2.0 mg/kg

Conversely, the toxicologist may have data on the toxicity of a drug expressed as mg drug per kg body weight and in this case wishes to know what the equivalent level in the feed would be in order to produce similar toxicologic effects. In this case the formula is given as:

$$\text{ppm in feed} = \frac{(\text{mg drug/kg body wt}) \times (\text{wt of animal in kg})}{(\text{wt of animal in kg}) \times (\text{percentage of body wt eaten as food/day})}$$

In the numerator the total number of mg of drug per animal is determined and in the denominator the amount of food eaten per day is calculated. The quotient is then mg drug/kg feed or ppm drug. However, inspection of the formula shows that by removing the weight of the animal from both the numerator and the denominator the formula is simplified to yield:

$$\text{ppm in feed} = \frac{\text{mg drug/kg body weight}}{\text{percentage of body wt eaten as food per day}}$$

Therefore, if the toxicologist knows what the toxicity of a drug or chemical is on a mg drug/kg body weight basis and can estimate the feed intake, then the equivalent exposure on a ppm basis can be calculated. In clinical situations the problem is encountered from a slightly different perspective. The clinical situation requires the toxicologist to determine, often using chemical analysis, the amount of chemical in the feed and then to make a judgment of whether or not the levels found are sufficient to cause the veterinary toxicologic problem under consideration.

Example 6: Assume that you know based on published information, that the toxicity of a new feed additive is 2 mg/kg body weight for young pigs. At this dose the pigs become anorexic. You are called in on a case where pigs being fed the new drug have become anorexic and are scouring. The person responsible for mixing the the feed claims to have added the appropriate amount to achieve a drug level of 10 ppm. However, based on a report of a chemical analysis you suspect the level is 30 ppm. Would 30 ppm be a high enough level to cause the problem? First you might determine what the feed level would be to give an exposure equivalent to 2 mg/kg. This can be determined using either of the two formulas given above. Assume that this case involves 10 pound pigs eating an amount of feed equivalent to 8% of their body weight/day. Calculate the level in the feed required to give an exposure of 2 mg/kg.

Method 1—

a.   ppm in feed = $\dfrac{(mg/kg) \times (wt\ of\ animal\ in\ kg)}{(wt\ of\ animal) \times (\%\ of\ body\ wt\ eaten\ as\ feed)}$

b. $= \dfrac{(2\ mg/kg) \times (10\ pounds \div 2.205\ pounds/kg)}{(10\ pounds \div 2.205\ pounds/kg) \times (.08)}$

c. $= \dfrac{(2\ mg/kg) \times (4.535\ kg)}{4.535\ kg \times 0.08}$

d. $= \dfrac{9.070\ mg}{.363\ kg}$

e. $= 24.98\ mg/kg \cong 25\ ppm$

*Method 2—*The problem can be solved more directly by using the simplified formula:

a.   ppm in feed = $\dfrac{toxicity\ of\ drug\ in\ mg/kg}{percent\ body\ wt\ eaten\ as\ feed}$

b. $= \dfrac{2\ mg/kg}{.08}$

c. $= 25\ ppm$

Since you have reason to believe that the level actually fed (30 ppm) exceeds the toxicity of 2 mg/kg or 25 ppm in feed, you would seriously consider the involvement of the drug in this instance.

Feed consumption by an individual animal will vary with body weight, ambient temperature, disease conditions, type of feed and a host of other conditions. However, it is necessary to have some estimate of feed consumption under normal conditions. The estimated feed consumption values presented in table 2 are guidelines and should be used with due caution, especially if you have reason to suspect that unusual conditions exist in a particular situation.

Occasionally the veterinary toxicologist suspects the toxicant was present in the drinking water. To calculate the exposure it is necessary to estimate the amount of water consumed. Table 3 gives the daily water consumption values for a variety of domestic animals. Water consumption can be even more variable than feed consumption. There can be a twelve-fold increase in water consumption by an individual animal during hot summer days compared to cold winter days. Also, the amount of water consumed during any one drinking will vary depending on whether or not the animal has continuous access to water or is only watered once per day. Considerable judgment must be exercised by the veterinarian when estimating water consumption for in-dividual animals in a specific environmental situation. Note in table 3 that most values are given for an individual animal of a specified body weight or for a specific physiologic condition. Some values are based on milk production or feed consumption. The poultry values are based on a unit of 100 birds.

Estimating Dosages When Exposure Is Based on Consumption of Green Forage That Has Been Sprayed

A difficult situation is encountered when the toxicologist is faced with a field problem involving "sick" or dead animals "associated" with the spraying of forages with a chemical. One must estimate the amount of forage eaten and make an estimate of the uniformity of the sprayed material on the forage. Short grass may be uniformly sprayed, whereas, tall weeds or grasses may have spray material concentrated at the top with little material reaching the lower portions of the plant.

Palmer and Radeleff (1969. The Toxicity of Some Organic Herbicides to Cattle, Sheep, and Chickens, ARS, Production Research Report No. 106) estimated that a high quality improved pasture would yield 0.1 pound (45 grams) of air-dry forage/square foot or about 2 tons per acre. Application rates of 1 pound of chemical/A would result in 10.4 mg chemical per square foot. (1 A = 43,560 square feet) They further assumed a forage consumption factor of 3 percent of body weight and total availability of the chemical (maximizes exposure). This results in an equivalent exposure of 7 mg/kg for each pound of chemical/A. (1 kg × .03 = 30 grams of forage consumed per kg body weight; 45 grams of forage from 1 square foot contains 10.4 mg or 30 grams contains 6.9 mg which rounds off to 7 mg.)

On a ppm basis the forage would be estimated to contain 230 ppm of chemical. [(1,000 gm/kg ÷ 45 grams) × (10.4 mg) = 230 mg/kg] Thus another useful rule of thumb is that *1 pound of chemical per acre results in an exposure in a grazing animal of approximately 7 mg of chemical per kg body weight.* Therefore, if a herbicide were applied at 2 pounds per acre and cows were allowed to graze the sprayed forage, the herbicide exposure would be approximately 14 mg/kg. If the no-effect exposure level is 300 mg/kg for the herbicide, then the toxicologist would rightly conclude that the herbicide would not be responsible for any adverse health effects seen in the cattle.

Conversion Factors

Table 4 contains some commonly used conversion factors or numeric constants frequently or occasionally needed in veterinary toxicology.

TABLE 2
Estimated Feed Consumption Rates for Animals Under Ideal Conditions.
Numbers Based on NRC Nutrient Requirement Data

| Animal | Body Weight | | Weight of Food Eaten per Day Expressed as Percentage of Body Wt. |
	Pounds	Kilograms	
Horse			
Mature	408	185	2.0
Weight	806	365	1.7
Work, moderate	1,203	545	1.6
	1,401	635	1.5
Colt			
Growing	199	90	3.1
Mature weight—270 kg	596	270	1.3
Growing	199	90	3.4
Mature weight—365 kg	408	185	2.3
	596	270	1.7
	806	365	1.2
Growing	199	90	3.8
Mature weight—545 kg	806	365	1.7
	1,203	545	1.0
Beef			
	300	136	2.3
	450	204	2.5
	650	295	2.4
	1,000	454	2.1
Dairy Cow			
Lactating and nonpregnant	770	350	1.4
	1,760	800	1.2
Last two months gestation	770	350	1.8
	1,760	800	1.6
Swine			
	10-25	4.5-11.3	8
	50	23	6.4
	100	45	5.3
	150	68	4.5
	200	91	4
Lamb			
	59	27	4.5
	99	45	3.9
Ewe			
Nonlactating	141	64	2.4
Lactating	141	64	3.9
Dog			
Adult	5	2.3	3.9
(Dry food)	15	6.8	2.8
	30	13.6	2.5
	70	31.8	2.5
	110	49.8	2.4
Dog			
Growing	5	2.3	7.8
(Dry food)	15	6.8	5.6
	30	13.6	5.0
	50	22.7	5.0

TABLE 2 (Cont.)

Animal	Body Weight		Weight of Food Eaten per Day Expressed as Percentage of Body Wt.
	Pounds	Kilograms	
Chicken			
	0.5	.23	14
	1.0	.45	11.4
	1.5	.68	9.7
	3.5	1.59	6.7
	5.5	2.50	5.0

TABLE 3
Estimated Water Consumption of Domestic Animals Under Normal Conditions

Animal and Condition	Consumption/Head/Day	
	Gallons	Liters
Horse	0.6 gal/100 pounds body weight	5.4 ℓ/100 kg body weight
Horse—lactating		4 ℓ H_2O/ℓ milk
Range cattle	10-12	38-45
Range cattle		3-8 ℓ/kg dry feed
Feeder calves	4-6	15-23
Finishing calves	8-10	30-38
Dairy cow—lactating	12-36	3-4 ℓ/ℓ of milk prod. 45-136
Dairy calves		
4- 8 weeks	1-1 1/2	3.8-5.6
12-20 weeks	2-4 1/2	7.6-17
6 months	4	15
Sow—pregnant	3 1/2-4 1/2	13-17
Sow—lactating	5-6	19-23
Swine—growing		
30 pound	0.6-1.0	2.3-3.8
60- 80 pound	0.8	3
75-125 pound	2.0	7.6
200-230 pound	1 1/2-3 1/2	5.7-13
Sheep		
Lamb	0.8	3
Ewe	1.0	3.8
Ewe lactating	1.5	5.7
Hens—nonlaying	5.0 gal/100 birds	19 ℓ/100 birds
Hens—laying	5-7 1/2 gal/100 birds	19-28 ℓ/100 birds
Chicken		
4 weeks	2.0 gal/100 birds	7.6 ℓ/100 birds
8 weeks	4.1 gal/100 birds	15.5 ℓ/100 birds
12 weeks	5.5 gal/100 birds	21 ℓ/100 birds

TABLE 4
Equivalents, Constants and Prefixes

Length

1 inch = 2.54 centimeters
1 foot = 30.48 centimeters
1 yard = 91.44 centimeters
1 furlong = 660 feet
1 rod = 16.5 feet
1 mile = 5280 feet
1 mile = 1609.3 meters
1 chain = 66 feet
1 centimeter = 0.3937 inch
1 meter = 39.37 inches
1 meter = 3280.8 feet
1 micron = 1×10^{-6} meter
1 micron = 1×10^{-3} = 0.001 millimeter
1 angstrom = 1×10^{-5} = 0.00001 micron

Area

1 acre = 43,560 square feet
1 acre = 4,047 square meters
1 hectare = 2.471 acres
1 hectare = 10,000 square meters
1 square mile = 640 acres

Weight

1 grain = 64.8 milligrams
1 ounce = 28.35 grams
1 ounce = 16 drams
1 pound = 453.59 grams
1 short ton = 2000 pounds
1 short ton = 907.18 kilograms
1 long ton = 2240 pounds
1 long ton = 1016.05 kilograms
1 metric ton = 1000 kilograms
1 metric ton = 2204.6 pounds
1 gram = 15.43 grains
1 kilogram = 2.205 pounds

Miscellaneous

Degrees Centigrade = ($^{\circ}$F — 32) x 0.55
Degrees Fahrenheit = ($^{\circ}$C x 1.8) + 32
1 Calorie = 0.003968 BTU
1 BTU = 252 Calories (Gram) (15°C)
1 atmosphere = 33.90 feet of water
1 atmosphere = 29.92 inches of mercury
1 atmosphere = 14.7 pounds/square inch
1 horsepower = 745.7 watts
1 gallon water = 8.3453 pounds

Capacity—Liquid

1 minim = 0.062 milliliters
1 ounce = 8 drams
1 ounce = 29.57 milliliters
1 dram = 3.697 milliliters
1 gill = 4 ounces
1 quart = 0.946 liters
1 quart = 256 drams
1 quart = 57.75 cubic inches
1 gallon = 3.785 liters
1 cubic foot = 7.48 gallons
1 cubic foot = 59.84 pints
1 cubic foot = 28.32 liters
1 bushel = 9.309 gallons
1 barrel (oil) = 42 gallons
1 barrel (US liquid) = 31.5 gallons
1 acre-foot = 3.259×10^{5} gallons
1 liter = 1.057 quarts
1 liter = 270.5 drams
1 liter = 33.81 ounces
1 liter = 0.264 gallons
1 liter = 61.03 cubic inches
1 liter = 1000 milliliters
1 teaspoon = 5 milliliters
1 tablespoon = 15 milliliters

Capacity—Dry

1 bushel = 8 gallons
1 bushel = 4 pecks
1 bushel = 35.24 liters
1 bushel = 1.24 cubic feet
1 cubic foot = 0.804 bushel
1 cubic foot = 28.316 liters
1 cubic foot = 25.714 quarts
1 peck = 8 quarts
1 quart = 1.101 liters
1 liter = 0.908 quarts
1 liter = 61.03 cubic inches
1 cubic meter = 35.314 cubic feet
1 cubic inch = 16.387 milliliters

TABLE 4 (Cont.)

Prefixes Applied to Metric System Units

Multiples	Prefix	Symbol
10^{12}	tera	T
10^{9}	giga	G
10^{6}	mega	M
10^{3}	kilo	k
10^{2}	hecto	h
10	deka	da
10^{-1}	deci	d
10^{-2}	centi	c
10^{-3}	milli	m
10^{-6}	micro	μ
10^{-9}	nano	n
10^{-12}	pico	p
10^{-15}	femto	f
10^{-18}	atto	a

Density of Dry Feed Ingredients*

Product	Pounds/cubic foot	Product	Pounds/cubic foot
Alfalfa meal	18	Oat, seed	30
Alfalfa pellets	42	Oat, ground	22
Barley, whole	41	Oat, rolled	21
Barley, ground	25	Pellets, 0.25 inch	39
Calcium carbonate	75	Phosphate	75
Corn, shelled	45	Rye, bran	17
Corn, ear chopped	35	Rye, middlings	42
Corn, meal	39	Salt, fine	75
Cottonseed oilmeal	38	Sorghum, seed	33
Dairy, concentrates	43	Soybeans, ground	30
Fishmeal	35	Soybeans, seed	47
Hay, loose	5	Soybean oilmeal	38
Hay, pressed	8	Tankage	49
Linseed oilmeal	29	Urea	38
Milk, powdered	20	Wheat, whole	49
Millet	39	Wheat, bran	13
Milo, seed	42	Wheat, ground	39
Milo, ground	34	Whey, dry	41
Molasses, feed	23		

*Source: Feed Manufacturing Technology, 1970.

DOSE-RESPONSE RELATIONSHIPS

Man and animals are born, mature, reproduce, grow old and die in an environment which constantly exposes them to potentially harmful chemicals and energy forms. To understand how life can be maintained under these conditions requires an understanding of the concepts of dose-response relationships, in other words, the level of exposure versus the magnitude of biological reaction.

Toxicologists developing new chemicals use dose-response relationships to determine whether a suitable margin of safety can be achieved. Pharmacologists use dose-response relationships to optimize dosage schedules to achieve desired therapeutic effects. Clinical and diagnostic toxicologists must understand dose-response functions in order to determine likelihood of poisoning associated with specific exposures to toxic substances.

In this chapter you will see how LD_{50} values are determined. While this may all seem complicated and perhaps unrelated to clinical toxicology, there are several items that should be kept clearly in mind. If you know how the LD_{50} is determined you will be better able to understand and interpret acute toxicity data. You will also gain an understanding of the rationale for determining dosage levels.

It must be recognized that the LD_{50} is a simple and crude measure of the toxicity of a compound. Crude, not in the sense of inaccuracy, but crude in the sense it is a measure of lethality. Lethality is the final, decisive dramatic toxic effect of a compound. Between no effect and lethality lies a wide spectrum of physiologic and pathologic changes.

It is possible in some instances to more precisely describe the dose-response relationships of nonlethal changes by using regression and correlation analysis.

The information presented in this chapter is only the tip of the iceberg representing the body of information on dose-response.

When an organism is exposed to a given dose of a toxicant or drug a variety of responses can occur. The exposure may be so low that no discernible biologic response occurs. Or the organism may respond with some measurable alteration in a biologic function such as altered liver enzyme activity, increase in heart rate or change in pupil size. At the extreme end the organism responds with a lethal decrease in function resulting in death. The same exposure in another similar organism may or may not result in the same intensity of biological response. Therefore, there are two major problems to consider in understanding dose-response relationships. First there is the basic phenomenon that for most toxicants the magnitude of biologic response is related to dosage. Generally, the higher the exposure the more intense the response. Therefore, it should be possible to mathematically define the relationship between dosage and response. Note, however, at this time the dose-response relationship has not been defined to be linear, curvilinear, logarithmic, cubic, etc.

The second major problem is that not all animals will respond to the same exposure to the same degree. Hence there is variation between subjects. To deal with this matter the dose-response relationship must contain a measure of variability which reflects the inherent differences in expected response between animals. Quantities such as standard deviations, variances or confidence intervals are used to define the boundaries or the expected variation in the dose-response relationship.

One of the better known uses of dose-response relationships deals with the determination of the LD_{50} or LC_{50} (leathal dose or lethal concentration). It is noteworthy to realize that the analytical techniques for determining an LD_{50} can be used for any biological response that can be considered to be a yes-no or binary (on-off, present-absent, 0-1) response. In a LD_{50} the binary response is determined by whether the subject is dead or alive. There can be no intermediate category; either each subject is dead or it is alive. Other biologic responses can be similarly classified if the experimenter can clearly define a separation point. For example, the experimenter might define the point as any blood pressure above 140 mm Hg as one category and any subject below 140 mm Hg is assigned to the other group. Then the dosage required to increase blood pressure above 140 mm Hg in 50 percent of the subjects can be calculated. The remaining problem is the intelligent selection of dosages which will facilitate obtaining the most information from a limited number of subjects. These and other points are illustrated in the following discussion.

Wagner and Johnson (1970) reported an experiment determining the LD_{50} of Dichlorvos® (2, 2- dihloro-vinyl dimethyl phosphate or DDVP) in young adult mice. The actual experiment used 270 females and 270 males. For the present purpose only the data for the females will be used. Table 1 presents the dosages and number of mice dying at each dosage. Ten females were tested at each dosage. Since the LD_{50} can be estimated from a plot of the raw data, the first step is to develop the graph shown in figure 1, which yields the sigmoid curve that commonly occurs in the biologic response of organisms to drugs. Notice that at both the low and high dose ends the response line is curved and in the center the line is straighter. Since it is known that often times the response is more linear (i.e., the response curve is straighter) with the logarithm of the dose than with the arithmetic value of the dose, the dose-response curve can be plotted on semilog paper as shown in figure 2. Plotting the response against the logarithm of the dose results in a steeper and straighter dose-response curve. However, there is still some curvature at the extremes. From both the curves an estimate of the LD_{50} is obtained. It is obvious from both graphs that the animals given less than 50 mg/kg (4 groups of 10) and those given 230 mg/kg or more (6 groups of 10) are not yielding very much useful information, especially re-

garding the determination of the LD_{50}. Namely, they either all survived or they were all killed. More about selecting doses later.

There are three frequently cited methods for determining the LD_{50} and a measure of variability: namely, Miller and Tainter (1944), Litchfield and Wilcoxon (1949) and Weil (1952). The Miller and Tainter method is fairly simple and requires logarithmic-probit paper. The LD_{50} is obtained as well as the standard error of the LD_{50}. The method of Litchfield and Wilcoxon is also a graphic method but is a little more complex in the use of nomographs which are designed to avoid the use of probits and logarithms. The method yields the LD_{50}, slope of the dose-response function and confidence limits. The method of Weil requires more calculations than the Miller and Tainter method, but is still straight forward. The Weil method depends on the use of published tables which define the response and certain numerical coefficients depending on the responses within each group, the number of groups and the size of each group. The published tables provide for groups of two, three, four, five, six, or ten subjects per drug level with the stipulation that four or more different dosage groups be used and each group be the same size. The LD_{50} and the 95 percent confidence interval of the LD_{50} are obtained.

Since it is unusual that enough animals (due to financial resources, space, time) are available for testing at numerous dosage levels, what is known that will help

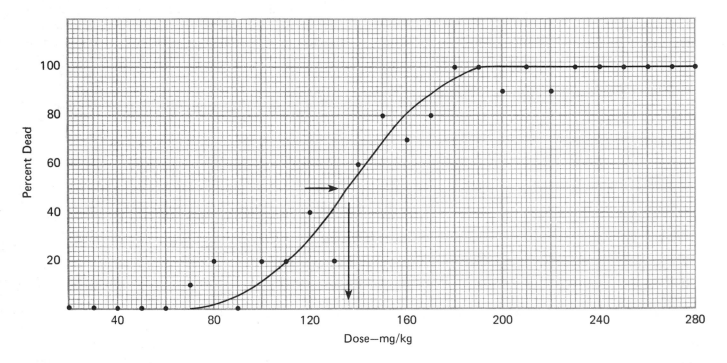

Figure 1. Dose-response curve for dichlorvos in mice using the data from table 1. Linear response (percent dead) is plotted against linear dose. The LD_{50} (arrow) is 136 mg/kg. (Adapted from the data of Wagner and Johnson, 1970).

TABLE 1
Deaths Occurring in Groups of 10 Mice Given
Dichlorvos at Levels from 20 to 280 mg/kg.

Dose	No. Dying per Group of 10	Dose	No. Dying per Group of 10
20	0	160	7
30	0	170	8
40	0	180	10
50	0	190	10
60	0	200	9
70	1	210	10
80	2	220	9
90	0	230	10
100	2	240	10
110	2	250	10
120	4	260	10
130	2	270	10
140	6	280	10
150	8		

(Adapted from Wagner and Johnson, 1970.)

select dosage levels that are likely to yield meaningful data?

A good place to start is to use successive dosages which follow a geometric progression; namely, $Y_N = Y_1 R^{N-1}$. Y_N is the nth dose, Y_1 is the first dose, R^{N-1} is the progression factor, and N is the ith consecutive dose. Although this appears complicated at first, you will find it to be straightforward if you will follow the calculations step by step as presented below. To see how this works, select an arbitrary first dose of 10 mg/kg and a geometric factor (R) = 2. The calculations follow as:

Dose 1 = 10 (specified)

Dose 2 = $Y_2 = Y_1 R^{2-1}$
Substitute: $Y_1 = 10, R = 2, N = 2$
for second dose.
$Y_2 = 10 \times 2^1$
$= 10 \times 2$
$= 20$

Dose 3 = $Y_3 = Y_1 R^{3-1}$
Substitute: $Y_1 = 10, R = 2, N = 3$
for third dose.
$Y_3 = 10 \times 2^2$
$= 10 \times 4$
$= 40$

Dose 4 = $Y_4 = Y_1 R^{4-1}$

Substitute: $Y_1 = 10, R = 2, N = 4$
for fourth dose.
$Y_4 = 10 \times 2^3$
$= 10 \times 8$
$= 80$

Therefore the four dosages would be 10, 20, 40, and 80 mg/kg. Note the R must be some value other than 0 or 1. If R = 3 and $Y_1 = 10$ then the dosage sequence is 10, 30, 90, 270. Another scheme for selecting dosages is to use a logarithmic relationship where the difference between the logarithm of any two successive dosages is a constant. In the two dosage series developed above (log 10 = 1, log 20 = 1.301, log 40 = 1.602, log 80 = 1.903; for dosage sequence 1 and for dosage sequence 2 the values are: log 30 = 1.472, log 90 = 1.954, log 270 = 2.431) the difference in the logs of two successive dosages in the first series is 0.301 (log 20 − log 10, or log 40 − log 20) and in the second series the differences is 0.477 (log 30 − log 10, or log 90 − log 30). Note that in the first case 0.301 is the log of 2, namely the value of R in the geometric progression and in the second case 0.477 is the log of 3, also the selected value for R.

For illustrative purposes assume that you are given a vial of Dichlorvos with no toxicity data and you want to determine the LD_{50}. You might begin by injecting two mice each with 1, 10, 100 and 1,000 mg/kg. From what is known you would expect the 1 and 10 mg animals to live, the 1,000 mg animal to die and the 100 mg animal may live or die. You have narrowed the dosage range (using eight mice) to 10-1,000 mg. If one or both of the 100 mg animals dies you would have even more information. Next you might try two mice at each of 50 and 500 mg/kg. The 500 mg will die and the 50 mg will most likely survive. From this you know, after using only twelve mice, that the LD_{50} lies between 50 and 500 mg. Selecting a dosage of $Y_1 = 50$ and R = 2 a dosage sequence of 50, 100, 200, 400 might be used. Other schedules that might be considred depending on different dosage choices in the range-finding experiments could be 20, 40, 80, 160, 320 mg/kg or 30, 60, 120, 240, 480 mg/kg. Using the information available in table 1 dose-response data can be obtained as shown in table 2 for the three dosage schedules developed above.

Using the above data, the LD_{50} will be calculated using the probit method of Miller and Tainter.

Using the method of Miller and Tainter requires either probit-percentage graph paper (fig. 3) or probit paper and a table of probits (table 3). Using the data in schedule I given in table 2, the dose-response curve is graphed in figure 3. Note that in order to keep the slope

TABLE 2
Lethality of Dichlorvos

Schedule I		Schedule II		Schedule III	
Dose	% Dead	Dose	% Dead	Dose	% Dead
50	0	20	0	30	0
100	20	40	0	60	0
200	90	80	20	120	40
400	100	160	70	240	100
		320	100	480	100

(Adapted from the data on Wagner and Johnson, 1970.)

positive the percent survivors is graphed for each dosage. The method used to handle the 0 percent and 100 percent extremes is to substitute 0.25 for 0 response and then divide by the number of animals per group and multiply by 100 to get the percentage (0.25 ÷ 10 × 100 = 2.5%) and (N − 0.25) ÷ N is used to substitute for 100 percent. (9.75 ÷ 10 × 100 = 97.5%). A line is drawn to best fit the data and the LD_{50} is determined by the dosage corresponding to the intersect at 50 percent (probit 5), which in this example is 135 mg/kg.

To obtain the SE (standard error) of the LD_{50}, first determine the dosage at probit 6 (P6 corresponds to 84%) and probit 4 (P4 corresponds to 16%). These two values (P6, P4) represent the mean ± one standard deviation. Substracting the smaller (P6) from the larger (P4) results in the numerical value of two standard

deviations (2s). The SE of the LD_{50} is calculated from the following:

$$S.E. = \sqrt{\frac{2s}{2N'}}$$

N' is the number of animals tested that *would be expected* to show effects between probits 6.50 and 3.50. In the example used, $N' = 20$ since only two groups of ten were tested between the dosages of 70 mg (P6.5) and 265 mg (P3.5). Therefore, SE of the $LD_{50} = 19.6$ mg/kg.

The Miller and Tainter method yields results with a minimum of calculation and time. If percentage-probit paper is available there is no need for a probit table and the most difficult calculation is determining a square root.

If the results of using dosage schedules II and III (table 2) are used to calculate the LD_{50} using the probit method the resulting LD_{50} values ± the SE are: schedule II = 120 ± 18 mg/kg and schedule III = 123 ± 21 mg/kg. The point that should be clearly perceived is that nearly the same LD_{50} value is obtained even though three different dosage schemes were used. It should also be noted that only four or five groups of ten female mice were required to determine the LD_{50}. While this is not very many mice, it is really apparent why more percise LD_{50} values are not determined for most compounds in domestic animals.

Now that you have seen how an LD_{50} dose-response is determined, turn your attention to differences in the

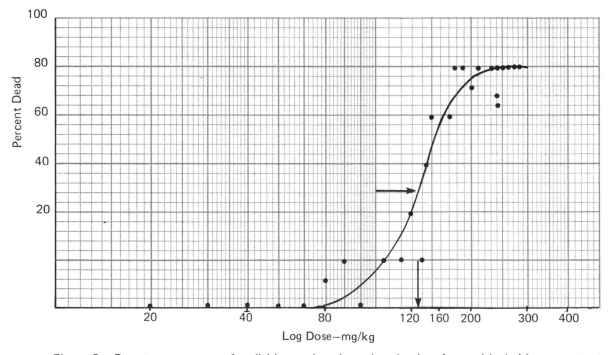

Figure 2. Dose-response curve for dichlorvos in mice using the data from table 1. Linear response (percent dead) is plotted against log dose. The LD_{50} (arrows) is 133 mg/kg. (Adapted from the data of Wagner and Johnson, 1970).

TABLE 3
The Probit Transformation

Response Rate	0.00	0.01	0.02	0.03	0.04	0.05	0.06	0.07	0.08	0.09
0.00	——	2.67	2.95	3.12	3.25	3.36	3.45	3.52	3.59	3.66
0.10	3.72	3.77	3.82	3.87	3.92	3.96	4.01	4.05	4.08	4.12
0.20	4.16	4.19	4.23	4.26	4.29	4.33	4.36	4.39	4.42	4.45
0.30	4.48	4.50	4.53	4.56	4.59	4.61	4.64	4.67	4.69	4.72
0.40	4.75	4.77	4.80	4.82	4.85	4.87	4.90	4.92	4.95	4.97
0.50	5.00	5.03	5.05	5.08	5.10	5.13	5.15	5.18	5.20	5.23
0.60	5.25	5.28	5.31	5.33	5.36	5.39	5.41	5.44	5.47	5.50
0.70	5.52	5.55	5.58	5.61	5.64	5.67	5.71	5.74	5.77	5.81
0.80	5.84	5.88	5.92	5.95	5.99	6.04	6.08	6.13	6.18	6.23
0.90	6.28	6.34	6.41	6.48	6.55	6.64	6.75	6.88	7.05	7.33
0.97	6.88	6.90	6.91	6.93	6.94	6.96	6.98	7.00	7.01	7.03
0.98	7.05	7.07	7.10	7.12	7.14	7.17	7.20	7.23	7.26	7.29
0.99	7.33	7.37	7.41	7.46	7.51	7.58	7.65	7.75	7.88	8.09

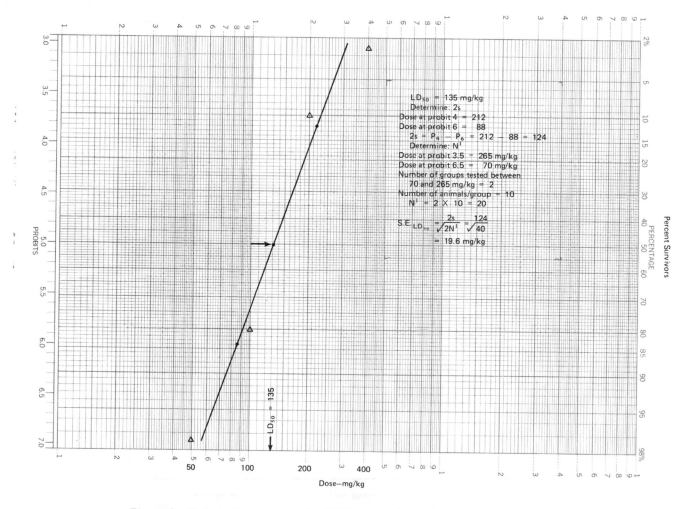

Figure 3. Dose-response curve plotted on probit (left verticle scale) and percentage (right verticle scale) paper for dosage schedule I in table 2.

shapes of dose-response curves. Figure 4 shows LD_{50} dose-response curves for several insecticides tested in several species. Note the difference in slopes. Some of the curves are steep suggesting that the dosage range between few deaths and many deaths is fairly restricted, while the more flat curves reflect compounds with much wider lethal dose ranges. This reflects differences in animal species resulting in variations in biologic response and difference in the compounds. The toxicologist needs to be aware of the extrinsic and intrinsic factors that influence biologic response to toxicants. For example, sex may influence response as basic as life versus death as reflected in LD_{50} values. Table 4 gives more examples.

A fuller understanding of the biologic mechanisms which might account for these differences can be ob-

TABLE 4
Effect of Sex on Acute Oral LD_{50} in Rats

Compound	LD_{50} (mg/kg)	
	Female	Male
Digitoxin	56	94
Trifluperidol	140	360
Dieldrin	119	213
Parathion	3.6	9

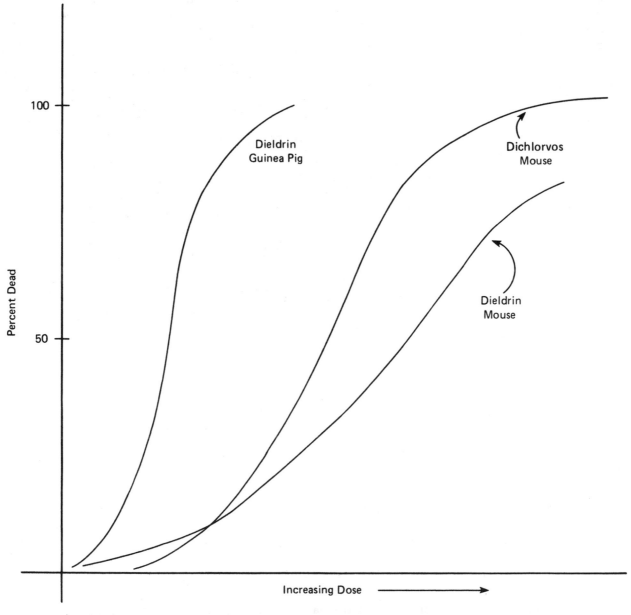

Figure 4. Examples of LD_{50} dose-response curves demonstrating differences in response slopes.

tained by comparing the rate of liver metabolism. Table 5 shows the faster metabolism of dieldrin by male rat liver.

The above illustrates the use of differences in dose-response effects that leads to answering basic questions that contribute to the understanding of biologic mechanisms.

Traditionally our concept of dose is in terms of mg/kg. Considering that at the actual site of action the biologic response may involve interaction of single molecules of toxicant with discrete subcellular components, then the computation of the LD_{50} (or other measure of effective dose) on the basis of numbers of molecules may be more illustrative. In table 6 the oral LD_{50} of several compounds in 20 gram mice is compared on a mg/mouse and molecules/mouse basis.

One of the major problems with this comparison is that differences in absorption rates or percent of the oral dose absorbed are not considered. However, it is another method of evaluating dose-response phenomena.

There are other methods of calculating dose-response functions that do not have the restriction of segregating each response into yes or no, present or absent categories. Regression analysis is very useful for several reasons. First, all of the data can be used. Second, there are fewer restrictions on dosage schedules allowing the use of this method for some types of clinical data. And third, the dose-response function is

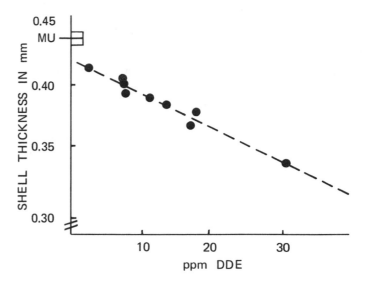

Figure 5. Example of a calculated linear regression dose-response function. (Adopted from Anderson, D. W. *et al.,* 1969. Significance of Chlorinated Hydrocarbon Residues to Breeding Pelicans and Cormorants. Canadian Field-Naturalist. 83:91-112.)

not limited to liner-linear or linear-log relationships. Curvilinear response such as quadratic or cubic are easily handled. An example of a linear regression dose-response function is shown in figure 5, which depicts the relationship between DDE residues and eggshell thickness in Doubled-crested Cormorants.'(Anderson *et al.,* 1969) This dose-response relationship shows that as the level of DDE residue increased then the thickness of the eggshell decreased in a predictable manner.

The more data available and the wider the exposure range over which data is available the better is the basis for both understanding the nature of the biologic response and being able to determine the likelihood of cause and effect in specific clinical situations. The factor limiting fuller use of dose-response functions is the limited number of dosage levels used in many toxicologic experiments.

TABLE 5
Sex Difference in Rate of Liver
Metabolism of C^{14}—Dieldrin

| Gender | Metabolism—(Dpm/g liver) | |
	One Hour	Six Hours
Male	1,200	10,500
Female	270	3,200

TABLE 6
Comparison of LD_{50} Values and Molecules in an LD_{50} for Compounds Tested in 20 Gram Mice

Compound	Mol. Wt.	LD_{50} mg/Mouse	Ratio*	LD_{50} Molecules/Mouse	Ratio*
Botulinum toxin	900,000	.01 mg	1	6.75×10^{12}	1
Tetrodotoxin	319	.0087 mg	.87	1.63×10^{16}	240
Parathion	291	.36 mg	3.6	7.452×10^{17}	110,400
DDT	352	6 mg	600	1.003×10^{19}	1,480,000

*Ratios relative to botulism toxin.

REFERENCES

Litchfield, J. T. and Wilcoxon, F. 1949. A Simplified Method of Evaluating Dose-Effect Experiments. *Journal of Pharmacology and Experimental Therapeutics.* 96:99-113.

Miller, L. C. and Tainter, M. L. 1944. Estimation of the ED_{50} and Its Error by Means of Logarithmic-Probit Graph Paper. *Proceedings of the Society of Experimental Biology and Medicine.* 57:261-64.

Wagner, J. E. and Johnson, D. R. 1970. Toxicity of Dichlorvos for Laboratory Mice—LD_{50} and Effect on Serum Cholinesterase. *Laboratory Animal Care.* 20:45-47.

Weil, C. . 1952. Tables for Convenient Calculation of Median-Effective Dose (LD_{50} or ED_{50}) and Instructions in Their Use. *Biometerics.* 8:249-63.

TOXICOKINETICS

Only selected aspects of toxicokinetics will be presented in this section. The advanced student is directed to the reference list for specific books which discuss in more detail the kinetics of drugs and foreign compounds.

Important Principles

Toxicokinetics involves the relationship between tissue concentration of a toxicant and time. In principle toxicokinetics is similar to pharmacokinetics. However, with toxicants the interest is in how long something will remain in the body as a contaminant, while with therapeutic agents the length of time that an effective drug level is maintained is of primary interest. Individuals involved in regulatory functions have a vested interest in chemical kinetics, be it a drug or toxicant, because of residue problems in meat, milk and eggs. It is not unusual to have a herd or flock quarantined because of excessive drug or chemical residues. The more that is known about the kinetics of a compound the better the advice that can be given in a specific situation.

The following discussion covers principles considered to be fundamental to the general knowledge of most veterinary students and veterinary clinicians.

With most toxicants the major factor determining the biologic impact on the animal is dose. Dose is highly important since most toxicants appear to be absorbed along concentration gradients. Therefore, if more toxicant is present at the membrane surface then more toxicant is absorbed through the membrane. Conversely, this relationship would not hold if the toxicant were absorbed via active absorption. In active absorption the rate of toxicant absorption would be limited to the amount of carrier substance and the amount of energy available.

The physical nature of the toxicant is also related to absorption. For example, finely divided lead has more surface area than the equivalent amount in one piece. This results in a larger surface area for dissolu-tion and absorption from the stomach and intestinal tract.

The route of exposure is also an important consideration. The most frequent route of exposure in clinical toxicosis is oral. This is with the exception of adverse reactions to parenterally administered drugs. Dermal absoprtion is usually limited to overdosing with insecticides used to treat ecto- or endoparasites. The inhalation route seems to be of practical significance primarily in cases of gas poisoning such as carbon dioxide, carbon monoxide or hydrogen sulfide. It is recognized that many herbicides, insecticides, and heavy metals can be absorbed from the respiratory tract. Rarely, however, does this result in recognizable clinical toxicosis unless the animal is housed or maintained in an area with a high ambient air level of the toxicant. For grazing animals clinical toxicosis is more likely to result from aerosol and particulate matter precipitating on and contaminating forage and resulting oral ingestion rather than from direct respiratory exposure.

With the exception of compounds such as strong acids and bases, most toxicants are absorbed from one site and moved or *translocated* to other sites within the body. Obviously then, the blood vascular system is directly involved. This means that with many toxicants analytical chemists can find the chemical in the blood of exposed animals. And in fact that is what is often done in poisoning cases to demonstrate the presence of specific toxicants. A word of caution, however, in interpreting the results of blood residue analyses. One must remember that in most cases the toxicant is not producing its biologic effect on the blood cells or plasms, but rather is acting at some other site such as the brain, myoneural junction, skin or liver. For this reason blood levels do not always correlate with severity of clinical signs. Blood levels will also vary with the time elapsed since exposure and with the amount of "tissue storage space" available for deposition of the toxicant. It is also possible in cases of low-level chronic exposure for tissue levels to build up sufficiently to cause poisoning while blood levels may be lower than observed with acute poisoning. Because of the above factors the toxicologist must often use a range of blood residue values in order to determine the significance of a single observation. This difficulty does not completely undermine the utility of blood residue chemistry. Blood samples can be routinely obtained from most animals under veterinary care and it is better to have a specimen with some degree of valid use than to have no specimen at all.

There is considerable range in the dynamics of tissue storage of individual toxicants. Some are metabolized rapidly, such as urea and some organophosphorus insecticides, while others such as lead may persist in bone for years. Both the specific tissue involved and the duration of storage vary with specific toxicants.

A few examples of tissue storage are presented here for illustration. Dieldrin is a chlorinated hydrocarbon insecticide. It is lipid soluble and accumulates in tissues with a high lipid content. Table 1 gives the tissue levels found in an animal fed 0.1 mg dieldrin/kg for fifty-five days. If the results were presented on the basis of the amount of lipid present in each tissue, then the distribution would be more uniform. The data are presented on a wet weight basis to illustrate the nonuniform distribution on a tissue or organ basis.

Toxicants are also eliminated from the body at different rates. Table 2 compares the rate of elimination of dieldrin and the herbicide 2, 4-D from the blood of animals. From table 2 it can be seen that the rate of removal from the blood varies over a wide range. This is of particular significance to the clinician since the animal in some cases may have eliminated most of the toxicant before the sample is obtained in a field investigation. Or the slower rate of elimination of a foreign chemical may require the prolonged mainte-

TABLE 1
Dieldrin Tissue Levels

Tissue	Dieldrin Residue—Wet-Weight Basis, ppm (parts per million)
Brain	0.050
Liver	1.968
Omental fat	2.321
Kidney	0.045
Adrenal gland	0.287
Spleen	0.028
Testicle	0.031
Blood serum	0.013

TABLE 2
Elimination of Dieldrin and 2, 4-D from Blood

Time after a Single Oral Dose	Residue in Blood (ppm) Dieldrin	2, 4-D
2 hours	0.025	100
6 hours	0.100	250
12 hours	0.100	200
24 hours	0.150	100
48 hours	0.175	5
4 days	0.100	0
8 days	0.060	0
16 days	0.040	0
22 days	0.025	0

nance of a contaminated herd or flock until the tissue residue is below regulatory actionable level.

Toxicokinetics

In this section several examples will be presented utilizing mathematical and graphic descriptions of the kinetics of toxicant excretion. The mathematical examples are worked out step by step such that if the reader will take the time to follow these through, a solid working knowledge should be achieved.

There are two types of kinetics involved, namely, zero-order and first-order. If a toxicant is eliminated at a *fixed amount* per day, then this is zero-order kinetics. This can occur when the toxicant elimination process is saturated and a fixed number of mg or gm are excreted per unit time.

The more usual situation is where first-order kinetics occur. In first-order kinetics a constant fraction of the toxicant present is eliminated per unit time. This means that when toxicant concentration is high, such as occurs after acute exposure, a large amount is initially eliminated per unit time. As the tissue toxicant concentration decreases then less actual toxicant (mg/time) is eliminated. Another way of stating this is to realize that if the initial level were 100 mg and it took ten days to reach 50 mg, then it would take an additional ten days to reach 25 mg. During the first ten days a total of 50 mg toxicant was excreted and during the second 10 days only 25 mg. In each case the amount excreted was a constant fraction (50%) of the value in the tissue at the start of the ten-day period.

There are several points to emphasize before going on. (1) Concentrate on understanding the concept of first-order kinetics as related to excretion of toxicants. Many toxicants are eliminated from animal tissues in a first-order manner. As will be shown later this type of first-order kinetic description of elimination of toxicants is an exponential function. (2) The concept of first-order kinetics will better enable the clinician to understand and explain the rationale for estimating the expected duration of a quarantine. (3) Up to this point the contaminated animal body has been assumed to consist of one compartment whose toxicant elimination function can be defined by a single component equation (function) or a simple exponential decay curve. As will be shown later it may be necessary to consider the animal body as consisting of two or more compartments with distinctly different excretion kinetics.

As a starting point assume the toxicant is eliminated in an exponential manner such as $C_R = C_i e^{-kt}$, where C_R is the remaining concentration, C_i is the initial concentration, e is 2.72 (base of natural logarithms), k is a rate constant for the particular tissue, toxicant and species, and t is the time in hours or days. From this relationship the half-life can be calculated. The half-life is defined as the amount of time required for the residue to decrease to 50 percent of the time zero level. Knowing the half-life value can be of some use when the clinician is dealing with a herd of animals quarantined because of excessive drug or toxicant residues. For example, if you find that the initial residue level is 10 ppm and ten days later the level has decreased to 7 ppm, you can calculate the constant "k" as follows:

Step 1: Use the assumed model of $C_R = C_i e^{-kt}$ to get

$$7 = 10e^{-10k}$$

Step 2: Divide both sides by 10.

$$0.7 = e^{-10k}$$

Step 3 Recall that equations of this form $(N = b^x)$ can be reduced to $\log_b N = x$, and therefore:

$$\ln 0.7 = -10k$$

Step 4: Since $\ln 0.7 = -0.3567$, therefore it follows that -0.3567 equals $-10k$

$$10k = 0.3567$$

and finally

$$k = 0.03567 = 0.036$$

Step 5: Thus the equation fitting the observed rate of excretion is

$$C_R = C_i e^{-0.036t}$$

with t expressed in days.

Since this type of mathematical expression is difficult to visualize a graphic representation is presented in figure 1 which shows the elimination curve associated with the specific equation given in step 5 above.

The next step is to calculate the half-life. Assume that the starting level is 10 ppm and you want to determine how many days are required before the level reaches 5 ppm. This is calculated as follows:

Step 1: Using the same data as above, the equation is:

$$C_R = C_i e^{-0.036t}$$

Given $C_R = 5$ or one-half the starting value of C_i which is 10, it follows that

$$5 = 10e^{-0.036t}$$

Step 2: Reduce the equation to:

$$.5 = e^{-0.036t}$$

Step 3: Using the relationship given above, this is further reduced to:

$$\ln 0.5 = -0.036t$$

Step 4 Since $\ln 0.5 = -0.69315$ the equation is solved for t as follows:

$$-0.69315 = -0.036t$$

$$t = \frac{0.69315}{0.036}$$

$$t = 19 \text{ days}$$

which is the half-life for this particular example.

This can be carried one step further. Assume that the residue level must reach 0.5 ppm before the animals can be sold for slaughter and the livestock owner wants *some indication* of how long the animals must be maintained before they would be expected to eliminate the

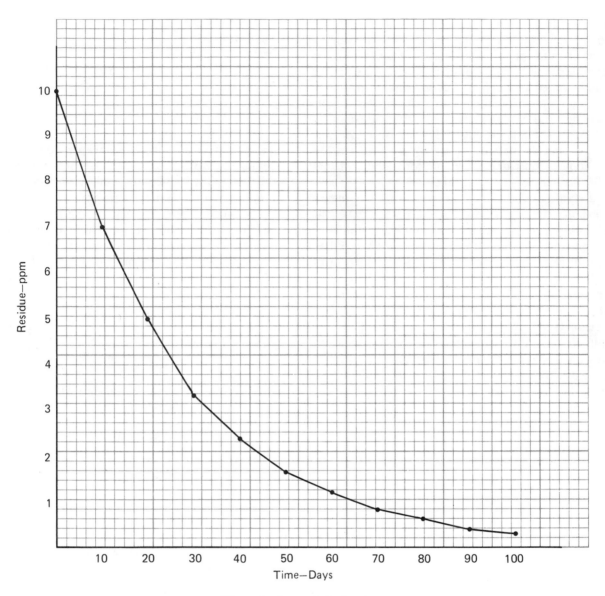

Figure 1. Rate of elimination.

foreign chemical to acceptable levels. This is calculated as follows:

Step 1:

$$C_R = C_I e^{-kt}$$

Given that $C_I = 10$, $C_R = 0.5$ and $k = 0.036$, solve for t

$$0.5 = 10e^{-0.036t}$$

Step 2:

$$0.05 = e^{-0.036t}$$

Step 3: Rewrite as in previous examples.

$$\ln 0.05 = -0.036t$$
$$\ln 0.05 = -2.99$$

Step 4:

Therefore $-2.99 = -0.036t$

and $t = \dfrac{2.99}{.036}$

        $t = 83$ days

Thus you would predict that about eighty-three days would be required for the animal to eliminate the foreign chemical under the assumed conditions. There are several reasons to be cautious when making these calculations. First, you assume that you have representative data. That is, that the analytical results obtained accurately reflect the level of contamination in the whole herd. If the animals sampled have unusually high or low values compared to the rest of the herd then the calculated time for elimination to acceptable levels will be in error. Secondly, you assume that you have reliable data, meaning that the analytical results accurately reflect the levels actually presented. Occasionally analytical results vary by 25-30 percent depending on the laboratory and the methods used. For this reason you want to present the results of your calculations as guarded predictions.

It is also assumed that the source of contamination has been eliminated, because if the herd is still being exposed to the toxicant you will be unable to accurately predict the rate of elimination.

The above examples were based on a single component exponential model. In some cases two or more exponential components are needed to adequately describe the elimination of a toxicant. For example, a single component model as used above describes the elimination of dieldrin from fat while a two component model is used to describe the elimination of dieldrin from blood. The two component model is of the form:

$$C = Ae^{-k_1 t} + Be^{-k_2 t}$$

Fitting such a model becomes much more complicated and is usually accomplished with computer techniques. When the model contains two or more components it essentially means that several dynamic biologic processes are involved which operate at different rates. For example, the normalized equation for the excretion of dieldrin in cows' milk is $C = .52e^{-.2t} + .48e^{-.012t}$. The resulting curve is shown in figure 2. Note the initial rapid decline, associated with the first term in the equation, followed by the slower decline, associated with the second term in the equation. The half-life associated with the first term ($.52e^{-.2t}$) is 3.5 days and for the second term ($.48e^{-.012t}$) is fifty- seven days.

An extreme case is found when the toxicant is initially stored in both soft tissue and bone. It has been found that to model, and thus be able to predict, the

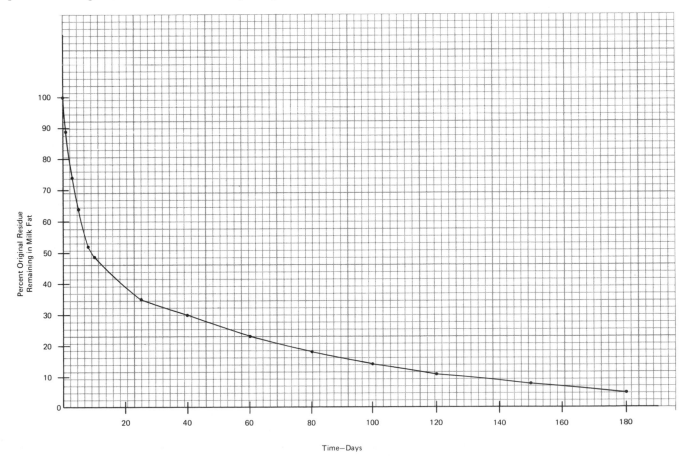

Figure 2. Elimination of dieldrin in cows' milk.

elimination of strontium from the body requires at least a four component exponential equation with a time span of several thousand days.

As more and better models become available the toxicologist, both clinical and environmental, will be better able to accurately describe the interaction of storage and elimination of foreign substances in biologic systems.

REFERENCES

Golstein, A., *et al.* 1974. *Principles of Drug Action.* 2nd ed. New York: Harper and Row.

Goodman, L. S., and Gilman, A. 1975 *The Pharmacological Basis of Therapeutics.* 5th ed. New York: MacMillan Publishing Co., New York.

Jones, L. M. 1965. *Veterinary Pharmacology and Therapeutics.* Ames, Iowa: Iowa State University Press.

Park, D. V. 1968. *The Biochemistry of Foreign Compounds.* Pergamon Press.

BIOTRANSFORMATION

In general the mammalian body attempts to modify the chemical structure of foreign compounds (xenobiotics) in order to reduce physiological activity of such drugs or chemicals and to enhance excretion.

Biotransformation usually results in the following:

1. Metabolites are more polar, less lipophilic and more water soluble.
2. The metabolite is often more highly ionized.
3. As a result of the first two changes, protein binding may be reduced, storage in fat is less likely, and reabsorption through biologic membranes such as renal tubules and intestinal epithelium is prevented.

Biotransformation may either enhance or reduce the toxicity of foreign compounds. When the toxicity of a chemical is reduced it is said to be detoxified. When the product of metabolism is more toxic than the parent compound the term "lethal synthesis" is often used, i.e., the body has produced a new chemical more detrimental to life processes than was the original. Examples of lethal synthesis include:

1. The conversion of fluoroacetate to fluorocitrate, which interferes with the tricarboxylic acid cycle.
2. The oxidation of the insecticide parathion to paraoxon, which is highly toxic.
3. The oxidation of relatively innocuous ethylene glycol to more toxic intermediates and to oxalic acid.

Types of Biotransformations

There are two major phases to foreign compound metabolism constituting four principal chemical mechanisms. (Parke, 1969) During Phase I, a chemical may acquire reactive groups such as OH, NH_2, COOH or SH. The major reactions are nonsynthetic in nature and include the following:

1. Oxidation: Hydroxylation, deamination, dealkylation, and sulfoxide formation are examples.
2. Reduction: Nitro reduction and addition of hydrogen are examples.
3. Hydrolysis: Splitting of ester and amide bonds are examples.

Phase II reactions are synthetic or conjugation reactions. A drug may combine directly with an endogenous substance, or may be altered by Phase I and then undergo conjugation. The endogenous substances commonly involved in conjugation reactions include glucuronic acid, amino acids (e.g., glycine), sulfates, acetates, and methyl groups.

Of the biotransformation mechanisms available, oxidation is a major mechanism. Hence, the importance of the microsomal mixed function oxidases which are described later in this chapter.

Specific chemical examples of biotransformation are given in figure 1. Many other specific transformations take place but figure 1 will serve to depict the chemical changes associated with some common metabolic changes.

Mechanism of Biotransformation

The principal site of biotransformation is the liver. Lesser activity is lodged in specific tissues such as the brain, kidney, intestinal mucosa and plasma. Within the liver, the hepatic endoplasmic reticulum, particularly the smooth endoplasmic reticulum, is the locus of most biotransformation activity. Biotransformation is catalyzed primarily by the microsomal mixed function oxidases, and biological oxidations constitute the majority of biotransformation reactions. These mixed function oxidases (MFO) lack substrate specificity, and will metabolize substances of quite varied chemical structure if they are lipid soluble. The MFO are active in metabolism of lipids, steroids, and foreign compounds.

Mechanism	Reaction

Oxidation

Hydroxylation

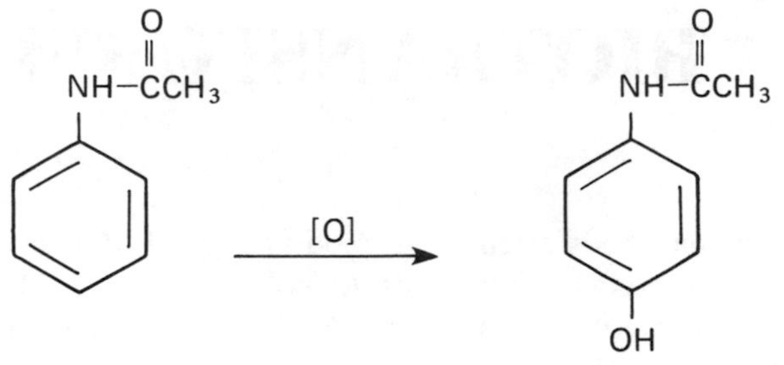

Acetanilid →[O]→ p-hydroxyacetanilid

Deamination

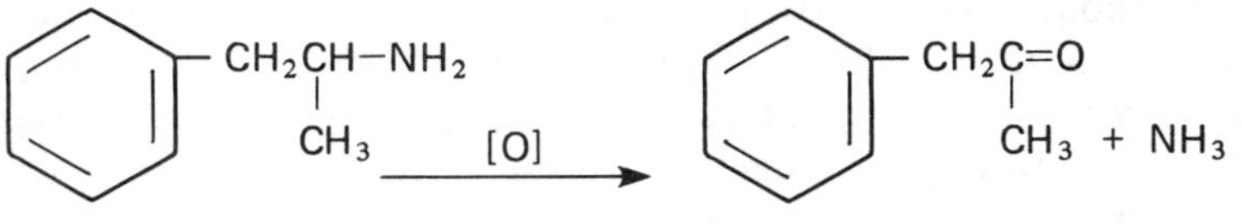

Amphetamine →[O]→ Phenylacetone + NH_3

Dealkylation

Acetophenetidin →[O]→ p-hydroxyacetanilid + CH_3CHO

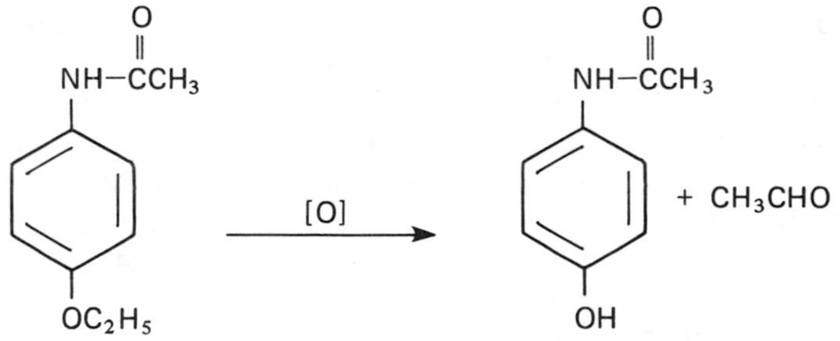

Sulfoxide Formation

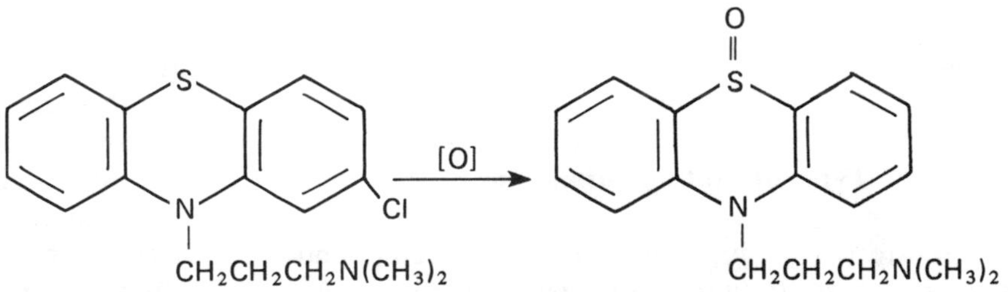

Chlorpromazine →[O]→ Chlorpromazine Sulfoxide

Figure 1. Chemical mechanisms of biotransformation.

Mechanism	Reaction

Oxidation

Desulfuration

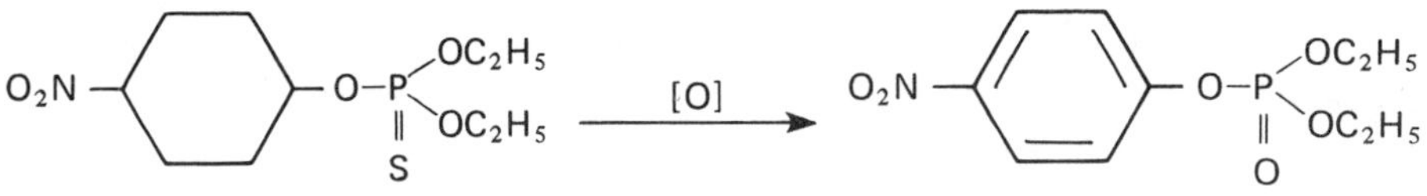

Parathion → Paraoxon

Reduction

Nitro Reduction

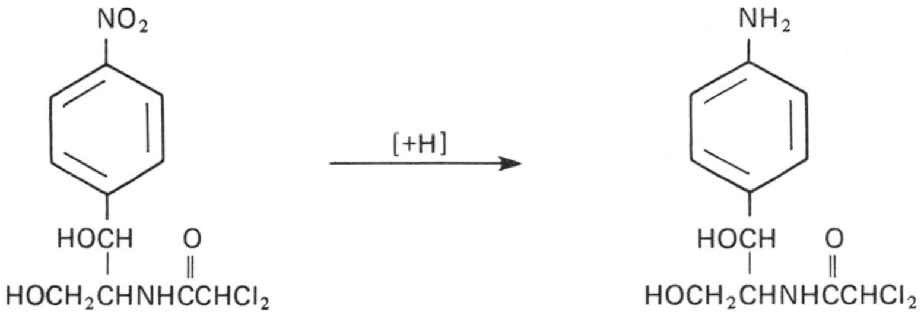

Chloramphenicol → Reduced Chloramphenicol

Hydrolysis

$(CH_3)_3N-CH_2CH_2-O-\overset{O}{\underset{\parallel}{C}}-CH_3 \xrightarrow{[H_2O]} (CH_3)_3N-CH_2CH_2OH + CH_3-\overset{O}{\underset{\parallel}{C}}-OH$

Acetyl Choline → Choline + Acetic Acid

Congugation

Glucuronides

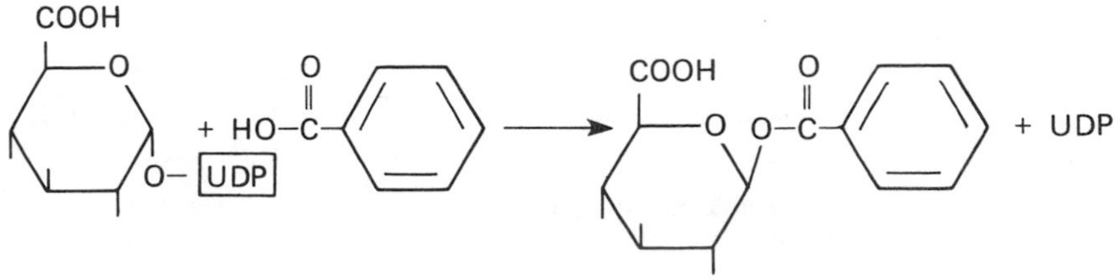

Uridine-Diphosphate Glucuronic Acid + Benzoic Acid → p-hydroxyacetanilid Glucuronide + UDP

Figure 1. (continued.)

The result is conversion of such compounds into more polar, less lipophilic metabolites for rapid excretion from the body.

Biological oxidation involves a common mechanism, hydroxylation, which is dependent on an oxidation-reduction (redox) system including $NADPH_2$ and "active oxygen." The "active oxygen" results from combination of the hemoprotein cytochrome P-450 with molecular oxygen (Camp, 1974; Goldstein, et al., 1974) Figure 2 depicts the major events theorized to occur in the electron flow pathway of the microsomal drug oxidizing system.

Microsomal enzymes may be induced to greater activity by continued exposure to certain drugs or chemicals.

Enzyme induction means that the microsomal enzymes have been stimulated to the extent that there is a higher rate of enzyme activity resulting in an increased rate of drug metabolism. This effect has been most extensively studied in the liver but also exists in other tissues. For example, placentas obtained from smoking women contain enzymes which metabolize 3, 4-benzpyrene while placentas from nonsmoking women do not possess this enzyme activity. Because of the drug metabolizing role of the liver, enzyme induction usually refers to liver activity, but it is important to recognize that enzyme induction is not limited to the liver.

Several days of exposure to a drug are required to increase enzyme activity and the effect may persist for one to four weeks after dosing is discontinued. The persistence of the effect varies with the drug, species and sensitivity of the analytical techniques.

The effects of enzyme induction in toxicology are manifested in several ways. In chronic toxicity studies the plasma drug level may be high during the first few days of administration and the animal may manifest side effects. But after a few days the plasma level decreases even though the same dosage is given daily. The decreased plasma level is a result of the drug stimulating the liver microsomal drug metabolizing enzymes which results in an increased rate of drug metabolism. Table 1 presents data which demonstrates

that a progressively higher dose must be given in order to maintain comparable plasma drug levels.

Another effect of enzyme induction is when one drug induces enzyme activity which increases the metabolism of a second drug. For example, barbiturates increase the rate of metabolism of the anticoagulate drug bishydroxycoumarin. This has clinical significance since it has been demonstrated that dogs maintained on phenobarbital and warfarin anticoagulate therapy may go into a hemorrhagic crisis a few days after the phenobarbital is withdrawn if the warfarin dosage is not decreased.

Drug induced enzyme activity may also increase the metabolism of natural body constituents. It has been demonstrated in laboratory animals that steroid metabolism could be affected by administration of exogenous drugs. The clinical importance of this effect is not well understood at the present time.

The effect of exogenous drugs increasing metabolism of natural body constituents has also been put to clinical use. The anticonvulsant diphenylhydantoin increases the metabolism of cortisol and has been used with some success in treating patients with Cushing's syndrome.

Another manifestation of enzyme induction in toxicology occurs when animals previously exposed to other drugs and environmental contaminants are used in an experiment to study the effects of a new compound. A number of the insecticides, which might be used in animal quarters, have been shown to increase drug metabolism. Also animals maintained on cedar shavings have been shown to have increased liver microsomal enzyme activity. The effect of pretreating rats with phenobarbital for five days on the LD_{50} of several organophosphorus insecticides is shown in table 2. Note that the LD_{50} values are increased in the phenobarbital pretreated animals, meaning that larger doses were required to produce death.

Since man and animals are continuously exposed to a wide variety of drugs and chemicals in their food and environment, considerable interest exists concerning the possible effects of environmental con-

TABLE 1

Drug Stimulated Liver Microsomal Enzyme Activity

| Day | Relationship Between | |
	Oral Drug Dosage	Plasma Drug Levels
1	100	118
8	100	14
21	200	43
30	300	120

TABLE 2

Phenobarbital Pretreatment Effects on LD_{50} in Rats

Organophosphorus Insecticides	Control	Phenobarbital Pretreated
Parathion	2.5	7.3
Systox	1.4	5.8
Delnan	17.2	118.7
Co-Ral	7.5	13.8

taminants on the metabolism of therapeutic drugs and natural body constituents. Using available techniques it appears at the present time that a certain threshold exposure level must be present before enzyme induction occurs. If this is the case then subthreshold exposure to environmental contaminants would not be expected to have any direct biologic impact on induced drug or natural body constituent metabolism.

Alteration of Biotransformation

Many factors can alter the biotransformation of drugs and chemicals, and the effect may be either enhancement or reduction of toxicity of the parent compound. The factors affecting biotransformation may be both biological and chemical as follows.

Species Differences

Marked differences among species metabolism of the same compound exist. Cats, lacking adequate glucuronyl transferase, form glucuronides poorly and are thus more susceptible to poisoning by materials such as benzoic acid and phenol. Rabbits have high levels of an enzyme active against atropine, and thus resist doses of atropine toxic to other species. Horses have greater amounts of plasma esterases active against succinylcholine than do cattle.

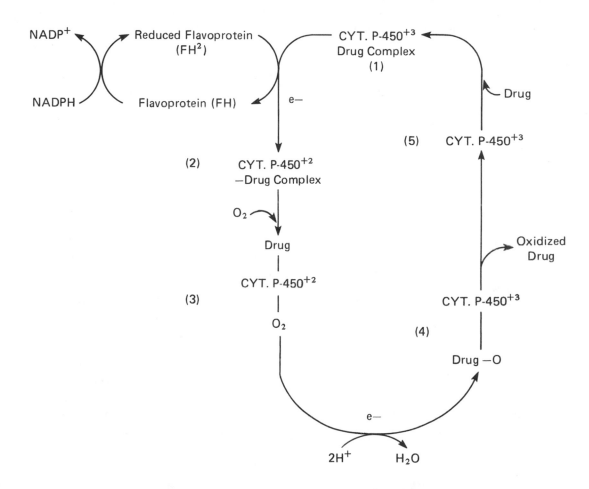

(1) Substrate (drug) combines with (ferric hemoprotein) P-450 to form Fe^{+3} drug complex.

(2) CYT P-450^{+3} drug complex undergoes a one-electron reduction to a CYT P-450^{+2} drug complex.

(3) Complex reacts with oxygen to form oxycytochrome P-450.

(4) Addition of another electron results in generation of water and oxidized drug.

(5) The "active oxygen" form of cytochrome P-450^{+3} drug complex decomposes into oxidized drug and oxidized P-450.

Figure 2. Electron flow pathway in the microsomal drug oxidizing system.

Genetic and Strain Differences

Within species, certain breeds or strains vary in ability to detoxify drugs. While Dutch rabbits have higher ability to metabolize amphetamine than do other breeds, their ability to metabolize 3, 4- benzpyrene is lower than for other breeds. Dalmatian dogs, lacking uricase, are less able to carry out purine metabolism. Shetland ponies appear to have as much as 25 percent less cholinesterase activity than do standard-sized breeds.

Age

New born animals are generally deficient in drug metabolizing enzymes, and this lack may persist for one to two months after birth. Very old animals, with depressed protein synthesis may also suffer the same deficit. Interactions with hormones at various ages may also be involved.

Sex

There is differential toxicity for certain foreign compounds between the sexes. Such differences have been recorded in rats for strychnine, parathion, paraoxon, warfarin, and hexobarbital. In cats and dogs, parathion is more toxic to the female.

Sex differences in metabolism are mainly observed after puberty and are probably largely related to hormonal influences.

Disease Conditions

In particular hepatic disease may interfere with optimum liver function. For example, warfarin may be more toxic in liver-damaged animals because metabolic conversion to less toxic metabolites is slower.

Nutritional Status

Nutritional deficiencies such as protein depletion, lack of cofactors and conjugating pools (e.g., methionine, ATP) may interfere with enzyme activity or synthesis. Interactions of dietary components with metabolizing enzymes or cofactors could also be involved.

Decreased Body Temperature

Lower temperatures slow the rate of enzyme-mediated reactions.

Route of Administration

Orally and intraperitoneally administered drugs pass initially through the liver where they are subjected to hepatic activity. Intravenous administration may rapidly spread chemicals to diverse sites including receptors and storage depots.

Time of Administration

Circadian rhythms, light, and seasonal influences may alter metabolic rate in relation to time of exposure to drugs. Thus, drug administration during a quiescent metabolic period may result in decreased biotransformation.

Interaction or Competition with Endogenous Substances

Steroids or decomposition products of other body systems may effect induction of microsomal enzyme systems.

Protein Binding in Plasma

This delays the amount of drug available for detoxication. Conversely, administration of a second drug which displaces the first may enhance metabolic transformation of the first drug.

Localization of Drug in Body Tissues

Storage in depots such as bone, fat, or muscle may delay biotransformation.

Enzyme Inhibition by Other Drugs

Drugs such as SKF 525A and chloramphenicol may depress the metabolsim of other drugs.

Enzyme Induction or Stimulation by Other Drugs

Previous or concurrent administration of a second drug may induce increased activity of microsomal enzymes and stimulate more rapid metabolism. This phenomenon is more fully explained under the topic of enzyme induction.

Both the toxicity of chemicals and the therapeutic efficacy of drugs may be influenced by biotransformation. In addition, alteration of metabolism may be used to rid the body of certain undesirable residues such as pesticides. One must carefully consider all of the factors involved in biotransformation when considering toxicologic diagnosis or drug therapy, since biotransformation may be either beneficial or detrimental to the animal.

REFERENCES

Camp, B. J. 1974. *Biotransformation of Drugs.* Second Biennial Veterinary Toxicology Workshop. College Station, Texas.

Goldstein, A.; Aronow, L.; and Kalman S. 1974. *Principles of Drug Action.* 2nd ed. New York: John Wiley & Sons.

Hildebrant, A., and Estabrook, R. 1971. Evidence for the participation of cytochrome 6_5 in hepatic microsomal mixed function oxidation reactions. *Arch. Biochem. Biophys.* 143:66.

Matsumura, F. 1975. *Toxicology of Insecticides.* New York: Plenum Press.

Parke, D. V.; Williams, R. T., 1969. Metabolism of toxic substances. *Br. Med. Bull.* 25:256—62.

St. Omer, V. V. E. 1975. *Veterinary Pharmacology Notes.* Columbia, Mo.: University of Missouri.

Sher, S. 1971. Drug enzyme induction and drug interactions: literature tabulation. *Tox. Appl. Pharm.* 18:780-834.

SAFETY TESTING

Millions of dollars are spent each year in assessing the safety and toxicity of new drugs for human and veterinary use, new agricultural chemicals such as herbicides and insecticides, new feed additives and, more recently, a wide variety of industrial chemicals. It has been the authors' experience that, in general, people are not knowledgeable about the testing that is done prior to release of a new product. In this chapter an overview of toxicity tests and testing procedures is provided. It is intended that the student gain some understanding and general awareness of the information that is being generated in toxicology today. This chapter represents an overview and not a protocol cookbook.

A protocol is the description of the toxicology tests that will be conducted on a given compound. Protocols may be general or specific. A general protocol would represent the variety of tests that would be conducted, while a specific protocol would provide more detail for an individual toxicology test and would be expected to contain information specifying specific drug formulation, vehicle, species of animals, number of animals per group, physiologic and biochemical determinations to be conducted, pathology procedures and data collection and reduction procedures. General protocols are available for safety evaluation, while specific protocols are developed within these general concepts to meet the needs for specific information on individual compounds.

Toxicology tests can be divided into two major groups. The first group includes the general tests for acute, subchronic and chronic toxicity. The second group are the special tests for specific effects on: reproduction; fertility; potentiation; teratogenicity; carcinogenicity; mutagenicity; skin, eye, muscle, subcutaneous or intramammary irritation; hemolysis; and behavior.

For compounds that may enter the general environment, toxicity testing will include studies using fish and birds.

General Principles

Regardless of the test involved there are some general principles and factors that influence the design and conduct of the study. The species of animals used is influenced by cost, availability, ease of handling, amount of known physiologic data, ability to reproduce in captivity, caging and housing requirements and known pharmacologic or physiologic peculiarities. The ideal choice is to select species that metabolize the compound in the same way as the target species. Target species means the species which will ultimately be exposed to the compound.

In general, rats and dogs are most commonly used. Other animals used include mice, rabbits, guinea pigs, hamsters and gerbils. Primates are frequently used although cost and availability limit their use. It is possible that miniature swine will someday become more common as public opinion and legislation cause a decline in the use of dogs. Problems with using larger species include physical size, housing and amount of compound required for long-term dosing.

On the one hand the compound being studied should be as chemically pure as possible. On the other hand the compound must be representative of the product as it will be used commercially. The toxicologist must always be aware of toxic contaminants.

If a solvent or vehicle is needed, then care must be taken so that the vehicle neither chemically alters the compound nor binds it in such a way that it is biologically inert. A vehicle control is also needed to ensure that observed changes are compound induced and not vehicle induced.

The most common route of exposure for general testing is oral. If the compound can be mixed in the feed, this is usually done for prolonged exposure studies. It is much more expensive to individually dose each animal daily. Animals should be dosed seven days per week. Variations include five and six-day exposures.

Allowing animals one or two days recovery every week may alter the toxicologic response.

Animals are observed daily for clinical signs. For the veterinarian these clinical signs represent the same types of responses and alterations associated with clinical medicine.

Dosages for subchronic, chronic and some special tests must be carefully selected. It is intended that a high dose be used that will result in definite clinical toxicosis. A middose will be used that produces mild toxicosis. The low dose is selected to approach the criteria of being the largest dose that does not cause toxicosis. It is no problem to select a very low dose that does not produce toxicity. However, the purpose of the low-dose group is to establish what level of exposure can be tolerated without causing adverse effects.

A common mistake made by the novice is to conduct interim sacrifices. That is to kill and necropsy a selected number of animals from each group at specified intervals. There is nothing inherently wrong with interim sacrifices if they are planned for in the original protocol. The problem with interim sacrifices occurs when, for example, a chronic twenty-four-month toxicity study is conducted in which each group has initially forty animals per group. If interim sacrifices are done at one, three, nine and twelve months the following two types of problems can occur. First, if only one to two animals per group are necropsied at each interim period then insufficient data is available for any meaningful statistical comparisons. If five or more animals are necropsied at the end of each interim period then at the end of twelve months the group size has been reduced to twenty or fewer subjects. The decrease in number of animals per group severely diminishes the chances of detecting low-level adverse reactions. If interim sacrifices are needed then additional animals should be added at the beginning of the experiment.

GENERAL TESTS

Acute Toxicity. This is the one test most commonly conducted on the widest variety of compounds. From this the LD_{50} or LC_{50} is determined. The route of exposure can be dermal, oral, inhalation, or parenteral with oral being the most common route. Acute toxicity refers to the effects obtained following a single exposure or multiple exposures during a twenty-four-hour period. The observation period is usually seven or fourteen days. If delayed deaths occur near the end of the observation period, the time should be lengthened. The data is interpreted using the methods in the chapter—**Dose-Response Relationships.** More than one species of rodents may be used. If the larger, more expensive

animals are used then the limited number of animals usually precludes determination of the LD_{50}; but rather estimates of the lethal dose or minimum toxic dose are obtained.

Subchronic Toxicity. This category refers primarily to results obtained following thirty to ninety days of exposure. Although, occasionally fourteen-day exposures are used. There is not general agreement as to call these studies subchronic, prolonged, three month, ninety day, six weeks or whatever. Probably the best and most accurate is to reference the toxictiy data by the number of days of exposure. A usual design would involve rats and dogs at three different dosage levels plus a control group. If rodents are used then thirty to forty animals equally divided by sex are used per group. If dogs or large animals are used then six to ten animals are used per group, again representing equal numbers of males and females.

Biochemic and hematologic determinations are made at intervals and all animals are necropsied. Other data collected includes weekly body weights, feed and water consumption and clinical signs.

Another use of subchronic tests is for range finding to determine dosages for chronic studies.

Chronic Toxicity. Chronic toxicity studies are conducted to determine the effects of continuous long-term exposure. A study lasting more than ninety days is referred to as a chronic study. In rodent chronic toxicity studies the toxicant exposure includes the greater portion of the expected life span of the species, often eighteen months in mice and twenty-four months in rats. If dogs or primates are used then the duration of exposure is usually twenty-four months unless there are overriding concerns. Some studies may last seven to ten years in these species. A chronic toxicity protocol will often include at least one rodent and one nonrodent species.

Usually three dose levels plus controls are used. Group sizes are similar to those employed in subchronic studies. Similar clinical observations are made as in subchronic studies.

SPECIAL STUDIES

Reproduction. A toxicant can have many effects on reproduction including: ovulation, conception, implantation, gestation, embryo development, fetal development, parturition, lactation and early postnatal growth. Usually a two or three successive generation rat study is conducted. The males and females are dosed for sixty days prior to mating and throughout gestation and lactation. The offspring (second and third generation) are dosed from weaning through the complete reproductive cycle including lactation. Some of the offspring from the first generation are mated to produce a second generation. Then some of the second generation are mated to produce the third generation. At each step the following information is obtained: fertility index, length of gestation, live births, stillbirths, survival at five days and at weaning, number of each sex, body weights, and gross abnormalities. Microscopic examinations may be done on selected offspring. Results of these experiments may also provide information on embryotoxicity and teratogenicity.

Teratology. A teratogen is a substance that produces nonlethal structural or functional changes in the fetus. If the change results in stillbirth or *in-uterio* death the effect is more properly called embryotoxic or fetatoxic. Examples of teratogenic responses are cleft palate, polydactia, retarded ossification, malformed ribs, renal agenesis and club feet. Test species commonly used include mice, rats and rabbits. The females are exposed after mating and only during the period of organogenesis (organ development). Mice and rats are dosed on days six to fifteen and rabbits on days six to eighteen of gestation. The objective is to administer the test compound only during the critical period when the basic embryonic tissues are differentiating into the fetal organs and tissues.

The fetuses are usually removed surgically from the dam one or two days before the end of gestation. Each fetus is examined for gross changes and special stains are used to examine skeletal and soft tissue development.

The tragic experience with thalidomide in the early 1960's greatly increased the interest in teratology. There are several important plant teratogens that are of veterinary importance. These are discussed in the chapter on **Plant Teratogens.**

Mutagenesis. Mutagenesis is the induction of DNA changes. There may be chromosomal alterations such as breaks or rearrangements, or the change can involve only one nucleotide pair that would be manifested as a change in phenotype.

The three types of mutagenic tests currently used are: a. dominant lethal, b. cytologic and, c. host-mediated microbial assay. In the *dominant lethal assay* treated and untreated males are mated with untreated virgin females. The males are usually treated with a single dose or multiple doses over a short period of time. The dosing is then discontinued and the males mated at weekly intervals. The females are necropsied before the end of gestation, for example, fourteen days postmating in mice, and evaluated for number of corpora lutea, implantation sites, dead fetuses and live fetuses. Dominant lethality is measured by preimplantation and/or postimplantation loss compared to untreated controls. Recall that the spermatogenic cycle takes seven to eight weeks to produce mature sperm. Consequently, depending on which matings result in dominant fetal lethality, it is possible to determine what stage in the spermatogenic cycle is sensitive to the drug.

Cytologic testing. This involves treating experimental animals with the test compound and then examining cells such as bone marrow, regenerating liver cells or germ cells for chromosome aberrations. In the *host-mediated assay* an indicator organism, for example a strain of Salmonella, is injected into the peritoneal cavity of a mouse or rat. The animal is administered the compound and after a period of time fluid is withdrawn from the peritoneal cavity. The microorganisms are then cultured and examined for mutagenic changes. The advantage of the *in vivo* host assay over the *in vitro* microorganism assay is that the host-mediated assay takes into account the metabolism of the potential mutagen by a host mammal. The host mammal may either metabolically activate a compound to an active mutagen or may detoxify a mutagen to a nonmutagenic compound. Comparing results of *in vivo* and *in vitro* tests provides valuable information on the mutagenic hazard of compounds for mammals.

Carcinogenicity. The veterinarian has a good understanding based on his training in pathology of the differences between benign and malignant tumors. Toxic substances can induce either benign tumors or malignant tumors in the form of either carcinomas (epithelial origin) or sarcomas (connective tissue origin). The debate in toxicology centers on the potential for chemically induced tumors to become malignant. At an earlier time the term "carcinogenic agent" was reserved for agents inducing malignant tumors. Today, there is a growing tendency to make the term all inclusive. Until more is known about tumor induction, growth and spread, the argument will probably not be resolved. The immediate impact of considering all tumorigenic agents, either benign or malignant, as carcinogenic agents is to reduce the number of drugs, industrial chemicals, agricultural chemicals and other agents that have had or potentially have important economic uses. On the one hand there is the definite need and desire to protect animal and human health and on the other hand not to overreact and be overly protective so as to seriously disrupt the production of food and fiber and raw and manufactured goods.

Carcinogenic studies are usually conducted in laboratory rodents, most frequently the mouse and rat. The exposure is usually for the life of the animal beginning at weaning, and sometimes, before; and continuing until the animal dies. In most instances the largest number of tumors occur during the last part of the life cycle. Consequently, it is necessary to start with a large number of animals per group so that a significant number live to "tumor bearing age." The point of lifetime studies is emphasized. A two-year exposure in dogs that were one.year old at the start, would not be a carcinogenic study if the results were negative after two years. If the study continued for seven to ten years in dogs then there would be increased confidence in the results.

The following comparisons are made between the drug treated groups and the control group: (1) Is there an increased incidence of tumors of a type seen in the normal control group? (2) Are there tumors occurring of a type not seen at all in the normal control group, and (3) Is there a combination of increased incidence of control group type tumors and occurrence of tumor types not found in the control group. It is important to know what types of tumors occur spontaneously in the species and strain of animals used. This information is available for commonly used animals.

A difficult and as yet unresolved question is the determination of the public health hazard associated with very low-level exposures to chemicals which are weak carcinogens even when administered at high levels to experimental animals. This is of particular interest in veterinary toxicology as related to residues of feed additives and agricultural chemicals.

OTHER TESTS

Hemolysis. Hemolysis tests are required for all formulations administered intravenously. The test involves obtaining a preinjection blood sample followed with a second sample taken one minute after injection. The plasma hemoglobin level is then determined in both samples.

Eye Irritation. Formulations intended for use in the eye or material which may inadvertently get into the eye are tested for ocular irritation. The material is placed in the conjunctival sac of one eye in an albino rabbit. The other eye serves as the control. The resulting tissue response of the eye and surrounding structures is scored at periodic intervals for up to seventy-two hours.

Skin Irritation. The test involves applying the compound to shaved skin on an albino animal, usually a rabbit. Sometimes the material is kept in place with an occlusive bandage. The severity of the skin response is scored at periodic intervals.

Other Irritation Tests. Drugs intended for intramuscular, subcutaneous or intramammary administration are tested for tissue irritation by evaluating degree of swelling, edema, hemorrhage, necrosis and milk leukocyte counts.

REFERENCES

Loomis, T. A. 1974. *Essentials of Toxicology.* Philadelphia, Pennsylvania: Lea & Feibiger.

Robens, J. F. 1973. FDA Requirements for Toxicity Testing of Veterinary Drugs. *Veterniary Toxicology* 15:27-34.

The Testing of Chemicals for Carcinogenicity, Mutagenicity and Teratogenicity. 1973. *Food and Drug Directorate.* Ottawa 3, Ontario, Canada KIA OL2: Tunney's Pasture.

DIAGNOSTIC TOXICOLOGY

An accurate diagnosis is the single-most important factor in dealing with animal toxicoses. Once the cause of a problem is known, specific treatment and prevention can be initiated. Prior to that time, however, the veterinarian is limited to supportive and symptomatic therapeutic measures. The toxicologic diagnosis is based upon a knowledge of pertinent criteria in the case, qualified laboratory evaluation of proper specimens, and intelligent interpretation of laboratory results in light of the circumstances associated with the problem.

Types of Diagnostic Criteria

The accurate diagnosis of toxicosis, like many other diseases, is made by utilizing information obtained from five types of criteria. These have been discussed by Burns (1961), Buck (1969), and Radeleff (1970). The five criteria include history, clinical signs, postmortem findings, chemical analyses, and laboratory animal tests.

It is important that diagnosticians refrain from making diagnoses on the basis of information obtained from only one criterion while neglecting to obtain or consider other criteria essential to making a proper diagnosis. These five diagnostic criteria are briefly discussed below.

History

A knowledge of the circumstances associated with poisoning is very useful and may provide a key for making a proper diagnosis. Much of a case history may have no bearing on the diagnosis, but important points may be gleaned from it. The presence of poisons such as rodenticides, insecticides, drugs, paints, fertilizers, petroleum products, and other chemicals on the premises, or a history of their having been used or available for animal exposure should be ascertained. One should be prepared to approximate the amount or degree of possible exposure to these chemicals. The feed and water supply should be carefully examined for the presence of toxic plants, molds, algae, fungi, or other toxicants.

When the practicing veterinarian desires to consult with a diagnostic laboratory or other colleagues in an effort to establish a diagnosis, certain fundamental information should be given: veterinarian's name and address; owner's name and address; species, breed, sex, age, and weight of the animal. When livestock and poultry are involved, additional important facts should be included: number of animals in the herd or flock; number affected; number that have died; course of events in hours or days; type of management; feeding program; history of past illnesses; and immunization records. Other factors which often guide the diagnostician are: (1) the length of time the animals have been on the last batch of prepared feed; (2) if the animals are on pasture, the type of pasture and whether or not trash, rubbish, old motors, or farm machinery are available to the animals; (3) detailed description of clinical signs; (4) detailed description of postmorten findings including negative observations; (5) the length of time since the animal was last observed before its death and its condition at the time of observation; (6) what medications were given, if any, how long before death, and the response; (7) a history regarding any spraying or otherwise treating for internal and external parasites.

In presenting a history involving small animals, certain specific factors should be included: (1) type of area in which the animal lives, whether city or farm; (2) did it roam at will or was it tied or maintained in the house; (3) the distance to the nearest dump, grain elevator, or other source of poison; (4) history of rodenticide or other pesticide use on the home premises; (5) history of treatment for parasites and immunizations within the past two or three weeks.

Although the history or circumstantial evidence is a very important aid in making toxicologic diagnoses, it should be kept in its proper perspective. A diagnosis should never be based on the history alone. Veterinarians have diagnosed herbicide poisoning, for example, on the basis of a history of 2, 4-D having been sprayed on a fence row or pasture thirty days before cattle losses occurred. Such diagnoses are usually made only after cursory attempts to make other diagnoses have failed. The history has greater value if it can be determined that animals have consumed or were definitely exposed to a particular agent. One should guard against such things as diagnosing lead poisoning simply because lead paint is found on the premises, or plant poisoning unless there is ample evidence that the prospective plant has been consumed in sufficient quantities to produce intoxication. Often the presence of toxic plants, although plentiful in a pasture, is not significant because the animals have not consumed them. Those plants which were actually the source of the poison may have been eaten and are no longer obvious. The history should be viewed as just one piece of the puzzle; other criteria must be present upon which to base a diagnosis.

Clinical Signs

To the clinician, signs of illness are of prime importance in making a diagnosis. They are equally important to the toxicologist. When observing clinical signs of disease, particular attention shoud be given to details. The slightest unusual sign seen by an astute observer may give a clue to identification of a toxic agent. For example, there are many toxic agents which affect the central nervous system (CNS). Yet, many different sequences of events may be observed. Rather than stating that an animal exhibited central nervous system symptoms, one should describe exactly how the animal acted. The term "CNS signs" is too vague to be of value in differential diagnosis. This is because nearly any animal will exhibit some type of CNS disturbance during some of the stages of illness before death. However, if one describes these signs in detail and reports the changes from beginning until termination, important clues may be supplied.

There are dangers in making a toxicologic diagnosis only on the basis of signs observed. First, there are only nine body systems responsible for clinical signs, but there are thousands of toxic agents to affect these systems. There are almost no pathognomonic signs of toxicoses. Yet, a particular sequence of events and the degree of severity of signs can be a key to a diagnosis. Second, when an investigator observes an animal with signs of illness or poisoning, he may see only one phase of the syndrome. He will not have seen what had happened prior to his arrival nor will he see what will happen after his brief observation.

Postmortem Findings

Gross and microscopic examinations will frequently reveal valuable evidence in suspected poisoning cases and, in most instances, should be done if one expects to make an accurate diagnosis. Some poisons produce extensive lesions, others only slight tissue alterations, and still others produce no observable morphologic changes.

Often, the lack of lesions is diagnostically as important as the presence of extensive changes. Frequently, the pathologic examination will reveal evidence suggestive of conditions other than poisoning. A postmortem examination must be performed if legal action is likely to occur.

Chemical Analyses

Chemical evidence is often an indispensable aid in diagnosing toxicologic problems. Used properly and in the right perspective, chemical analyses may provide the single-most important diagnostic criterion. There are limitations, however, to the value of chemical analyses. Rarely should chemical results be used alone in making a diagnosis. Positive chemical data plus history, clinical signs, and postmortem findings may provide evidence to arrive at an accurate diagnosis. One should never request a chemistry laboratory to simply "analyze for poisons" because an animal died of unknown causes. There are thousands of toxic chemicals and plants and analysis for all of them would be impossible not only because of the limited amount of sample available but also because the cost would be prohibitive. Also, there are many toxic plants and even some chemical agents for which no chemical analytical procedures are available.

Although there are some toxicologic tests suitable for the veterinary hospital or clinic laboratory, many procedures for toxicologic analyses are complicated, time-consuming, and require expensive equipment. Unfortunately, many of the screening qualitative tests for toxicants are not worth the time it takes to perform them. An example is the Reinsch test for arsenic and mercury. When performed by an inexperienced individual, this test is worse than no test at all. Several metals such as arsenic, mercury, and antimony will give a positive reaction to this test. Also, sulfur and other elements found in biological specimens will give false positives with the Reinsch test. Thus, in our experience, unless a laboratory is adequately staffed and equipped for analytical chemistry procedures, little significance can be placed on toxicologic screening tests. False-positive or false-negative results can be disastrous, especially when one considers that a majority of toxicoses involve potential litigations. One can find himself in an embarrassing position when he is unable to rely upon his analytical procedures in making a toxicologic diagnosis. Perhaps a certain amount of screening and preliminary tests can be performed by a veterinary clinic for the sole purpose of aiding in treatment rationale but relying upon subsequent chemical confirmation by a qualified toxicology laboratory.

The minimum equipment necessary for an analytical chemistry-toxicology laboratory includes an atomic absorption spectrophotometer, a colorimeter or ultraviolet spectrophotometer, and a gas-liquid chromatograph or a thin-layer chromatograph. Facilities for ashing or digesting specimens such as a perchloric acid hood and a muffle furnace should be available as well as analytical balances, specialized glassware, and other routine analytical chemistry laboratory equipment. The cost of equiping such a laboratory would be prohibitive to all except a large group practice or hospital.

Laboratory Animal Tests

Laboratory animal testing is used only to a limited extent by the practitioner but may be valuable to the diagnostic toxicologist. It involves the administration of suspected toxic material to a susceptible animal and observing the effects. Usually it is better to administer the suspected material to the same species of animal as was originally affected. Positive results may be very valuable in establishing a diagnosis. However, negative results do not always indicate that poisoning did not occur because many factors may be involved in the natural case that are unkown or cannot be duplicated experimentally. Also, animals of the same species vary greatly in their susceptibility to a given toxic agent.

Laboratory animal testing is an important procedure, especially when one is dealing with fungal, bacterial, and plant toxins in animal feeds. In order to confirm that a particular chemical found in feed is a toxic agent, one must be able to extract it from the feed and reproduce the condition in a test animal.

Submitting Specimens for Laboratory Evaluation

When submitting specimens to a diagnostic laboratory, certain considerations should be made. The importance of supplying a complete account of history, symptoms, and lesions with specimens submitted for laboratory evaluation cannot be overemphasized. Such information will enable the toxicologist to intelligently select toxicants for which to make analyses. This is especially important when a test for the toxicant originally suspected proves negative. A chemist still has the opportunity to test for other poisons if adequate specimens have been submitted.

The choice of specimen is important in making a chemical analysis. Specimens should be taken free of chemical contamination and debris and should not be washed because of the possibility of removing residues of the toxic agent or of contaminating the specimen with the water. Keep in mind that one is often dealing with trace amounts of a particular chemical, and even the slightest contamination may produce erroneous results. Tissue specimens should be frozen and packaged to arrive at the laboratory while still frozen. Serum and blood should not be frozen but kept refrigerated. Always package specimens from the various organs separately. Use clean glass or plastic containers that can be tightly sealed. Always label each specimen with the owner's name, animal name or number, and tissue or specimen in the container. Never add preservatives such as formalin to specimens unless there is a specific reason for doing so and such information is included along with the specimen. Always send more material than you think is necessary. It is easier to throw away excess specimen than to obtain more specimen after the carcass has been discarded.

Serum cations and enzymes may be very helpful in the diagnosis of certain toxic and metabolic conditions. To obtain meaningful results, several general rules for collection and preservation of serum should be followed. Always collect blood with clean equipment and transfer it to clean vials or tubes. Avoid excessive aspiration pressure, splashing, or time lag during collection to minimize hemolysis. Make every effort to avoid trauma to the unclotted or clotted sample. Allow sufficient time for the blood to clot and begin to retract, usually about one hour. Always try to remove serum from the clot within two hours. This may be done by carefully pouring serum off the retracted clot or by centrifugation. After the serum is separated from the clot, it can be frozen and transported with ice.

Specimens that should be submitted from a live animal include 5 ml of serum with clot removed; 10 ml of whole blood; 50 ml of urine; and 200 grams of bait, vomitus, or other such materials.

Specimens that should be submitted from a dead animal include:

Serum—whole blood (if available)	10 ml
Urine	50 ml
Liver	100 gm
Kidney	100 gm
Body fat	100 gm
Brain (entire—1/2 frozen; 1/2 formalin)	
Rumen or stomach contents	500 gm

Plastic bags, newspaper, canned ice, and cardboard are good materials to use for transporting specimens to a laboratory for examination. Liquids such as blood, urine, stomach contents, and water should be shipped in a glass or heavy plastic container that can be sealed. Wrap each labelled specimen well in newspaper and package for mailing unless they can be delivered in person which, of course, is the most desirable. Always wrap the specimens individually for mailing so that the contents cannot leak and contaminate other mail or other specimens.

When submitting feeds, silage, and forages, it is often advisable to send enough material to feed a guinea pig or rabbit for one to two weeks. In most instances, 100 ml of water is sufficient for chemical analysis. However, if organic insecticides are suspected, at least one gallon of water is necessary. One to two pints of silage, hay, and feed are sufficient for most chemical analyses.

If one is in doubt about proper tissues for analysis or availability of confirmatory tests, much time, effort, and confusion can be avoided by placing a telephone call to the laboratory.

Specimens for Diagnosis of Specific Toxicants

The procedures for sending in specimens as outlined under the heading, "Submitting Specimens for Laboratory Evaluation," are suitable for the detection of most toxicants. There are instances, however, where special considerations regarding chemical analysis and pathologic evaluation are required. Some specific examples for specific toxicants are given in table 1 and summarized in table 2.

Interpretation of Laboratory Results

Interpretation of the significance of chemical data should be done carefully, taking into consideration other evidence presented with the case. Positive chemical findings are not always evidence of intoxication, nor are negative findings always indicative that a toxicosis did not occur. For example, finding chlorinated hydrocarbon insecticides in the fatty tissues of an animal only indicates that the animal was exposed to the pesticide, not that the insecticide produced a toxicosis. On the other hand, failure to find certain organophosphorous insecticides in the body tissues would not guarantee that the animal had not been poisoned by such a chemical. In the case of most chlorinated hydrocarbon insecticides, the animal may store a considerable amount of the chemical in its tissues without apparent harmful effects. With organophosphorous compounds, the body may metabolize them so rapidly that they are not detectable by chemical analysis.

In summary, it is imperative that a thorough history be obtained, that astute observations be made, and that intelligent questions be asked. The veterinarian should apply the professional skills that only he possesses in determining the signs of illness and in performing a thorough postmortem examination. Properly prepared tissue specimens and other suspected material should be sent without undue delay to a qualified laboratory for chemical and histopathologic examination. All information that can be obtained regarding the case should accompany the specimens to the laboratory. Cooperation and communication with the laboratory can usually result in a rapid, proper diagnosis.

BIBLIOGRAPHY

Buck, W. B. 1969. Laboratory Toxicologic Tests and Their Interpretation. *JAVMA* 155:1928-41.

Burns, P. W. 1961. Clinical Diagnosis in Veterinary Toxicology. Proceedings. *A.C.V.T.* pp. 5-12.

Radeleff, R. D. 1964. *Veterinary Toxicology*. 1st ed. Philadelphia, Pennsylvania: Lea & Febiger. pp. 33-37.

TABLE 1

Specimens Required for Specific Tests

Poison or Analysis Requested	Specimen Required	Amount of Specimen Desired	Comments
Ammonia	Whole blood or serum	5 ml	Frozen (1-2 drops of saturated HgCl$_2$ may be used
	Rumen contents (composite)	100 gm	instead of freezing rumen contents)
	Urine	5 ml	
ANTU	Stomach and intestine contents	200 gm	Can be detected only within 12-24 hours after ingestion
	Liver	200 gm	
Antimony, Arsenic, or Selenium	Liver	50 gm	
	Kidney	50 gm	
	Feed	100 gm	
	Stomach contents	100 gm	
	Rumen contents	100 gm	
	Urine	50 ml	
Calcium, Magnesium, Potassium, or Sodium	Serum	2 ml	Serum must NOT be hemolyzed; separate clot before transit
	Feed	25 gm	
	Brain	5 gm	
	Spinal Fluid	1 ml	
Carbon monoxide	Whole blood	15 ml	
Chloride	See sodium above		
Chlorinated hydrocarbon insecticides	Brain (cerebrum)	One-half of brain	Must not be contaminated with hairs or stomach contents; preferable to use chemically clean glass jars; avoid plastic containers; wrap specimens in clean aluminum foil
	Stomach contents	100 gm	
	Rumen contents	100 gm	
	Liver	50 gm	
	Body fat or	100 gm	
	Blood*	10 ml	*Blood samples can be analyzed most rapidly
	Kidney	50 gm	
Copper, Nickel, Iron, Cobalt, or Chromium	Kidney	50 gm	
	Liver	50 gm	
	Whole blood	10 ml	
	Feces	100 gm	
Cyanide	Whole blood	10 ml	Freeze specimen promptly in air-tight container
	Liver	50 gm	
	Forage, silage	100 gm	
	Other materials	100 gm	

47

TABLE 1 (Cont.)

Poison or Analysis Requested	Specimen Required	Amount of Specimen Desired	Comments
Ethylene glycol	Serum	10 ml	
	Kidney (in formalin)	Whole organ	One kidney, both in small animals
	Urine	10 ml	
Fluoroacetate	Stomach contents	All available	Frozen
Strychnine	Liver	50 gm	
	Kidney	One whole	
	Urine	50 gm	
	Other materials	100 gm	
Fluorides	Bone	5 gm	Representative of whole skeleton
	Water	100 ml	
	Forage	100 gm	Representative sample
	Soil	100 gm	
	Urine	50 ml	
Herbicides (Diquat, Paraquat, 2, 4D)	Weeds	100 gm	See also chlorinated hydrocarbons, organophosphate insecticides
	Urine	50 ml	
	Rumen contents	200 gm	
Nitrates or Nitrites	Water	50 ml	
	Forage, silage	100 gm	
	Whole blood (methemoglobin)	10 ml	
	Other materials	100 gm	
Carbamates or Organophosphorus insecticides	Feed	100 gm	Normal control animals blood, urine, stomach contents or rumen contents very valuable as reference
	Stomach contents (composite)	50 gm	
	Rumen contents (composite)	50 gm	
	Urine	50 ml	
	Blood (heparinized)	10 ml	
	Brain (refrigerated or frozen)	Half of cerebrum	
Oxalates	Fresh forage	6-8 plants	Do NOT chop plants; freeze promptly
	Kidney (in formalin)	Whole organ	One kidney, both in small animals
Phenols	Stomach contents	500 gm	Pack in air-tight container
	Rumen contents	500 gm	
	Other materials	200 gm	
Sulfa drugs, Antibiotics, Arsenicals, or Phenothiazines	Feed	50 gm	
	Other materials	50 gm	

TABLE 1 (Cont.)

Poison or Analysis Requested	Specimen Required	Amount of Specimen Desired	Comments
Phosphates	Serum	5 ml	
	Bone	25 gm	
	Other materials	100 gm	
Lead,	Urine	10 ml	
Thallium, or	Kidney	50 gm	
Mercury	Liver	50 gm	
Urea	Feed	100 gm	All specimens should be frozen
	Other materials	500 gm	
	See also ammonia		
Warfarin	Whole blood	5 ml	
	Feed	100 gm	
	Liver	100 gm	
	Other materials	100 gm	
Zinc	Liver	50 gm	
	Kidney	50 gm	
	Other materials	100 gm	

TABLE 2
Specimens to Submit for Diagnostic Toxicology

	Stomach or rumen contents (frozen)	Liver—frozen (100 gm)	Kidney—frozen (100 gm)	Kidney—formalin fixed	Brain—1/2 frozen	Brain—1/2 formalin fixed	Heparinized blood (10 ml)	Serum (no hemolysis) (2 ml)	Urine (20 ml)	Bone	Feed—1 quart	Body fat (100 gm)	Suspect material or bait	Milk (200 ml)	Feces	Forage	Fresh plants in plastic bag	Kidney—1/2 in alcohol	Water (100 ml)
Ammonia	*						*	*											
ANTU	*	*																	
Arsenic	*	*	*						*		*								
Calcium								*		*	*								
Carbon monoxide							*												
Chloride (see sodium)																			
Carbamates (see organophosphates)																			
Chlorinated hydrocarbon insecticides	*	*	*		*						*	*	*	*					
Copper		*	*				*				*				*				
Cyanide		*					*									*			
Ethylene glycol				*				*	*										
Fluoroacetate (1080)	*	*	*										*						
Fluorides								*	*						*				
Fuel oils	*																		
Herbicides (synthetic organic)	*												*						
Lead	*	*	*				*			*	*								
Magnesium								*			*								
Mercury		*	*	*	*	*			*										
Mycotoxins	*										*								
Nitrates/nitrites	*							*								*			*
Organophosphates	*				*			*			*								
Oxalates				*													*		
Phenols	*												*						
Phenothiazines		*						*			*								
Phosphates								*		*	*								
Phosphorus	*												*						
Pindone (pival)		*											*						
Poisonous plants																	*		
Potassium								*											
Prussic acid (see cyanide)																			
Salt/sodium					*	*		*			*								
Strychnine	*	*							*				*						
Sulfa drugs				*														*	
Thallium		*	*						*										
Urea (see ammonia)											*		*						
Warfarin	*	*						*					*						
Zinc		*	*					*			*								

MANAGEMENT AND TREATMENT OF TOXICOSES

Introduction

Animal toxicoses may be either acute or chronic in nature. The speed of onset and degree of involvement may dictate, in part, the therapeutic and prophylactic measures used. In many situations the veterinary physician is presented with an animal having acute, serious clinical disorders, often with no direct history of exposure to toxicants. To properly manage toxicologic emergencies, a *modus operandi* is proposed as follows:

1. Institute emergency and supportive therapy necessary to maintain a living subject.
2. Establish tentative clinical diagnoses upon which to base rational therapy.
3. Institute appropriate remedial and antidotal procedures.
4. Obtain confirmation of the chemical or agent responsible as quickly as possible.
5. Determine as nearly as possible the source of toxicant responsible.
6. Educate the client to the hazards of such toxicants and instruct him in the avoidance of these instances in the future.

This section deals primarily with the supportive, remedial and antidotal features used in veterinary toxicology.

Factors Influencing Toxicity

Toxicologic exposures may be influenced or altered by both animal factors and chemical factors. Animal factors include age, species, state of health, and plane of nutrition. Chemical factors include particle size, solubility, toxicity, absorption, excretion rate, affinity for body tissues or fluids, and interaction with other drugs.

Young animals, lacking development of metabolic pathways, are usually more susceptible to toxicants. Old or debilitated animals are likewise more susceptible to

poisoning. Liver or kidney insufficiency may enhance toxicity due to poor metabolism or slow excretion of toxicants. Gastrointestinal inflammation, blockage, or reduced peristalsis allows increased absoprtion of poisons. Alterations in gastrointestinal pH can change the ionization of drugs or chemicals and influence their absorption. Presence or absence of food in the stomach affects the toxicity of certain compounds.

Nonionized chemicals of smaller particle size and high solubility are generally absorbed more rapidly. Once absorbed, fat solubility may partition a compound to decrease its toxicity but increase its retention. Urinary pH affects the degree of ionization and, consequently, the rate of excretion of drugs and chemicals. Other drugs may potentiate a toxicant by decreasing plasma binding or inhibiting metabolism.

Rate and duration of exposure to a compound as well as route of entry must be considered. Exposure can be acute and massive or small, repetitive, and cumulative. However, both situations can result in acute or chronic clinical disease. Common routes of entry are respiratory, alimentary, and cutaneous. Vapors or small particles are rapidly absorbed by the lungs. The GI tract is the most common route of exposure in small animals. Cutaneous exposure depends on the integrity of the skin as well as the ability of a chemical to penetrate intact epidermis.

A multiplicity of factors and interactions may then be available to influence the toxicity of a material. The correct application of therapy is best accomplished when as many of the circumstances as possible are available for consideration.

Emergency and Supportive Therapy in Toxicologic Situations

Acute intoxicants commonly affect the nervous, gastrointestinal, hepatic, renal, and cardiovascular systems. Life-saving measures are generally aimed at maintaining vital functions in these areas.

Telephone Instructions

Initial contact with a potential poisoning case may be via telephone. At this point, any questions or instructions should be clear and calm. Several pertinent questions and instructions may aid in preparation of the client and the veterinarian for therapy and diagnosis. Suggested steps for the telephone include the following:

1. Attempted determination of this case as a poisoning. If no clinical signs are present, ask for the owner's identification of the material to which the animal was exposed as well as the approximate amount. Ideally, a reading of generic name and antidotal procedures would be in order. The route of exposure should be determined.

2. If vomition has not occurred and the patient is asymptomatic, emesis may be induced with a teaspoonful of table salt in the back of the animal's mouth or by administration of 1 teaspoonful of hydrogen peroxide orally. If vomiting does not occur within five to ten minutes, the animal should be submitted immediately to a veterinarian. Any vomitus should be saved. *Do not* recommend induction of vomiting for oily or corrosive materials. If dermal or ocular exposure has occurred, have the animal flushed with large amounts of water.

3. Advise prompt submission of the animal, vomitus or bait, and any containers or labels to the veterinarian responsible for the case.

Therapeutic Preparations

Initial preparations for toxicologic emergencies include availability of equipment. Table 1 lists recommended instruments and equipment for toxicologic

TABLE 1
Equipment for Toxicologic Emergencies*

1. Mechanical respirator
2. Stomach tubes of several sizes
3. Endotracheal tubes of several sizes
4. Aspirator bulbs or large syringes
5. Venostomy kit (for locating veins hard to find or for animals with low blood pressure)
6. Intravenous catheters and stylets
7. Miscellaneous: syringes, needles, urinary catheters, thermometers, stethoscope

*Adapted from Kirk (1971)

emergencies. Of particular importance are facilities for restraint, respiration, gastric evacuation, and intravenous therapy.

Appropriate antidotes with clearly marked indications and dosage should be available. The major detoxicant and antidotal compounds for veterinary use are listed in table 2. After the initial clinical examination and determination of vital signs, emergency supportive and detoxication therapy can be instituted.

Supportive Procedures

Supportive measures depend on the clinical difficulties in the animal. These include (1) prevention of convulsions, (2) maintenance of respiration, (3) maintenance of temperature, (4) treatment for shock, (5) correction of electrolyte and fluid loss, (6) control of cardiac dysfunction, and (7) alleviation of pain.

Convulsions may be readily controlled by induction of light anesthesia with ultrashort barbiturates (e.g., thiopental). One must keep in mind that barbiturates are respiratory depressants and may aggravate the respiratory embarrassment induced by some toxicants. Newer products for controlling convulsions, such as inhalation anesthetics, diazepam, methocarbamol, and glyceryl guiacolate may be of more benefit in specific instances of chemically induced convulsions. Combinations of muscle relaxants and anesthetic agents or tranquilizers may be as effective and much safer than barbiturates alone.

Respiratory maintenance depends either on mechanical assistance in air exchange or upon chemical stimulation of the respiratory reflex. Since many toxicants kill by virtue of respiratory paralysis or depression, assistance in ventilation may be life-saving. Conversely, excessive ventilation may induce respiratory alkalosis and complicate other aspects of supportive therapy.

The use of analeptics should be avoided unless judged absolutely essential since it is difficult to maintain a balance between analeptics and certain other controls such as anesthesia.

Both hypothermia and hyperthermia may be induced by various toxicants. Attention to changes in body temperature and the prompt appropriate correction may influence susceptibility to the toxicant, speed of metabolic degradation, and rate of dehydration in an affected animal.

Therapy for shock, electrolyte and fluid loss, cardiac dysfunction, and pain is an important facet in the survival of an intoxicated patient. Extensive literature is available in each of these important topics and the clinician is well advised to apply appropriate methods in the correction of such deficits induced by poisoning.

TABLE 2
Antidotes and Therapeutic Agents for Veterinary Toxicology

Antidote	Dosage	Route	Use	Comments
Acid, acetic 6%	4 ml/kg 25 ml/kg	Oral Intraruminal	Neutralize acids Counteract NPN toxicosis	Most effective before animal is recumbent.
Ammonium chloride	SA* 0.2-0.5 gm LA** 5-30 gm	Oral Oral	Urinary acidifier and strontium toxicosis	Administer in water solution, q.i.d.
Amphetamine sulfate	SA 0.5-1.0 mg/kg LA 100-300 mg/kg	SC, IV, IP SC	Barbiturate overdose	Do not repeat within 60 minutes. Reliable only for instances of mild depression.
Antivennin crotalidae (wyeth)	Use as directed			
Apomorphine	Dog 0.5-1.0 mg/kg	IV, SC, IM	Emetic	Safe dosage not established for cats.
Arsanilic acid	.02% in diet	Oral	Prevent selenium toxicosis	CAUTION: 0.02% in diet in absence of selenium could induce chronic organic arsenical toxicosis.
Ascorbic acid	SA 250-500 mg	IV, SC	Overcome methemoglobin in nitrite and aniline poisoning. Capillary integrity in coumarin anticoagulant toxicosis.	
Atropine sulfate	0.2-0.5 mg/kg in all species	IV, SC, IM	Cholinesterase inhibitors	Must repeat in 4-6 hours or as needed. Effect is diminished with repeated dosages. Give 1/4 dose IV, balance SubQ, and allow 15-20 minutes for full atropinization. Use in combination with oximes for organophosphorus insecticides only.
Batyl alcohol	Bovine: 10 ml of a 10% olive oil soln. daily for 5 days	SC	Bracken fern toxicosis	Use in conjunction with blood transfusion.
Bicarbonate, sodium	100 mg/kg/day	Oral	Gastric lavage for dinitrophenol, ethanol and turpentine	DO NOT use for acid poisons, may cause CO_2 tympany.

* Small animals
** Large animals

TABLE 2 (Cont.)

Antidote	Dosage	Route	Use	Comments
BAL (see dimeracaprol)				
Calcium				
Ca borogluconate 23%	LA 250-500 ml	IV, SC	Hypocalcemia	Administer slowly, monitor cardiac rate and rhythm.
Ca gluconate 10%	SA 5-30 ml	IV	Hypocalcemia	Slow IV administration.
Ca EDTA (see EDTA)				
Ca hydroxide 0.15%	SA 25-100 ml	Oral	Oxalate ingestion	
Charcoal, activated	SA 5-50 gm	Oral	Adsorbant	Best oral detoxicant available.
	LA 250-500 gm			Difficult to handle. Administer in water slurry.
Chlorides (sodium or ammonium salts)	SA 0.5-1.0 gm/day	Oral	Hasten excretion of bromides	Give for 2-4 days.
Copper glycinate	Cattle 60-120 ml	SC	Molybdenosis	Inject in dewlap. May cause local reaction.
Copper sulfate	SA 20-100 ml of a 0.2-0.4% soln.	Oral	Gastric lavage for inorganic phosphorous	
Copper sulfate	1-5% in salt	Oral	Prophylaxis of molybdenum toxicosis	
Deferoxamine	20 mg/kg	IM	Iron toxicosis	Human dosage given.
	40 mg/kg	IV	Iron shock	Dosage not established for animals.
Demerol	15 mg/kg	SC	Narcotic analgesic	Not for use in cats.
Dimeracaprol (BAL in oil)	5 mg/kg t.i.d.	IM	Arsenic, mercury	Best if given prior to onset of clinical signs. Drop dosage to 3 mg mg/kg after first day. Continue 4-10 days.
Diphenylthio-carbazone	Dog 70 mg/kg t.i.d.	Oral	Thallium	Administer for 6 days. Watch closely. May initiate toxicosis by rapid thallium mobilization.
Doxapram	3-5 mg/kg	IV	Barbiturate overdose	Repeat as necessary.
EDTA (edathamil calcium disodium)	110 mg/kg/day in 4 divided doses for 5 days	IV, SC	Lead toxicosis	Give initial dose IV, then subcutaneously as 10 mg/ml in 5% dextrose.
Ethanol (20%)	5 ml/kg	IV	Ethylene glycol, methanol	Repeat every 6-8 hours for up to 48 hours.
Ferrocyanide (sodium salt)	SA 0.3-0.5 gm	Oral	Copper salts	

TABLE 2 (Cont.)

Antidote	Dosage	Route	Use	Comments
Glyceryl guiacolate (33% soln.)	110 mg/kg	IV	Strychnine toxicosis	Repeat as needed.
Glycerol monoacetate	0.1-0.5 mg/kg given hourly to total 2-4 mg/kg	IM, IV	Fluoroacetate (1080)	Effective only if given prior to onset of clinical signs. Available only from chemical supply houses.
Levallorphan tartrate	Dog 0.1-0.5 mg	IV	Morphine	Use only in acute poisoning.
Magnesium oxide	Dogs 1-5 gms Foals 10-15 gm Calves 10-15 gm LA 20-30 gm	Oral	Acids	
Milk of magnesia (magnesium hydroxide)	SA 1-15 ml LA 20-30 ml	Oral	Acids	
Methylamphetamine	Horses 0.1-0.2 mg/kg	IV	Phenothiazine tranquilizers	
Methocarbamol (10% soln.)	Dogs 150 mg/kg (Range 40-300 mg/kg)	IV	Strychnine	Give to effect. Repeat half dose as needed.
Methylene blue	8.8 mg/kg	IV	Methemoglobinemia (Nitrate, nitrite, chlorate, aniline derivatives)	Repeat therapy may be needed, especially in ruminants. Combine with a sympathomimetic drug to prevent fall in blood pressure.
Mineral oil	Dogs 5-15 ml Cats 2-6 ml LA 1-3 liters	Oral	Cathartic for oil soluble toxins	
Molybdenum	Sheep 100 mg NH_4 molybdate/day	Oral	Copper toxicosis	Treat for 3 weeks.
Nalorphine	Dog 5-10 mg	IV	Morphine overdose	Do not repeat if respiration is not satisfactory.
Neostigmine	SA .022 mg/kg	SC	Curare	If given IV, administer very slowly.
	LA .022 mg/kg	SC, or IV	Scopalomine, Jimson weed	
Nitrite (1%) Thiosulfate (20%) (sodium salts)	Nitrite 16 mg/kg Thiosulfate 30-40 mg/kg	IV IV	Cyanide	Repeat only once. If additional treatment is required, use only thiosulfate.
Oximes	See pralidoxime chloride			
Oxygen	Pure oxygen with 5% CO_2	Inhalation	Carbon monoxide	Do not overventilate.

TABLE 2 (Cont.)

Antidote	Dosage	Route	Use	Comments
Penicillamine	15-50 mg/kg	Oral	Lead, mercury, copper chelation therapy	Side effects are vomiting, anorexia. Dosage based on human data.
Pentobarbital	28-mg/kg	IV	Sedative, anticonvulsant	Dosage is approximate. Give to effect.
Pentylenetetrazol (10% soln.)	SA 10-20 mg/kg LA 1,000-3,000 mg	IV	Analeptic	Repeat at 30 minute intervals as needed.
Permanganate, potassium (1:10,000 soln.)	2-4 ml/kg	Oral	Alkaloids, phosphorous	Strong solutions may damage stomach.
Potassium chloride	Dog 2-6 gm/day	Oral	Thallium	Use in combination with diphenylthiocarbazone.
Pralidoxine chloride (2-PAM)	SA 20-50 mg/kg LA 25-50 mg/kg	IV, IM IV	Cholinesterase regeneration in organophosphate toxicosis	Give slowly IV. Maximum dose is 500 mg/min.
Propranolol	0.5 mg/kg	IV, IM	Digitalis glucosides, oleander	Repeat as needed to control cardiac arrhythmia.
Protamine sulfate (1% soln.)	1-1.5 mg/mg heparin	IV	Heparin antagonism	Slow IV injection.
Protopam	(See pralidoxime)			
Sodium sulfate	SA 2-25 gm LA 250-1,000 gm	Oral	Saline cathartic	Use a 20% solution. May be combined with activated charcoal.
Tannic acid	SA 200-500 mg in 30-60 ml water	Oral	Alkaloid inactivation	Not for use with cocaine, nicotine, physostigmine, atropine and morphine.
Tannic acid	LA 5-25 gm in 2-4 liter water			Not to be left in stomach. Remove by emesis or catharsis.
Thiamin	Horses 100-200 mg t.i.d.	SC	Bracken fern toxicosis	Continue therapy for 14 days.
Thiosulfate (sodium salt 20% soln.)	LA 30-40 mg/kg	IV	Inorganic arsenic poisoning	Continue therapy for 3-4 days.
Vitamin K_1 and/or menadione	1 mg/kg	IV, IM, Oral	Coumarin anticoagulants hemorrhagic mycotoxicoses	Therapeutic effect is within 60 minutes. Early parenteral therapy may be followed by oral therapy for 4-5 days.

DETOXICATION PROCEDURES

Detoxication procedures generally follow these basic steps:

1. Removal of the source of the toxicant.
2. Prevention of further absorption of a toxicant.
3. Inactivation and elimination of absorbed toxicant.

Removal of the Source of Toxicant

Obviously physical separation of animals from toxicants or potential toxicants is necessary to prevent additional exposure. Collection of suspected baits, vomitus, trash or feeds will not only prevent reaccess of affected animals, but alleviates additional animals coming in contact with suspected toxicants. If a specific toxicant cannot be identified, a complete change in location (pasture, feedlot, kennel) as well as feed, water, and utensils may be advisable until adequate diagnostic procedures are completed.

If removal cannot be accomplished (e.g., confinement housing, no alternate pastures), then careful cleanup of the premises should be attempted. One must also be cautious against changing circumstances so drastically as to induce new problems as well (e.g., sudden change in feed ration which can initiate digestive disturbances).

Prevention of Further Absorption

Since exposure to toxicants in veterinary medicine is mainly oral or dermal, and because unsuccessful outcome of poisoning often results from the effects of continued absorption, methods for removal of toxic materials from the gastrointestinal tract and skin are of paramount importance.

Gastrointestinal Tract

If ingestion has occurred recently, much of the toxicant may still be in the stomach. Keep in mind that some toxicants (e.g., alcohol) may be absorbed directly from the stomach. In many cases, vomition occurs as a result of toxic effects of a chemical or plant, but this may result in only partial emptying of the stomach. Furthermore, in certain species such as horses and ruminants, vomition is not a viable option for gastric emptying.

If an hour or more has elapsed since ingestion, it is prudent to assume that a large portion of toxicant will also be in the small intestine.

The methods generally employed to decrease absorption from the gastrointestinal tract include (1) emesis, (2) gastric lavage, (3) containment in an inabsorbable form, (4) catharsis, and (5) direct removal.

Emesis. Emesis is most effective in dogs, cats and swine. Usually emesis is of limited benefit if performed more than four hours after ingestion. Induction of emesis is contraindicated in the following instances:

1. Ingestion of corrosive agents.
2. Ingestion of volatile hydrocarbons and petroleum distillates.
3. Unconscious or semicomatose patients, or those animals without an active cough reflex.
4. Convulsant poisons, unless convulsions are controlled.

Central emetics which act on the chemoreceptor trigger zone are most effective. These include apomorphine and syrup of ipecac. Apomorphine is quite reliable and may be used in dogs at 0.05 to 0.10 mg/kg intravenously, intramuscularly, subcutaneously, or subconjunctivally. The upper dosage may produce prolonged vomiting and some CNS depression. Apomorphine is not generally recommended for cats. Syrup of ipecac, 10-20 ml orally in the dog is an effective emetic, although less reliable and slower in onset of emesis than is apomorphine.

Other emetics which act orally are recommended as follows:

1. Copper sulfate: 25 to 75 ml of a 1% solution. Do not use for poisons that damage the gastroenteric tract.
2. Ground mustard seeds: 2 to 4 teaspoonfuls in a cup of hot water.
3. Sodium chloride: 1 to 3 teaspoonfuls in a cup of warm water.
4. Hydrogen peroxide: 5 to 25 ml orally. Repeat if no response in five to ten minutes.

Gastric Lavage. Gastric lavage is done in an unconscious or anesthetized animal. An appropriate endotracheal tube is placed to prevent aspiration and to ensure that the lavage tube is not introduced into the lungs since anesthetized animals lack both the esophageal reflex and the cough reflex. Use the largest bore stomach tube possible and use a tube with a fenestrated tip which aids in prevention of plugging with particulate gastric contents. Lower the head of the animal at a 30° angle and introduce approximately 10 ml/kg body weight of lavage fluid either by gravity or gentle pressure. Aspiration or gravity is then used to remove the lavage fluid. Repeat several times or until lavage is clear and free of particulate matter. Lavage fluids used may be tap water or saline solution.

A specialized form of lavage, known as enterogastric lavage may be of greater benefit than gastric lavage for oral toxicant removal. The entergastric lavage technique results in removal of the entire contents of the gastrointestinal tract. A standard gastric lavage is performed. Simultaneously, a moderately high warm-water enema is performed. The lavage tube is left in place, and mild digital pressure is maintained on the anus. This results in retrograde filling of the intestine. The digital pressure is maintained until clear water flows from the gastric lavage tube. Details and equipment for this technique are in the literature. (Frey, 1974)

Depending on the type of lavage used, it is usually appropriate to instill inactivating agents with the last washing and allow that solution to remain in the gastroenteric tract. The use of activated charcoal and/or a saline cathartic is recommended and is explained in more detail later in this section.

Physical removal of toxicants from equine and ruminant patients is complicated by the design of the alimentary canal. Gastric lavage and emesis are neither safe nor effective in these animals. Catharsis with nonabsorbable oils or with saline purgatives are recommended. Irritant or stimulant laxatives are not advocated for poisoned animals. Surgery may be utilized for removal of toxins from the rumen which can represent a sizeable reservoir of toxicant to be considered. The decision for a rumenotomy must be governed by the nature of the toxicant, conditions of exposure, and evaluation of the animal as a surgical risk.

Gastrointestinal Containment in an Inabsorbable Form. Of extreme importance in toxicology therapy is the prevention of absorption of those toxicants which cannot be removed physically. Basically three options are available:

1. Formation of an insoluble precipitate or complex.
2. Ion trapping.
3. Adsorption.

The first of these methods (complexation) involves the use of agents which can prevent the dissolution of a toxin or which can preferentially form an insoluble complex. Some examples include (a) sulfate used to form insoluble complexes such as lead sulfate or barium sulfate; (b) calcium ion used to complex with anions such as oxalates or oak tannins; (c) chelating agents which can complex with a variety of metallic poisons. Oral decontaminants are given in table 2. This table also includes agents which may neutralize or chemically inactivate certain toxicants.

Ion trapping is the use of pH manipulation for the prevention of absorption across a membrane. Maintaining the toxicant in an ionized state will prevent absorption. Thus alkalinization or acidification of the alimen-

tary tract may aid in therapy. The greatest difficulty is the great buffering capacity of the alimentary fluids, making pH manipulation at this site difficult to achieve and maintain.

Adsorption therapy is the process of physical binding of toxicant molecules to an inabsorbable carrier which is eliminated from the intestinal tract. Of all the adsorbents available (including "universal antidote") the single-most effective by far for a wide range of toxicants is activated charcoal. It is the residue from destructive distillation of vegetable origin organic matter. It is porous, low in ash content, and high in surface area (100 sq m/gm). Activated charcoal is effective for virtually all chemicals (except cyanide). The efficacy of adsorption is not reduced by acidity or alkalinity of the toxicant and adsorbed material is generally retained throughout the entire alimentary tract.

Activated charcoal should not be used simultaneously with other drugs, since it may decrease their efficacy and at the same time be reduced in its detoxicant potency. One gram of activated charcoal has been shown to adsorb from 300 to as much as 1,800 mg of various drugs.

Table 4 is a listing of some toxicants known to be effectively adsorbed by activated charcoal. Recommended dosage for various animals are given in table 2.

Activated charcoal is the adsorbent and detoxicant of choice when a poisoning is suspected, but a specific toxicant is not known. In most cases, it is the adsorbant of choice for verterinary toxicology therapy.

Cathartics may be used to hasten removal of toxicants from the alimentary tract. This is particularly important in horses, cattle, and sheep. Generally, mineral oil (nonabsorbable oil) or sodium sulfate are the preferred cathartics. Dosages are given in table 2.

Skin. Removal of dermal exposure to toxicants may be accomplished by thorough washing with water containing a small amount of detergent. Oil based preparations or hydrocarbon solvents may penetrate intact skin and increase absorption. Clipping of the hair may be necessary to accomplish rapid and complete removal of chemicals.

Inactivation and Elimination of Absorbed Toxicants

Antidotal Therapy. Prompt use of an effective antidote for specific toxicants is an ideal way of inactivating such toxicants. Unfortunately, the number of specific antidotes is small compared to the array of real and potential toxicants. Specific systemic antidotes and their dosages are listed in table 2. In addition, table 3 cross-references the toxicants and refers to specific antidotes detailed in table 2. Additional details for specific therapy are given in appropriate chapters for individual toxicants.

Antidotal therapy is accomplished by a number of mechanisms as follows:

1. The antidote may complex with a toxicant, rendering it inert. Examples are the heavy metals which are chelated by EDTA, and arsenic which complexes with dimercaprol.

2. The antidote accelerates metabolic conversion of toxicant to a nontoxic product. For example, nitrite ion and thiosulfate ion complex with cyanide to form cyanmethemoglobin and thiocyanate respec-

TABLE 3

Guide to Antidotal and Therapeutic Measures for Veterinary Toxicants

Toxicant	Useful Drugs Indexed in Table 2
Acids	Magnesium oxide, milk of magnesia
Alkalis	Acetic acid
Alkaloids	Potassium permanganate or tannic acid or charcoal
Ammonia (urea)	Acetic acid, calcium borogluconate
Arsenic	Dimercaprol, thiosulfate
Barbiturates	Doxapram; pentylenetetrazol; amphetamine
Barium	Sodium sulfate or magnesium sulfate
Bromides	Chloride salts
Bracken fern	Batyl alcohol (bovine) or thiamin (horse)
Carbamate insecticides	Atropine, charcoal
Carbon monoxide	Oxygen
Chlorates	Methylene blue; ascorbic acid
Chlorinated hydrocarbon insecticides	Pentobarbital; charcoal
Cholinesterase inhibitors	Atropine; pralidoxime; charcoal
Copper	Molybdenum; penicillamine; ferrocyanide
Coumarin anticoagulants	Vitamin K_1, menadione
Curare	Neostigmine
Cyanide	Nitrite and thiosulfate
Digitalis glycosides	Propranolol, atropine
Ethylene glycol	Ethanol, bicarbonate
Fluoroacetate	Glyceryl monoacetate, pentobarbital
Heparin	Bicarbonate, deferoxamine
Lead	EDTA, BAL, Penicillamine, sodium sulfate
Mercury	Dimercaprol, thiosulfate, penicillamine
Methanol	Ethanol
Molybdenum	Copper sulfate, copper glycinate
Nitrate—nitrite	Methylene blue, ascorbic acid
Organophosphorus insecticides	Atropine, pralidoxime, charcoal
Oxalates	Calcium hydroxide, calcium gluconate
Petroleum distillates	Mineral oil; sodium sulfate
Phenols and cresols	Bicarbonate, charcoal; mineral oil
Phenothiazine derivatives	Methylamphetamine
Phosphorous	Copper sulfate, permanganate; charcoal
Snake (crotalid) venom	Antivenin
Selenium	Arsanilic acid
Strychnine	Apomorphine, charcoal, pentobarbital, methocarbamol, glyceryl guiacolate
Strontium	Calcium borogluconate, ammonium chloride
Thallium	Diphenylthiocarbazone, potassium chloride
Urea, NPN	Acetic acid; calcium borogluconate
Warfarin	See coumarin anticoagulants

TABLE 4
Some Substances Adsorbed by Activated Charcoal

Organics	Metals
Alcohol	Antimony
Atropine	Arsenic
Barbiturates	Lead
Camphor	Mercury
Cocaine	Phosphorus
Digitalis	Silver
Ipecac	Tin
Methylene blue	
Morphine	
Nicotine	
Organophosphorus insecticides	
Oxalate	
Penicillin	
Phenol	
Salicylates	
Strychnine	
Sulfonamides	

tively, both of which are relatively nontoxic compared to free cyanide.

3. The antidote may block formation of a toxic metabolite from a less toxic precursor. A recent development has been the use of ethyl alcohol to compete with alcohol dehydrogenase and block the formation of oxalic acid from ethylene glycol.

4. The antidote may accelerate the excretion of toxicant. The presence of sulfate ion, for instance, aids in rapid elimination of excess copper in the ruminant.

5. The antidote may compete with the toxicant for essential receptors. For example, vitamin K competes with coumarin anticoagulants for receptors involved in formation of the prothrombin complex.

6. An antidote may block receptors responsible for a toxic effect. A familiar example of this mechanism is the antimuscarinic effect of atropine against cholinesterase inhibitors.

7. The antidote may restore normal function by repairing or bypassing the effect of a toxicant. This mechanism is illustrated by the use of methylene blue in the correction of methemoglobinemia.

In addition, agents which accelerate or depress the metabolic conversion of toxicants may either increase or decrease the effect of the toxicant. For example, if a metabolite is more toxic than a parent compound (e.g.,

organothiophosphates converted to organophosphates) then a metabolic inhibitor could alleviate the toxicity. However, if the parent compound (e.g., warfarin) is more toxic than its metabolites then metabolic inhibitors may enhance the toxicity of warfarin.

Other aspects of drug interactions such as enzyme induction and displacement from plasma protein binding may markedly alter what was expected. Thus, knowledge of drug interaction is an additional important aspect of antidotal therapy.

Elimination of Absorbed Poisons. The animal body handles foreign compounds in one of the following ways:

1. Excretion (kidney, enterohepatic, milk, sweat, saliva and lungs).
2. Biotransformation.
3. Storage (bone, fat, hair).

The route of excretion most adaptable to therapeutic manipulation is renal excretion. Most alterations in renal excretion are based on diuresis and/or urinary pH. In some cases, a specific renal tubular transport mechanism may be of value for tubular secretion, but this route is mainly limited to endogenous toxins.

Enhancing renal excretion depends first on glomerular filtration of the toxicant. As such, only materials of limited molecular size which are not protein bound will be filtered. Thus, increasing the ratio of free/bound toxicant and augmenting the glomerular filtration rate will result in more toxicant being passed into the tubular lumen. Increased glomerular filtration is accomplished by diuresis, using either osmotic diuretics (e.g., mannitol) or chemical diuretics (e.g., furosemide).

Once in the tubule, a toxicant may be either excreted in the urnie or resorbed back through the tubule. Reabsorption is prevented when the molecule is more polar, less lipophilic, and ionized. Polarity and lipophilia are often altered by the animal's metabolism. Ionization may be influenced by the pH of the blood and urine. Ionization of an acid toxicant (proton donor) occurs when the medium is alkaline relative to the dissociation constant of the drug. Ionization of a basic drug (proton acceptor) occurs when the medium is acidic relative to the dissociation constant for that drug. To utilize urinary manipulation one must know if a toxicant is acidic or basic and the value of its pKa (dissociation constant). In general, alkaline urine enhances acidic drug excretion and vice versa.

A complete discussion of pH, pKa, and ionization relationships, if desired, may be found in many modern biochemistry or pharmacology texts.

Extracorporeal dialysis (the artificial kidney) is being used with increasing frequency in human toxicology. In certain intoxications (barbiturates, bromides, salicylates) the use of dialysis may be vital to survival.

A large number of toxicants are known to be dialyzable. Among these are barbiturates, sedatives, alcohols, glycols, antibiotics, metals, halides, endogenous toxins (e.g., ammonia, lactic acid), and some alkaloids and glycosides. More complete listings are being developed each year.

Peritoneal dialysis may be an alternative to consider in toxicology therapy, especially if renal function does not allow for effective urinary manipulation. Peritoneal dialysis is inexpensive and effective for removal of endogenous toxins when toxic renal failure occurs. In addition, many of the exogenous toxicants may be removed by peritoneal dialysis. This area needs additional consideration and research in veterinary medicine.

Some comment should be made on the manipulation of body systems to remove unwanted residues such as pesticides and antibiotics from food producing animals. This aspect of toxicologic management is in its infancy. Presently, chelating agents, such as penicillamine, may be used to deplete residues of heavy metals from tissue and bone. The accelerated removal of copper from liver in ruminants is enhanced by administration of molybdenum, and the presence of arsenic aids in elimination of excess selenium. Residues of chlorinated hydrocarbon insecticides in body fat may be excreted more rapidly if animals are fed phenobarbital so that the liver is induced to greater metabolism and biliary excretion of insecticide. In addition, low energy diets with depletion of body fat may enhance insecticide elimination.

As new compounds are developed and used, additional work may be essential to prevent unacceptable residues in the food animal population.

REFERENCES

Arena, J. 1970. *Poisoning: Toxicology—Symptoms—Treatments*. 2nd ed. Springfield, Illinois: Charles C. Thomas, Publisher.

Arena, J. M. 1974. *Poisoning. Toxicology, Symptoms, Treatments*. 3rd ed. Springfield, Illinois: Charles C. Thomas, Publisher.

Aronson, A. 1971. General Approach to the Treatment of Poisonings. In *Current Veterinary Thearpy IV*. R. W. Kirk, ed. Philadelphia: W. B. Saunders Company.

Aronson, A. L. 1973. Emergency and General Treatment of Poisonings. In *Current Veterinary Therapy V*. R. W. Kirk, ed. Philadelphia: W. B. Saunders.

Bailey, E. M., and Szabuniewicz, M. 1975. Treatment of Strychnine Poisoning Using Glyceryl Guiacolate Ether. *VM/SAC* Feb. 1975:170-74.

Cashman, T. H., and Shirkey, H. C. 1970. Emergency Management of Poisoning. *Pediatric Clinics of North America* 17:525-33.

Corby, D. G.; Fischer, R. H.; and Decker, W. J. 1970. Re-evaluation of the Use of Activated Charcoal in the Treatment of Acute Poisoning. *Pediatric Clinics of North America* 17:545-56.

Frye, F. L. 1974. Enterogastric Lavage in Small Animal Practice. *VM/SAC* July 1974:835-36.

Harrison, W. A.; Lipe, W. A.; and Decker, W. J. 1972. Apomorphine Induced Emesis in the Dog: Comparison of Routes of Administration. *JAVMA* 160:85-86.

Jackson, L. L.; and Lundvall, R. L. 1970. Observations on the Use of Glyceryl Guiacolate in the Horse. *JAVMA* 157:1093-95.

Kirk, R. W. 1971. *Current Veterinary Therapy IV*. W. B. Saunders Company, Philadelphia.

Szabuniewicz, M.; Bailey, E.; and Wiersig, D. 1971. Treatment of Some Common Poisonings in Animals. *VM/SAC*. 66:1197-1205.

Yaffe, S. J.; Sjoqvist, F.; and Alvan, G. 1970 Pharmacological Principles in the Management of Accidental Poisoning. *Pediatric Clinics of North America* 17:495-507.

MEDICAL-LEGAL TOXICOLOGY

The pursuit of the law has a purpose similar to that of veterinary medical science—the ascertainment of the facts, the truth. The tools used in the law are different from those of veterinary medicine. Both professions seek to make diagnostic judgments, and both professions turn their attention to prognoses. A lawsuit is the public forum in which the legal profession works, much as the laboratory or the clinical office is the forum in which the veterinary practitioner works.

A practicing veterinarian frequently is called upon to participate in his professional capacity in medical-legal proceedings. He may be a direct party in the proceeding, having been sued for alleged negligence or malpractice; he may sue for damages to his professional reputation or practice; he may be involved in trying to obtain payment of fees charged. As a party to such proceedings, he may also appear as a witness. In those proceedings the practicing veterinarian may give testimony both in his professional capacity and as a lay observer of fact.

When the practicing veterinarian testifies in his professional capacity, he serves as an expert witness. The expertise of this witness comes from his training, his knowledge and his experience. They permit him to offer his opinions, again, in his professional capacity.

The practicing veterinarian much more frequently will be called upon to participate in medical-legal proceedings as an expert witness, which is as if the practicing veterinarian were called upon to be a teacher of the court and the jury. The greater the training in the specific area of concern in the medica-legal proceeding, such as veterinary toxicology, the greater weight that can be attached to the opinions of the expert witness in veterinary medicine.

The Witness

Anyone who knows facts can be called upon to testify as to what he knows. He is a witness. Normally he is called upon to testify as to what he personally has seen or done, not what he has heard others say that they have seen or done. For a witness to testify as to what others may have seen or done is called "hearsay," and may be excluded testimony. Normally a witness does not give his own opinion, for that function is left to a jury, or to a judge who sits as a trier of fact instead of a jury.

Unlike the ordinary witness who testifies to what he has seen or done, the expert witness is allowed to draw his conclusions, both on the basis of what he has seen or done, and on the basis of his training, education, experience and other qualifications. An expert witness may know nothing of the facts at issue, but he can give his opinion, in some instances, as sufficient hypothetical facts are put to the expert for his assumption. Then the opinion rests upon the assumptions made. As a functioning expert witness, the veterinary medical practitioner may make use of instructive tools, such as models, pictures, charts and diagrams.

The initial qualification of an expert witness is determined by the court, on appropriate examination by the attorney who calls the expert witness to testify. Thereafter, the weight given to the expert's opinion will depend upon the credibility which the testimony compels. An attorney opposing the party whose counsel called the expert witness may attempt to discredit the expert on the basis of inadequate or improper qualifications. The discrediting of the expert witness can focus on his academic performance, such as course failures. The opposing attorney may ask about the motivating interests of the expert witness, if it appears that he may be testifying other than for professional purposes.

If errors were made in the observations of the testifying expert, in the work that he did, or in the nature of the assumptions which the expert was asked to make, those errors can be brought to the attention of the expert, in order to question the conclusions reached. It is not uncommon that the attorney asking questions of an expert witness, in an extremely narrow range of technical material pertaining to the case, may be highly knowledgeable to the point of embarrassing the expert witness.

Availability

The Constitution of the United States and of most states provides for compulsory process to summon the testimony of witnesses. Expert witnesses cannot be compelled to perform services. Once they have performed services, however, then their opinions can be compelled for testimonial purposes. Expert witnesses, like all other witnesses, may be subpoenaed to testify. No subpoena can be ignored, without peril of criminal punishment. A witness will be compensated for his expenses in attending a lawsuit, as those expenses are provided by statute. They generally do not provide for professional compensation, on subpoena costs. Nevertheless, an expert witness is entitled to a fee commensurate with his expertise. That fee should be agreed upon between the attorney and the expert witness before they conclude their understanding of the work which the expert witness will provide at the instance or request of the attorney.

If a subpoena issues to require the attendance of an expert witness at a trial, normally the court would not expect the expert to be donating his services, without compensation. It is a general professional obligation of a practicing veterinarian to share the fruits of his knowledge, training and experience, and he should do so consonant with professional ethics and the demands of his practice. It may be one of the more important services which the practicing veterinarian may give to his client, to provide testimony and assistance to the veterinarian's client's attorney, in representing the best interests of the client. It is not always in the best interests of the client to "support his story;" facts must be faced, and that is the job which the attorney, as well as the veterinarian, have been hired to perform.

Evidence

Certain precautions should be taken for an expert witness to present his evidence, of a technical nature, in the most effective manner. If an expert does not take care to educate the court and the jury, then he has failed in his professional calling in the medical-legal proceeding. In the judicial, administrative or legislative forum—any of these may be legal proceedings—some rules of evidence may be prescribed. The attorney, working with the practicing veterinarian, should give guidance to the expert witness on the rules of evidence which must be followed. Normally those rules include:

1. Do not volunteer information. It will be drawn from you by questions, so that your answers can be complete without rambling.

2. Whenever it is necessary for you to use technical language, explain it. Do not assume that the court and jury understand jargon or technical terms.

3. Do not be dogmatic. No one is required to accept your opinions. They are worth only what they can compel by the reasoning you employ, the methods you undertook and the qualifications you bring to the witness chair.

4. Know your subject well; prepare thoroughly for all of the aspects which you will cover in your testimony.

5. Be objective. Do not hesitate to say, "I do not know," when that is an honest answer. Short answers are normally preferable to long answers; "Yes" or "No" are better answers than the complicated ways of saying the same thing. However, when a simple or direct answer is not scientifically justifiable, you should be given the opportunity to explain your answer.

6. Expect questions on direct examination to elicit your opinions, and the work which is the basis for those opinions, or the assumptions upon which you rest your opinions. Leading questions cannot be permitted on direct examination, although they can be used on cross-examination.

7. If you refer to specific published works, you should be prepared to defend them, if you accept them as authoritative. On cross-examination you can expect to have your opinions, work and qualifications tested by reference to published works.

8. Records, analyses and the results of experiments, tests or work can be introduced, if those records have been maintained by you in the regular course of your business, or under your supervision and control.

9. You may refer to notes for your testimony; if you do so, they may be inspected by the attorney who will cross-examine you.

Privileged Information

If you have been retained by an attorney to assist him in the preparation of a client's case, your direct communication with that attorney may be confidential. If so, then such communication cannot be discovered without the permission of the client. Certain privileges are respected by the statues of the states of the United States and of the federal government as well. These include:

1. Communications between an attorney and his client.

2. The work product of the attorney and his expert assistants, in many cases.

3. Communications between a husband and wife.

4. Communications between a doctor and a patient, in most cases; although this has been established for human medicine, it is not granted to the veterinarian-client relationship.

5. Communication between a minister and a parishioner.

6. The constitutional privilege against self-incrimination.

When you are involved in a medical-legal proceeding, you should not divulge information regarding the work you have done without the permission of your client and his attorney. Formal methods of discovery are available to obtain the benefit of the work you have done, where permitted by law.

Professional Malpractice

To avoid having a lawsuit brought against you in your capacity as a practicing veterinarian, certain precautions should be taken. Your professional activity should be conducted in a thorough, systematic manner. You should not expect that frequent claims will be brought against you if you have conducted your professional activity in keeping with the ethics of the veterinary medical profession and using the scientific methods accepted as of the time.

Those cases brought to your clinical attention, involving the poisoning of an animal, frequently may result in legal action. In those instances it is important that as the attending veterinarian you make a complete clinical examination, do thorough necropsy, sample and prepare specimens for laboratory study in an acceptable manner, as well as use conservative and recognized therapeutic measures. It is vital that you maintain records of the history, clinical signs, postmortem changes, therapeutic measures, and the dates of your involvement in the case. See further the chapters on **Diagnostic Toxicology and Management and Treatment of Toxicoses.**

Some classical means for inviting lawsuits include:

1. Missing a diagnosis.

2. Giving erroneous treatment.

3. Ignoring current veterinary literature.

4. Ignoring drug precaution statements.

5. Critizing your colleagues, without justification.

6. Failing to keep adequate records.

7. Ignoring clients.

8. Giving optimistic prognoses when they are unwarranted.

9. Failing to advise clients when you intend to be absent from your practice.

10. Failing to explain the risks and hazards associated with treatment.

11. Failing to carefully select, train and supervise assistants.

12. Extending your practice beyond the limits of your qualifications and training.

13. Failing to maintain your equipment in good, clean condition.

14. Making diagnoses and prescriptions without adequate information and history obtained.

15. Failing to conduct thorough postmortem examinations when indicated.

16. Failing to use careful laboratory techniques.

17. Avoiding the use of acceptable methods of diagnosis and treatment.

18. Failing to follow the advice of your lawyer and your malpractice insurance carrier.

Feed-Related Toxicants

IODINE

Elemental iodine is classed as a rare element, occurring in the earth's crust as about 1 part per 15 million. The chief sources of iodine are seaweed and a nitrate-bearing rock known as Chilean Caliche. Cuprous iodide occurs in nature as the mineral "marshite" but the discovery of iodine itself was incidental to the manufacture of nitrates for gunpowder from seaweed ash by Napoleon's scientists in the early 19th century. Prior to that time, seaweed and other marine forms had been used strictly on an empirical basis since ancient times as a treatment for goiter, long before iodine was known or the nature of the disease understood.

Iodine is an essential element that has its entire functional significance through its presence in thyroid hormones. Manifestations of iodine deficiency are those of deficient supply of these hormones to the organism. An enlargement of the thyroid, or goiter, must be regarded as a final common expression of a number of separate and distinguishable disease processes, of which one of these is an absolute iodine deficiency. Therefore, iodine is a *Generally Recognized as Safe* (GRAS) food ingredient for man and animals.

Source

Many different compounds containing iodine have been used as therapeutic agents in medicine and veterinary medicine. Salts of iodine, such as potassium and sodium iodide have been used for the treatment of granulomatous infections such as soft tissue lumpy jaw, caused by *Actinobacillus lignierisi* and footrot, caused by *Spherophorus necrophorus*. An organic iodide, ethylene diamine dihydriodide (EDDI), is recommended as a feed additive for livestock and poultry, but not dairy cattle in production. (Feed Additive Compendium, 1976) Table 1 summarizes the recommended oral levels and indications for use of EDDI in livestock and poultry.

A warning statement associated with the use of EDDI for livestock in general is as follows: "Do not administer to animals showing symptoms of acute respiratory conditions; treatment levels should not be administered to animals whose milk will be used for human consumption . . . treat animals with caution until tolerance is determined, because of variation

TABLE 1
Recommended Oral Levels of EDDI

Animal	Use Level	Indications
Cattle	50 mg/head/day in feed or salt continuously	Prevent footrot, soft tissue lumpy jaw and nutritional source of iodine
	400-500 mg/head/day for 2-3 weeks (not to dairy cattle in production)	Treatment of footrot, soft tissue lumpy jaw, and mild respiratory infections by action as an expectorant
Sheep	12 mg/head/day continuously	Prevent soft tissue lumpy jaw
Swine	250-500 mg/day for 7 days	Aid in control of respiratory difficulties by loosening mucus and congestion in the upper respiratory tract
Turkeys and chickens	one-fourth lb/ton of feed (125 ppm) for 5-7 days	An aid in the removal of mucus from the upper respiratory tract following treatment for chronic respiratory disease

in susceptibility to iodides." (Feed Additive Compendium, 1976)

The minimum dietary requirements of iodine for man and other species is quite variable and depends entirely upon the diet and region. Apparently, the adult human requirement is from 100-200 μ/day and the rat requires from 1-2 μ/day. The estimated body requirements for livestock and poultry are given in table 2. (Underwood, 1971)

TABLE 2
Estimated Minimum Requirements of Iodine

Animal	Body Weight (lbs)	Iodine Requirement (μ g/day)
Poultry	5	5-9
Swine	150	80-160
Sheep	110	50-100
Dairy cow (in production)	1,000	400-800

(Underwood, 1971.)

Toxicity

There is a wide range between the toxic dose and the minimum daily required dose of iodine in animals and man. It has been estimated that a dose 14,000-56,000 times that of the daily iodine requirement has been consumed by humans while only producing minimal signs of toxicosis. (Informatics, Inc., 1973) Similar findings have been reported in cattle, sheep and other domestic animals. Table 3 summarizes the acute toxicity of various salts of iodine to laboratory animals.

The toxicity of EDDI to livestock and poultry has not been systematically studied. Buck and Rosiles, 1975, distributed sixteen apparently healthy beef steers, weighing approximately 500 pounds each, into four groups of four animals per group and fed EDDI in their ration. Dosages of 0, 50, 500, and 1,000 mg EDDI per head per day were fed for twenty-one days, after which all animals, except the controls, were given 50 mg per head per day for an additional seventy days. The EDDI was mixed with a basal concentrate ration. The animals were fed all of the concentrate they would eat plus alfalfa hay *ad libitum* two times per day. All animals given 1,000 and 500 mg EDDI/head/day manifested its expectorant action in the form of a translucent nasal discharge which became yellowish and opaque after five to seven days and which was accompanied by a mild intermittent nonproductive cough. Such signs became apparent after five to eight days in the 1,000 mg/head/day group, between six to ten days in the 500 mg/head/day group, and continued throughout the remainder of the twenty-one-day high-level feeding period. The above signs subsided significantly within two days after the EDDI exposure was reduced to 50 mg/head/day. Those animals given 50 mg/head/day exhibited slight nasal discharge and mild cough in an occasional animal, beginning from about two weeks of exposure through-

TABLE 3
Acute Toxicity of Iodine Salts to Laboratory Animals

Substance	Animal	Route	Dosage (mg/kg BW)	Measurement	Reference
KIO_3	Mice	IP	136 ±5	LD_{50}	Webster et al., 1957
KIO_3	Mice	Oral	1,177 (not fasted)	LD_{50}	Webster et al., 1957
KIO_3	Mice	Oral	531 (fasted)	LD_{50}	Webster et al., 1957
KIO_3	Guinea pig	Oral	400 (fasted)	LD_{50}	Webster et al., 1959
KIO_3	Dog	Oral	200-500	Min. LD	Webster et al., 1966
KI	Mice	IP	1,177 ±30	LD_{50}	Webster et al., 1957
KI	Mice	Oral	2,068	LD_{50}	Webster et al., 1957
KI	Mice	Oral	1,862 (fasted)	LD_{50}	Webster et al., 1957
KI	Rat	IV	285	Lethal dose	Stecker et al., 1968
$NaIO_3$	Mice	IP	119 ±4	LD_{50}	Webster et al., 1957
$NaIO_3$	Mice	IV	108 ±4	LD_{50}	Webster et al., 1957
$NaIO_3$	Mice	Oral	505 (fasted)	LD_{50}	Webster et al., 1957
$NaIO_3$	Dog	IV	200	Lethal dose	Stecker et al., 1968
NaI	Mice	IP	1,690 ±85	LD_{50}	Webster et al., 1957
NaI	Mice	IV	1,500	LD_{50}	Webster et al., 1957
NaI	Mice	Oral	1,650 (fasted)	LD_{50}	Webster et al., 1957
NaI	Rat	IV	1,300	LD_{50}	Stecker et al., 1968

out the three-month feeding trial. Excessive lacrimation was not observed in any of the animals being fed the various levels of iodine, nor in the controls. There was no statistically significant difference in body temperatures and in mean body weight gains of any of the animals on the various levels of iodine versus the controls. All animals in all groups gained an average of 1.7 pounds per day during the experimental period.

The serum protein bound iodine (PBI) levels and total serum iodine levels for the four groups of animals described in the above study are presented in figures 1 and 2, respectively. Although peak mean total serum iodine levels averaged 1,600 μg/100 ml after two weeks of EDDI exposure to 1,000 mg/head/day, the levels rapidly diminished when exposure was reduced from 1,000 mg to 50 mg/head/day. No clinical signs of tox-

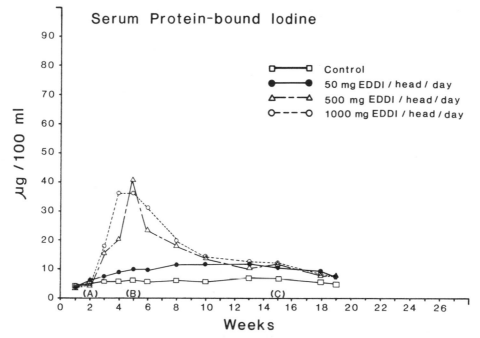

Figure 1. Serum protein-bound iodine. (A = exposure started, B = all groups except controls given 50 mg/head/day, C = exposure stopped.)

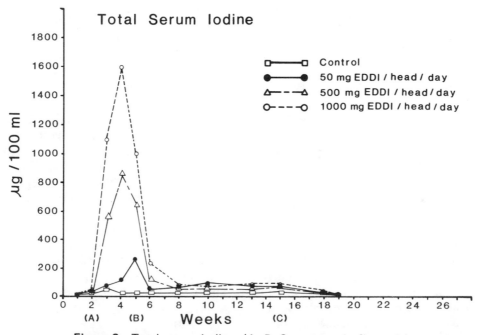

Figure 2. Total serum iodine. (A, B, C, same as in figure 1.)

icosis or statistically significant differences in the following parameters were noted: packed RBC volume, hemoglobin percent, WBC count, neutrophil count, lymphocyte count, serum glutamic oxalacetic transaminase, serum creatinine, plasma fribrinogen, and total serum protein. The authors concluded that except for signs reflecting the expectorant action of EDDI, no adverse effects were noted.

In another study, Buck, 1970, fed EDDI to two 500-600 pound beef calves for a total of eighty days, according to the schedule in table 4. After the dosage level reached 5,000 mg/head/day, the animals would occasionally refuse to eat their EDDI contaminated feed.

TABLE 4
Schedule of EDDI Fed to Beef Cattle

| No. of Days Dosed | Dosage (mg/head/day) | |
	Animal 1	Animal 2
21	1,000	2,000
20	3,000	4,000
17	5,000	6,000
17	7,000	8,000
5	20,000	20,000

(Buck, 1970.)

Subsequently, the dose was given via gelatin capsule orally. The first subjective clinical sign was a bilateral sero-mucoid nasal discharge occurring intermittently throughout the experiment beginning after seven days of exposure to 1,000 and 2,000 mg/head/day, respectively. The discharge became progressively more pronounced as the levels of iodine were increased. After the levels of exposure were increased to 4,000 and 5,000 mg/head/day, respectively, an occasional cough was noted. This cough became consistently present after the 20,000 mg/head/day level of exposure was begun. Minor skin changes were noted at the 4,000 mg/head/day level in the form of scaliness on the dorsum of the neck and a slight amount of sloughing of the epidermis appearing in the form of dandruff. This change became more pronounced at 8,000 mg/head/day and was very evident at 20,000 mg/head/day, at which time there was considerable scaling of the epidermis over the neck, whithers, ears, brisket, shoulders, back, and on the tail head. A slight degree of hair loss was evident at the termination of the experiment. Within two weeks after discontinuing the exposure to iodine, the skin changes had disappeared and the animals appeared normal.

Six-week-old Holstein bull calves were fed calcium iodate ($Ca(IO_3)_2$) added to a basal diet at the rate of 0,

10, 25, 50, 100 and 200 parts per million for periods of time ranging from 112-144 days. (Newton et al., 1974) The calves weighed approximately 83 kg at the beginning of the experiment and ranged from 159 to 122 kg at the end of the experiment. Calculated on the basis of mg of iodine per head per day, and assuming that a calf will eat 2.5 percent of his body weight, those animals on the 50 ppm dosage consumed approximately 105 mg/head/day at the beginning and 265 mg/head/day by the end of the experiment. Those animals on the 200 ppm diet consumed approximately 415 mg/head/day at the beginning of the experiment and 795 mg/head/day by the end of the experiment. If one considers that EDDI, the most common source of iodine as a feed additive, consists of approximately 80 percent iodine by weight, then the calves on the 50 ppm diet, at the beginning of the experiment consumed an equivalent of 131 mg/head/day of EDDI and 331 mg/head/day by the end of the experiment. Those animals on the 200 ppm diet consumed an EDDI equivalent of 520 mg/head/day at the beginning of the experiment and an EDDI equivalent of 994 mg/head/day by the end of the experiment. These workers reported that the minimum toxic iodine level for calves was near the 50 ppm level (equivalent to 131-331 mg/head/day) as evidenced by slightly depressed weight gains and feed intake. They also noted slightly increased adrenal and thyroid gland weights in most of the animals given iodine. At the end of the approximate four-month feeding trials, the control animals had serum iodine concentrations ranging from approximately 11-18 mcg/100 ml. Those on 10 ppm iodine diet had approximately 100 mcg/100 ml; on 25 ppm, 225 mcg/100 ml; 50 ppm, 405 mcg/100 ml; 100 ppm, 512-830 mcg/100 ml; and on 200 ppm, 1,516 mcg/100 ml.

Forty lambs, averaging 30 kg each, were distributed into ten groups of four animals each and given various levels of EDDI and KI at dosages ranging from 94 mg/head/day to 785 mg/head/day for a total of twenty-two days. The dosages were given via gelatin capsules orally in the nondiluted form. The lowest treatment levels at which an adverse effect was noted, as evidenced by decreased body weight gain, occurred in the groups consuming 393 mg/head/day of KI and 562 mg/head/day of EDDI. This dosage is forty-seven times the FDA recommended feeding level of EDDI to sheep as an aid in the prevention of soft tissue lumpy jaw (12 mg/head/day). These workers measured the total iodine concentration in the serum of the four animals given 375 mg of EDDI per day. On day fifteen of exposure, the concentration ranged from 1,215-4,058 mcg/100 ml. One week after exposure was discontinued, the serum levels ranged from 36-194 mcg/100 ml. (McCauley et al., 1973)

In summary, the nutritional requirement for iodine by most animals and humans are in the general range of 0.5-1 μg per pound body weight. The recommended continuous feeding level for the prevention of disease states such as soft tissue lumpy jaw and footrot are about 50-100 times the recommended nutritional requirement; the level that would be expected to produce clinical signs of excessive exposure when fed continuously is about 1,000 times the nutritional requirement for cattle and other livestock. The lethal doses for the various species of livestock and humans have not been delineated. However, the single acute lethal dose must certainly be above 20-50,000 times the recommended daily nutritional requirement.

Mechanism of Action

Iodine metabolism and thyroid function are closely linked, since the only known metabolic role is the synthesis of thyroid hormones—thyroxine and triiodothyronine. Iodine metabolism thus consists essentially of the synthesis and degradation of the thyroid hormones and the reutilization or excretion of the iodine so released. (Underwood, 1971) After consumption of either inorganic or organic iodine, it is rapidly and almost completely absorbed from the gastrointestinal tract in the ionic form, although some of the iodinated amino acids are slowly, and to a much less extent, absorbed as such.

Iodine is excreted mainly in the urine, with smaller amounts being present in the feces and sweat. The salivary glands have the capability of removing iodine from amino acids and recycling it via saliva through the GI tract. The biological half-life of iodine for most animals and human is quite rapid, in the neighborhood of six to ten hours.

The thyroid gland has an efficient capacity for trapping iodine in its process of iodinization of the amino acids thyroxine, thyronine, 3, 5, 3-triiodothyropyruvic acid and 3-monoiodotyrosine.

Considerably more has been written concerning the nutritional requirements of iodine than concerning its toxicity. Nutritionally, the entire functional significance of iodine can be accounted for through its presence in the thyroid hormones. The manifestations of iodine deficiency are those of a deficient supply of these hormones to the organism. The rate of energy exchange and the quantity of heat liberated by an organism is elevated in hyperthyroidism and reduced below normal in hypothyroidism. The iodine containing thyroid hormone(s) is essential for growth during early life in all mammals and birds. A deficiency of iodine results in a type of dwarfism known as cretinism which may be associated with goiter and mental retardation. Iodine deficiency in domestic animals is manifested by stunted growth but may not necessarily be associated with visible presence of goiter. Iodine deficiency is associated not only with mental sluggishness and apathy, but also emotional instability, nervousness, and irritability, accompanied by muscle tremors and hyperactive sweat glands. Other manifestations of iodine deficiency in domestic animals and man include failure to develop normal sexual vigor, delayed maturation of genitalia, and failure of the production of ova. Reproductive failure is often the outstanding manifestation of iodine deficiency in domestic animals. Fetal developemnt may be arrested at any stage, leading either to early death and resorption, to abortion and stillbirth, or to live birth of weak, hairless fetuses, often associated with prolonged gestation and retention of fetal membranes. (Underwood, 1971)

In addition to its metabolic functions, iodine appears to have some additional peculiar effects on the mammalian system which has enabled it to be used as a therapeutic agent. Taken orally, salts of iodine, whether inorganic or organic (such as KI or EDDI) have an expectorant action via stimulation of the vagus nerves in the GI tract (Boyd et al., 1945). Thus, iodides have been recommended for use as expectorants in cattle as an aid in the treatment of mild respiratory infections by action as an expectorant. EDDI apparently has less irritating effects on the gastrointestinal system than does KI or other salts. It is also more stable when mixed with feeds or livestock minerals than are many of the other iodine compounds. McCauley et al., (1972), have empirically questioned the use of EDDI as an expectorant for the treating of respiratory infections in cattle. They noted in connection with three field observations that animals receiving therapeutic or greater levels of EDDI (380-1,700 mg/head/day) had a high incidence of concomitant respiratory tract infections and certain reproductive problems. This report is of questionable validity because serum iodine levels ranged from 103-524 μg/100 ml, which are below the levels reported by Buck and Rosiles, (1975), that were not associated with evidence of iodine toxicosis (1,600 μg/100 ml) and those of Rosiles et al., (1975), that were not associated with increased severity of clinical infectious bovine rhinotracheitis infection in cattle being fed EDDI.

Another property of iodine is its specific antifibrotic effect. Various iodine compounds, especially KI and EDDI, are effective in the treatment of granulomatous conditions, such as soft tissue lumpy jaw. This action is apparently due to iodine's capacity to penetrate fibrotic tissue. On the other hand, high levels of iodine may also enhance the inflammatory process. (Stone and Willis, 1967)

Clinical Signs

Clinical signs of iodism in most animal species involve increased secretions of the respiratory tract fluid with an accompanying intermittent nonproductive cough. As the amount or time of exposure is increased, the eyes, skin, joints, hematopoietic and, ultimately, reproductive systems are involved.

The most prominent early signs of iodine exposure are those of its expectorant effect: increased seromucoid nasal discharge with an accompanying intermittent cough, followed by lacrimation and skin changes. In cattle, the skin of the dorsum, neck, ears, brisket, shoulders, and head of the tail become scaly due to sloughing of the epidermis. This phenomenon gives the appearance of a severe case of dandruff. If animals are exposed to very high levels of iodine for a prolonged period of time, other signs may include lameness of the knee and hock joints in a low percentage of the animals affected. In chickens, very high levels of iodine in the diet (2,500 ppm) have been associated with cessation of egg production.

Clinical signs of iodidism disappear rapidly after exposure is discontinued, even though animals have been exposed to massive levels of iodine. Likewise, serum concentrations of iodine rapidly disappear when exposure is discontinued. (Buck and Rosiles, 1975)

Diagnosis

The fairly rapid development of a syndrome manifested by a sero-mucoid nasal discharge, intermittent nonproductive coughing and perhaps excessive lacrimation, together with a history of having a continuous exposure to high levels of iodine are sufficient to warrant a tentative diagnosis of mild iodidism. In cattle, serum levels of iodine may reach 1,600 μ /100 ml in animals manifesting only an increased nasal discharge and occasional coughing. If clinical signs include lacrimation, scaling of the epidermis, and joint related lameness, one can expect the iodine exposure to be considerably higher than is recommended for therapeutic purposes. In such an event, the total serum iodine concentrations may reach 4-5,000 μ /100 ml or greater.

One must keep in mind, however, that once iodine exposure is discontinued, the blood levels decrease rapidly to near background levels within a matter of a few days. Background levels of total serum iodine in cattle usually range below 25-50 μ /100 ml.

Treatment

Since iodine is rapidly mobilized and excreted from the tissues, the best treatment is removal of the iodine source.

BIBLIOGRAPHY

Boyd, E. M.; Blancher, M. C.; Copeland, J. S.; Jackson, S.; and Stevens, M. 1945. The Effect of Inorganic Iodides Upon Respiratory Tract Fluid. *Canad. J. Res.*, 23:195-205.

Buck, W. B. 1970. *Organic Iodine Toxicity in the Bovine.* Unpublished report. Vet. Diag. Lab., Ames, Iowa: Iowa State University, pp.1-5.

Buck, W. B., and Rosiles, R. 1975. *Safety Evaluation of Ethylenediamine Dihydriodide as a Cattle Feed Additive. Unpublished report. Vet. Diag. Lab., Ames, Iowa: Iowa State University, pp.1-14.*

Feed Additive Compendium. 1976. Minneapolis: Miller Pub. Co., pp. 198-201.

Informatics, Inc. 1973. *Scientific Literature Reviews on Generally Regarded as Safe (GRAS) Food Ingredients—Iodine and Iodine Salts.* PB 223-849, Prepared for the Food and Drug Administration, distributed by National Tech. Inf. Serv., U.S. Dept. of Commerce, pp. 1-82.

McCauley, E. H.; Johnson, D. W.; and Alhadj, I. 1972. Disease Problems in Cattle Associated with Rations Containing High Levels of Iodide. *Bovine Practicioner.* Nov., pp. 22-27, 55.

McCauley, E. H.; Linn, J. G,; and Goodrich, R. D. 1973. Experimental Induced Iodide Toxicosis in Lambs. *Am. J. Vet. Res.,* 34:65-70

Newton, G. L.; Barrick, E. R.; Harvey, R. W.; and Wise, M. B. 1974. Iodine Toxicity: Physiological Effects of Elevated Dietary Iodine on Calves. *J. Anim. Sci.,* 38:449-55.

Rosiles, R.; Buck, W. B.; and Brown, L. N. 1975. Clinical Infectious Bovine Rhinotracheitis in Cattle Fed Organic Iodine and Urea. *Am. J. Vet. Res.,* 36:1447-53.

Stecher, P. G.; Windholz, M.; and Leahy, D. S., eds. 1968. *Merck Index,* 8th ed. Rathway, N.J., pp. 1713.

Stone, O. J., and Willis, C. J. 1967. Iodine Enhancement of Inflammation—Experimental with Clinical Correlation. *Texas Reports of Biol. and Med.,* 25:205-213.

Underwood, E. J. 1971. *Trace Elements in Human and Animal Nutrition,* 3rd ed. New York: Academic Press, pp. 281-322.

Webster, S. H.; Rice, M. E.; Highman, B.; and Von Oettingen, W. F. 1957. The Toxicology of Potassium and Sodium Iodates: Acute Toxicity in Mice. *J. Pharmacol. and Exptl. Therap.,* 120:171-78.

Webster, S. H.; Rice, M. E.; Highman, B.; and Stohlman, E. F. 1959. The Toxicology of Potassium and Sodium Iodates, II; Subacute Toxicity of Potassium Iodate in Mice and Guinea Pigs. *Toxicol. and Appl. Pharmacol.,* 1:87-96.

Webster, S. H.; Stohlman, E. F.; and Higman, B. 1966. The Toxicology of Potassium and Sodium Iodates, III; Acute and Subacute Oral Toxicity of Potassium Iodate in Dogs. *Toxicol. and Appl. Pharmacol.,* 8:185-92.

UREA AND NONPROTEIN NITROGEN

Ammonia toxicosis results when animals ingest compounds which release excessive quantities of ammonia into the gastrointestinal tract with a resultant hyperammonemia. All species of domestic animals are susceptible to poisoning by ammonium salts. Only ruminant animals are normally poisoned by the more complex amides and excess high protein feedstuffs. This chapter deals primarily with urea toxicosis in ruminants, but the basic mechanism of ammonia toxicosis is the same in all mammals. Animals differ in susceptibility to poisoning from orally ingested amides because of dissimilarities in gastrointestinal digestion and metabolism.

Source

Ammonium salts, especially ammonium nitrate, and solutions containing ammonia and anions such as nitrate and phosphate, and sometimes urea, are common commercial fertilizer components. Farm animals may drink liquid fertilizers if available; cattle and sheep have been known to ingest dry granular fertilizers containing ammonium salts and urea, usually when animals have access to open bags or piles of spilled fertilizers in fields. Ammonium chloride is used to reduce the incidence of urolithiasis in cattle and sheep at respective daily doses of 0.75-1.5 and 0.25 ounces per animal, and as an expectorant in swine. Monoammonium phosphate, and to a lesser extent, diammonium phosphate, have been used as sources of nonprotein nitrogen (NPN) in ruminant rations.

Urea and other nonprotein nitrogen compounds are used as substitutes for natural protein in ruminant feeds. Although urea and related compounds are considered to be feed ingredients, if not used properly and under certain nutritional conditions, they can become toxicants that are highly lethal. This section will be concerned primarily with urea, since problems associated with its use have been the most prominent.

Nonprotein nitrogen (NPN) for ruminant feeding is derived primarily from urea and ammonium salts.

While most nitrogen substitution is from urea, a number of products containing NPN are available as follows:

1. Feed Urea—feed grade urea is a dry granular product containing approximately 45% nitrogen (equivalent to 281% protein). When this product is used in livestock feed the level of NPN must be shown on the label, and sufficient feeding directions and caution statements must also be included.

2. Feed Grade Biuret—feed grade biuret results from the controlled pyrolysis of urea. It would normally contain approximately 230% equivalent crude protein.

3. Gelatinized Starch-Urea Product—this product is obtained by mixing urea and a finely ground grain together and processing it under conditions of moisture, pressure, and high temperature. The resulting product can then be used as a source of energy and the NPN in commercial feeds. (trade name—Starea).

4. Urea Phosphate—an acidic crystalline urea product containing 17.3% urea and 19.9% phosphorous. It is freely soluble in water dissociating to urea and phosphoric acid.

5. Diammonium Phosphate—contains at least 17% nitrogen and 20% phosphorous. It may be used in ruminant feeds as a source of these nutrients in amounts that supply not more than 2% of equivalent crude protein in the total daily ration.

6. Ammonium Polyphosphate Solution—this product is commonly used to add nitrogen and phosphorous to liquid feed supplements. It must contain not less than 9% nitrogen and 13% phosphorous, and must be used to supply not more than 2% of equivalent crude protein in the total animal diet.

7. Ammoniated Rice Hulls—obtained by the treatment of ground rice hulls with monocalcium

phosphate and anhydrous ammonia under conditions of temperature and pressure. This product can be used in beef cattle feeds as a surce of NPN and fiber at a level not to exceed 20% of the total ration.

8. Ammoniated Cottonseed Meal—obtained by the treatment of cottonseed meal with anhydrous ammonia under pressure. It can be used in the feed of ruminants as a source of NPN in an amount not to exceed 20% of the total ration NPN.

9. Ammonium Sulfate—results from the neutralization of sulfuric acid with ammonia. It must contain not less than 21% nitrogen and not less than 24% sulfur. It can be used in ruminant feeds as a source of these two nutrients in an amount that supplies not more than 2% of the equivalent crude protein in the total daily ration.

10. Monoammonium Phosphate—contains not less than 9% nitrogen and 23% phosphorus. It can be used as a source of these two nutrients in ruminant feeds in an amount that supplies not more than 2% of equivalent crude protein in the total daily ration.

The available nitrogen, phosphorous, and protein equivalence of NPN sources should be known when considering the role of NPN in toxicity or nutrition for the bovine. Table 1 lists the nitrogen, phosphorous, and protein equivalence of some common NPN sources.

TABLE 1
Some Characteristics of NPN Sources

Compound	Content N%	P%	Protein Equivalent %
Urea—pure	46.7	0.0	292
Urea—feed grade	45.0	0.0	281
Biuret—pure	40.8	0.0	255
Biuret—feed grade	37.0	0.0	230
Monoammonium phosphate	12.0	27.0	75
Diammonium phosphate	21.0	23.0	131
Ammonium polyphosphate	10.0	15.0	62
Ammonium sulfate	21.0	0.0	131

NPN is generally supplied to ruminants as (1) feed supplements for mixing or blending, (2) range block or cubes for free-choice access, and (3) liquid supplements commonly combining molasses and urea in a controlled access system such as "lick-tanks" or float- controlled tanks.

Urea is generally recommended in ruminant rations at a rate of approximately 3 percent of the grain ration or about 1 percent of the total ration. A third general rule is that NPN should constitute no more than one-third of the total nitrogen in the ration. More recently, however, formulations increasing these levels have been recommended and appear to be in general use.

Biuret is recommended in ruminant rations at levels approximating 3 percent of the total ration. Ammonium chloride may be used at a rate of 0.75-1.5 ounces for cattle and 0.25 ounces for sheep/head/day to reduce urolithiasis. Diammonium phosphate may be used to furnish about one-third of the nitrogen requirements for ruminants.

Toxicity

The toxicity of urea and other NPN formulations is dependent upon their hydrolysis to ammonia. Cattle and other ruminants are the most susceptible because their rumen contains urease and is an ideal environment for hydrolysis of urea, releasing carbon dioxide and ammonia. Horses are mildly susceptible to urea but are more susceptible to ammonium salts. Monogastric animals are not susceptible to urea poisoning but are susceptible to poisoning by ammonium salts.

Circumstances which usually result in urea toxicosis often involve (1) improper mixing or formulation of NPN rations; (2) feeding urea to ruminants unaccustomed to NPN or animals which have been starved; (3) using high levels of urea in rations low in energy and protein and high in fiber; and (4) giving animals free access to a palatable source of urea concentrate.

In ruminants, urea usually is lethal at 1-1.5 gm/kg body weight; 0.3-0.5 gm/kg may be toxic. Urea phosphate usually is toxic at 1 gm/kg. Ammonium salts and diammonium phosphate may be lethal at 1-2 gm/kg (Singer, 1969).

In horses, urea is lethal at approximately 4 gm/kg body weight (Hintz et al., 1970). Ammonium salts may be lethal at 1.5 gm/kg body weight.

In monogastric animals, urea and biuret have very low toxicity. Ammonium salts are toxic at approximately 1.5 gm/kg body weight (Bicknell, 1965).

Urea toxicity Varies with the age of ruminant animals. The very young ruminant has very low susceptibility because its rumen flora have not developed. After rumen development, the younger animals appear to be more susceptible than older animals. Cattle and sheep adapt to the feeding of urea rather quickly but also quickly lose their adaptation. By slowly increasing the amount of urea fed, the ruminant can tolerate as much as 1 gram urea/kg body weight daily. In practice, however, the feeding of very high levels of urea may be dangerous because animals may go off feed during adverse weather conditions or digestive upsets and quickly lose their tolerance for urea. Then after coming back on full feed, they may be poisoned by the high levels of urea.

The toxicity of NPN products depends in part on the form of NPN. Figure 1 depicts the comparative toxicity of various forms of NPN for ruminants.

Some predisposing factors for ammonia toxicosis in ruminants include (1) fasting, (2) high roughage diets, (3) lack of adaptation to high NPN diets, (4) high ruminal pH, (5) high rumen and body temperature, (6) dehydration or low-water intake, and (7) hepatic insufficiency.

It is often imperative to be able to calculate the concentration of urea in a feed. Pure urea equals 292 percent protein equivalent; however, commercial urea equals 262-280 percent protein equivalent. Thus, 1 pound of pure urea is equivalent to 2.92 pounds of NPN protein. If a label indicates 64 percent protein from urea, the concentration of urea is 64/292 equals 22 percent urea. If a feed contains 10 percent urea, the NPN protein is $10 \times 2.92 = 29.2$ percent.

Mechanism of Action

Urea hydrolysis to ammonia and carbon dioxide is catalyzed by the ruminal emzyme urease. Urease has a temperature optimum of 49° C and a pH optimum of 7.7-8.0. Furthermore, sufficient urease is available to rapidly hydrolyze large amounts of introduced urea so that peak ammonia levels are attained within one-half to two hours. Unfortunately the ruminant needs as much as several days to adapt fully to incorporation of additional ammonia into microbial protein.

Toxicosis from NPN formulations results from the absorption of NH_3 from the gastrointestinal tract. Ammonia from urea and ammonium salts is absorbed into the bloodstream more rapidly when rumino-reticulum pH is high (8.0 or above). An alkaline reaction also enhances urease-ureolysis to NH_3 and CO_2. At a pH of 6.5 or below, the ammonia is primarily in the form of ammonium ion ($NH_4{}^+$) and, thus, would not readily be absorbed through the gastrointestinal wall.

NPN salts such as ammonium sulfate, ammonium acetate and urea phosphate are highly acidic. Acid ruminal conditions favor both a slowing of urease activity and a shift in nitrogen equilibrium toward the ammonium ion. Thus, the acidic NPN products may be both safer and more efficient as well as protecting against any urea included in the diet.

As excess ammonia formed in the rumen is absorbed across the rumino-reticular wall, the liver attempts to convert the ammonia, via the urea-orinithine cycle, into urea. The urea formed can then be excreted in the urine, recycled back across the ruminal wall, or secreted in saliva. When the detoxication process is overwhelmed and blood ammonia reaches 1 to 2 mg/dL clinical signs of ammonia toxicosis develop. The interrelationships of

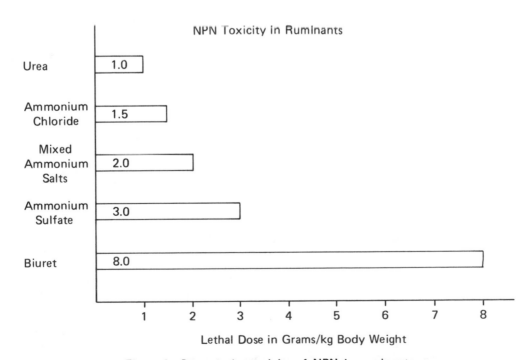

Figure 1. Comparative toxicity of NPN in ruminants.

NPN, nitrogen metabolism, and ammonia toxicosis are depicted in figure 2.

Although alkalosis of the rumen occurs during urea toxicosis, a systemic alkalosis does not occur. In fact, a metabolic acidosis develops. Lloyd (1970) has shown that blood pH drops from 7.4 to 7.0 at the time of urea-induced death. There is an apparent inhibition of the citrate cycle with resulting compensatory anaerobic glycolysis. Highly significant increases in packed cell volume, blood ammonia, blood glucose, blood urea nitrogen, serum potassium and phosphorus, blood lactate, SGOT, SGPT, and rumen pH occur during urea toxicosis in cattle and sheep. There are concomitant decreases in blood pH and urine excretion. Death probably is due to hyperkalemic cardiac blockage and cessation of respiration (Lloyd, 1970).

Some workers have theorized that since urea is hydrolyzed to ammonia in the rumen, it follows that it would be eructated by the ruminant and aspirated into the respiratory tract, causing irritation and increased susceptibility to respiratory infections. While it is true that urea is hydrolyzed into ammonia under normal conditions of digestion, over 99 percent of the released ammonia is in the form of NH_4OH which is nongaseous. Also, that NH_3 which is present is soluble in the liquid portion of the rumen contents and would also be nongaseous.

Clinical Signs

Toxicosis usually occurs in ruminants when ammonia concentrations reach 80 mg/100 ml in rumen fluid and 2 mg/100 ml in serum or whole blood. The

NPN—Protein Relationships

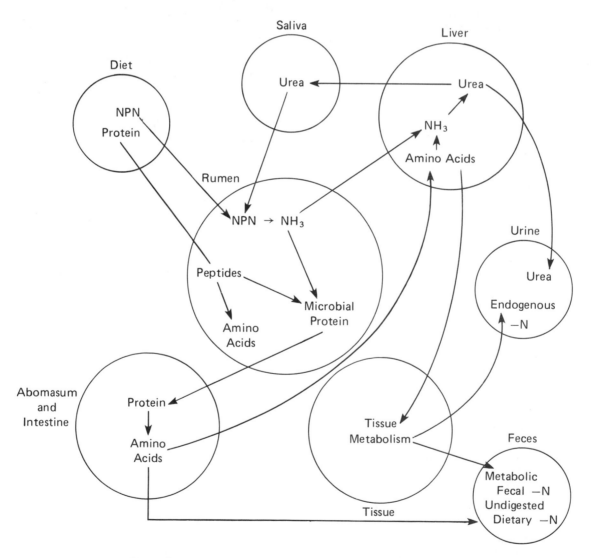

Figure 2. Nonprotein nitrogen and protein interrelationships.

clinical course of urea toxicosis usually is rapid and acute, from ten minutes to as much as four hours after consumption. Clinical signs, include frothy salivation, grinding of the teeth, and kicking at the abdomen indicating abdominal pain. There usually is polyuria, muscle tremors, incoordination, weakness, forced rapid breathing, bloat, violent struggling and bellowing, and terminal tetanic spasms. There often is a marked jugular pulse. Respiration often is forced and rapid. Toward the terminal stages, vomiting is especially common in sheep. Hyperthermia and anuria usually are evident just prior to death.

Physiopathology

Upon opening the rumen of an animal which has recently died of urea toxicosis, one occasionally can detect the odor of ammonia. There are no characteristic lesions of urea-NPN poisoning. Pulmonary edema, congestion, and petechial hemorrhages are rather common findings. There may be a mild bronchitis, and commonly rumen ingesta is found in the trachea and bronchi, especially in sheep. There may be a catarrhal gastro-enteritis.

Ruminal pH of 7.5 or greater at necropsy is indicative of urea or NPN toxicosis. However, several hours of postmortem autolysis may cause acid conditions to reoccur in the rumen. In addition, animals consuming high carbohydrate diets may not develop ruminal alkalosis even though ammonia concentration is high. This is thought to be due to increased lactic acid production associated with high carbohydrate diets.

Animals dead of urea toxicosis often are extremely bloated, and the carcass appears to decompose quite rapidly. Body tissues taken for diagnostic purposes should be obtained from an animal which has recently died. As a carcass is allowed to decompose, the breakdown of the natural protein in the tissues and stomach contents will result in a buildup of ammonia, which would tend to lead one diagnostically astray.

Diagnosis

Diagnosis of urea or NPN poisoning is based on the history of acute illness following consumption of feed containing urea or other NPN formulations. It usually is very important that the feed be analyzed for urea content and calculations be made to determine the possibility of poisoning under the conditions of consumption. If the clinical signs and necropsy findings are compatible with urea toxicosis, the diagnosis may be confirmed by analysis for ammonia in whole blood, serum, ruminal fluid, and urine. The specimens should be frozen immediately and thawed only at the time of analysis or preserved by the addition of saturated mercury chloride to stop enzymatic action on the natural protein. If the specimens are not frozen or preserved, proteolytic enzymes will break down the amino acids and tissue proteins, releasing ammonia. Thus, the longer a cadaver decomposes, the higher will be the ammonia content.

In most cases of urea poisoning, the rumen ammonia content will be greater than 80 mg/100 ml and may be as high as 200 mg/100 ml. It is important to take samples from several areas in the rumen and reticulum for ammonia analysis because it is possible that an animal may die before the urea that has been consumed has a chance to evenly distribute throughout the rumen and reticulum. Blood or serum ammonia nitrogen concentrations between 2-4 mg/100 ml or greater would be compatible with a diagnosis of NPN (ammonia) poisoning.

Conditions that may be confused with urea toxicosis include acute encephalitic diseases such as thromboembolic meningoencephalitis and polioencephalomalacia, grain engorgement, acute nitrate and cyanide poisoning, organophosphorus and chlorinated hydrocarbon insecticide poisoning, and enterotoxemia.

Treatment

The best treatment for urea poisoning is to give several gallons of cold water orally. As much as 5-10 gallons should be given to an adult cow.

If 6 percent acetic acid or vinegar is available, up to 3 gallons should be given along with the cold water. The rationale is that water lowers the rumen temperature and dilutes the reacting medium, while the acetic acid lowers rumen pH (preventing ammonia absorption) and also supplies carbon skeletons needed by rumen bacteria. Urea intoxicated animals should be watched closely for at least twenty-four hours after treatment or apparent recovery, since an occasional relapse of clinical signs may occur.

Occasionally poor growth and increased incidence of disease has been associated with consumption of urea or NPN supplements in cattle. At present, there appears to be little published information supporting this claim.

One must remember that NPN is a substitute for natural products and that a high level of management is required for its safe and effective use. When formulating rations containing urea, care must be taken to consider the other nutrients lost when NPN replaces a natural protein. Chief among these are a loss of phosphorous, vitamin A and possibly some trace minerals as well as some loss of metabolizable energy if only nitrogen is supplied. The age of ruminants should be considered when feeding NPN products. It is accepted by many nutritionists and physiologists that full rumen function for NPN utilization may not be attained until animals weigh approximately 500 pounds, and high urea diets are not fully utilized until that time.

Stressed animals (e.g., recently shipped, sick, castrated, vaccinated, etc.) may utilize urea poorly. Inconsistent feeding, with poorly controlled release of ammonia may also depress the efficiency of NPN products.

Urea feeding does not appear to interfere with reproductive performance, provided other aspects of the diet are adequate. Recent work indicates that pregnant sheep experimentally poisoned by urea still had live fetuses at the time of death; and the blood and tissue ammonia nitrogen values for the fetuses were lower than for the dams. (Kirkpatrick *et al.,* 1973)

A technique has recently been developed to calculate the efficiency with which urea may be utilized when considering various types of rations. This technique is known as the Urea Fermentation Potential. For those interested, additional details are available. (Burroughs *et al.,* 1972)

From the evidence available, NPN products appear to be safe and effective when formulated and used properly in animals capable of optimum nutritional response.

BIBLIOGRAPHY

Balestri, P. L.; Rindi, P.; and Biagni, M. 1971. Chronic Urea Intoxication in Dogs. *Experientia.* 27:811-12.

Bicknell, E. J. 1965. Experimental Ammonia Toxicosis in the Pig. Unpublished Ph.D. Thesis. Lansing, Michigan: Michigan State University.

Buck, W. B. 1969. Laboratory Toxicologic Tests and Their Interpretation. *JAVMA* 15:x928-41.

Buck, W. B. 1970. Diagnosis of Feed-Related Toxicoses. *JAVMA* 156:1434-43.

Burroughs, W.; Trenkle, A. H.; and Vetter, R. L. 1972. Proposed New System of Evaluating Protein Nutrition of Feedlot Cattle. Iowa State University of Science and Technology. pp. 1-19.

Carver, L. A., and Pfander, W. H. 1973. Urea Utilization by Sheep in the Presence of Potassium Nitrate. *J. Animal Sci.* 36:581-587.

Carver, L. A., and Pfander, W. H. 1974. Some Metabolic Aspects of Urea and/or Potassium Nitrate Utilization by Sheep. *J. of Animal Sci.* 38:410-16.

Dougherty, R. W., and Cook, H. M. 1962. Routes of Eructated Gas Aspiration in Cattle—A Quantitative Study. *Am. J. Vet. Res.* 23:997-1000.

Helmer, L. H., and Bartley, E. E. 1971. Progress in the Utilization of Urea as a Protein Replacer for Ruminants. A Review. *J. of Dairy Sci.* 54:25-51.

Hintz, H. F.; Lowe, J. E.; Lowe, A. J.; and Visek, W. J. 1970. Ammonia Intoxication Resulting from Urea Ingestion by Ponies. *JAVMA* 157:963-66.

Horn, H. H. and Mudd, J. S. 1971. Comparison of a Liquid Supplement of Nonprotein Nitrogen with Urea and Soybean Meal for Lactating Cows. *J. Dairy Sci.* 54:58-64.

Hutson, J. E.; Shelton, M.; and Breuer, L. H. 1974. Effect of Rate of Release of Urea on its Utilization by Sheep. *J. Animal Sci.* 39:618-28.

Kedlor 230 Feed Compound for Ruminant Feeding Programs. The Dow Chemical Co., Midland, Michigan.

Kirkpatrick, W. C.; Roller, M. H.; and Swanson, R. V. 1973. Hemogram of Sheep Acutely Intoxicated with Ammonia. *Am. J. Vet. Res.* 34:587-89.

Kromann, R. P.; Joyner, A. J.; and Sharp, J. E. 1971. Influence of Certain Nutritional and Physiological Factors on Urea Toxicity in Sheep. *J. Animal Sci.* 32:732-39.

Lloyd, W. E. 1970. Chemical and Metabolic Aspects of Urea-Ammonia Toxicosis in Cattle and Sheep. Ph.D. Thesis. Ames, Iowa: Iowa State University.

Morris, J. G., and Payne, E. 1970. Ammonia and Urea Toxicoses in Sheep and Their Relation to Dietary Nitrogen Intake. *J. Agric. Sci., Camb.* 74:259-271.

Parkins, J. J.; Hemingway, R. G.; and Brown, N. A. 1973. The Increasing Susceptibility of Sheep to Dietary Urea Toxicity Associated with Progressive Liver Dysfunction. *Res. Vet. Sci.* 14:132-34.

Ritchie, N. S.; Parkins, J. J.; and Hemingway, R. G. 1972. Urea Phosphate. A Dietary Source of Nonprotein Nitrogen with Low Potential Toxicity to Ruminants. *Br. Vet. J.* 128:LXXVII-LXXXI.

Singer, R. H. 1969. Acute Ammonium Salt Poisoning in Sheep. M.S. Thesis. Ames, Iowa: Iowa State University.

Tillman, A. D. 1973. Nonprotein Nitrogen in the Feeding of Cattle. *Bovine Pract.* 8:9-19.

Webb, D. W.; Bartley, E. E.; and Meyer, R. M. 1972. A Comparison of Nitrogen Metabolism and Ammonia Toxicity from Ammonium Acetate and Urea in Cattle. *J. Animal Sci.* 35:1263-70.

Yelverton, C. C.; Roller, M. H.; and Swanson, R. N. 1975. Ammonium Nitrogen in Fetuses of Urea- Treated Sheep. *Am. J. Vet. Res.* 36:191-92.

WATER DEPRIVATION— SODIUM SALT

Water deprivation—salt poisoning, is a condition primarily seen in swine and poultry but is also occasionally encountered in ruminants under husbandry practices in which high levels of sodium ion are consumed without adequate consumption of water. In swine and poultry, the term "salt poisoning" is a misnomer since the condition does not occur unless there has been water deprivation. Therefore, we prefer to refer to this condition as water deprivation—sodium toxicosis.

Source

Most of the discussion in this section will be limited to the syndrome as it is seen in swine, which seems to be the most susceptible species of our domestic mammals. Any husbandry practice which results in a limited water intake may precipitate the problem. This may be due to a mechanical problem with automatic waterers or neglect on the part of the caretaker when animals are being hand watered. Other causes of reduced water intake include (1) medication of water with antibiotics, sulfonamides, and other drugs, making it unpalatable; (2) frozen water supply; (3) faulty automatic water heaters; (4) overcrowding; and (5) placing animals in a strange environment where the water supply is unfamiliar to them, as may occur at weaning.

Although a limited water intake is the primary factor in water deprivation—sodium ion toxicosis, the level of salt in the feed influences the amount of water required. Even when feeds contain the proper levels of salt, usually 0.5-1 percent, toxicosis may occur if water is withheld or intake reduced. With ample water intake, a ration may contain as much as 13 percent salt with no apparent harmful effects, although animals will urinate excessively. Unusual husbandry practices, such as the feeding of brine or whey, garbage and kitchen wastes which contain 3-4 percent salt, may produce the classic form of this disease. It is important to understand that the sodium ion, whether in the form of chloride salt, carbonate, or sulfonamide, is the offending agent along with reduced water intake.

The feeding of poultry a wet mash made with brine or whey is an excellent method of producing this condition. In cattle and sheep, feeding grain or protein supplement mixed with a high percentage of sodium salt to limit its intake has also resulted in salt poisoning in these species. When this happens, the water supply may be some distance from the feeding area.

Toxicity

The toxicity of the sodium ion is directly related to the amount of water intake. Thus, feeder pigs may suffer from water deprivation—sodium ion poisoning when the feed contains as little as 0.25 percent salt, provided there is no water intake. On the other hand, levels of 2-3 percent and even 13 percent salt in the feed may not produce poisoning if water is available and it is consumed. Optimally, swine feeds should contain 0.5-1 percent salt with plenty of freshwater available at all times.

Poultry also are susceptible to the sodium ion if water intake is restricted. Problems usually occur in hot weather or in very cold weather when freezing of the water supply occurs. Poultry can withstand a maximum of 0.25 percent sodium chloride in their drinking water regardless of the feed level. Wet mash containing 2 percent sodium chloride has caused poisoning in ducklings. Salt in wet mash seems to be more toxic than in dry feeds.

Cattle and sheep have been poisoned on high concentrations of salt in feed and water, especially in range conditions in which a high percentage of mineral is added to feed and there is concomitant limited water intake. Sheep can tolerate 1 percent salt in the drinking water but 1.5 percent may be toxic. Some nutritionists recommend that drinking water should contain no more than 0.5 percent total salts for any species of livestock. The acute toxic dose of sodium chloride for the pig, horse, and cow appears to be approximately 2.2 gm/kg body weight and in the sheep about 6 gm/kg body weight. This is dependent, however, upon water intake. In the dog, 4 gm/kg sodium chloride may be lethal.

Mechanism of Action

The mechanism of water deprivation—sodium toxicosis has not been clearly established. Presented here is a theory held by some authorities. The normal levels of sodium in the blood plasma are reported to be between 135 and 155 mEq/1 (mean 143.3 ± 6.52). Cerebrospinal fluid sodium levels are slightly lower, 135 to 150 (mean 139.6 ± 5.17) mEq/1. (Osweiler and Hurd, 1974) Between these two biologic compartments there exists a dynamic relationship. Sodium passes from the plasma to the cerebrospinal fluid passively. However, the transport from cerebrospinal fluid to plasma is a dynamic relationship requiring energy and is, therefore, called active transport. With limited water intake, dehydration occurs in the body. Due to this dehydration, the sodium level in the blood compartment rises to 150-190 mEq/1 or greater. Due to this increased concentration, sodium passively crosses into the cerebrospinal fluid and achieves levels of 145-185 mEq/1 or greater. Sodium at these levels inhibits anaerobic glycolysis. Inhibition of glycolysis results in reduced energy production. With the reduced energy production, the high level of sodium in the brain is prevented from going back into the blood because this is an active transport mechanism and no energy is available for this active transport. With water intake or kidney excretion of sodium, the blood level of sodium returns to normal. However, the high brain level of sodium is maintained because the sodium is trapped in this compartment due to the lack of energy. With the combined effects of increased fluid in the blood and high levels of sodium in the brain, there exists an osmotic gradient between the blood and the brain resulting in edema in this compartment. With edema, we have the resulting clinical signs of the water deprivation—sodium ion toxicosis syndrome. The preceding is only a good theory and has not been experimentally confirmed. It does not explain why in swine there is a selective attraction of eosinophils to the cerebral area.

It is important to realize that the sodium ion is the offending agent in this syndrome. Sodium propionate, acetate, carbonate, etc., will produce the same disease syndrome as sodium chloride if there is water deprivation. High concentrations of salt will cause gastroenteritis and dehydration.

Clinical Signs

In swine, the initial signs may be increased thirst, pruritus, and constipation. These rarely are seen by the herdsman. After one to five days of water deprivation, intermittent convulsive seizures are manifested which become more frequent until they are continuous or until the animal becomes recumbent and comatose. Affected animals may be blind and deaf and oblivious to their surroundings. They will not eat or drink nor respond to external stimuli. They often wander aimlessly, push against objects, circle, or pivot around a front or rear limb. A characteristic convulsive seizure occurs with the pig sitting on its haunches, drawing his head backwards and upward in a jerking motion, finally falling over on its side in clonic-tonic seizures and opisthotonus. Terminally, pigs usually lie on their side, paddling in a comatose condition.

In a group of affected animals, all of these signs may be observed at any one time because the progression of the syndrome varies with each individual animal.

Poultry suffering from water deprivation—sodium ion toxicosis manifest excessive thirst, respiratory distress, discharge of fluid from the beak, wet feces, and paralysis of the limbs.

In cattle, both the alimentary tract and the central nervous system are affected. There may be vomiting, diarrhea, abdominal pain, anorexia, and mucus in the feces. There may be a constant polyuria and a nasal discharge. The neurologic signs include blindness and convulsive seizures followed by partial paralysis and knuckling of the fetlocks. Animals usually die within twenty-four hours of the appearance of clinical signs. A characteristic sequelae to salt poisoning in cattle is the dragging of the rear feet while walking and, in more severe cases, knuckling of the fetlock joints. This appears to occur without pain to the animal, although it may be damaging to the tendons, peripheral nerves, and tissues involved.

Physiopathology

In swine but not in other species, a characteristic but mysterious attraction of the circulating eosinophils for the cerebrovascular and meningeal areas occurs. During the acute stages of the syndrome (first forty-eight hours) the circulating eosinophils disappear from the blood vascular system. If the animal dies during this period, the eosinophils will be found clogged around the vessels within the cerebral cortex and the adjacent meninges. If the affected pig lives three to four days, the eosinophils apparently leave the cerebral area, returning to the blood vascular system. If the animal dies during this period, no eosinophils will be present in the cerebrovascular area. However, the spaces where they once were will be evident.

Gross postmortem changes in both swine and cattle may include some form of gastric inflammation and ulceration. In swine, pinpoint ulcers filled with blood are commonly seen in cases involving high levels of salt in the feed. There may be marked congestion of the gastric mucosa. It should be understood, however, that such a lesion is not infrequent in apparently normal pigs. There may be a fluid, dark feces or animals may be constipated. In cattle, there may be edema of the skeletal muscles and hydropericardium. Often, no gross lesions are present upon necropsy.

Microscopic changes are characteristic in swine and are the single-most important criteria for establishing a diagnosis of this condition. The lesions occur in the deep layers of the cortex and the adjacent white matter. The initial change is an infiltration of the meningeal and cerebral blood vessels by eosinophils. This is referred to as eosinophilic meningoencephalitis. Concomitantly, there is an increase in vascularity due to endothelial proliferation in the deep layers of the cerebral cortex and the adjacent white matter. The increased vascularity with surrounding eosinophils is often very prominent. In addition, there is often an increase in the number of histiocytes or gitter cells in the white matter adjacent to the deep layers of the cortex. If the animal dies early in the syndrome, the perivascular cuffing with eosinophils is very prominent. If the animal lives two to three days after the onset of signs, the eosinophils disappear from the brain and reappear in the blood, leaving spaces around the vessels. There often is vacuolization and breakup of the continuity of the tissue in the junction of the cortex and white matter. This is a reflection of edema or early necrosis and malacia. In cattle, similar lesions are present but without the eosinophilic involvement.

Diagnosis

It is important to obtain a history of limited water intake. This may, however, be a very difficult task because the animal caretaker rarely is willing to admit that the husbandry practices have resulted in a limited water intake. Therefore, the clinician must depend upon clinical signs, course of events, and the specific syndrome that is characteristic of this condition. If an adequate description of clinical signs and course of events has been obtained, the probability of this condition will be evident. Laboratory confirmation procedures include the analysis of serum and cerebrospinal fluids and cerebral tissue for sodium concentrations. Levels above 160 mEq/1 in both serum and CSF and 1,800 ppm in cerebral tissue are sufficient to make a tentative diagnosis. CSF sodium concentrations will usually be higher than serum concentrations by about 5 mEq/1 (Osweiler and Hurd, 1974) and cerebral tissue concentrations may be from 2,000-3,000 ppm (Furr, 1976).

Confirmation of a diagnosis is dependent upon finding the characteristic microscopic or histopathologic changes in the cerebral cortex.

There are several disease conditions similar to water deprivation—sodium ion toxicosis in swine. Pseudorabies may present a similar central nervous system disturbance. This condition can be differentiated by histopathologic changes in the brain and by inoculation of nerve tissue in the rabbit. Nonspecific viral encephalomyelitic conditons also produce distinctly different lesions in the brain. Chlorinated hydrocarbon insecticides cause clinical signs identical to water deprivation—sodium ion toxicosis. Chemical identification of the insecticide in the body tissues can aid in differentiation. The clinician should keep in mind that other diseases such as enterotoxemia or gut edema and mulberry heart disease may be confused with water deprivation syndrome, although this is a relatively infrequent occurrence.

Treatment

Treatment of water deprivation—sodium ion toxicosis is nonspecific and may be futile. If affected animals are given small amounts of fresh water at frequent intervals, recovery may occur within four or five days. Usually, about 50 percent of those affected die regardless of the treatment. Diuretics and anticonvulsants have been recommended but have not given dramatic results.

Case History 1

An Iowa farmer weaned fifty-six pigs at the age of four weeks by removing their mothers from the hoghouse leaving the pigs behind. He also opened some small trap doors leading to an outside pen which contained an automatic waterer. He removed some troughs from the hoghouse in which the pigs had previously been watered, expecting the pigs to go outside to get water from the automatic waterer. He continued to feed the pigs a pelleted complete starter ration containing 0.25 percent sodium chloride.

No attempt was made to show the pigs where the automatic waterer was located. Three days later, three pigs were noticed in convulsive seizures. They would sit on their haunches, lifting their head upward and backward in a jerking motion and fall over in a tonic-clonic seizure. Within twelve hours, a total of fifteen pigs were exhibiting various clinical signs ranging from intermittent convulsive seizures, pushing their heads in a corner, circling, to lying on their side in a continuous paddling motion. Realizing that the pigs perhaps had not found the waterer, the farmer put a trough in the outside pen and filled it with water. Immediately the pigs drank the water. Within an hour, an additional fifteen to twenty animals were exhibiting convulsive seizures. During the course of the next twenty-four hours, twenty-five died. The remainder slowly recovered during the next week.

Necropsy examination of three of the dead pigs revealed numerous small (1-2 mm) gastric ulcers filled with clotted blood. One pig had a large area (5-6 cm diameter) of hyperemia in the fundus of the stomach. No other gross lesions were apparent.

Cerebrospinal fluid specimens were taken from the lumbosacral junction of two affected pigs. Blood samples were taken from the medial canthus of the eye and allowed to clot for serum analysis. The cerebrospinal fluid samples averaged 185 mEq sodium/l, and the sera averaged 180 mEq sodium/l. Microscopic examination of the cerbral cortex revealed severe perivascular cuffing by eosinophils of the blood vessels in the meninges and cerebral cortex of two pigs. There was also increased vascularity and glial proliferation at the junction of the cerebral cortex and white matter. Microscopic examination of the cerebral area of the third pig revealed no eosinophilic infiltration, but large spaces around the vessels were evident. There was also edema and early malacia at the junction of the cerebral cortex and underlying white matter.

Case History 2

An Iowa farmer had 140 black Angus steers weighing about 700 pounds each which had been in a bromegrass pasture. He decided to start feeding them grain in a self-feeder. The feed formulation consisted of 7,400 pounds of cracked corn, 400 pounds of 34 percent natural protein supplement, and 800 pounds of salt. The ration was placed in the self-feeder, and the steers were given free access to it. The feeder was placed approximately one-half mile from the only water source, a creek which was in the pasture. Four days later, thirty animals were affected with bloody diarrhea and symptoms of a central nervous system disorder, including convulsions, ataxia, and posterior weakness with prominent knuckling of the fetlocks. One steer became vicious and belligerent. Approximately forty of the animals were found in the creek, down, unable to rise, and many drowned in the muddy water. The following day, most

of the animals were slow to rise and walked stiffly. Several tended to drag the rear feet and knuckle at the fetlocks. Some excessive overextension (goose-stepping) was seen. Diarrhea, while not prominent, was observed; and many animals were covered posteriorly with feces.

Because of severe postmortem decomposition, no necropsies were performed. Serum electrolyte levels were determined from one affected animal: sodium, 158.7 mEq/l; potassium, 7.48 mEq/l; calcium, 11.25 mg/100 ml; and magnesium, 3.2 mg/100 ml.

Since the animals had never been fed grain prior to this episode, the high salt content apparently had been added to decrease the palatability and, thus, reduce intake. However, the amount of salt added was not sufficient to do this. Since the animals manifested ataxia and dehydration, along with the diarrhea, there is a possibility that there was a complication of grain engorgement. Analysis of a feed specimen indicated the presence of approximately 11 percent sodium chloride.

BIBLIOGRAPHY

Blood, D. C., and Henderson, J. A. 1968. *Veterinary Medicine*. 3rd ed. Baltimore: The Williams & Wilkins Co., pp. 782-85.

Buck, W. B. 1969. Laboratory Toxicologic Tests and Their Interpretation. *JAVMA* 155:1928-41.

Clarke, E. G. C., and Clarke, M. L. 1967. *Garner's Veterinary Toxicology*. 3rd ed. Baltimore: The Williams & Wilkins Co., pp. 61-66.

Furr, A. A. 1976. Cerebral Tissue Sodium Levels Associated with Water Deprivation in Swine. Unpublished data.

Osweiler, G. A., and Hurd, J. W. 1974. Determination of Sodium Content in Serum and Cerebrospinal Fluid as an Adjunct to Diagnosis of Water Deprivation in Swine. *JAVMA*. 164:165-7.

Smith, D. L. T. 1957. Poisoning by Sodium Salt—A Cause of Eosinophilic Meningoencephalitis in Swine. *Amer. J. Vet. Res.* 18:825-50.

———. 1970. Sodium Salt Poisoning. In *Diseases of Swine*. 3rd ed. H. W., Dunne. ed. Ames, Iowa: The Iowa State University Press. pp. 772-79.

Todd, J. R.; Lawson, G. H. K.; and Dow, C. 1964. An Experimental Study of Salt Poisoning in the Pig. *J. Comp. Path.* 74:331-37.

Industrially-Related Toxicants

FLUORIDE

Fluoride toxicosis is usually encountered as chronic fluorosis in herbivores, especially dairy cattle. An acute condition can occur following ingestion of high levels of certain fluorine compounds, but this is uncommon.

Source

Fluorine is usually found in nature in the combined fluoride form. In chronic fluorosis the common sources of fluoride are (1) forages subjected to airborne contamination in areas near industrial plants that heat fluorine-containing materials to high temperatures and expel fluorides; (2) drinking water with high fluoride levels; (3) feed supplements and mineral mixtures with high fluoride contents; and (4) vegetation grown on soils of high fluoride level. In cases of acute fluoride toxicosis, the source is more likely to be one of the following: sodium fluoroacetate (1080) used as a rodenticide (see fluoroacetate); sodium fluorosilicate, also a rodenticide; sodium fluoride used as an ascaricide in swine; or water, vegetation, or feeds containing extremely high fluoride levels.

Industrial sources of fluorides commonly include those which process the mineral ores of iron or aluminum and those which produce fertilizers and mineral supplements from fluoride-bearing phosphate rock. Defluorinated phosphate is classified as phosphate which contains no more than 1 part of fluoride for each 100 parts phosphate. Exposure of livestock results when the fluorides emitted settle on the vegetation around such operations. Such exposures are mainly oral and primarily encountered in herbivores. Direct inhalation does not contribute significantly to total fluoride accumulation in livestock.

Organic forms of fluoride (fluoroacetate and fluorocitrate) may be formed in some forage and grain crops grown in areas contaminated by atmospheric fluoride. Thus far, no toxicologic consequences have been reported, although some naturally occurring fluoroacetate containing plants are known to be toxic (see fluoroacetate).

Animals normally ingest low levels of fluoride throughout their lives. Factors governing an animal's reaction to fluoride ingestion include the following: (1) level or amount of fluoride ingested; (2) duration of ingestion time; (3) type and solubility of fluoride ingested; (4) age of the animal during ingestion; (5) level of nutrition; (6) stress; and (7) individual biologic response.

Fluoride is cumulative in the animal body as long as constant or increasing amounts are ingested. Chronic toxicity may result from prolonged ingestion of sufficiently high levels.

In general, the following levels of sodium fluoride calculated in parts per million fluoride for the total dry ration can be ingested over a normal life span without adverse effects on the normal animal: dairy heifers and cows, up to 30; beef cows, up to 40; sheep, up to 50; swine, up to 70; horses, up to 90; turkeys, up to 100; and chickens, up to 150. Tolerances are higher over shorter time intervals, such as normal fattening periods of 180 days for cattle and 70 days for sheep. Under these conditions, cattle and sheep can safely ingest up to 110 parts per million.

Fluoride tolerances have usually been expressed as the concentration in the diet assumed to be a constant exposure. Recent work (Suttie et al., 1972) has indicated that intermittent exposures to levels in excess of the tolerances may cause increased severity of bone and tooth lesions, even if the yearly average is within tolerance limits. This is particularly important since under field conditions exposure is rarely constant.

Tolerances for compounds such as calcium fluoride and those of similar solubility would be higher than for sodium fluoride. The fluorides from industrial sources are the same order of toxicity as sodium fluoride.

Mechanism of Action

Soluble fluoride is passively absorbed in the gastrointestinal tract. Approximately half of the fluoride absorbed is excreted rapidly in the urine by glomerular filtration. The remaining half is stored in the calcified tissues, mainly bone. From 96 to 99 percent of retained fluoride is sequestered in bones and teeth where it interacts with the hydroxyapatite of bone mineral.

Fluoride accumulates in calcified tissue with both duration and rate of fluoride intake. If fluoride exposure ceases, bone fluorides will be depleted very slowly over a period of months or years. Normal adult bovine bones may contain from 1,000 to 1,500 ppm fluoride on a dry fat-free basis.

Fluoride will accumulate to some degree in the bones of fetuses from fluoride exposed dams, but has not been shown toxicologically significant in that regard. The primary effect of fluorine is thought to be a delaying and alteration of normal mineralization of the pre-enamel, predentine, precementum, and preskeletal matrices.

Excess fluoride intake produces dental fluorosis by affecting the teeth during development. Specific ameloblastic and odontoblastic damage seems to be caused by high fluoride intake and varies directly with the levels consumed. Faulty mineralization results when the matrix laid down by damaged ameloblasts and odontoblasts fails to accept minerals normally. Once a tooth is fully formed, the ameloblasts have lost their constructive ability and the enamel lesions cannot be repaired. Odontoblasts can produce secondary dentine to compensate for fluorotic deficiencies.

The dental lesions of chronic fluorosis are accentuated by the rapid wear of the affected cheek teeth, especially if coarse, abrasive feeds are fed.

Oxidation of organic material in the teeth involved results in brown or black discoloration, which is observed in dental fluorosis.

There are two schools of thought concerning the pathogenesis of fluorotic bone lesions. One theory relates high fluoride levels to osteoblastic activity which leads to inadequate matrix and defective, irregular mineralization. Others believe that bone lesions are related to the replacement by fluoride ions of hydroxyl radicals in the hydroxyapatite crystal structure of bone substance. This results in a decrease in crystal lattice dimensions.

The pathologic results of skeletal fluorosis include dissociation of normal sequences of osteogenesis, acceleration of bone remodeling, production of abnormal bone (exostosis, sclerosis) and in some cases accelerated resorption (osteoporosis).

Clinical Signs

Either acute or chronic fluoride intoxication can be observed clinically. *Acute* fluoride toxicity usually results from accidental ingestion of extremely large amounts of fluorine-containing compounds. In these cases, clinical signs may develop as soon as one-half hour after ingestion. Common signs are excitement, clonic convulsions, incontinence of urine and feces, stiffness, weakness, loss of weight, drop in milk production, excessive salivation, nausea, vomiting, severe depression, cardiac failure, and death.

Chronic fluorosis is much more common in livestock and is manifested almost entirely by signs involving the hard tissues of the body. This condition is quite insidious in nature and may be confused with a chronic debilitating disease such as degenerative arthritis. The clinical picture in chronic fluorosis is complicated by variations in the factors mentioned under *Toxicity* and by the fact that there may be a time lapse between ingestion of elevated levels of fluoride and the appearance of clinical signs. Animals ingesting high fluoride levels at the time of development of the permanent teeth may show dental lesions. (figs. 1 and 2) The enamel may be mottled, and the teeth may appear brown and unevenly worn.

As dental lesions develop, clinical signs may include difficult mastication, periodic decrease in feed intake, slow growth and poor performance secondary to reduced feed intake, and lapping of water (evidence of dental pain).

The bone lesions of fluorosis are manifested as hyperostosis, enlargement, and roughening of the involved bones (fig. 3). These lesions appear first bilaterally on the medial surfaces of the proximal one-third of the metatarsal bones. As the condition progresses, the mandible, metacarpals, and ribs become involved. These lesions can result in spurring and bridging at joints and a subsequent lameness.

Skeletal lesions result in the intermittent lameness characteristic of chronic fluorosis. Appendicular lameness, arched back, and generalized stiffness may all be seen at various times. Affected animals typically show brief periods of remission. Experienced examination by palpation may result in detection of skeletal lesions before they are grossly visible.

The hair coat may become dry and roughened and affected animals decrease in weight and milk production. The major economic losses caused by chronic fluorosis are due to the general unthriftiness of the animals rather than to death.

Physiopathology

Dental lesions in chronic fluorosis range from slight mottling of enamel to definite erosion of enamel with staining and pitting. There exists the following positive relationship between dental fluorosis in certain incisors and the degree of wear of certain molars and premolars:

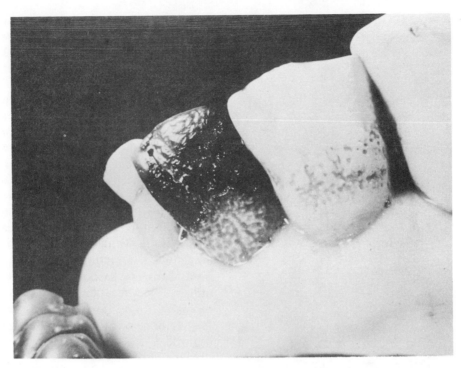

Figure 1. Dental lesions of chronic bovine fluorosis. Enamel hypoplasia and staining is evident.

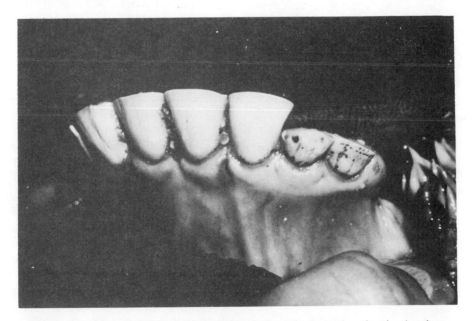

Figure 2. Dental effects of intermittent fluoride ingestion in the bovine. There is enamel hypoplasia and excessive wear in incisors 3 and 4, corresponding to fluoride exposure during formation of those teeth.

first incisor and second molar; second incisor and third molar; third incisor and second premolar. This relationship is based on the concurrent formation and eruption of incisor and cheek teeth.

Fluorotic bone lesions appear first on the medial aspects of the proximal one-third of the metatarsals. They may also appear on the metacarpals, mandible, and ribs. Affected bones appear enlarged and chalky white and have a roughened periosteal surface. Lesions are diffuse and bilateral in nature. Some spurring and bridging of joints may occur in advanced cases. Fluorosis does not cause direct involvement of articular surfaces.

Histopathologic examinations of affected bones

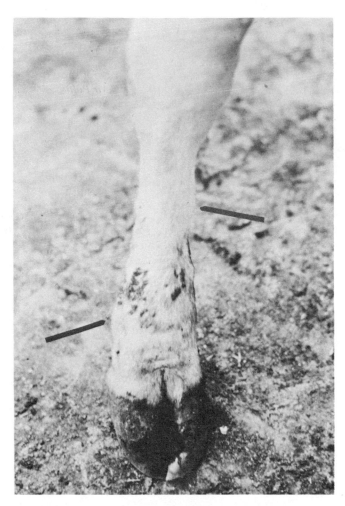

Figure 3. Skeletal effects of chronic bovine fluorosis. Note the location and extent of excess new bone formation (exostosis) as indicated by the arrows.

show many changes. Among these are thickened cortical substance due to periosteal hyperostosis, uneven mineralization, zones of immature bone, reabsorption on the endosteal surface, and excessive osteoid tissue.

The primary lesion associated with acute fluoride poisoning is a severe gastroenteritis.

Diagnosis

Accurate diagnosis of fluorosis is based primarily on knowledge of exposure to fluorides, dental lesions in susceptible animals, skeletal fluorosis, intermittent lameness, and evidence of elevated fluorides in bone. Other procedures are supportive and confirmatory.

Diagnostic aids in chronic fluorosis involve analysis of skeletal and dental tissues and excretions for fluorine levels as well as radiographic and microscopic examinations of bony structures.

Urine analysis for fluoride levels is a commonly used test. Experiments have shown that two to six-year-old dairy cattle showing moderate signs of fluorosis void urine containing about 15-20 ppm of fluoride as compared to about 2-6 ppm for normal cattle. Urine fluoride may be used to approximate fluoride exposure in the recent past. It may be somewhat elevated in animals carrying a high concentration of skeletal fluoride.

Bone specimens obtained by either biopsy or necropsy are also analyzed for fluoride. Bones usually sampled are metatarsal, metacarpal, rib, pelvis, and mandible because good data for comparison are available. Techniques have been developed which allow for biopsy of ribs or coccygeal vertebrae. It is most important when interpreting fluoride analyses to note the bone sampled and the location of samples from that bone. Cancellous bone is normally higher in fluoride than is cortical bone. Some investigators prefer to use proximal, middle and distal transverse sections from long bones while others utilize the sawdust obtained by sectioning a bone longitudinally. Results are usually expressed as ppm of dry fat-free bone or as ppm of bone ash. In general, bone ash values are approximately one-third higher than dry fat-free values.

Fluorotic dairy cows have been found to carry 3,000 to 5,000 ppm fluoride in their bones. Normal levels for cattle would be in the range of 400 to 1,200 ppm.

Histopathologic and radiographic examination of bones has been used to detect bone lesions.

Feed and water consumed by the suspect animals should be analyzed for fluoride.

Treatment and Prevention

No substances are known to completely prevent the toxic effects of ingested elevated levels of fluorides. Some products can counteract and reduce the effects of high fluoride levels. Aluminum sulfate, aluminum chloride, calcium aluminate, calcium carbonate, and defluorinated phosphate have been successfully used to reduce the toxic effects of fluoride.

If animals must ingest a material of high fluoride content, it is wise to dilute it with feed of low content. For example, if cattle must drink water which is high in fluoride, be sure the roughage they are fed has a low fluoride level.

The seed or grain of crops do not accumulate fluorides as do roughages.

REFERENCES

Blood, D. C., and Henderson, J. A. 1967. *Veterinary Medicine.* 3rd ed. Baltimore: The Williams & Wilkins Co.

Fluorosis Subcommittee. 1974. Effects of Fluorides in Animals. Washington, DC: National Academy of Sciences.

Greenwood, D. A.; Shupe, J. L.; Stoddard, G. E.; Harris, L. E.; Nielsen, H. M.; and Olson, L. E. 1964. Fluorosis in Cattle. Special Rep. No. 17, Utah Agr. Exper Sta.

Shupe, J. L. Alther, E. W. 1966. The Effects of Fluorides on Livestock, with Particular References to Cattle. In *Handbook of Experimental Pharmacology*. vol. XX/1. *Pharmacology of Fluorides*. F. A. Smith, Sub-ed. New York: Springer-Verlag.

Shupe, J. L. 1971. Clinical and Pathological Effects of Fluoride Toxicity in Animals. Ciba Foundation Symposium Sept. 13-15.

Shupe, J. L., and Olson, A. E. 1971. Clinical Aspects of Fluorosis in Horses. *JAVMA* 158:167.

Shupe, J. L.; Harris, L. E.; Greenwood, D. A; Butcher, J. E.; and Nielsen, H. M. 1963. The Effect of Fluorine on Dairy Cattle. V. Fluorine in the Urine as an Estimator of Fluorine Intake. *Am. J. Vet. Res.* 24:300.

Suttie, J. W., and Faltin, E. C. 1971. Effect of a Short Period of Fluoride Ingestion on Dental Fluorosis in Cattle. *Am. J. Vet. Res.* 32:217.

Suttie, J. W. 1969. Air Quality Standards for the Protection of Farm Animals from Fluorides. *J. Air Pollution Assoc.* 19:239.

Suttie, J. W., and Kolstad, D. L. 1974. Sampling of Bones for Fluoride Analysis. *Am. J. Vet. Res.* 35:1375.

Suttie, J. W., and Faltin, E. C. 1973. Effects of Sodium Fluoride on Dairy Cattle: Influence of Nutritional State. *Am. J. Vet. Res.* 34:479.

Suttie, J. W.; Carlson, J. R.; and Faltin, E. C. 1972. Effects of Alternating Periods of High- and Low-Fluoride Ingestion on Dairy Cattle. *J. Dairy Sci.* 55:790.

Suttie, J. W. 1967. Vertebral Biopsies in the Diagnosis of Bovine Fluoride Toxicosis. *Am. J. Vet. Res.* 28:709.

POLYBROMINATED BIPHENYLS

A large scale disaster occurred in Michigan in 1973, when a polybrominated biphenyl (PBB) compound was accidently mixed in animal feed. Normally, the PBB, used as a fire retardent, was supplied in red bags and labelled "Firemaster." The feed ingredient magnesium oxide was supplied in brown bags and labelled "Nutrimaster". Due to a red bag shortage the PBB was sold in brown bags and subsequently was confused with "Nutrimaster" because of the similarity in names.

Initially most of the involved feeds were dairy feeds intended to contain magnesium. Later other feeds become contaminated when prepared in the contaminated mixers, storage bins, transfer augers and so on. (Dunckel, 1975)

Clinical Signs

Milk production and feed consumption decreased by 50 percent over a twenty-day period. The cows were afebrile with some lameness, increased frequency of urination and some lacrimation. When the feed was changed, the anorexia regressed but milk production did not improve significantly. A large number of cows came back into estrus suggesting early embryonic resorptions.

Cows continued to lose weight and hematomas developed in 10 percent of the cows. Hoofs became elongated in about 30 percent of the cows. Alopecia with thickened skin was noted over the thorax, neck and shoulder. Cows exposed during the last trimester had prolonged gestation and dystocia. Udder development was retarded and calves were often dead or died soon after birth. Metritis was common and milk production negligible. A number of cows died. (Jackson and Halbert, 1974)

Physiopathology

Lesions included hemorrhagic necrotic hepatitis, fatty metamorphosis (liver), amyloidosis (liver) and varying degrees of interstitial nephritis. SGOT levels were elevated in terminally ill cows. BUN, WBC and packed cell volumes were generally within acceptable limits.

PBB residues occur in body fat, milk fat and eggs. The tolerances set in November 1974 were milk and meat, 0.3 ppm and eggs and finished feeds, 0.05 ppm.

The half-life of PBB in milk fat is estimated to be twelve weeks. Cows contaminated at levels of 200-400 ppm require an estimated 120 weeks to decline to the 0.3 ppm tolerance. (Detering et al., 1975)

Treatment

No useful treatment has been identified. Because of the long-term residue problem and the apparent long-term damage to acutely affected animals a massive disposal and cleanup program was undertaken. The following number of animals were destroyed and buried: 18,000 cattle from 172 herds, 3,500 swine from 32 droves, 1,200 sheep from 16 flocks and 1,500,000 birds from 92 flocks.

In addition, 788 tons of feed, 3,000 pounds of butter, 18,000 pounds of cheese, 34,000 pounds of dry milk and 5,000,000 eggs were buried.

As late as 1975, 37,000 cattle representing 286 herds contained PBB residues in milk or body fat. Some owners continued to suspect adverse health effects. Subsequently, teams of toxicologists and FDA personnel surveyed the health status of the herds and found the prevailing health problems to be unrealted to the presence of the low level of PBB. (Mercer et al., 1976)

It is not unexpected to have people ascribe all subsequent health problems to a previously identified cause. Particularly when the cause is as dramatic as occurred here. It behooves the practicing veterinarian to encourage livestock owners to seek professional help in identifying the causes of each specifc health problem. The veterinarian should also encourage vigilence in maintaining good husbandry and management and not let feeding or sanitation programs decline because of suspected disease problems or the possibilities of financial reimbursements. One must not forget that other causes of disease, decreased weight gain or production and reproductive failures are still present.

REFERENCES

Detering, C. N.; Prewitt, L. R.; Cook, R. M.; and Fries, G. F. 1975. On the Rate of Excretion of Polybrominated Biphenyls by Lactating Holstein. *J. Animal Science* 41:265 (Abstract).

Dunckel, A. E. 1974. An Updating on the Polybrominated Biphenyl Disaster in Michigan. *J. American Veterinary Medical Association* 167:838-41.

Jackson, T. F., and Halbert, F. L. 1974. A Toxic Syndrome Associated with the Feeding of Polybrominated Biphenyl Contaminated Protein Concentrate to Dairy Cattle. *J. American Veterinary Medical Association* 165:437-139.

Mercer, H. D.; Buck, W. B.; Furr, A.; Teske, R. H.; Meerdink, G. L.; Fries, G. F.; and Condon, R. J. 1976. A Report on the Herd Health Status of Dairy Cattle Exposed to Polybrominated Biphenyls. Unpublished report.

POLYCHLORINATED
BIPHENYLS

Not too many years ago the clinical veterinary toxicologist was concerned almost exclusively with animal toxicoses involving deaths and overt illness. The major probelm was to identify the offending chemical substance, find the source of exposure and make recommendations regarding treatment. In recent years another type of problem that is much more insidious has confronted the veterinary toxicologist and veterinary practitioner. This newer problem involves the low-level contamination of meat, milk and egg-producing domestic animals. The contamination is of significance because of existing state and federal regulations which prohibit the marketing of food products containing residues over certain levels. The levels may be specified as either a legal tolerance or an interim actionable level.

Examples of toxicants involved include numerous organochlorine insecticides such as DDT, aldrin-dieldrin, heptachlor and chlordane; the polychlorinated biphenyls; mercury and numerous therapeutic drugs.

From the toxicologist's point of view the contamination of food producing animals occurs in one of two ways. The most obvious situation occurs when an animal or a herd of animals is overtly poisoned and some deaths or pronounced clinical toxicoses occur. The surviving animals are then obviously contaminated. The length of time during which the chemical residues may exceed acceptable levels depends on the specific toxicant involved and the time ranges from hours to months.

A second situation resulting in contamination of food producing animals occurs in the absence of any overt toxicosis. That is, the livestock producer has no clue as to how or when the animals were exposed and the animals fail to show any clinical signs suggestive of poisoning. The first notice that the animals are contaminated with some chemical substance occurs when the producer receives a letter or phone call informing him that the products he has marketed or is marketing contain excessive residues. In these cases it is often impossible to positively identify the source since the source may have involved exposure while the animals were on another pasture or in another feedlot.

Polychlorinated biphenyls have occasionally been involved in excessive residue problems.

Source

Generally, polychlorinated biphenyls are referred to by the abbreviation PCB. The general structure of PCB's is shown in figure 1 along with the structure of p, p'DDT. The similarity in chemical structure of PCB's and DDT led to considerable confusion in the chemical analysis of DDT prior to 1966. Residue chemists now use modified chemical techniques to adequately separate DDT and its metabolites from PCB residues in biologic samples.

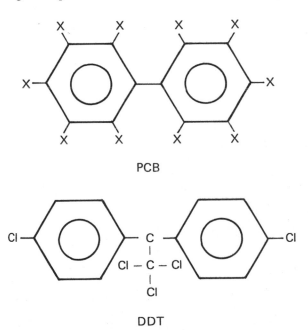

Figure 1. The chemical structure of polychlorinated biphenyls (PCB) and p,p'DDT. The PCB molecule contains chlorine atoms at one or more of the sites designated "x" in the figure.

PCB's were first described in 1881 and commercial production achieved in 1929. PCB's have been used as nonflammable oils in transformers, condensers and paints. They have also been used in some closed heat transfer systems. Other applications include use as plasticizers, flame retarders, pressure sensitive adhesives, agents to increase chemical oxidation resistance, agents to increase strength of fiberglass resins, and as electrical insulators.

One reason PCB's are used is because of their chemical stability. They are chemically inert, not hydrolyzed by water and resist alkalis, acids and corrosive chemicals. Their boiling points range from 278 to 415° C. They are destroyed when exposed to 800°C for ten seconds or 1000° C for three seconds. Because of their stable chemical properties PCB's tend to persist when released into the open environment.

PCB production peaked at 74 million pounds in 1970 in the United States. About 60 percent of the total PCB production was used in closed system electrical and heat transfer systems, 25 percent for plasticizers, 10 percent for hydraulic fluids and lubricants and less than 5 percent for all other uses. Sales in the United States have been voluntarily reduced and currently are limited to use in confined systems. The manufacturer has also provided disposal facilities for waste and used PCB's in order to help prevent unwise disposal into the general environment.

The commercial PCB products are a mixture of compounds and individual products are usually specified by the percent chlorine. In the United States the major registered trade name for PCB compounds is Aroclor. The commercial PCB compound is usually identified by the name Aroclor followed by a four digit number. The first two digits specify the type of compound while the last two digits specify the percent chlorination. For example, Aroclor 1242 contains 42 percent chlorine while Aroclor 1254 contains 54 percent chlorine. The first two digits (12) specify the compound as a polychlorinated biphenyl. In other areas of the world PCB trade names include Kanechlor, Phenochlor, and Clophen.

Toxicity

At the present time there is very little experimental information on the acute and chronic toxicity of PCB's in domestic animals. The acute toxicity appears to decrease as the percent chlorination increases, although the relationship between the toxicity of individual PCB's and percent chlorination is not absolutely clear. The toxicity seems to increase with percent chlorination for mallards, pheasants, bobwhite and Japanese quail, while an opposite trend was observed for domestic chickens. The difference may be due to contaminants present in the technical compounds used in the different studies.

Mammals and birds tend to retain more of the highly chlorinated biphenyls than the lesser chlorinated portion of the commercial mixtures. Recent work has also shown that some of the commercial PCB formulations contain other types of chlorinated compounds that are more toxic than the PCB.

The LC_{50} toxicities for birds appear to be of the order of 100-400 ppm depending on the percent chlorination and the duration of feeding. In small laboratory rodents the subacute, multiple dose LD_{50} is in the range of 30-300 mg/kg.

The major impact of PCB's in veterinary medicine has been in excessive tissue residues rather than in acute deaths; although, both in the United States and in Japan field episodes have occurred which resulted in clinical illness and death in poultry.

Feeding levels of 100 ppm PCB to poultry results in fat residue levels of 280-500 ppm which is many times higher than the 5 ppm actionable level. These residues occurred in the absence of clinical deaths.

The results of several investigations of PCB poisonings in domestic animals have been reported. Dairy cattle were exposed as a result of eating silage stored in concrete silos treated with PCB. The ultimate magnitude of this problem is presently unkown, but could conceivably be a larger problem than presently documented. In other cases animal feedstuffs were contaminated during manufacture as a result of leaks in heat transfer systems.

The dairy cow also eliminates PCB in the milk fat. Milk residues plateaued after forty to sixty days of feeding at a constant level. Milk fat PCB residues were 45 ppm after thirty days of feeding 200 mg Aroclor 1254/cow/day. Milk fat PCB residues were of the order of 5-10 ppm in the cases involving PCB treated silos. When silage feeding from the PCB contaminated silos was discontinued the milk fat residues decreased to 1-3 ppm.

PCB's are more toxic to mink than to rats, mice or birds. The relative toxicity is inversely related to the percentage of chlorine in the PCB for Aroclor 1221, 1242, and 1254. Dietary levels of 30 ppm PCB result in anorexia, bloody stools, fatty liver, kidney degeneration and hemorrhagic gastric ulcers. Levels of 30 ppm PCB result in complete reproductive failure in mink and is lethal when fed for three to six months. Tissue residue levels in mink that died averaged 11 ppm in brain, 4-5 ppm in liver and 2-6 ppm in kidney, spleen, lung, muscle, and heart. Dietary levels of 10 ppm PCB for four months, 10 ppm PCB plus 10 ppm DDT for two months or 10 ppm PCB plus 0.5 ppm dieldrin for four months significantly decreased body weight gains in female mink. (Aulerich et al., 1973)

Feeding of coho salmon by-products to mink has resulted in mortality and severe reproductive failures. The coho salmon were found to be contaminated with 10-15 ppm PCB, 0.3 ppm mercury, 18 ppm DDT and 0.12 ppm dieldrin. Major reproductive and mortality problems developed when mink were fed a diet containing 30 percent coho salmon canning by-products for three months or less. Subsequent studies have implicated PCB, as well as, suggesting a PCB-chlorinated hydrocarbon insecticide interaction.

Human dietary exposure is estimated at only 0.1 μg/kg/day.

Mechanism of Action

The major lesion is the generalized edema which suggests that PCB's somehow increase cell permeability. Some suggest that the primary effect is on the heart resulting in hydropericardium. Pulmonary edema and general systemic edema is then secondary to decreased cardiac function. A detailed cellular or enzymatic mode of action has not been postulated.

In the boar a single dose of 100 mg Aroclor 1254/kg body weight or ten daily doses of 10 mg Aroclor 1254/kg body weight reduced the urinary excretion of estrogen and dehydroepiandrosterone. (Platonow et al., 1972) The mechanism and impact on reproductive performance is unknown.

Clinical Signs

In the bird a depressed growth rate occurs at the lower levels of exposure. There is possibly a two to three-day transient stasis of the gut. The pericardial and pulmonary edema result in gasping in birds. Advanced stages include droopiness, ruffled feathers, weakness and deaths.

In mammals there may be pustules formed on the skin and pigmentation along with generalized weakness.

Physiopathology

The physiopathology of PCB toxicosis in poultry includes swelling and hemorrhages of the kidney, varying degrees of centrilobular liver degeneration, small spleen, hydropericardium, generalized abdominal and subcutaneous edema, depressed growth and decreased hemoglobin values. The lesions are similar to those observed in chick edema disease, a condition caused by chlorinated dioxins.

In mammals the pathology involves follicular pyodermatitis (chloracne) and liver atrophy and necrosis. PCB's also stimulate the smooth endoplasmic reticulum (SER) and increase the activity of drug metabolizing enzymes. PCB's appear to be better enzyme inducers than DDT and dieldrin. The no-effect level for enzyme

induction in rats and rabbits is on the order of 1-10 mg/kg and is 0.1 mg/kg in Japanese quail.

PCB's cause a chemical porphyria with an increased fecal excretion of coproporphyrin and protoporphyrin. PCB's in sufficient quantities are embryotoxic and when injected into eggs will cause edema and beak deformities in chick embryos.

The nervous system is also affected. There is impaired motor function, decreased motor-nerve conduction velocity and loss of large nerve fibers. Some animals experience convulsive seizures prior to death. Whether this is a direct effect on the brain or secondary to liver damage is unclear.

One of the more PCB sensitive mammals may turn out to be the mink. Reports suggest that PCB levels of a few ppm significantly decrease reproductive success in mink.

Diagnosis

A positive diagnosis will require chemical identification of PCB residues in body fat or liver tissues. Only limited data is available on tissue levels reported from dead animals. Also PCB's represent a wide variety of compounds and consequently tissue residues associated with lethality may be expected to vary. Levels in livers of dead chickens have varied from 200-2,900 ppm and in the brain levels varied from 70-700 ppm.

Treatment

Both birds and mammals slowly eliminate PCB residues. The residue half-life in hens is probably four weeks or longer. In most cases of high-level contamination, the most economic solution is humane slaughter and disposal rather than maintaining the birds on a clean diet for an extended period of time.

The kinetics of PCB excretion in milk of dairy animals has been described. It was found that residues of Aroclor 1254 were eliminated at the same rate as the DDT metabolite DDE. A two component first-order equation adequately described the rate of elimination. The equation was given as $C = 0.52e^{-0.25t} + 0.48e^{-0.008t}$ where C is concentration, e is the base of natural logarithms and t is time in days. The equation was normalized for an initial unity concentration. The first component represents an excretion rate with a half-time of 2.7 days. This represents a more rapid elimination of approximately 52 percent of the initial residue. The second component represents a slower rate of excretion of the remaining 48 percent of the residue with a half-time of eighty-six days. Assuming an initial milk fat residue of 25 ppm the time required for the milk fat residue to decline to 5 ppm can be estimated using the above equation and is found to be about 110 days.

The feeding of charcoal and phenobarbital did not significantly increase the rate of elimination of PCB or DDE residues.

With the increased responsibility for drug and chemical residues being placed on the livestock producer and the veterinarian, the author suggests that veterinary practitioners consider encouraging livestock producers to begin saving samples of feed and feedstuffs such as salt and minerals. This could be accomplished by livestock producers saving a quart jar sample of every batch of feed that is fed. The samples could be disposed of one month after the animals were marketed. In the case of poultry the samples would be saved until the broilers are marketed or the hens are done laying eggs and are marketed. For dairymen the samples could be disposed of after one year. It is probably unrealistic to expect very many producers to take the time to do this, and yet almost any currently practicing clinical toxicologist could cite cases where access to such feed samples would have been very helpful. The cost would be minimal since ordinary quart glass jars and tape labels would be all that is required. The properly labelled stored samples would be invaluable in legal cases involving determination of responsibility for contaminated feed.

REFERENCES

Aulerich, R. J.; Ringer, R. K.; and Iwamoto, S. 1973. Reproductive Failure and Mortality in Mink Fed on Great Lakes Fish. *J. Reprod. Fert., Suppl.* 19:377-89

Anonymous. 1973. If All the Sea Were PCB. *Fd. Cosmet. Toxicol.* 11:131-44.

Fries, G. F. 1972. Polychlorinated Biphenyl Residues in Milk of Environmentally and Experimentally Contaminated Cows. *Env. H. Persp.* 1:55

Harris, J. R., and Rose, L. 1972. Toxicity of Polychlorinated Biphenyls in Poultry. *JAVMA* 161:1584.

Heath, R. G.; Spann, J. W.; Kreitzer, J. F.; and Vance, C. 1970. Effects of Polychlorinated Biphenyls on Birds. Proceedings XV International Ornithological Congress.

Kuratsune, M.; Yoshimura, T.; Matsuzaka, J.; and Yamaguchi, A. 1972. Epidemiologic Study on Yusho, a Poisoning Caused by Ingestion of Rice Oil Contaminated with a Commercial Brand of Polychlorinated Biphenyls. *Env. H. Persp.* 1:119.

McCann, J. 1972. High PCB's Cause of Mink Decline. *Biomed. News.* October.

National Swedish Environment Protection Broad 1970. Report of PCB Conference, Stockholm, Sweden. Research Secretariat, Solna. September 19.

Platonow, N. S.; Liptrap R. M.; and Getssinger, H. . 1972. The Distribution and Excretion of Polychlorinated Biphenyls (Arochlor 1254) and Their Effect on Urinary Gonadal Steroid Levels in the Boar. *Bulletin of Environmental Contamination and Toxicology.* 7:358-65.

Van Gelder, G. A., and Teske, R. H. 1974. Biological Impact of Polychlorinated Biphenyls with Emphasis on Veterinary Aspects. *Veterinary Toxicology* 16:109-11.

Vos, J. G. 1972. Toxicology of PCB's for Mammals and for Birds. *Env. H. Persp.* 1:105.

CRUDE OILS, FUEL OILS AND KEROSENE

Source

Crude oil or petroleum distillates ranging from diesel oil to gasoline have occasionally caused illness and death in domestic animals and children. Pollution of rangeland with crude oil has been commonly associated with oil exploration and production activities. (McConnell, 1957 and Monlux et al., 1971) Although uncommon in today's enlightened age, kerosene and other petroleum distillates have been used for the treatment of digestive upsets in ruminants and other animals. Petroleum distillates are often used as carrier agents for insecticides. Sometimes they are applied to animals dermally for the treatment of external parasites. In children accidental swallowing of kerosene and other petroleum distillates is not uncommon.

Toxicity

All animals are susceptible to oil toxicosis, but problems are more commonly seen in cattle, horses and children.

In a study using cattle, Rowe et al., 1973, found that when multiple doses of oil were given, the minimum total dosages resulting in aspiration pneumonia and subsequent death were 48 ml/kg, 56 ml/kg and 74 ml/kg respectively for sweet crude, kerosene and sour crude. In each case dosage was divided over a period of seven days. "Sweet" crude is a term for raw crude oil relatively high in gasoline, naphtha and kerosene, whereas "sour" crude is a term describing raw crude oil relatively low in gasoline, naphtha and kerosene, but high in gas oil, lubricating distillates, residue and sulfur.

The toxicity of crude oil appears to correlate with the relative content of kerosene, naphtha and gasoline.

Mechanism of Action

The toxicity of crude oils and kerosene appears to be directly correlated with its aspiration hazard and its irritant activity on pulmonary tissue. The most serious consequence of crude oil or kerosene ingestion is aspiration pneumonia due to aspiration of the oil. Microorganisms in the respiratory tract or carried into the lungs by the oil may also be important in the final outcome. (Rowe et al., 1973) Factors such as ability of an oil to induce vomiting or bloat may contribute to the likelihood that a particular oil will be aspirated. Abnormal eructation may mistakenly introduce oil into an open glottis.

Other effects of crude oils, but not kerosene, include bloat and vomiting.

Clinical Signs

In cattle those animals receiving "sweet" crude oil frequently develop immediate bloat and rapid death. After bloat is relieved by intubation it does not reoccur. Vomition also occurs with sweet crude toxicosis, but not with sour crude or kerosene poisoning.

Shivering and incoordination associated with early signs of pneumonia are common. Usually animals eventually develop pneumonia which becomes increasingly intense leading to death. Anorexia and subsequent weight loss over a period of several days to weeks are common. The appearance of oil or kerosene in the feces may occur after one to two weeks, however, dry-formed feces may be observed in animals consuming kerosene.

Signs of central nervous system derangement including incoordination, shivering, head shaking and mental confusion have been reported in calves and children suffering from kerosene and crude oil toxicosis. This effect may be due to low molecular weight hydrocarbons.

Physiopathology

Animals suffering from crude oil or kerosene toxicosis often have significantly decreased blood glucose levels, probably because they are anorectic and debilitated. All significant blood chemical and hematologic changes are associated with the development of pneumonia. These include hemoconcentration, as evidenced by increased PCV and hemoglobin, and increased BUN and serum transaminase enzymes. A leucocyte response characterized by initial leucopenia, followed within two or three days by a relative increase in neutrophils, but with a depressed total WBC count have been reported by Rowe *et al.,* 1973.

Lesions of foreign-body pneumonia are the most usual necropsy finding. This is often accompanied by localized pleuritis and in severe acute cases by hydrothorax. The distribution of pulmonary lesions is usually bilateral and include the caudoventral apical, cardiac, cranioventral diaphragmatic and intermediate lobes. The affected portions are dark purple, consolidated, and in animals surviving several days after aspiration, contain multiple abscesses. Oil may be grossly visible in pulmonary tissue. In those animals lingering for quite some time after exposure, large encapsulated pulmonary abscesses may be present. Animals that have consumed kerosene or "sweet" crude oil may contain ulcerations and raised yellowgreen plaques approximately 1 cm in diameter in the ventral tracheal mucosa.

Oil or kerosene will usually be visible in the gastrointestinal tract.

Diagnosis

The history, clinical signs and physiopathologic changes are of primary importance in establishing a diagnosis. One can mix a pint of stomach contents with warm water in a one liter container and shake it. If oil or kerosene is present, it will float to the surface. Sometimes the identity of an oil can be established using infrared spectrophotometry.

Treatment

Treatment of animals suffering from crude oil or kerosene toxicosis is an exercise in frustration. At best it can only be symptomatic, utilizing CNS and cardiac stimulants, intravenous fluid and electrolytes, antibiotics and blood transfusions. If treatment is initiated soon after consumption of the oil, attempts should be made to empty the stomach, followed by purgatives and demulcents.

If oils or kerosene have been applied to the skin, they can be removed using detergents.

REFERENCES

Burns, P. *Toxicology Notes.* School of Veterinary Medicine, College Station, Texas.

Clarke, E. G. C., and Clarke, M. L. 1967. *Garner's Veterinary Toxicology.* Baltimore: The Williams and Wilkins Co., pp. 292-93.

McConnell, W. C. 1957. Oil Field Problems Confronting the Veterinarian. *Vet. Med.* 52:159-63.

Monlux, A. W.; Schoeppel, R. J.; Pearson, C. C.; and Waller, G. R. 1971. The Effects of Oil Field Pollutants on Vegetation and Farm Animals. *JAVMA* 158:1379-90.

Rowe, L. D.; Dollahite, J. W.; and Camp, B. J. 1973. Toxicity of Two Crude Oils and of Kerosene to Cattle. *JAVMA* 162:61-66.

Plant-Related Toxicants

CYANIDE

Source and Toxicity

Cyanide, hydrocyanic acid, or prussic acid are all terms relating to the same toxic principle. This is one of the most rapid-acting poisons available to mammals. It is present as inorganic salts, as a naturally occurring glycoside in certain plants, or as free HCN.

Cyanides are used in industry for metal cleaning, electroplating, and chemical synthesis. Compounds containing cyanide are used as rodent or vermin killers and for legal execution of criminals in some states. HCN is commonly used as a fumigant.

A number of common plants may accumulate large quantities of cyanogenetic glycoside which hydrolyze to form free HCN. Of chief agricultural importance are the sorghums, sudan grass, and corn. Other species with characteristic high HCN potential are flax, lima beans, cherry, apple, peach, and apricot. A more complete listing of cyanogenetic plants will be found in table 1.

TABLE 1
Plants with Cyanogenetic Potential

Hoecus lunatus	velvet grass
Hydrangea spp.	hydrangea
Linum spp.	flax
Lotus corniculatus	birdsfoot trefoil
Phaseolus lunatus	lima bean
Prunus spp.	cherries, apricots, peach
Pyrus malus	apple
Sambucus canadensis	elderberry
Sorghum spp.	Sudan grass, Johnson grass
Suckleya suckleyana	poison suckleya
Trifolium repens	white clover
Triglochin maritima	arrow grass
Vicia sativa	vetch seed
Zea mays	corn

Under natural conditions the hydrolysis of cyanogenetic glycosides in plants is inhibited since the degradative enzymes of plants which can cause release of cyanide from the glycoside are kept spatially separated from the glycoside in intact plant cells.

Upon wilting, frosting, or stunting of the plant, free HCN may be released as a result of plant cellular damage which allows enzymatic degradation of the glycoside. Thus consumption of cyanogen-containing plants which possess glycosidase enzyme will initiate release of HCN when maceration occurs in the digestive tract. Figure 1 depicts the changes which occur in the release of free cyanide. Remember that β-glycosidase is a *plant* enzyme and that it is specific for the β-glycoside linkage of the cyanogenic glycoside. Note also that hydroxynitriles are degraded by an enzyme, but they may also dissociate nonenzymatically.

Plant cyanogenic glycosides and β-glycosidase are both genetically controlled by a dominant gene. It is possible to selectively breed plants with low cyanogenic potential; in many case, such as the modern *Sorghum spp.*, this has been done.

In addition to the cyanide-producing ability of a plant, other factors of toxicity should be considered. Most cyanogenic activity is located in leaves and/or seeds of plants, and the potential for high glycoside levels is greatest in immature and rapidly growing plants. Conditions such as drought, wilting or frosting which damage the plant may allow for more rapid combination of glycoside and enzyme, thus greater toxicity.

Ingestion of the glycoside by ruminants with the subsequent action of rumen microflora may release HCN from the glycoside. This release is also accomplished by the acid medium of the monogastric stomach as maceration of plants occur. Salts of cyanide (*e.g.*, KCN) also hydrolze readily to form free cyanide. Fertilizers (*e.g.*, calcium cyanamide) may contain a cyanogenic potential.

Plants of the mustard family (*Cruciferae*) may contain thiocyanates or 1-5-vinyl-2-thiooxazolidone as glycosides. These substances inhibit the production of thyroid hormone resulting in hyperplastic goiter and symptoms of hypothyroidism (table 2). Lambs from ewes fed goitrogenic rations may be born dead or sluggish or may have enlarged thyroids. The formation of

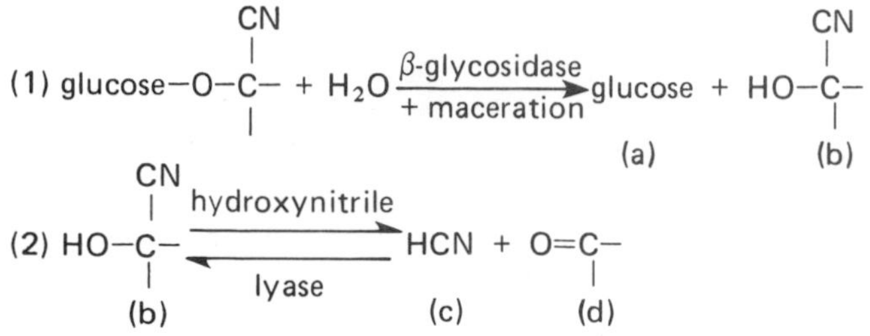

(1) glucose—O—C— + H₂O $\xrightarrow[\text{+ maceration}]{\beta\text{-glycosidase}}$ glucose + HO—C—

(a)   (b)

(2) HO—C— $\underset{\text{lyase}}{\overset{\text{hydroxynitrile}}{\rightleftharpoons}}$ HCN + O=C—

(b)   (c)   (d)

Figure 1. Schematic representation of cyanide release from cyanogenic plants. (1) glycoside is hydrolyzed by plant β-glycosidase to yield glucose (a) and hydroxynitrile (b); (2) hydroxynitrile (b) is dissociated enzymatically to free HCN (c) and a ketone or aldehyde (d).

thiocyanate in the liver of animals receiving low levels of cyanides (*e.g.,* from flaxseed) may also be a toxic factor. The goiter produced is responsive to iodine therapy.

Cyanide ion is readily absorbed orally or parenterally, and percutaneous prolonged exposure could produce toxicity. HCN gas in concentrations above 50 to 60 ppm in air may be absorbed in sufficient quantity to cause poisoning.

Small amounts of cyanide can be tolerated by animals, since the body has a mechanism for detoxication and excretion of cyanide (see Mechanism of Action). Sheep are able to metabolize approximately 22 mg/50 kg body weight per hour. Animal and dosage factors that influence toxicity include:

1. the size and type of animal.
2. the speed of ingestion
3. the type of food ingested simultaneously with the cyanogen
4. presence of active degradative enzymes in the plant and in the animals' digestive tract
5. ability to detoxify cyanide

Mechanism of Action

The cyanide ion reacts readily with ferric (trivalent) iron of cytochrome oxidase. This reaction forms a cyanide cytochrome oxidase complex which is quite stable.

TABLE 2
Plants Containing Goitrogenic Compounds

Brassica spp.	includes rape seed, mustard, kale, broccoli, cabbage and turnip
Glycine max	soybean
Linum usitatissimum	flax

When iron is maintained in the trivalent state, electron transport stops and the chain of cellular respiration is brought to a halt. Thus cyanide causes a cellular hypoxia or *cytotoxic anoxia* (see fig. 2). As a result, hemoglobin cannot release its oxygen to the electron transport system. The clinical appearance, then, is of bright red (oxygenated) blood which cannot be utilized by the cells. Cytochrome oxidase is most concentrated in those tissues which carry on a high rate of oxidative metabolism (*e.g.,* CNS and cardiac muscle).

As cyanide reaches the aortic and carotid bodies, the effect of hypoxia is reflected in the respiratory system. There is rapid depression of cerebral, hypothalamic, and midbrain activity in that order. The brain stem and hence, the respiratory center is not as rapidly affected. Heart rate initially increases and then slows progressively over several minutes. The heart may continue to beat several minutes after respiration ceases.

Cyanide detoxication occurs when endogenous thiosulfate combines with cyanide to form thiocyanate which is excreted in the urine. This reaction is catalyzed by the enzyme rhodanese. The natural detoxication is somewhat limited by the availability of endogenous thiosulfate.

Clinical Signs

Cyanide is a potent, rapidly acting poison. Animals will commonly be found dead, since clinical signs last only a few minutes after ingestion.

Clinical effects, when seen, occur in rapid succession. Initially there is excitement and generalized muscle tremor. Pronounced polypnea and dyspnea follow. There may be salivation, lacrimation, and voiding of feces and urine. The animal goes down, gasps for breath, and may have clonic convulsions due to anoxia. The pupils are dilated; mucous membranes are bright. The characteristic blood color is a bright cherry red.

A condition potentially related to cyanide or nitrile metabolism in plants is the Equine Sorghum Cystitis-

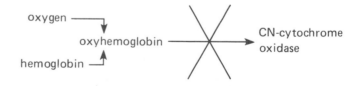

Figure 2. Oxyhemoglobin cannot release oxygen for electron transport in the cytochrome system since the cyanide-cytochrome oxidase complex will not function in electron transport.

Ataxia syndrome. This is observed in horses grazing *Sorghum* sp. or hybrid sudan pastures. Clinically there is urinary incontinence, posterior incoordination and cystitis. Pathologic lesions include myelomalacia of the lower spinal cord. In pregnant mares there may be abortion, and foals from sudan grazed mares may have musculoskeletal deformities such as articular ankylosis or arthrogryposis.

The cause is postulated to be either a chronic low-level exposure to cyanide with resultant degenerative CNS lesions, or production of a lathyrogenic principle (nitrile related amino acid).

Physiopathology

The only consistent postmortem changes in animals poisoned by cyanide are those relating to the oxygenation of the blood. Mucous membranes are pink and appear well oxygenated. The blood itself is a bright cherry red color and often clots slowly or not at all. Subendocardial and subepicardial hemorrhages associated with violent death and terminal anoxia are seen. The abomasum and intestine are congested and may contain petechial hemorrhage. Congestion of the lungs and trachea occurs. The smell of "bitter almond" may be present in fresh rumen contents.

There are indications that chronic exposure to sublethal amounts of cyanide in dogs and man may result in multiple foci of degeneration and/or necrosis of the central nervous system. Generally cyanide poisoning encountered in veterinary medicine is peracute to acute and neither gross nor microscopic lesions are consistently seen.

Diagnosis

A diagnosis of cyanide poisoning should be considered whenever animals consuming cyanogenetic plants or cyanide salts are affected acutely with signs of oxygen starvation and bright colored blood or mucous membranes.

Chemical confirmation of cyanide poisoning can be accomplished either directly or indirectly. Proper preservation of samples for analysis is imperative. Forage, blood, rumen contents, liver and muscle tissue may be submitted for laboratory diagnosis. All samples should be quick-frozen as soon as possible and maintained in a frozen state until analysis. Immersion in 1-3 percent mercuric chloride is also satisfactory. This prevents further hydrolysis of the cyanogenetic plant to free HCN and subsequent loss of the gaseous HCN.

Levels in plant material in excess of 20 mg/100 ml (200 ppm) are significant levels. A simple test for cyanide in plant material is available (table 3). Low levels of cyanide found in the tissue are significant as chemical evidence of cyanide poisoning.

Other conditions which may initially be confused with cyanide poisoning are nitrate poisoning in cattle, pulmonary adenomatosis or emphysema, and urea poisoning. The blood is chocolate colored in nitrate poisoning. Lesions and respiratory sounds should identify adenomatosis. Urea poisoning is suggested by the history and by prominent nervous signs and ammoniacal rumen odor.

Treatment

Therapy is directed at splitting of the cytochrome-cyanide bond and subsequent rapid removal of a cyanide complex. The cyanide-cytochrome complex is broken by the addition of sodium nitrite with the formation of methemoglobin which competes with cytochrome oxidase for the cyanide ion and cyanmethemoglobin is formed. Thiosulfate then reacts with cyanide, under influence of the enzyme rhodanese, to form thiocyanate which is readily excreted in the urine. A recommended therapeutic regimen is the intravenous administration of a mixture of 1 ml of 20 percent sodium nitrite and 3 ml of 20 percent sodium thiosulfate, giving 4 ml of this mixture per 45 kilograms body weight. Commercial solutions for treatment of prussic acid poisoning are available.

Some beneficial effect has been shown for cobalt salts administered for cyanide poisoning. However, the nitrite and thiosulfate remains most effective.

TABLE 3
Test for Cyanogenetic Material in Plants

1. Prepare "picrate paper" by wetting filter paper with a solution of 5.0 grams sodium bicarbonate and 0.5 gram picric acid in 100 ml water.
   a. Solution keeps indefinitely.
   b. Dried papers keep a few days.

2. Crush suspect plant or rumen contents and place in water in a test tube or jar that can be corked.

3. A few drops of chloroform and sulfuric acid added will hasten autolysis.

4. Suspend strips in a bottle after moistening it.

5. Heat to 30-35° C (86°-95° F).

6. A brick red color on paper indicates cyanide.
   a. A well-marked color within a few minutes is significant.
   b. A mild reaction in one to several hours is not of much concern.

Control and Prevention

Several factors may influence the cyanide potential of forage crops. (1) Soils high in nitrogen and low in phosphorous favor a higher cyanogenetic potential. (2) Drought, frosting or wilting of the plants may result in a release of cyanide from the glycoside or a buildup in glycoside levels. (3) Age of the plants is important. Young, green plants have the highest cyanide potential, but this drops off rapidly after pollination occurs and seed sets. Regrowth of cyanogenetic pasture should not be grazed until a heighth of two feet has been attained. (4) Leaves are typically higher in cyanide potential than are stalks. Properly cured hay and silage usually lose a majority of cyanogenetic potential. However, if levels are extremely high at cutting, a second sample should be checked prior to feeding.

REFERENCES

Adams, L. G.; Dollahite, J. W.; Romane, W. M.; Bullard, T. L.; and Bridges, C. H. 1969. Cystitis and Ataxia Associated with Sorghum Ingestion by Horses. *JAVMA.* 155:518.

Bellamy, D. *et al.* 1968. Anaerobiosis and the Toxicity of Cyanide in Turtles. *Comp. Biochem. Physiol.* 24:543-48.

Blood, D. C., and Henderson, J. A. 1963 *Veterinary Medicine.* 2nd ed. Baltimore: The Williams & Wilkins Co.

Bohosiewicz, M. *et al.* 1965. Cyanide Poisoning in Livestock. *Medycyna. Wet.* 21:616-18.

Clarke, E. G., and Clarke, M. L. 1967. *Garner's Veterinary Toxicology.* The Williams & Wilkins Co.

Dashkovskii, A. I. 1968. Dynamics of the Oxygen Content in Animal Tissue During Sodium Cyanide Poisoning and Experimental Study of Temperature Changes in the Polarographic Diffuse Current. *Farmakol. Toksik.* 31:486-89.

Kingsbury, J. M. 1964. *Poisonous Plants of the United States and Canada.* Englewood Cliffs, N.J.: Prentice-Hall, Inc.

Prichard, J. T., and Voss, J. L. 1967. Fetal Ankylosis in Horses Associated with Hybrid Sudan Pasture. *JAVMA.* 150:871.

Rentsch, G. 1967. Toxic Reactions of Methylene Blue in the Whole Animal. *Helv. Physiol Pharmacol. Acta.* 25: CR216-17.

Rose, C. L. *et al.* 1965. Cobalt Salts in Acute Cyanide Poisoning. *Proc. Soc. Exp. Biol. Med.* 120:780-83.

Rump, S. *et al.* 1968. Effects of Centrophenoxime on Electrical Activity of the Rabbit Brain in Sodium Cyanide Intoxication,. *Int. J. Neuropharm.* 7:103-13.

Sanchez, F. *et al.* 1966. Detoxication of Cyanides by Cobalt Compounds. *Renta. Patron. Biol. Amin.* 10:99-123.

Smith, A. M. *et al.* 1963. Neuropathological Changes in Chronic Cyanide Intoxication. *Nature* 200:179-81.

Subcommittee on Food Protection. 1973. Toxicants Occurring Naturally in Foods. Washington, DC: National Academy of Sciences.

Van Kampen, K. R. 1970. Sudan Grass and Sorghum Poisoning of Horses. A possible Lathyrogenic Disease. *JAVMA.* 156:629.

NITRATES, NITRITES, AND RELATED PROBLEMS

Source

The nitrate ion is both a product and a reactant in the chain of animal and plant interrelationships. Atmospheric nitrogen (N) utilized by nitrogen-fixing bacteria is converted to nitrate (NO_3^-). The nitrate is used by plants to form plant protein. Vegetable protein is either utilized by animals to form animal protein or is returned by decay to the soil. Animal metabolic waste (urea and ammonia) is then converted to nitrites and/or ammonia and, thence, to nitrogen to begin the cycle again. As long as proper balance in this cycle is maintained, no problems are encountered.

Nitrate or nitrite toxicity occurs most commonly from plant or water sources. Fertilizers (*e.g.,* ammonium nitrate or potassium nitrate) are sources of high nitrate to either plants or animals. Nitrates may be present at varying levels in water, plants, animal wastes, and chemicals.

Nitrate in Water

Nitrates and nitrites are water soluble. Thus, nitrate added to soil may be leached away, moving with ground water into the water table. Decaying organic matter, nitrogen fertilizers, animal wastes, silage juices, and soil high in nitrogen-fixing bacteria may be sources of contamination to a well or reservoir. The likelihood of high levels is much greater when the source is nearby. Nitrates are generally highest in the water supply in periods after high surface runoff such as spring snow melts or heavy rains. Ponded water which collects feedlot or fertilizer runoff may contain toxic levels of nitrates. Nitrates are not excessive in ponds with abundant algae or other plant growth, the plant growth apparently utilizing the excess nitrate. The most common source of contamination to wells is surface water, usually in shallow, poorly cased wells. Deep, drilled wells occasionally contain excess nitrates also.

Plant Nitrates

Abnormal accumulation of nitrate in plants is influenced by a number of factors. The most important of these are the following:

1. Species of plant (see table 1).
2. Content and form of nitrogen in the soil. Soils high

TABLE 1
Common Plants Known to Accumulate Nitrate

Weeds	
Amaranthus spp.	✓pigweed
Chenopodium spp.	lamb's quarters
Cirsium arvense	Canada thistle
Datura spp.	Jimsonweed
Helianthus anuus	wild sunflower
Kochia scoparia	fireweed
Malva parviflora	cheeseweed
Melilotus officinalis	✓sweet clover
Polygonum spp.	smartweed
Rumex spp.	dock
Salsola pestifer	Russian thistle
Solanum spp.	nightshades
Sorghum halepense	Johnson grass
Crop Plants	
Avena sativa	oats
Beta vulgaris	beet
Brassica napus	rape
Glycine max	soybean
Linum usitatissimum	flax
Medicago sativa	alfalfa
Secale cereale	rye
Sorghum vulgare	Sudan grass
Triticum aestivum	wheat
Zea mays	corn

in nitrate content or ammonia levels supply nitrate more readily to plants.

3. Soil conditions which favor nitrate uptake: adequate moisture for uptake; acid soils favor nitrate absorption; low molybdenum; sulfur deficiency; phosphorus deficiency; low temperature (55° F); soil aeration.
4. Drought conditions.
5. Decreased light. Light is required to maintain activity of the enzyme nitrate reductase.
6. Herbicide treatment with phenoxyacetic herbicides. The 2,4-D herbicides are plant hormones which favor increased growth rate and nitrate accumulation in early stages.

Nitrates accumulate in vegetative tissue, not in fruits or grain. The accumulation of nitrates is usually greatest in the stalk and less in the leaves. Levels are most elevated just prior to flowering and drop off rapidly after pollination occurs and grain or fruit sets.

When silage is made from high nitrate forages, the anaerobic fermentation in the silo results in reduction of some of the nitrates to oxides of nitrogen. These oxides are seen as pungent, yellowish brown gases. Upon reaction with air, the main product is nitrogen dioxide (NO_2) and some nitrogen tetraoxide (N_2O_4). Levels may accumulate to 150 ppm in such a silo. This gas is heavier than air and forms a yellowish brown fog. It may travel down silo chutes and ducts, collecting in low places or tight buildings in sufficient concentration to kill livestock. The production of gas commences within a few hours after ensiling and reaches a maximum in one and one-half to two days.

Toxicity

Both acute and chronic poisoning may occur. Acute poisoning may be expected when forage nitrates exceed 1.0 percent nitrate (dry weight basis) or 1,500 ppm nitrate in water.

Recent work (Dollahite and Rowe, 1974) indicates that water containing 2,000 ppm nitrate can be fed at 10 percent of body weight to cattle for as long as seventeen days with no indication of acute toxic effects. However, 3,000 ppm given to cattle for three days resulted in death from acute nitrate poisoning. Concentrations of nitrate ranging from 2 to 4 percent have occasionally been tolerated by ruminants, although such values have extremely high potential for acute toxicosis.

The effects of feed and water levels are additive, and both must be considered when evaluating a nitrate problem. Reports on the lethal dose of nitrate to ruminants are rather variable and probably reflect differences in nutritional status, method of administration, and the type of nitrate compound used. An approximate LD_{50} in cattle of 1 gm/kg body weight has been reported. (Crawford et al., 1966)

Ruminants have been shown to tolerate higher levels of nitrates when dosage is spread throughout the feeding period or mixed with the total diet. When nitrate is fed continuously, animals become adapted to higher nitrate concentrations and may be able to utilize a portion of dietary nitrate as nonprotein nitrogen. (Emerick, 1974; Murdock, 1972) Tolerance to nitrate in ruminants increased by high quality diets with readily available carbohydrate.

Nitrate toxicity does not appear to be altered and is not enhanced by simultaneous feeding of urea.

The amount of nitrite present may influence the toxicity of forage or water, especially for monogastric animals. Monogastric animals are generally quite tolerant to nitrate, there being no mechanism for rapid reduction to the more toxic nitrite. Nonruminants are approximately ten times more susceptible to oral nitrite than to nitrate, while ruminants are some two to three times more sensitive to nitrite than nitrate. (Emerick, 1974)

Nitrogen in feeds and water may be expressed in various ways (table 2). These distinctions must be remembered when evaluating nitrogen toxicity data.

The hemoglobin of pregnant women has been reported more susceptible to methemoglobin formation. (Turner and Kienholz, 1972) Fetal and neonatal hemoglobin is considered more susceptible to methemoglobin formation and may bind nitrite more firmly. The gastric hypochlorhydria of human infants predisposes to bacterial habitation in the upper gastrointestinal tract, allowing increased nitrate reduction to nitrite. (Steyn, 1959) In addition, the fetus has a lower level of the enzyme (diaphorase) responsible for reoxidation of nitrite to nitrate in the body. These conditions and changes are not well established in domestic livestock but could have a bearing on toxicity to fetal or newborn animals.

Levels or doses of nitrate used in attempts to produce chronic poisoning have been extensively reviewed. (Turner and Kienholz, 1972; Emerick, 1974; Murdock, 1972; Ridder and Oehme, 1974) The bulk of evidence indicates that sublethal effects are extremely rare and difficult to verify. When present, the clinical signs usually reflect a lowered degree of acute toxicosis.

Subacute or chronic nitrate poisoning has been described as causing various problems. Chief among these are poor growth rate, abortion, infertility, vitamin A deficiency, goiter, and increased susceptibility to infection. Experimental evidence to substantiate many of these claims is lacking.

Nitroso Compounds

The nitroso compounds, including N,N-dimethylnitrosamine, N-methyl-N-nitrosourea, and N-methyl-N,-nitor-N-nitrosoguanidine, are alkylated oxides of nitrogen. They have been found in prepared foods such as smoked herring, smoked sausage, and bacon at concentrations of from 0.5-9.0 μg/kg as well as occurring naturally in plants and foods from localized areas of the world. (Magee, 1971; Low, 1974)

The nitroso compounds are recognized tumor inducers in experimental animals and have been used experimentally to cause neoplasia of the stomach, skin, brain, spinal cord, and subcutaneous tissue. From 2.5-9.0 mg/kg has been used to induce tumors in experimental animals. Newborn rats are more susceptible CNS tumor development than adolescent or adult animals. A synergistic effect from polycyclic hydrocarbons and tumor formation has also been noted. Natural cases of carcinogenicity caused by nitroso consumption have not been recorded.

Acute toxic effects of nitroso compounds can occur, but few spontaneous outbreaks of acute clinical poisoning have occurred. The nitrosos have been associated with liver necrosis in sheep when present at 30-100 ppm in fish meal protein supplement. However, most concern over nitroso compounds has been from potential carcinogenic activity of low levels in food or feed supplies.

Nitrosamines may be formed from secondary or tertiary amines in combination with nitrite at pH ranging from 1 to 3.4. Dimethylnitrosamine formation appears proportional to dimethylamine concentration and to the square of the nitrite concentration. Thus, questions have been raised regarding the formation of nitroso compounds in the stomach when naturally occurring secondary and tertiary amines are present concurrently with nitrites. While nitrosation of secondary amines in the mammalian stomach has been shown, more complete assessment of any hazard must be preceded by accurate dose-response data and determination of potential exposure.

Mechanism of Action

Nitrate ion itself is not particularly toxic. However, nitrite ion, the reduced form of nitrate, is readily absorbed and is quite toxic. Ruminants and herbivores can readily reduce nitrate to nitrite and toxicosis may occur. The nitrite ion oxidizes ferrous iron in hemoglobin to the ferric (trivalent) state forming methemoglobin. As such, methemoglobin cannot accept molecular oxygen. The result is hypoxia or anoxia due to poorly oxygenated blood.

Thyroid function may be influenced by nitrate in some species. The rat and sheep are apparently susceptible to nitrate interference with thyroidal iodine uptake, whereas this effect has not been demonstrated for cattle and dogs. (Ridder and Ochme, 1974) Several monovalent ions including nitrate have been shown capable of interfering with iodine uptake by the thyroid. In addition, there is adaptation to the antithyroid effect of nitrate, so that thyroid function returns to normal after two to four weeks of nitrate exposure.

TABLE 2

Nitrate and Nitrite Expressions and Factors for Converting from One Designation to Another

Form of Expression	Chemical Formula	Molecular or Atomic Weight	Conversion Factor from One Designation to Another			
			N = 1	NO_2 = 1	NO_3 = 1	KNO_3
Nitrate-Nitrogen	$NO_3^- - N$	14	1.0	0.30	0.23	0.14
Nitrite-Nitrogen	$NO_2^- - N$	14	1.0	0.30	0.23	0.14
Nitrate	NO_3^-	62	4.4	1.34	1.00	0.61
Nitrite	NO_2	46	3.3	1.00	0.74	0.64
Potassium Nitrate	KNO_3	101	7.2	2.20	1.63	1.00
Sodium Nitrate	$NaNO_3$	85	6.1	1.85	1.37	0.84

Examples: 1. 1.0% $NO_3 - N$ = 4.4% NO_3^- or 7.2% KNO_3

2. 1.0% NO_3^- = 0.23% $NO_3 - N$ or 1.63% KNO_3

3. 1.0% KNO_3 = 0.61% NO_3^- or 0.14% $NO_3 - N$

4. 100.0 ppm NO_3^- = .01% NO_3

5. 2.0% NO_3 = 20,000 ppm

Some apparent interrelationships of nitrate-nitrite with vitamin A have been suggested. Nitrite under acidic conditions is capable of destroying carotene and vitamin A. Nitrate does not have this effect in nonruminants. (Emerick, 1974)

In ruminants, neither nitrate nor nitrite appear to destroy vitamin A or carotene in the rumen. Prediction of vitamin A or carotene destruction in the abomasum is difficult because of the limited and varied amounts of nitrite that may reach the acidic medium of the stomach. Agreement among workers on the question has not been reached. It appears that the majority of recent evidence does not support nitrate-induced vitamin A destruction in ruminants as a clinically significant problem.

Clinical Signs

Acute poisoning usually occurs within one-half to four hours after ingestion of high nitrate feed or water. Under certain conditions, clinical signs of poisoning may not be apparent until animals have consumed nitrate-containing forages for five to eight days. Clinical signs become apparent when methemoglobin levels reach 30 to 40 percent, and death ensues at about 80 to 90 percent methemoglobin. This may be greatly influenced by the stress and exertion to which an animal is subjected.

The direct irritant action of nitrates may cause salivation, vomiting, diarrhea, and abdominal pain. Frequent urination may be an early sign. These signs are most common when the nitrate is not of plant origin. The most characteristic and likely signs are those referable to anoxia. Dyspnea, cyanotic mucous membranes, and rapid weak pulse are cardinal signs. The blood is typically dark brown or "chocolate" colored. Muscle tremors, weakness, ataxia, and low tolerance to exercise are observed. Animals may appear relatively unaffected until forced to move about. There may be terminal anoxic convulsions. Death usually occurs within twelve to twenty-four hours but may be within several hours if nitrate levels were high or if nitrite ion was involved.

Dietary nitrate may be detrimental to thyroid function by inhibiting iodine uptake by that gland. Low or moderate levels of nitrates have been associated with signs of vitamin A deficiency. This may be related to thyroid function or to some other factor. Ruminal destruction of vitamin A does not appear to be significant in such cases. At any rate, vitamin A supplementation will alleviate the signs.

Abortions are often ascribed to high dietary nitrate. A "lowland abortion" syndrome in cattle has been related to consumption of weeds high in nitrates. Elimination of the weeds reduced the abortion problem.

Many suggestions of problems resulting from chronic low-level nitrate or nitrite intake are the result of field observations. Controlled experimental work has not verified poor growth, poor rate of gain, infertility, abortion, thyroid deficiency, or significant vitamin A depletion as clinically significant nitrate effects. Field observations have many times failed to delineate other variables from which the same chronic effects might arise. For example, high nitrate forages are often poor quality and have low vitamin A or carotene content. Nitrate contaminated wells are also often contaminated with bacteria, sulfates, or other minerals.

One must be extremely careful in assessing only nitrate as the cause of poor performance in livestock unless exhaustive clinical and laboratory studies are done.

Physiopathology

The characteristic and consistent finding in animals poisoned by nitrate or nitrite is dark brown ("chocolate") blood with staining of tissues as well. Mucous membranes are cyanotic. Petechial and/or ecchymotic hemorrhages may be observed on serous surfaces. Congestion of the rumen or abomasum does occur.

Nitrite and methemoglobin disappear rapidly from blood. (Watts et al., 1969) Nitrate or nitrite levels will remain stable for up to forty-eight hours if plasma or serum is separated from the cells. Under conditions of low exposure to nitrate, serum nitrate and nitrite levels would be expected to range below 25 μ/ml and 0.75 μ/ml, respectively. Methemoglobin may be stabilized in blood for forty-eight hours by diluting blood 1:20 with phosphate buffer, pH 6.6. Fluctuations in serum nitrite may be correlated with changes in methemoglobin level.

Urinary excretion of nitrate and nitrite occurs when sublethal doses of nitrate are consumed. Urinary nitrite is stable for up to forty-eight hours in stored urine.

Diagnosis

Nitrate and nitrite levels in the rumen or stomach contents, plasma, serum, urine, forage, and water may be examined. Samples mailed or held overnight should be frozen. The finding of high nitrite levels in feed or ingesta, correlated with methemoglobinemia, elevated serum nitrite, and proper clinical signs, is sufficient for a diagnosis of nitrate poisoning.

Several other toxicants may be confused with nitrate poisoning (table 3). A simplified test for nitrates in water or forage is described in table 4. Commercial test kits are also available.

TABLE 3
Comparison of Clinical Effects of Common Toxicants Which May Be Confused with Nitrates (Nitrites)

Toxicant	Blood Color	Mechanism	Treatment	Physical Characteristic
Nitrate (Nitrite)	Brown	Methemoglobin	Methylene blue	
Sodium Chlorate	Brown	Methemoglobin	Methylene blue	
Silo Cases (Nitrous Dioxide; Nitric Oxide)	Slight brown	Slight methemoglobin	Methylene blue; Ca gluconate	About same density as air
Cyanide	Cherry red	Anticytochrome oxidases	Nitrite-thiosulfate	
Carbon Dioxide	Dark	Displaces oxygen	Oxygen; fresh air	Heavier than air
Carbon Monoxide	Bright red	Carbon monoxide hemoglobin (stable)	Fresh air; oxygen + 5% CO_2; thionine solution	Lighter than air

Treatment

Therapy is aimed at restoring the iron in hemoglobin to the divalent state. To do this, methylene blue is added to the system. It is rapidly reduced to leukomethylene blue and then serves as the reducing agent to convert methemoglobin (Fe_{+3}) to hemoglobin (Fe_{+2}) as follows:

$$
\begin{array}{ccc}
\text{NADPH} & \text{Methylene Blue (Ox)} & \text{Hemoglobin Fe}^{+2} \\
\text{NADP} & \text{Leukomethylene Blue (Red)} & \text{Methemoglobin Fe}^{+3}
\end{array}
$$

It may be seen that overpowering the system with methylene blue will also produce methemoglobinemia. The suggested dosage is 2 mg/lb body weight administered in a 2 to 4 percent solution. This may need to be repeated, since absorption of nitrate from a full rumen can continue. Mineral oil given via a stomach tube will counteract the caustic action of nitrate salts and help to speed elimination. For forage nitrate poisoning, purging with saline cathartics and control of bacterial nitrate reduction with intraruminal antibiotics and 3-5 gallons of cold water may be beneficial.

Case History 1

Twenty-seven head of yearling feeder cattle were placed in a western drylot and were fed a poor-grade baled sudan-sorghum cross known as "Sweet Sorg" at a rate of 3 lbs/head twice/day for five days. On the sixth day, 6 lbs/head were fed at a single feeding at evening time. The following morning, eight head were found dead. No other animals were exhibiting signs of toxicity.

Postmortem examination revealed a dark carcass with dark, nonclotted blood in the dilated vessels.

The veterinarian suspected prussic acid and submit-ted a sample of the sudan-cross plants for laboratory analysis at Iowa State University. No cyanide was present, but analysis revealed 12 percent nitrate (NO_3^-) on a dry matter basis.

Case History 2

A marginal farmer in northwestern Iowa had about thirty head of shorthorn-cross cows, heifers, and calves in less-than-good condition. He was feeding a poor quality alfalfa hay, ear corn, and water. He put four heifers in the barn lot and watered them at noon when they appeared alright. At 4 p.m., all four animals were

TABLE 4
A Qualitative Field Test for Detection of Nitrate or Nitrite

Nitrate

1. Add 0.5 gram diphenylamine in 20 ml of water.
2. Add sulfuric acid q.s. to 100 ml. Cool the resulting solution and store in a brown bottle.
3. Mix equal parts of the stock solution and 80 percent sulfuric acid.
4. Test suspect material by dropping one drop of reagent on the cut surface of the plant.
5. A color change from green to blue is a positive reaction indicating more than 2 percent nitrate.

Nitrite

1. Reagents needed are: (a) sulfanilic acid (0.5 gram in 150 ml of 20 percent glacial acetic acid) and (b) alphanaphthylamine hydrochloride prepared by dissolving (with heat) 0.2 gram of the salt in 20 percent glacial acetic acid.
2. Add 2 ml of unknown to a test tube. Then add 2 ml of sulfanilic acid, followed by 2 ml alphanaphthylamine. A pink to red color is positive for nitrites. The solutions applied to cut surfaces of plants in the same order will give a pink to red reaction if positive.

down in convulsions. The veterinarian arrived and adminstered atropine. Within five minutes, three died. The fourth was given some sodium thiosulfate and sodium nitrate IV. This animal was not as severely affected and recovered.

The veterinarian described their blood as a very dark, chocolate brown. The same hay and feed had been fed all winter to the cows with no apparent harm.

A sample of rumen contents from one dead heifer and water from the well, from which the water was taken to give the four heifers, were submitted to our laboratory for nitrate analysis. Samples from three nearby wells were also submitted for analysis. The rumen contents contained 1,230 ppm NO_3^-. The water from the well in question and the other three wells contained the following:

Sample #1 contained 2,840 ppm NO_3^-
Sample #2 contained   73 ppm NO_3^-
Sample #3 contained   512 ppm NO_3^-
Sample #4 contained   161 ppm NO_3^-

All four wells were dug wells about 3 feet in diameter and about 50 feet deep. They were not capped or sealed. The homestead was in a natural basin with the four wells adjacent to a long-established barn lot. It was apparent that surface drainage could easily contaminate them.

The nitrate levels of these wells were followed for several months, and the levels of NO_3^- remained quite high. Several wells on nearby farms contained NO_3^- levels from 200-500 ppm.

REFERENCES

Asbury, A. C., and Rhode, E. A. 1964. Nitrite Intoxication in Cattle: The Effects of Lethal Doses of Nitrite on Blood Pressure. *Amer. J. Vet. Res.* 25:1010-13.

Bjornson, C. B. 1964. Sources of Nitrate Intoxications in North Dakota. *N. D. Farm Res.* 23:16-20.

Blood, D. C., and Henderson, J. A. 1963. *Veterinary Medicine.* 2nd ed. Baltimore: The Williams & Wilkins Co.

Bloomfield, R. A.; Garner, G. B.; and Mahrer, E. 1961. Effect of Dietary Nitrate on Thyroid Function. *Science* 134:1690.

Case, A. A. 1957. Some Aspects of Nitrate Intoxication in Livestock. *JAVMA* 130:323.

Committee on Nitrate Accumulation. 1972. Accumulation of Nitrate. Washington, D.C.:National Academy of Sciences.

Crawford, R. F.; Kennedy, W. K.; and Davison, K. L. 1966. Factors Influencing Toxicity of Forages That Contain Nitrate When Fed to Cattle. *Cornell Vet.* 56:1-17.

Crowley, J. W.; Jorgensen, N. A.; Kahler, L. W.; Salter, L. D.; Tyler, W. J.; and Finner, M. F. 1974. Effect of Nitrate in Drinking Water on Reproductive and Productive Efficiency of Dairy Cattle. Tech. Report WIS. WRC. 74-06.

Davison, K. L.; Hansel, W.; Krook, L.; McEntee, K.; and Wright, M. J. 1964. Nitrate Toxicity in Dairy Heifers. I. Effects on Reproduction, Growth, Lactation, and Vitamin A Nutrition. *J. Dairy Sci.* 47:1065-73.

————. 1965. Responses in Pregnant Ewes Fed Forages Containing Various Levels of Nitrate. *J. Dairy Sci.* 48:968-77.

Divan, R. J.; Reed, R. E.; Trautman, R. J.; Pistor, W. J.; and Watts, R. E. 1962. Experimentally Induced Nitrite Poisoning in Sheep. *Amer. J. Vet. Res.* 23:494-96.

Dollahite, J. W., and Rowe, L. D. 1974. Nitrate and Nitrite Intoxication in Rabbits and Cattle. *Southwestern Vet.* 27:246.

Emerick, R. J. 1974. Consequences of High Nitrate Levels in Feed and Water Supplies. *Fed. Proc.* 33:1183.

Fowler, M. E. 1967. *Clinical Veterinary Toxicology.* University of California, Davis. Unpublished.

Goodman, L. S., and Gilman, A. 1965. *The Pharmacologic Basis of Therapeutics.* 3rd ed. New York: Macmillan Publishing Company.

Hanway, J. J.; Herrick, J. B.; Willrich, T. L.; Bennett, P. C.; and McCall, J. T. 1963. The Nitrate Problem. Spec. Rep. No. 34, Iowa State U. Coop. Exten. Serve. in Agricul. and Home Ec., Ames, Iowa.

Jainudeen, M. R.; Hansel, W.; and Davison, K. L. 1965. Nitrate Toxicity in Dairy Heifers. Endocrine Responses to Nitrate Ingestion During Pregnancy. *J. Dairy Sci.* 48:217-21.

Jones, L. M. 1965. *Veterinary Pharmacology and Therapeutics.* 3rd ed. Iowa State University Press.

Kaemmerer, K. 1965. Nitrate and Nitrite Poisoning of Geese by Mineral Fertilizers. *Arch. Geflugelk.* 29:161-74.

Kearly, E. O. 1964. Nitrate Metabolism in the Ruminant. *Proc. Amer. Coll. Vet. Toxicol.*

Kelly, S. T.; Oehme, F. W.; and Hoffman, S. B. 1974. Effect of Chronic Dietary Nitrates on Canine Thyroid Function. *Toxicol. Appl. Pharm.* 27:200.

Kingsbury, J. M. 1964. *Poisonous Plants of the United States and Canada.* Englewood Cliffs, New Jersey: Prentice-Hall, Inc.

Lewis, D. 1951. The Metabolism of Nitrate and Nitrite in Sheep. *Biochem. J.* 49:149.

London, W. T. 1967. An Attempt to Produce Chronic Nitrite Toxicosis in Swine. *JAVMA* 150:389-402.

Low, H. 1974. Nitroso Compounds: Safety and Public Health. *Arch. Environ. Health* 29:256.

Magee, P. N. 1971. Toxicity of Nitrosamines: Their Possible Human Health Hazards. *Food Cosmet. Toxicol.* 9:207-18.

Mitchell, G. E.; Little, C. O.; and Hayes, B. W. 1967. Preintestinal Destruction of Vitamin A by Ruminants Fed Nitrate. *J. Anim. Sci.* 26:827-29.

Moeschlin, S. 1965. *Poisoning, Diagnosis and Treatment.* New York: Grune and Stratton.

Murdock, F. R.; Hodgson, A. S.; and Baker, A. S. 1972. Utilization of Nitrates by Dairy Cows. *J. Dairy Sci.* 55:640.

Olson, J. R.; Oehme, F. W.; and Carnahan, D. L. 1972. Relationship of Nitrate Levels in Water and Livestock Feeds to Herd Health Problems on 25 Kansas Farms. *VMSAC* 67:257.

Ridder, W. E., and Oehme, F. W. 1974. Nitrates as an Environmental, Animal, and Human Hazard. *Clinical Toxicol.* 7:145.

Seerley, R. W.; Emerick, R. J.; Embry, L. B.; and Olson, O. E. 1965. Effect of Nitrate or Nitrite Administered Continuously in Drinking Water for Swine and Sheep. *J. Anim. Sci.* 24:1014-19.

Simon, J. 1959a. Prevention of Noninfectious Abortion in Cattle by Weed Control and Fertilization Practices on Lowland Pastures. *JAVMA* 135:315.

————. 1959b. The Effect of Nitrate or Nitrite When Placed in the Rumens of Pregnant Dairy Cattle. *JAVMA* 135:311.

Sinclair, K. B. *et al.* 1967. Nitrite Toxicity in Sheep. *Res. Vet. Sci.* 8:65-70.

Steyn, D. G. 1959. The Problem of Methemoglobinemia in Man with Special Reference to Poisoning with Nitrates and Nitrites in Infants and Children. Fifth International Convention on Nutrition and Vital Substances, Constance, Germany.

Stoewsand, G. S.; Anderson, J. L.; and Lee, C. Y. 1973. Nitrate-induced Methemoglobinemia in Guinea Pigs: Influence of Diets Containing Beets with Varying Amounts of Nitrate, and the Effect of Ascorbic Acid and Methionine. *J. Nutrition* 10:419.

Tillman, A. D. *et al.* 1965. Nitrate Reduction Studies with Sheep. *J. Anim. Sci.* 24:1140-46.

Turner, C. A., and Kienholz, E. W. 1972. Nitrate Toxicity Feedstuffs. Nov. 27:28-30.

Wang, L. C. *et al.* 1961. Metabolism of Nitrate by Cattle. *Biochem. J.* 81:237-42.

Watts, H.; Webster, M,; Chappel, A.; and Leaver, D. 1969. Laboratory Diagnosis of Nitrite Poisoning in Sheep and Cattle. *Aust. Vet. J.* 45:492.

Winter, A. J. 1962. Studies on Nitrate Metabolism in Cattle. *Amer. J. Vet. Res.* 23:500-05.

OAK POISONING

Source

The oaks are woody, perennial plants with varying habitat and wide geographic distribution. They range in size from shrubs to tall trees. More than sixty species are found in nearly all areas of the United States and Canada.

Oaks are recognized by their simple, alternate leaves with irregularly rounded lobes and by the acorn. The acorn is a matured, tricarpellate, inferior ovary subtended by a "cup" of many reduced, overlapping, scale leaves, Oaks are divided into two groups: white oaks and black oaks, depending on maturation characteristics of the acorn. (Kingsbury, 1964)

The oaks belong to the genus *Quercus sp.* (Family Fagaceae). Literature reports most commonly describe poisoning from *Q. gambelii* or *Q. havardii.*

Toxicity

Both white oaks and black oaks have been shown toxic to livestock. There apparently is wide variance in the toxicity of oaks in a given area. Changes in climatic conditions, habitat, and nutrition of susceptible animals may influence the onset of poisoning. Mature oak leaves are as toxic as the bud and bloom stage. However, in the southwestern United States toxicity usually is associated with the early spring appearance of leaves which are browsed by cattle and sheep. (Dollahite, 1961) In the midwest and northeast areas of the United States, oak poisoning occurs most often when acorns are consumed by cattle on fall pastures. Seasons of high rainfall with resultant softening and sprouting of acorns may contribute to the incidence of oak poisoning. While cattle are commonly involved clinically, sheep, goats, rabbits, and guinea pigs are susceptible.

The toxic principle in oak buds and acorns has been ascribed to a polyhydroxyphenolic moiety of oak tannin known as gallic acid (gallotannin). The tannin content of oak leaves is highest when shin oak plants are most toxic to range animals. (Pigeon *et al.,* 1962) The toxicity is not appreciably reduced by freezing or drying. (Dollahite, 1961) Lesions in rabbits similar to those produced by *Quercus havardii* have been demonstrated after feeding of a water-extracted oak tannin.

Mechanism of Action

The exact mechanism of oak poisoning is not known. As a class, tannins are considered to be heptatotoxic. (Arena, 1970) In addition, the commonly held property of precipitation of proteins may be a factor in the toxic action of tannins. (Jones, 1967)

Oak tannins given to rabbits (Camp *et al.,* 1967) produced elevations in serum glutamic oxalacetic transaminase (SGOT), serum glutamic pyruvic transaminase (SGPT), blood urea nitrogen (BUN), and packed cell volume (PCV). The changes observed are suggestive of heptatotoxic and nephrotoxic properties in oak tannin.

Clinical Signs

Clinical disease from oak poisoning is most often seen in cattle, occasionally in sheep, and rarely in horses. Both adult cattle and calves may be affected. Onset of signs is gradual with anorexia, dullness, rumen atony, and constipation as the initial signs. (Hulbert and Oehme, 1968) Dark, hard feces covered with a film of mucus initially may change during the course of poisoning to the black, tarry or fluid consistency of hemorrhagic enteritis. Elevation of the lumbar spine is a common feature. Affected animals become weak and prostrate after three to seven days.

Icterus, hematuria, dehydration, and elimination of large volumes of dilute urine are characteristic of advanced stages of the disease. Animals with advanced signs rarely recover. Occasionally, abortions have been observed associated with acorn consumption.

Physiopathology

Oak-poisoned animals have elevations in SGOT, SGPT, BUN, PCV, and hemoglobin.

In a series of eight cases presented in 1974 at the University of Missouri Veterinary Clinic, the clinico-pathological characteristics of subacute and chronic oak toxicosis were examined. In addition to elevations of blood urea nitrogen (45-320 mg/dL) there was a consistent hyperphosphatemia (7.0-20.3 mEq/L) and a corresponding hypocalcemia (3.5-4.2 mEq/L). This response agrees with the observation made by others that hyperphosphatemia and hypocalcemia are sequelae to renal insufficiency.

Urine specific gravity is low, and the urine may contain blood as well as granular and hyaline casts. At necropsy, gross lesions are reflected in four categories: (1) gastroenteritis, (2) hemorrhages, (3) edema, and (4) renal lesions.

Gastroenteritis is observed as mucoid to hemorrhagic and involves the terminal intestine most severely. Some degree of colonic hemorrhage and edema may be seen. Subserosal petechial or ecchymotic hemorrhages are distributed over the surface of the gastrointestinal tract. Acorns are not always found in rumen contents of poisoned animals. Subcutaneous edema is present over the pelvic limbs and along the ventral body wall. Ascites and hydrothorax are characteristic lesions. Gelatinous, blood-tinged edema occurs regularly around the kidneys and may infiltrate to the mesentery, mesorectum, and mesometrium.

The liver is occasionally pale and mottled but is not consistently involved grossly. Subserosal hemorrhages may be found throughout the abdominal cavity, over the gastrointestinal tract, and beneath the endocardium and epicardium. In addition, the kidney contains numerous petchial to ecchymotic subcapsular hemorrhages.

Renal lesions reflect a nephrosis. The kidney is enlarged, pale, and contains scattered hemorrhages. Microscopic lesions in the kidney are characteristic but not pathognomonic. Coagulative necrosis of the proximal convoluted tubules is a prominent feature. In addition, there is sloughing of necrotic tubules into the tubular lumen to form a pink-staining, solid mass of material apparently composed of epithelial cells and protein. (Smith, 1959) The numerous dilated distal convoluted tubules observed are indicative of a regenerating epithelium in a kidney excreting dilute urine.

The lesions of oak poisoning are quite similar to changes observed in both swine and cattle poisoned by *Amaranthus retroflexus* (pigweed). (Osweiler, 1969) Any relationship to a similar toxin in *A. retroflexus* is a possibility which should be investigated.

Diagnosis

The gradual onset of anorexia, gastrointestinal atony, and signs of renal disease in ruminants consuming oak buds or acorns should be considered a potential oak-poisoning case. Examination for appropriate clinical pathologic or gross pathologic lesions will further reinforce a tentative diagnosis. The characteristic microscopic lesion in formalin-fixed tissue is highly suggestive of oak poisoning. However, care must be exercised to separate a potential poisoning due to *A. retroflexus* from those caused by oak. Tannins could be identified in urine, but this procedure may not be of value in time to correct a clinical situation. Furthermore, many plants contain tannins and this in itself would not prove oak poisoning.

Treatment

Animals should be removed from further access to oak. Stimulation of the ruminal and intestinal motility with oils or ruminatorics may be of value. Parenteral fluids to correct dehydration and probable acidosis would be helpful. The usual precautions in administration of fluids to renal insufficient animals should be followed. (Hulbert and Oehme, 1968)

A preventive ration of 10-15 percent calcium hydroxide in a grain ration has been used with some success where exposure to oak cannot be avoided. (Dollahite *et al.*, 1966)

REFERENCES

Arena, J. M. 1970. *Poisoning: Toxicology-Symptoms-Treatments.* 2nd ed. Springfield, Illinois: Charles C. Thomas, Publisher.

Camp, B. J.; Steel, E.; and Dollahite, J. W. 1967. Certain Biochemical Changes in Blood and Livers of Rabbits Fed Oak Tannin. *Am. J. Vet. Res.* 28:290-92.

Cedervall, Anne; Johansoon, H. E.; and Jonsson, L. 1973. Acorn Poisoning in Cattle. *Vet.-Med.* 25:639-44.

Clarke, E. G. C., and Cotchin, E. 1956. A Note in the Toxicity of the Acorn. *The Brit. Vet. J.* 112:13539.

Dollahite, J. W.; Pigeon, R. F.; and Camp, B. 1962. The Toxicity of Gallic Acid, Pyrogallol, Tannic Acid, and *Quercus havardii* in the Rabbit. *Am. J. Vet. Res.* 23:1264-66.

Dollahite, J. W. 1961. Shin Oak (*Quercus havardii*) Poisoning in Cattle. *Southwestern Vet.* 15:198-201.

Dollahite, J. W.; Housholder, G. L.; and Camp, B. J. 1966. Effects of Calcium Hydroxide on the Toxicity of Post Oak (*Quercus Stellata*) in Calves. *JAVMA* 148:908-12.

Hulbert, L., and Oehme, F. 1968. *Plants Poisonous to Livestock*. 3rd. ed. Manhattan, Kansas: Kansas State University Press.

Jones, L. M. 1965. *Veterinary Pharmacology and Therapeutics*. 3rd ed. Ames, Iowa: Iowa State University Press.

Kingbury, J. M. 1964. *Poisonous Plants of the United States and Canada*. Englewood Cliffs, New Jersey: Prentice-Hall, Inc.

Osweiler, G. D.; Buck, W. B.; and Bicknell, E. J. 1969. Production of Perirenal Edema in Swine with *Amaranthus retroflexus*. *Am. J. Vet. Res.* 30:555-56.

Pigeon, R. F.; Camp, B. J.; and Dollahite, J. W. 1962. Oral Toxicity and Polyhydroxyphenol Moiety of Tannin Isolated from *Quercus havardii* (Shin Oak). *Am. J. Vet. Res.* 23:1268-70.

Smith, H. A. 1959. The Diagnosis of Oak Poisoning. *Southwestern Vet.* 13:34-36.

OXALATE

Source

The salts of oxalic acid are found both in nature and as products of human endeavor. Oxalic acid itself (HOOCCOOH) is rarely encountered as a toxicity problem. The salts of oxalic acid, primarily potassium oxalate, are found in household and industrial products such as rust removers, bleaches, and tanning compounds.

A common source of oxalates to livestock are plants, especially those of the family Chenopodiaceae and the genus Rumex. A listing of plants containing soluble oxalate salts is found in table 1. Other plants, especially the Araceae, contain large amounts of calcium oxalate crystals (table 2).

TABLE 1
Plants Which Contain Large Amounts of Soluble Oxalates

Amaranthus spp.	pigweed
Beta vulgaris	beet, mangold
Chenopodium album	lamb's quarters
Halogeton glomeratus	√ halogeton
Oxalis spp.	sorrel, soursop
Portulaca oleracea	purslane
Rheum rhaponticum	rhubarb
Rumex spp.	sorrel, dock
Salsola kali	Russian thistle
Sarcobatus vermiculatus	√greasewood

TABLE 2
Plants Which Cause Local Irritation Upon Chewing

Alocasia spp.	alocasia
Arisaema spp.	jack in the pulpit
Caladium spp.	caladium
Calla palustris	wild calla
Colocasia spp.	elephants-ear
Dieffenbachia spp.	dumbcane
Philodendron spp.	philodendron
Symplocarpus foetidus	skunk cabbage
Xanthosoma spp.	caladium

Several fungi, including certain species of *Aspergillus* and *Penicillium* are capable of producing oxalates which may contribute to a nephropathy in livestock.

Small animals and poultry may encounter oxalate poisoning indirectly via consumption of ethylene glycol in antifreeze. Ethylene glycol (HO—CH$_2$CH$_2$—OH) after ingestion is oxidized to form oxalic acid which can exert its effects similar to other oxalates.

The plant oxalates are the primary source of poisoning to cattle and sheep. This is a major problem in the western states as a result of *Halogeton* and *Sarcobatus* (greasewood) ingestion. The same problem may occur infrequently from other oxalate-containing plants. As much as 10 to 30 percent oxalic acid equivalent (dry weight basis) may be present in such plants.

James (1966) cites evidence that there are two forms of soluble oxalates in plants. One form is associated with plants having a cell sap of approximately pH 2 and the oxalate is present as potassium acid oxalate. This chemical form is characteristically found in the family Oxalidaceae. The second type of oxalate is primarily sodium oxalate, associated with plants having a cell sap of approximately pH 6, and is characteristic of plants in the family Chenopodiaceae.

Oxalate content is highest in the leaves, followed by the seeds, with the lowest levels in the stems.

Ruminants can consume large amounts of plant oxalates, apparently because the oxalates are metabolized to a large extent in the rumen. However, if oxalate is directly introduced into the abomasum, the ruminant responds similarly to a monogastric animal. If sheep and cattle graze slowly, they can consume twice as much halogeton as an animal getting one single lethal dose.

If large amounts of oxalate are consumed by ruminants, three consequences are possible.(1) The oxalate may be destroyed in the rumen; (2) it may combine with free calcium in the rumen and be excreted in the feces; or (3) be absorbed in the bloodstream to affect tissue and serum calcium. Rumen pH is higher than normal in ruminants receiving oxalate-containing plants. This may be related to the possible breakdown of oxalate to bicarbonate and carbonates. Animals receiving sublethal levels of halogeton may develop hypocalcemia, and blood levels of calcium may decrease to 20 percent of normal in sheep dying of halogeton poisoning.

Toxicity

Sheep may be poisoned by as little as 0.55 percent of body weight of soluble oxalate when on full feed. For sheep which are starved or deprived of water, less than 0.1 percent of the body weight is lethal. Smaller quantities will cause poisoning if rapidly ingested. The non-fatal toxic dose of sodium oxalate for adult horses is approximately 200 gm/day for eight days.

Mechanism of Action

After entrance into the systemic circulation, oxalates are believed to exert their influence in the following manner. Oxalates are able to combine with calcium ion to form insoluble calcium oxalate. This results in a functional hypocalcemia with tetany in acute cases or derangement in bone growth or milk production from lower levels of intake. A second problem is that oxalate may crystallize in the vasculature and infiltrate vessel walls causing vascular necrosis and hemorrhage. A third problem is renal tubular blockage and necrosis due to lodging of insoluble calcium oxalate in the tubules. This leads to anuria, uremia and electrolyte disturbances.

Complete evaluation of the changes induced by oxalate poisoning from halogeton plants suggests that hypocalcemia and renal damage are not the primary causes of death. James (1968) suggests that oxalate interference with carbohydrate metabolism, particularly succinic dehydrogenase inhibition may be a significant factor in death from halogeton-induced oxalate toxicosis.

Clinical Signs

Clinical signs may appear within two to six hours after ingestion of oxalate-containing plants. There is slight to moderate colic, depression, and muscular weakness. The gait is irregular and the head droops downward. Affected animals are restless and may get up and down frequently. Such animals initially lag behind the flock or herd. Weakness proceeds rapidly to prostration. The animals may become semicomatose with the head and neck pulled around to one side in a posture resembling milk fever in cattle. Rapid, labored breathing and blood-tinged froth and fluid around the mouth are observed. Bloat and frequent urination may occasionally be seen.

In some cases, convulsions presumed due to hypocalcemia may be seen. Serum calcium is depressed and blood urea nitrogen may be slightly elevated. Death from acute poisoning occurs within nine to eleven hours after initial symptoms.

Physiopathology

In acute oxalate poisoning, consistent changes in clinical chemistry values include moderate to marked hypocalcemia, hyperphosphatemia, hypernatremia, and hyperkalemia. Elevations in serum glutamic oxalacetic transaminase (SGOT), serum glutamic pyruvic transaminase (SGPT), lactic dehydrogenase, and blood urea nitrogen are also observed. Plasma pH increases within the first two hours of acute clinical signs. As signs progress and affected animals become terminal, blood pCO_2 increases and pO_2 decreases.

Ascites and hydrothorax are common findings upon gross examination. There are diffuse hemorrhages on the serous membranes, especially the anterior portion of the rumen and other forestomachs. The mouth and esophagus may be filled with blood-tinged froth. There is severe mucosal hemorrhage in the rumen, petechiation of the fundic portion of the abomasum, and edema of the anterior-ventral rumen wall. Partially digested plants may be present in the rumen. Gastrointestinal lymph nodes are enlarged and edematous. The respiratory tract appears moderately congested, and the bronchial tree is filled with blood-tinged froth.

The kidneys are pale, edematous, and swollen. The capsule peels easily and fluid oozes from the cut surface. A yellow, striated appearance may be present in the renal cortex. These striations are most prominent at the corticomedullary junction. This corresponds to the area of oxalate crystal accumulation as seen microscopically. The striking histopathologic lesion is the collection of birefringent oxalate crystals in the renal tubules. There is a pronounced dilatation of the renal tubules related to these crystals. These crystals may also be found in the walls of ruminal vessels and the vessels of the brain.

Diagnosis

Diagnosis is based on history, clinical signs and necropsy lesions, confirmed by the finding of oxalate crystals in kidneys or vasculature. The clinical syndrome appears similar to milk fever, starvation hypocalcemia, or grain overload. Ruminal pH is elevated in oxalate poisoning but depressed in grain overload. Lactation tetany (milk fever) does not involve such marked lesions as does oxalate poisoning.

Treatment and Prevention

After clinical signs appear, treatment is of little value. Calcium gluconate given IV may provide temporary relief but is not curative. Urinary acidifiers are probably of little value once signs are apparent. The use of saline-glucose solutions to produce diuresis and to combat alkalosis is rational, if not entirely effective, supportive therapy.

Control

Control of oxalate poisoning in ruminants is directed at preventing the intake and absorption of toxic quantities of oxalate-containing plants. Under range conditions, halogeton is the plant most likely to cause problems. Overseeding with suitable grasses will aid in competitive control of halogeton. Areas of high halogeton concentration should not be grazed during drought or periods when sheep are hungry.

Phenoxyacetic herbicides may be used to control the plant or may be combined with mechanical methods such as mowing or scalping. However, this must be combined with a positive reseeding and control program.

Supplemental feeding with dicalcium phosphate is of prophylactic value where exposure cannot be avoided. The use of 1/4 pound per sheep daily of pelleted alfalfa containing 5 percent dicalcium phosphate has been recommended. A free choice mixture of 75 pounds salt and 25 pounds dicalcium phsophate may also be used. These should be used only when animals are exposed to high levels of oxalate, since continued use may upset the Ca:P balance.

Any plant high in soluble oxalates is a potential problem if consumed in sufficient quantity. An awareness of those plants which may cause poisoning is necessary for prevention and/or accurate diagnosis.

REFERENCES

See next section (Ethylene glycol).

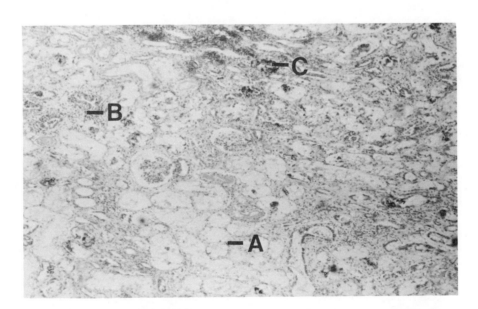

Figure 1. Microscopic appearance of renal cortex depicting (A) dilated tubules with hydropic epithelium, (B) focal accumulation of inflammatory cells, and (C) oxalate crystals.

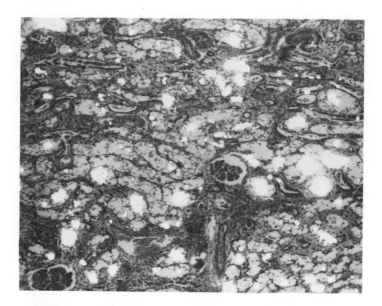

Figure 2. Microscopic appearance of renal cortex under partially polarized light. Note the prominent oxalate crystals and the hydropic tubular epithelium.

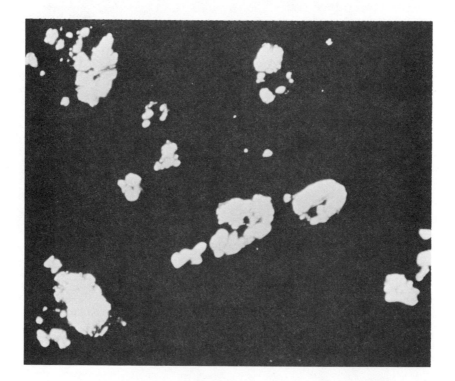

Figure 3. Microscopic appearance of oxalate crystals in renal cortex under fully polarized light.

ETHYLENE GLYCOL (ANTIFREEZE)

Source

Ethylene glycol (EG) is widely used as an industrial solvent, rust remover, and coolant. The most hazardous source to livestock and pets is its availability as a common antifreeze coolant for automobile engines. Poisoning from ingestion of antifreeze or chemical preparations containing ethylene glycol is most common in dogs and cats. Occasionally, swine or poultry may be affected. The effects of ethylene glycol are similar in most monogastric animals and poultry. Dogs most commonly are affected due to their less-than-discriminatory eating habits. Seasonal incidence appears to correspond to the times when antifreeze is being added or drained (*e.g.,* spring and fall).

Toxicity

Cats are quite susceptible to ethylene glycol poisoning, 2-4 ml/kg causing clinical signs and death. Dogs may be poisoned by 4-5 ml/kg while 7-8 ml/kg will be toxic to poultry.

Mechanism of Action

There are two routes by which ethylene glycol may affect animals. Initially, the glycol may enter the CSF and act directly on the CNS to produce a narcotic or euphoric effect. Later, clinical signs are associated with metabolism of the glycol to oxalic acid with subsequent formation of calcium oxalate. This may cause hypocalcemia due to its complexing with calcium. Renal tubular blockage with development of uremia is observed from one to three days after ingestion.

The complete mechanism of EG toxicosis is still controversial. Metabolism to oxalic acid may account for as little as 2 percent of the total dose (Pneumarthy and Oehme, 1975) and there is evidence for metabolic intermediates of EG being toxic. However, the success of early treatment with competitive inhibitors of EG metabolism (ethyl alcohol, pyrazol) would support the idea that a majority of the toxicity is from metabolites of EG. The formation of oxalate with subsequent inhibition of carbohydrate metabolism as proposed for oxalate poisoning may also play a role in toxicosis and death.

Clinical Signs

Shortly after ingestion of ethylene glycol (one to six hours), affected animals may vomit and become ataxic and incoordinated. Anorexia may be observed. Rapid heart rate and polypnea may be early signs. Animals often survive the initial poisoning signs and may return to near normal within twelve hours. However, there is recurrence of more serious signs usually around twenty-four hours after ingestion. These are characterized by vomiting, anorexia, dehydration, weakness, ataxia, convulsions, coma, and death.

If a large amount of EG (in excess of 6 ml/kg body weight) is consumed, signs may be acute and the entire course of illness will be no longer than twelve to thirty-six hours. Such animals become depressed, comatose, and acidotic. Occasional vomiting may occur. Acute poisoning terminates before uremia develops, but marked changes in urine flow, electrolytes, and acid-base balance may occur.

Animals which survive longer than twenty-four to thirty-six hours will develop signs of uremia. Vomiting, anorexia, depression and coma progress over a two to seven- day period. There may be oliguria or complete anuria, and there is usually a progressive increase in blood urea nitrogen as well as hyperkalemia and acidosis. Urinalysis reveals hematuria, albuminuria, and casts. Urine sediment may contain small birefringent oxalate crystals, best observed under polarized light.

Physiopathology

Gastritis or enteritis is common in dogs and cats poisoned by ethylene glycol. The gastric mucosa may be dark brown with hemorrhages in the mucosa. Hyperemia and edema of the lungs are seen. The kidneys are pale and streaked with gray or yellow, especially near the corticomedullary junction.

Histopathologic findings are consistent and characteristic in animals dying of ethylene glycol poisoning. Pale yellow birefringent (rosette-shaped) oxalate crystals are found in the convoluted renal tubules. Inflammatory response to the crystals is not usually seen. Renal tubules may be dilated and lined with flattened tubular epithelium. Birefringent, polarizing crystals are found in the adventitia and perivascular spaces of the blood vessels in the brain. Pulmonary hyperemia and edema are present in the lungs of dogs poisoned by ethylene glycol.

Diagnosis

Ethylene glycol poisoning is difficult to diagnose from clinical signs alone. Encephalitis, concussion, acute nephritis, garbage poisoning, uremia, foreign-body ingestion, leptospirosis, and acute gastritis have been confused with ethylene glycol poisoning. When a dog or cat is presented with signs of emesis, ataxia, convulsions, diarrhea, normal or subnormal temperature, and evidence of renal failure or uremia, ethylene glycol poisoning should be among the diagnoses considered.

Ethylene glycol may be determined chemically in body fluids by a colorimetric test. A histochemical method is available for demonstration of calcium oxalate in tissues following EG toxicosis. (Roscher, 1974)

A simple method for detection of oxalate crystals in tissue or impression smears of kidney is to place the slide on a microscope stage under low light. Then place one polarizing lens above and one below the microscope stage (Lens from polarized sunglasses are adequate for this). Turn one lens slowly until the light coming through the microscope is obliterated. The calcium oxalate crystals will be visible as bright rosette-shaped areas in a dark background (see figure 3).

Treatment

Once clinical signs (especially relating to renal failure) are advanced, treatment is usually of no avail. Rational therapy consists of (1) elimination of any remaining poison from the GI tract, (2) control of convulsions, (3) prevention or control of pulmonary edema, and (4) maintenance of proper fluid and electrolyte balance. Convulsions are controlled with pentobarbital sodium.

Calcium borogluconate is given as a 10 percent solution intravenously at the rate of 10-15 ml/30 pound body weight each day in three divided doses. Prednisolone (0.5 mg/lb) is used to combat shock and pulmonary edema. Fluid therapy should not include potassium until urine flow or BUN is established. Half-strength saline and 5 percent glucose may be used to establish urine flow.

Administration to dogs of 5.5 ml/kg body weight of 20 percent ethyl alcohol intravenously and 8 ml/kg body weight of 5 percent sodium bicarbonate intravenously has been used by some (Szabuniewicz et al, 1975; St. Omer et al, 1976) while others have advocated the intraperitoneal administration of ethanol and bicarbonate (Beckett and Shields, 1971). In addition, Szabuniewicz et al (1975) markedly improved survival by early oral administration of activated charcoal.

In cats, intraperitoneal therapy with 5 ml/kg of 20 percent ethanol and 6 ml/kg body weight of sodium bicarbonate has been used by Penumarthy and Oehme (1975) who noted an apparent irritating effect from intraperitoneal administration of bicarbonate. In dogs, Beckett and Shields (1971) indicated no serious irritation by intraperitoneal bicarbonate while St. Omer et al (1976) observed moderate to marked pain associated with intraperitoneal administration of bicarbonate.

Convalescent animals should receive a bland low protein diet which does not place undue stress on the kidneys.

REFERENCES

Anonymous. 1958. Reducing Livestock Losses from Halogeton Poisoning in the Western States. USDA Pub. PA-321.

Beckett, S. D., and Shields, R. P. 1971. Treatment of Acute Ethylene Glycol (Antifreeze) Toxicosis in the Dog. *JAVMA* 158:472-76.

Binns, W., and James, L. F. 1960. Halogeton and Other Oxalic Acid Poisonings. Proceedings, American College of Veterinary Toxicologists. pp. 5-8.

Blood, D. C., and Henderson, J. A. 1963. *Veterinary Medicine.* 2nd ed. Baltimore: The Willimas & Wilkins Co.

Blood, F. R. 1965. Chronic Toxicity of Ethylene Glycol in the Rat. *Food Cosmet. Toxic.* 3:229-34.

Borden, T. A. 1968. Treatment of Acute Ethylene Glycol Poisoning in Rats. *Invest. Urol.* 6:205-10.

Hagler, L., and Herman, R. H. 1973. Oxalate Metabolism. *Am. J. Clin. Nutrition* 26:1073.

Jakoby, W. B., and Bhat, J. V. 1958. Microbial Metabolism of Oxalic Acid. *Bact. Rev.* 22:75-80.

James, L. F. 1968. Serum Electrolyte, Acid-Base Balance, and Enzyme Changes in Acute *Halogeton glomeratus* Poisoning in Sheep. *Canadian J. Com. Med.* 32:539.

————. 1966. Oxalate Metabolism in Sheep and Its Effect on the Anion-Cation Balance. Ph.D. Thesis. Utah State University, Logan, Utah.

James, L. F., and Butcher, J. E. 1972. Halogeton Poisoning in Sheep: Effect of High-Level Oxalate Intake. *J. Anim. Sci.* 35:1233.

James, L F.; Street, J. C.; and Butcher, J. E. 1967. *In Vitro* Degradation of Oxalate and of Cellulose by Rumen Ingesta from Sheep Fed *Halogeton glomeratus. J. Anim. Sci.* 26:1438-44.

James, L. F.; Street, J. C.; Butcher, J. E.; and Binns, W. 1968. Oxalate Metabolism in Sheep: I. Effect of Low-Level *Halogeton glomeratus* Intake on Nutrient Balance. *J. Anim. Sci.* 27:718-23.

James, L. F.; Street, J. C.; Butcher, J. E.; and Shupe, J. L. 1968. Effect of *Halogeton glomeratus* on pH Values in Rumen of Sheep. *Am. J. Vet. Res.* 29:915-18.

————. 1968. Oxalate Metabolism in Sheep: II. Effect of Low-Level *Halogeton glomeratus* Intake on Electrolyte Metabolism. *J. Anim. Sci.* 27:724-29.

Kersting, E. J. *et al.* 1965. Ethylene Glycol Poisoning in Small Animals. *JAVMA* 146:113-18.

————. 1966. Experimental Ethylene Glycol Poisoning in the Dog. *Am. J. Vet. Res.* 27:574-82.

Kingsbury, J. M. 1964. *Poisonous Plants of the United States and Canada.* Englewood Cliffs, New Jersey: Prentice-Hall, Inc.

Kirk, R. W. 1968. *Current Veterinary Therapy.* 3rd ed. Philadelphia: W. B. Saunders Company.

Marshall, V. L.; Buck, W. B.; and Bell, G. L. 1967. Pigweed (*Amaranthus retroflexus*): An Oxalate-Containing Plant. *Am. J. Vet. Res.* 28:888-89.

Moeschlin, S. 1965. *Poisoning, Diagnosis, and Therapy.* New York: Grune and Stratton.

Mundy, R. L.; Hall, L. M.; and Teague, R. S. 1974. Pyrazole as an Antidote for Ethylene Glycol Poisoning. *Toxicol. Appl. Pharm.* 28:320.

Osweiler, G. D., and Eness, P. G. 1972. Ethylene Glycol Poisoning in Swine. *JAVMA* 160:746.

Penumarthy, L., and Oehme, F. W. 1975. Treatment of Ethylene Glycol Toxicosis in Cats. *Am. J. Vet. Res.* 36:209.

Riddell, C. *et al.* 1967. Ethylene Glycol Poisoning in Poultry. *JAVMA* 150:1431-35.

Roscher, A. A. 1974. A New Histochemical Method for the Demonstration of Calcium Oxalate in Tissues Following Ethylene Glycol Poisoning. *Am. J. Clin. Path.* 55:99.

Shupe, J. L. *et al.* 1969. Additional Physiopathologic Changes in *Halogeton glomeratus* (Oxalate) Poisoning in Sheep. *Cornell Vet.* 59:41-55.

Srivastava, S. K., and Krishnam, P. S. 1959. Oxalate Content of Plant Tissues. *J. Sci. Indus. Res.* 18:146-48.

Stoddart, L. A.; Baird, G. T.; Stewart, G.; Markham, B. S.; and Clegg, H. 1951. The Halogeton Problem in Utah. Utah State Agr. Coll. Exten. Serv. Bull. No. 250.

St. Omer, V. V.; Green, R. A.; Zumwalt, R. W.; and Dallman, M. J., 1976. Use of Dimethyl Sulfoxide in the Treatment of Experimental Ethylene Glycol Toxicosis in Dogs. Unpublished Data.

Szabuniewicz, M.; Bailey, E. M.; and Wiersig, D. O., 1975. A New Approach to the Treatment of Ethylene Glycol Poisoning in Dogs. *The Southwestern Veterinarian* 28:7-11.

Underwood, F., and Bennett, W. M. 1973. Ethylene Glycol Intoxication. *JAVMA* 226:1453.

Willson, B. J., and Wilson, C. H. 1961. Oxalate Formation in Moldy Feedstuffs As a Possible Factor in Livestock Toxic Disease. *Am. J. Vet. Res.* 22:961-69.

PERIRENAL EDEMA

(*Amaranthus retroflexus* Poisoning)

A distinct disease syndrome of swine, and sometimes cattle, called perirenal edema occurs during the summer and early fall months. Its onset is associated with gaining access to pastures containing *Amaranthus retroflexus* (redroot pigweed). Typical signs of the disease develop five to ten days after ingestion of the toxic plant. The condition is characterized by weakness, trembling, and incoordination followed by knuckling of pastern joints and paralysis of hind limbs. Sternal recumbency is a characteristic posture of affected pigs. Death usually takes place within forty-eight hours of the onset of clinical signs. The characteristic lesion is retroperitoneal edema of the perirenal connective tissue. Kidneys are pale brown and may show petechial or ecchymotic hemorrhages beneath the capsule.

Source, Toxicity, and Mechanism of Action

Perirenal edema is attributed to ingestion of excessive amounts of a common weed, *Amaranthus retroflexus,* commonly called redroot pigweed.

McNutt (1953) studied edema disease of swine and reported an occasional lesion characterized by a thickened and edematous renal capsule separated from the ischemic kidney by considerable amounts of blood-stained fluid. Perirenal edema was listed as a synonym for edema disease. Christensen (1955) reported a syndrome characterized clinically by acute illness with signs of ataxia, dyspnea, cyanosis, and edema. Surviving animals were affected with signs of uremia, polydipsia, polyurea, edema, and hemorrhage around the kidneys. Bennett (1964) summarized the clinical, pathologic, and etiologic factors considered relevant to edema disease. He mentioned edema of the stomach wall as the most prominent lesion, although edema was also common in the mesenteric folds of the spiral colon, eyelids, ears, subcutaneous tissues of the face, and the ventrolateral abdominal wall. Occasionally, edema of the capsule of the kidney was observed with the capsule separated from the kidney by a substantial amount of blood-tinged fluid. The kidney appeared ischemic, and the

perirenal fluids jelled upon exposure to air. (Bennett, 1964; McNutt, 1953)

Larsen *et al..* (1962) reported on a perirenal edema syndrome of swine. The lesions and clinical course resembled that reported by Buck *et al.* (1966), but no specific toxic etiology was suggested. The role of hemolytic strains of *Escherichia coli* has been established as a factor in edema disease in swine. However, reports indicating a direct relationship between edema disease and perirenal edema were not found.

Perirenal edema occurs during the summer months of July, August, and September. The most commonly affected group of swine are those weighing between 30 and 125 lbs. The clinical history usually includes sudden access of pigs to pasture or green plants after a period of confinement. The clinical signs of perirenal edema usually appear from five to ten days after access to pasture. *A. retroflexus,* is a member of the family Amaranthaceae. It is a common weed (Kingsbury, 1964) which tends to grow in abandoned hog lots, fence rows, or waste areas throughout North America. The coarse stem reaches a height of 3 to 5 feet by late July or early August and is topped by a large, rough inflorescence. It has been found to contain as much as 30 percent oxalic acid on a dry weight basis. Lack of hypocalcemia and infrequent occurrence of oxalate crystals in renal tubules does not substantiate oxalate as the toxic principle. (Osweiler *et al.,* 1969)

A. retroflexus is a known nitrate accumulator, but the perirenal edema disease bears no resemblance to nitrate or nitrite toxicosis.

The quantitative toxicity of *A. retroflexus* is not known. However, swine having free access to the plant consume it readily, even when their normal diet is available. Clinical signs may become evident as early as three days after initial ingestion.

The toxic principle in *A. retroflexus,* although not identified, appears to be specific for renal tubules. Early development of cloudy swelling, and hyaline degeneration is followed by coagulative tubular necrosis with sloughing of necrotic cells to form eosinophilic granular casts. In severe toxicosis, there is rupture of tubular

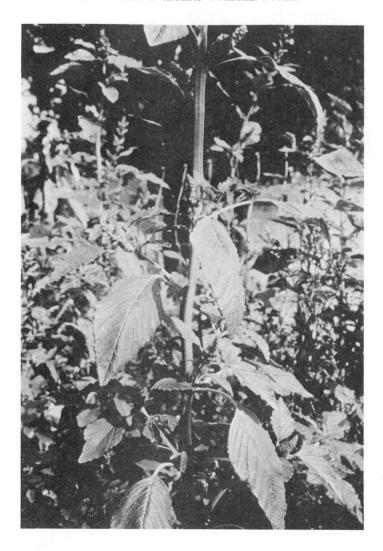

Figure 1. Vegetative growth of *Amaranthus retroflexus* (Pigweed).

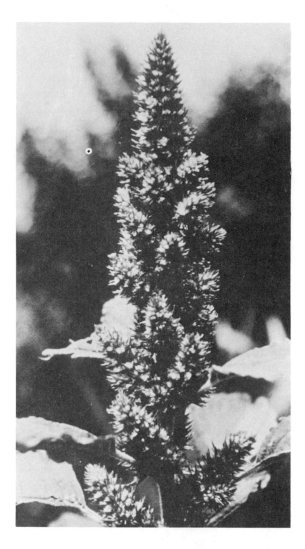

Figure 2. Characteristic inflorescence of *Amaranthus retroflexus* (Pigweed).

basement membranes with movement of glomerular filtrate to the surface of the kidney. This movement is the probable cause of the perirenal edema and associated retroperitoneal edema.

As a consequence of severe renal disease there are elevations in blood urea nitrogen, serum creatinine, and serum potassium. The electrocardiograph of affected swine is characteristic of pigs with experimentally induced hyperkalemic heart failure. (Osweler, 1968) The changes include bradycardia, a wide and slurred QRS complex, and an increase in magnitude and duration of the T wave. The probable cause of death is hyperkalemic heart failure.

Clinical Signs

Clinical signs appear suddenly five to ten days after the pigs are allowed access to pasture containing pig-

weeds. Initial signs are weakness, trembling, and incoordination. The disease progresses rapidly to knuckling of the pastern joints and finally to almost complete paralysis of the hind limbs. The affected pigs usually maintain an attitude of sternal recumbency followed by coma and death. (fig. 3) If disturbed while in sternal recumbency, attempts to walk are characterized by a crouching gait or dragging their hind limbs. The temperature is usually normal and the eyes are bright. Death usually occurs within forty-eight hours of the onset of clinical signs, but affected swine may live from five to fifteen days with progression from signs of acute nephrosis to those of chronic fibrosing nephritis. In affected herds, new cases may appear for as long as ten days after removal from the source. Kidneys from animals which survive acute *A. retroflexus* often have chronic lesions of interstitial fibrosis and dilated tubules with flattened tubular epithelium. Many such swine appear clinically normal.

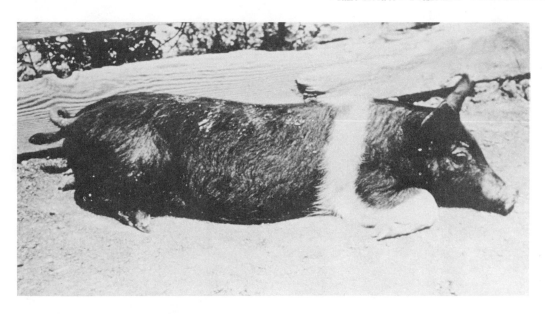

Figure 3. Attitude of sternal recumbency and pareisis assumed by pigs with *A. retroflexus* poisoning.

Occasionally, a syndrome of chronic wasting with abdominal enlargement is seen in swine having access to *A. retroflexus*. Large quantities of dilute urine are voided. Necropsy examination usually reveals large subcapsular accumulations of blood, fibrin and fluids with a small fibrotic kidney at the center. This chronic lesion is most often seen in late summer or early autumn when *A. retroflexus* is rather mature.

Morbidity ranges from less than 5 percent in some herds to 50 percent in others, and the mortality is usually about 75 to 80 percent in those clinically affected.

A. retroflexus toxicosis has been reported several times in cattle. The clinical signs, course of the disease, gross lesions and microscopic lesions are strikingly similar to those seen in oak (acorn) poisoning. The renal medulla may be relatively free of damage in oak toxicosis as contrasted to the damage induced by *A. retroflexus*. Examination of pastures and rumen contents for evidence of exposure to oak or acorns is essential to diagnosis.

Physiopathology

Gross postmortem findings invariably include edema of the connective tissue around the kidneys. (fig. 4) The amount of fluid in the perirenal area varies, at times occupying the greater portion of the abdominal cavity. In pigs which have a clinical course longer than twenty-four to thirty-six hours, there may be considerable blood in the edematous fluid, giving the appearance upon cursory examination of greatly enlarged, hemorrhagic kidneys. However, on incision of the le-

sion, a normal-sized but pale kidney is found. In addition to perirenal edema, there may also be edema of the ventral abdominal wall and the perirectal area. The thoracic and abdominal cavities may contain a transparent, clear, or straw-colored fluid, sometimes as much as one liter. The kidneys are usually of normal size but pale with areas of hyperemia extending into the cortex. They may occasionally be enlarged, congested, and contain ecchymotic hemorrhages in the cortex. The edema is in the perirenal connective tissue, and the kidney capsule remains normal.

The histologic lesions of affected swine were characterized by hydropic degeneration and coagulative necrosis of both proximal and distal convoluted tubules. (fig. 5) Glomeruli may be shrunken and apparently increased in cellularity. There may be dilatation of Bowman's capsules. Tubular proteinaceous casts are numerous in the distal and collecting tubules. (fig. 6) Often, single necrotic tubules appeared among comparatively unaffected tissue.

Swine affected clinically with signs of perirenal edema experience large increases in serum potassium. Blood urea nitrogen and serum creatinine are also increased in pigs fed pigweed.

Diagnosis

The diagnosis of perirenal edema in swine is not difficult. Affected pigs have a history of having been turned from a drylot onto a pasture containing a heavy growth of pigweed within ten days before the appearance of signs of illness.

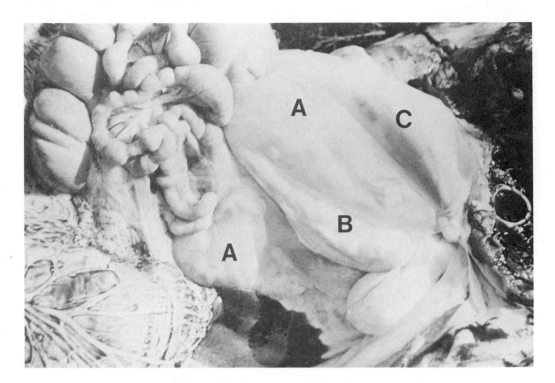

Figure 4. Gross lesions of perirenal edema. Note the extensive retroperitoneal perirenal edema (A), edema around the terminal colon (B), and in the ventral abdominal wall (C).

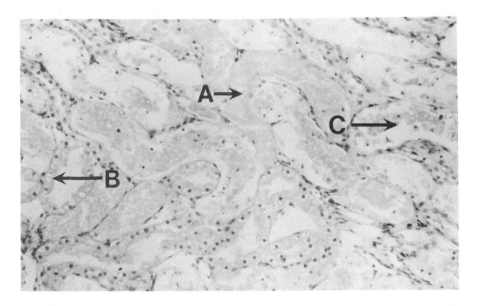

Figure 5. Microscopic renal lesions in the acute phase of perirenal edema. (A) Coagulative tubular necrosis, (B) hydropic degeneration, and (C) desquamation of necrotic cells are apparent in affected kidneys.

Posterior weakness, sternal recumbency, and normal temperature are found in most pigs with perirenal edema. Death usually occurs within forty-eight hours. Postmortem lesions are consistently characterized by edema in the perirenal tissue.

There are other conditions that have been confused with the perirenal edema syndrome. Infectious cystitis, resulting in hydronephrosis, may produce edema of the perirenal tissue and signs similar to those of perirenal edema. The well-known entity in feeder pigs, edema

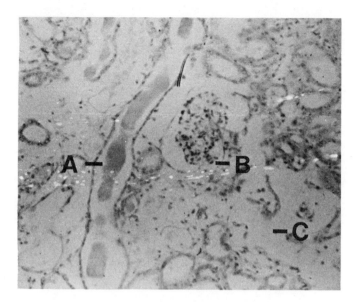

Figure 6. Microscopic renal lesions in subacute perirenal edema. Note the eosinophilic tubular casts (A), dilatation of Bowan's capsule (B), and confluence of renal tubules due to ruptured basement membranes (C).

disease, resembles perirenal edema; but marked mesenteric edema, gastric edema, and the hemorrhagic form of edema disease have not been observed in pigs with perirenal edema. The edema of the perirenal tissue that is characteristic of perirenal edema has rarely been observed in swine affected with edema disease. Acute toxicosis from ethylene glycol with subsequent oxalate nephrosis will cause perirenal edema grossly indistinguishable from *A. retroflexus* toxicosis. Ethylene glycol toxicosis is easily distinguished by histopathological examination of kidney tissue. Fungal nephrotoxins (see mycotoxins) may result in a lesion of perirenal edema. Examination of the feed supply and circumstances of exposure to plants will assist in differentation.

In cattle, the clinical course and lesions of *A. retroflexus* toxicosis are very similar to those of acorn (oak) poisoning. Careful examination for exposure to oak versus *A. retroflexus* is essential since reliable chemical analysis is not used in diagnosis of either condition.

Treatment and Prevention

Specific treatment of this condition has not been established so far. Immediate removal of the pigs from the weed pasture as soon as signs are seen is the only definite recommendation that can be made at this time. Pigs that have been confined to a drylot should not be allowed access to graze pastures containing a heavy

growth of *A. retroflexus*. Pigs raised on pastures with access to the offending weed seem to be resistant to the disease. This suggests that such pigs either avoid eating the toxic weed or they are accustomed to the weed and do not eat it in sufficient quantity to produce the clinical problem or develop resistance to the toxic principle(s).

In light of the recent findings that the cause of death in perirenal edema is associated with cardiac arrest due to hyperkalemia, it seems rational that management of hyperkalemia may be suitable treatment for this condition. Mineral-corticoid hormones may facilitate potassium excretion and sodium retention. Intravenous administration of a 10 percent solution of calcium gluconate may cause the ECG manifestations to return to normal. Welt (1966) recommends the use of infusions of carbohydrate with or without insulin to promote the movement of potassium into cells. He also recommends the use of exchange resins such as sodium-cycle resins administered by rectum or orally.

REFERENCES

Bennet, P. C. 1964. "Edema Disease," In *Disease of Swine.* 2nd ed. H. W. Dunne, ed. Ames, Iowa: Iowa State University Press, p. 612.

Buck, W. B.; Preston, K. S.; and Abel, M. 1965. Common Weeds as a Cause of Perirenal Edema. *ISU Vet.* 28:105.

Buck, W. B.; Preston, K. S.; Abel, M.; and Marshall, V. L. 1966. Perirenal Edema in Swine. A Disease Caused by Common Weeds. *JAVMA* 148:1525.

Christensen, N. O. 1955. VII International Congress of Comparitive Pathology Report. Cited in Larsen, H. E.; Aalund, O.; and Nielson, K. 1962. Perirenal Edema in Pigs. *Nordisk Vet. Med.* 14:33.

Egyed, M., and Miller, A. 1963. Nitrate Poisoning in Cattle Due to Feeding on *Amaranthus retroflexus Refuah Vet.* 20:167-69.

Jeppesen, Q. E. 1966. Bovine Perirenal Disease Associated with Pigweed. *JAVMA* 149:22.

Kingsbury, J. M. 1964. *Poisonous Plants of the United States and Canada.* Englewood Cliffs, New Jersey: Prentice-Hall, Inc.

Larsen, H. E.; Aalund, O.; and Nielson, K. 1962. Perirenal Edema in Pigs. *Nordisk Vet. Med.* 14:338.

Marshall, V. L.; Buck, W. B.; and Bell, G. L. 1967. Pigweed (*Amaranthus retroflexus*): An Oxalate-Containing Plant. *Am. J. Vet. Res.* 28:888-89.

McNutt, S. H. 1953. Edema Disease. *Adv. Vet. Sci.* 1:301.

Osweiler, G. D. 1968. Toxicologic Effects of Redroot Pigweed (*Amaranthus retroflexus*) in Swine. M.S. Thesis, Library, Iowa State University Ames, Iowa.

Osweiler, G. D.; Buck, W. B.; and Bicknell, E. J. 1969. Experimental Production of Perirenal Edema in Swine with *Amaranthus retroflexus*. *Am. J. Vet. Res.* 30:557-66.

Stuart, B. P.; Nicholson, S. S.; and Smith, J. B. 1975. Perirenal Edema and Toxic Nephrosis in Cattle: Associated with the Ingestion of Pigweed. *JAVMA* 167:949-50.

Welt, L. G. 1966. Water, Salts, and Ions. Agents Affecting Volume and Amposition of Body Fluids. In *Pharmacologic Basis of Therapeutics*. 3rd ed. L. S. Goodman and A. Gilman, eds. New York: The McMillan Co., p. 789.

PLANT TERATOGENS

In recent years the teratogenic effects of plants has been recognized. Some of the more important plants associated with livestock ranges are reviewed here. Much of this material has been abstracted from a paper published by R. F. Keeler in Clinical Toxicology 5:529-65, 1972.

PLANTS KNOWN TO BE TERATOGENIC

Leucaena and Related Plants

Leucaena is a legume known to be toxic to livestock when consumed in large quantities, but still it is an adequate forage for livestock. Ruminants are least susceptible. The toxic principle is mimosine (B-N- [3 hydroxy-4 pyridone]—α-aminopropionic acid), an amino acid. Teratogenic effects observed in swine and rats include increased fetal resorptions and polypodia of forelimbs.

Loco Plants

Certain members of the *Astragalus* and *Oxytropis* genera when ingested by livestock produce a disease called locoism. The signs include a peculiar gait, holding the head high, nervousness and unawareness of surroundings.

Loco plants also give rise to congenital deformities in sheep characterized by excessive carpal flexure and contracted tendons. Some animals have anterior flexure and hypermobility of the tarsal joint. The effects result from plant ingestion at almost any period during gestation. Feeding sheep the synthetic osteolathyrogen (aminoacetonitrile, AAN) produces similar but not identical deformities. Efforts to isolate AAN from loco plants have failed, leaving open the identification of the active principle.

Lupine and Other Genera Containing Quinolizidine Alkaloids

Acute toxicosis with quinolizidine alkaloids is a common toxicoses of sheep on western ranges in the United States. Cattle are less severely affected. The clinical signs include nervousness, difficult breathing, loss of muscular control, excess salivation, convulsions, coma and death.

Ingestion of lupine by cows during gestation is responsible for marked congenital deformities known as "crooked calf disease." This disease is characterized grossly by congenital deformities of the skeletal system including arthrogryposis, torticollis and scoliosis. Cleft palate also occurs.

In lambs congenital defects involve the forelimbs and the lambs are described as being "buck kneed."

Chemical analysis of plants have identified the alkaloid anagyrine and an isomer thermopsine as probable teratogens. The availability of a diagnostic test on lupines for these alkaloids would help in predicting grazing hazard prior to allowing animals access to the plants.

Plants involved include: *Lupinus sericeus* (Silky lupine); *Lupinus caudatus* (Kellogg's spurred lupine); *Thermopsis montana; Sophora arizonica; Sophora stenohylla* and *Cytisus scoparious* (Scotch broom).

Background on Plant Alkaloids

Many plants contain alkaloids, with some surveys indicating 5-10 percent of plant species may be involved. More than 5,000 alkaloids have been identified and given names. The toxicity of most of these is not known. Alkaloids of similar structure are commonly found in closely related plants. Toxic alkaloids produce a strong physiologic reaction in animals. The principal properties of alkaloids are: they are basic in reaction and form salts with acids, are generally water insoluble but are extractable with organic solvents and they are bitter in taste. They are a heterogeneous group of complex compounds containing nitrogen, usually in heterocyclic and/or aromatic ring structure.

The alkaloid content of plants usually varies little with growing season, climate and availability of water. Alkaloids are distributed throughout the plant and consequently, most parts of the plant may be dangerous for livestock.

Some examples of plant alkaloids and the plants involved are given below (see Kingsbury, 1964, pp. 17-59 for more information on plant poisonous principles).

Alkaloid Class	Plant Genus	Common Name
Tropane	*Datura*	Jimsonweed
	Atropa	Bellodonna
Pyrrolizidine	*Senecio*	Groundsel
		Senecio
Pyridine	*Conium*	Poison hemlock
	Nicotiana	Tobacco
Isoquinoline	*Sanguinaria*	Bloodroot
Indole	*Claviceps*	Ergot
Quinolizidine	*Lupinus*	Bluebonnet
		Lupine
	Sophora	Mescalbean
		Frijolita
Solanum (Steroid Alkaloid)	*Solanum*	Nightshades
Veratrum (Steriod Alkaloid)	*Veratrum*	False hellebore
Polycyclic Diterpenes	*Aconitum*	Monkshood
	Delphinium	Larkspur

Veratrum

The work of Binns, James, Shupe and Keeler at the USDA Poisonous Plant Research Laboratory, Logan, Utah has shown the cause of cyclopian lambs to be due to ingestion of *Veratrum californicum* (false hellebore, skunk cabbage) on the fourteenth day of gestation. This plant has been responsible for epidemics of cyclopian lambs on sheep ranches in Idaho. Until the cause was identified in 1973, there was concern among

sheep ranchers that it might be related to bad genetic stock.

Cyclopian abnormalities range from normal eyes and a short upper jaw to true cyclopia with a single medial eye, shortened upper jaw, protruding lower jaw and a skin covered proboscis above the single eye. Hydrocephalus and abnormal pituitary glands are observed. Many affected ewes have prolonged gestations. Three active compounds have been identified and shown to be teratogenic.

Tobacco

It is known that injections of nicotine will cause fetal resorptions in rabbits and mice. Skeletal defects also occur in mice if females are injected during the second week of gestation. Nicotine is also teratogenic in the chick embryo.

Crowe (1969) observed 300 pigs from sixty-four litters on five different farms that were born with skeletal defects. The sows had access to tobacco stalks during gestation. The malformations included twisting of the fore and hind limbs and dorsal flexure of hind limb digits.

Menges *et al.* (1970) reported on a tobacco-related epidemic of congenital deformities of swine. Forty percent (40%) of the offspring of sows with access to tobacco stalks during the first thirty days of gestation were malformed. The malformations were similar to those reported by Crowe.

Crowe and Swerczek (1974) expanded their observations to include 1,000 deformed pigs farrowed by 200 sows on thirteen farms in Kentucky. They confirmed experimentally that either tobacco leaf filtrate, tobacco stalks or tobacco stalk juice induced congenital arthrogryposis when ingested by sows between days four and fifty-three of gestation. The specific teratogenic agent in tobacco is not known. The clinical incidence appears to be related to heavy fertilization.

OTHER SUSPECTED TERATOGENIC PLANTS

Many plants are suspected of being teratogenic. In some cases the evidence is based on clinical field observations and for others on laboratory animal data.

Some clinical evidence suggests that ingestion of jimsonweed will cause arthrogryposis in swine. (Leipold *et al.*, 1973) Other plants suspected of causing arthrogryposis in swine include poison hemlock (*Conium maculatum*) and wild black cherries (*Prunus serotina*).

Alkaloids of the pyrrolizidine class have caused liver lesions in young rats born from treated mothers.

The fruit of the tropical tree akee (*Blighia sapida*)

contains a hypoglycemic compound that is teratogenic in rats. The fruit is eaten by man and if improperly prepared it retains the active agent, a cyclopropane amino acid. While this plant may not represent a threat to livestock there are other plants containing cyclopropane amino and fatty acids that may prove to be hazardous.

The autumn crocus (*Colchicum autumnale*) contains the alkaloid colchicine. All classes of livestock have been poisoned. Colchicine is an agent widely used in genetic studies to inhibit mitosis at the metaphase. A variety of soft tissue and skeletal deformities have been observed in mice.

REFERENCES

Crowe, M. W., and Swerczek, T. W. 1974. Congenital Arthrogryposis in Offspring of Sows Fed Tobacco (*Nicotiana tabacum*). *American Journal of Veterinary Research* 35:1071—73.

Crowe, M. W. 1969. Skeletal Anomalies Associated with Tobacco. *Modern Veterinary Practice* 50:54.

Keeler, R. F. 1972. Known and Suspected Teratogenic Hazards in Range Plants. *Clinical Toxicology* 5:529-65.

Leipold, H. W.; Oehme, F. W.; and Cook, J. E. 1973. Congenital Athrogryposis Associated with Ingestion of Jimson Weed by Pregnant Sows. *Journal of American Veterinary Medical Association* 162:1059-60.

Menges, R. W.; Selby, L A.; Marienfeld, C. J.; Aue, W. A.; and Green, D. L. 1970. A Tobacco-Related Epidemic of Congenital Limb Deformities in Swine. *Environmental Research* 3:285-302.

Anthelmintics

PHENOTHIAZINE

Source

Phenothiazine is frequently used as an anthelmintic for many species of livestock, especially ruminants. Derivatives of phenothiazine are widely used as tranquilizers in medicine and veterinary medicine. Chlorpromazine is the most notable example. Other phenothiazine tranquilizers include promazine, perphenazine, mepazine, trimeprazine, trifluomeprazine, propiopromazine.

Toxicity

Of the domestic animals, the horse is most susceptible to phenothiazine poisoning, followed by the dog, other carnivores and swine. Ruminants and birds are least susceptible. Cattle are more susceptible than goats, with sheep being the least susceptible of all domestic animals. The young and debilitated are more susceptible to toxic effects of phenothiazine. Digestive disturbances such as impaction, constipation and atony promote absorption of the phenothiazine metabolites (oxidation products) and thus increase its toxicity.

Several types of toxic syndromes have been associated with phenothiazine. They include photosensitization, hemolytic anemia, nervous symptoms and abortion. Photosensitization especially accompanied by keratitis is common in calves, but has also occurred in swine, goats, sheep, horses and other animals. Hemolytic anemia is especially common in horses. Central nervous system aberrations are frequently encountered with phenothiazine poisoning in swine and occasionally in horses and cattle. Abortion has been reported in sheep and other animals when phenothiazine is given during the last three weeks of gestation.

The acute toxic dose of phenothiazine varies with the species, physical condition and other factors such as age and state of health. Sheep usually tolerate 160 grams, but have been poisoned on as little as five grams. Cattle six to twelve months of age have tolerated 100 grams for three consecutive days without ill effects. A single dose of 250 grams had slight toxic effects to a young calf. The feeding of one gram per hen per day for eighty-five days produced only loss in weight and lowered egg production in chickens. Swine may tolerate as much as 2.2 g/kg body weight, but as little as 0.5 g/kg body weight has produced poisoning. The horse may be poisoned on 15 grams and 30 grams may be lethal. The toxic dose in the dog is less than the therapeutic dose.

Mechanism of Action

Phenothiazine sulfoxide produced in the alimentary tract is normally detoxified in the liver. When phenothiazine is given in high doses or when predisposing liver damage has occurred, detoxification is not rapid enough to prevent accumulation of the sulfoxide in aqueous humor and development of light sensitization of the cornea and nonpigmented areas of the skin. The degree of sensitization reflects the ability of the liver to detoxify phenothiazine sulfoxide. Sheep are resistant because of greater efficiency in converting phenothiazine sulfoxide to leucophenothiazone and leucothionol.

Hemolytic anemia is especially common in phenothiazine poisoning in horses and dogs. Metabolic derivatives of phenothiazine have a hemolytic effect. It is possible that this effect is due to diphenylamine impurities in the phenothiazine preparation rather than to phenothiazine itself. A dietary deficiency of thiamine apparently increases the susceptibility of dogs to phenothiazine induced hemolysis. Animals on a high protein diet appear to be less susceptible to this effect.

Abortions occur in sheep and goats exposed to phenothiazine during the last three weeks of pregnancy. This may be due to a direct effect upon the fetus.

The metabolic products of phenothiazine excreted by the kidneys are colorless at first, then turn brick red. This is due to oxidation of the metabolic products, leucophenothiazine, and leucothionol, to phenothiazine (red) and thionol (red), respectively. This phenomenon is not an indication of a toxic effect.

Clinical Signs and Physiopathology

As a rule sheep and goats tolerate therapeutic doses of phenothiazine. When toxicosis occurs photosensitization characterized by swelling of the ears, muzzle and bilateral keratitis is characteristic. Young lambs exposed to toxic levels of phenothiazine exhibit ataxia, circling, nystagmus, opisthotonos, and high mortality. As noted above, abortion may occur in animals exposed during late pregnancy. Photosensitization including bilateral keratitis is also a characteristic sign in cattle.

Horses are very susceptible to phenothiazine and exhibit weakness, anorexia, fever, hemolysis, icterus, anemia, hemoglobinuria, oliguria, colic, constipation and diarrhea. Poultry suffering from phenothiazine toxicosis also exhibit photosensitization and keratitis resulting in blindness. There is usually weight loss, decreased egg production and reduced hemoglobin levels.

Signs of poisoning in swine often involve the central nervous system manifested by incoordination, prostration, opisthotonos and circling. Mortality is usually low. Other signs include dermatitis, photosensitization, typhlitis (cecitis) and colitis. Poisoning in carnivora results in absence of deep tendon reflexes of extremeties. Initially there is a peculiar gait which is followed by complete paralysis.

Postmortem changes include subcutaneous edema, and corneal opacities in those animals suffering photosensitization effects. The tissues may be stained with blood pigment associated with hemolysis or light colored organs may be pale due to anemia. The liver and kidneys may have degenerative changes and be very dark colored. Urine and milk often turn red when exposed to air, as noted above.

Diagnosis

A history of phenothiazine administration a few days prior to, or having been fed on a continuous level and associated with typical clinical signs and postmortem changes is sufficient to warrant a presumptive diagnosis of phenothiazine poisoning. Chemical analysis of tissues has very little diagnostic value since it is already known that animals have been exposed and that phenothiazine or its metabolites would be present.

Some disease conditions which must be differentiated from phenothiazine toxicosis include copper poisoning, especially in sheep; plant and chemical photosensitization; hemolytic diseases, such as anaplasmosis and piroplasmosis; and diseases of the central nervous system in swine such as water deprivation and chlorinated hydrocarbon insecticide poisoning.

Treatment

Treatment of phenothiazine poisoning can only be directed toward prevention and alleviation of clinical signs. To prevent phenothiazine poisoning one should refrain from administering such compounds to young or weak and debilitated animals, especially those with evidence of liver injury. Animals that are weak, emaciated, on a low protein and calcium diet, in late pregnancy or suffering secondary infections should be exposed to phenothiazines cautiously. Such precautions may not be practical, however, since phenothiazine is used as an anthelmintic and such animals may be in poor, run-down condition. Phenothiazine should not be administered to dairy cows because of the coloring effect on the milk, to bulls because of the possibility of lowered fertility, and in combination with other drugs such as organophosphorous insecticides.

Animals suffering with phenothiazine photosensitization should be kept out of direct sunlight. Those with anemia should be given a blood transfusion and other blood-building therapeutic agents.

REFERENCES

Blood, D. C., and Henderson, J. A. 1968. *Veterinary Medicine.* 3rd ed. Baltimore: The Williams & Wilkins Co., pp. 798-99.

Clarke, E. G. C., and Clarke, M. L. 1967. *Garner's Veterinary Toxicology.* Baltimore: The Williams & Wilkins Co., pp. 145-49.

Radeleff, R. D. 1970. *Veterinary Toxicology.* 2nd ed. Lea & Febiger pp. 255-57.

Antibacterials

NITROFURANS

The nitrofurans are synthetic compounds that are used as bacteriostats and coccidiostats. They are yellow-colored powders or crystals that are generally sparingly soluble in water.

Source

Nitrofurazone (5-nitro-2-furaldehyde semicarbazone) is recommended as a coccidiostat for chickens at the dosage rate of 50-150 g/ton of feed. It has been used as an aid in the control of certain forms of swine enteritis at the rate of 500 g/ton of ration. It has also been marketed as a water mix to make a suspension in the drinking water of chickens and swine at dosage levels of 302 and 416 mg/gal, respectively. Individual daily doses that have been recommended are: dogs, 10-25 mg/kg; swine, 20-50 mg/kg; lambs and kids, 7 mg/kg. Various solutions and powders have been used to treat topical, uterine, and mastitic infections.

Nitrofurantoin (N-[5-nitro-2-furfurylidene]-1-aminohydantoin) is a nitrofuran that possesses low water solubility but is absorbed and excreted rapidly. It has been utilized in the treatment of chronic respiratory and urinary tract infections of horses and small animals at doses of 4.4 mg/kg every eight hours. Nihydrazone (acetic acid 5- [nitrofurfurylidene]hydrazide) has been used for the treatment of a variety of bacterial and protozoal infections in poultry at the level of 100 g/ton of feed.

Nifuraldezone (5-nitro-2-furaldehyde semioxamazone) is recommended for the treatment of bacterial scours of calves at daily doses of 30 mg/kg. Furaltadone (5-morpholinomethyl-3-[5-nitrofurfurylideneamino]-2-oxazolidinone) is a moderately soluble compound that is used in the intramammary treatment of bovine mastitis.

Furazolidone (3[5-nitrofurfurylideneamino]-2-oxazolidinone) has been used in the treatment of bacterial enteritides of swine at dosages of 100-300 g/ton of feed and for the control of coccidiosis of chickens, turkeys, and rabbits at levels of 7.5-200 g/ton. Baby pigs have been dosed with 100 mg/head/day.

Mechanism of Action

Studies with mammalian tissue slices and bacterial cultures indicate that the nitrofurans inhibit several enzymes that are responsible for aerobic oxidation of glucose and other carbohydrate intermediary substrates, i.e., pyruvate, succinate, glycerol, and lactate. This explains the predominance of neurological symptoms, since the brain possesses relatively high requirements for aerobic oxidation of glucose. Other metabolically active tissues that are reportedly affected are the testes, kidney, and liver.

Toxicity, Clinical Signs, and Physiopathology

The toxicity of nitrofurans appears to be related to the rate of absorption from the gut and, in part, to the degree of water solubility. Humans often develop hypersensitivities to the compounds, but it is also common for some species to develop a tolerance to drug side effects.

Nitrofurazone caused the death of calves within five days when dosed continuously at the rate of 30 mg/kg of body weight. A continuous dose of 15 mg/kg produced hyperirritability and convulsions within nineteen days and death by the twenty-seventh day. A continuous dose of 10 mg/kg produces varying degrees of toxicosis and depresses weight gains, but a dose of 5 mg/kg appears to be tolerated by calves. The LD_{50} of nitrofurazone for laboratory rats and mice, however, appears to be within the range of 380-590 mg/kg; and symptomatology includes hyperirritability, tremors, weakness, convulsions, and respiratory arrest. Rats fed 0.1 and 0.2 percent in feed for five weeks and rhesus monkeys dosed with 300 mg/day failed to produce clinical, hematologic, or histologic changes; rats fed at levels of 0.4 percent of the drug in the feed for five weeks appeared cachectic and hyperexcitable. Daily intravenous dosing to dogs caused hepatitis with dullness, diarrhea, and vomiting when the dose was equal to or more than 2.2 mg/kg. Single oral doses of 150-200 mg of nitrofurazone/kg of body weight to young chicks caused depression of hyperexcitability with convulsions within four hours. Ducklings are relatively sensitive, with a level of 0.022 percent (200 g/ton) in the feed causing 50 percent mortality. Nitrofurazone has been withdrawn from the market for human use because of toxicities and sensitivities.

Nitrofurantoin, being used as a systemic drug, would appear more apt to cause toxicosis; but there is a paucity of information on the toxicology of the drug in veterinary medicine. In humans, toxic symptoms are frequent and include vomiting, diarrhea, neuritis, sensitization, nephritis, and hemolytic anemia. Demyelination of peripheral nerves was found during necropsy.

Furazolidone and nihydrazone have not been commonly reported as causing toxicosis, perhaps due to their relatively poor absorbability from the gut. Furazolidone at the continuous level of 400 g/ton reportedly caused a chronic neuritis in chickens.

Furaltadone, a relatively soluble nitrofuran, has not been incriminated in toxicosis, perhaps since its use is restricted to intramammary infusions. It reportedly has caused toxic polyneuritis in humans after oral doses of 20 mg/kg and above had been given for several weeks.

Nifuraldezone has not been reported as causing toxicosis; but when doses of 54-72 mg/kg, approximately twice the recommended therapeutic dose, were given to dogs, they exhibited vomiting, anorexia, ataxia, and spastic paralysis.

Diagnosis

Diagnosis of nitrofuran toxicosis may be difficult. A history of nitrofuran therapy with symptoms of CNS disturbances may justify a tentative positive diagnosis, which may be substantiated by a chemical analysis of the ration. Chemical analyses of tissues for drug residues are not applicable due to the rapid degradation and excretion from the body. Most cases of toxicosis involve drug misuse such as overdosing and utilizing drugs for nonrecommended uses of species.

Treatment

The initial treatment should include withdrawal of the drug. Other treatments are symptomatic and may include correction of uremia, dehydration, or starvation.

Case History

A Wisconsin veterinary practitioner dispensed Nitrofurazone WD, 1,500-mg tablets, Vet-A-Mix, Inc. Each tablet contained 1,500 mg nitrofurazone, and recommended daily dosages on the label were 7 mg/kg for kids and lambs and 20-50 mg/kg for swine; there were no recommendations for use in calves. The practitioner prescribed 1,500 mg b.i.d., or a daily dose of *ca.* 100 mg/kg, for the treatment of calf scours on three farms. Most treated calves displayed convulsions and hyperirritability within twelve hours. Lead poisoning was suspected as a cause on two farms and confirmed on one farm but was neither confirmed nor disproved on the other farm. Medication was discontinued on the third farm after the second day. Animals were force-fed milk, and by the third day three of six had recovered from convulsions and scours. This case exemplifies an example of drug misuse, *i.e.,* unapproved drug therapy and an unusually high dosage.

REFERENCES

Carson, T. L. 1972. Toxicology of Nitrofurazone. Term paper, Vet. Path. 590, Iowa State University.

Deichmann, W. B., and Gerarde, H. W. 1969. *Toxicology of Drugs and Chemicals.* New York: Academic Press.

Garner, R. J. 1967. *Veterinary Toxicology.* Glascow, Scotland: The University Press.

Jones, L. M. 1965. *Veterinary Pharmacology and Therapeutics.* Ames, Iowa: Iowa State University Press.

Lloyd, W. E. 1965. From Vet-A-Mix, Inc. Files, Shenandoah, Iowa.

SULFONAMIDES

Source

Sulfonamides are bacteriostatic synthetic compounds that are widely utilized in veterinary medicine in the therapeusis of bacterial infections. In recent years, they have been used prophylactically in livestock rations. They are white powders that are sparingly soluble in water but very soluble in alkaline and strong acid solutions.

Toxicity and Mechanisms of Action

Sulfonamide toxicosis is most prevalent in dogs, cats, poultry, and baby calves following individual dosing or therapeutic applications in feed. Three types of syndromes have been noted. An acute "drug shock" is frequently observed when sulfonamide solutions are rapidly injected intravenously. A second chronic condition results from renal tubule obstruction by sulfonamide crystals. The third syndrome is a hypersensitivity that appears as an anaphylactoid reaction following extended and repeated dosings; both asthmatic and urticarial symptoms have been reported.

The mechanisms of action appear to be variable. The cause of acute toxicity is unknown. Rapid intravenous infusions of sodium sulfonamide solutions to cattle cause mydriasis, ataxia, blindness, collapse, and possibly death; but the toxicosis is not related to the relatively high alkalinity (pH 9.0-11.4) of the solutions. Large parenteral or oral doses to dogs and man have reportedly caused emesis, ataxia, spastic paralysis, epileptiform convulsions, and diarrhea which may be controlled with pentobarbital. Sulfonamides potentiate the action of curare, and it is postulated they may act on both the central nervous system and motor nerve end plates.

The chronic, or renal form, of sulfonamide poisoning is related to the solubility of sulfonamides and their metabolites. Sulfonamides are amphoteric, being relatively insoluble in slightly acid aqueous solutions and increase in solubility as the pH increases. Therefore, crystal formation in kidney tubules is most common in carnivores, which produce an acid urine. Sulfonamides are metabolized to varying degrees, usually to the conjugated or acetylated form. With the exceptions of the pyrimidine sulfonamides, *i.e.,* sulfamethazine, sulfamerazine, and sulfadiazine, the acetylated forms readily pass through biological membranes but are less soluble in urine and other aqueous solutions than the parent compounds.

High excretion rates increase kidney crystal formation. Sulfathiazole has been discontinued for use in humans due to the fact that its rates of acetylation and excretion are high and the drug often caused toxicosis. Finally animals which are dehydrated or lack adequate water intake are prone to chronic toxicosis. Most cases result from overdosing animals individually or in the feed to animals which have limited water supplies or high fluid loss due to diarrhea. It is almost impossible to induce chronic renal damage in mammals from the dosing of sodium salts in drinking water *ad lib,* since strong concentrations are unpalatable.

Hypersensitivity, a third type of toxicosis, has been observed in cattle which had previously received therapeutic doses of sulfamethazine orally and were being injected intravenously with a solution of sodium sulfamethazine. These anaphylactoid reactions apparently are not necessarily specific and may be due to cross-immunogenic reactions. Other sulfonamides reportedly have caused urticaria and hives in cattle and horses. It is plausible that "drug fever," seen occasionally with sulfonamide drugs, is an elicitation of hypersensitivity.

Sulfonamides can also cause several secondary metabolic reactions when given for long periods at therapeutic or lower doses. The compounds interfere with iodine metabolism, are goitrogenic, and may cause hyperplasia of the thyroid and reduced thyroid funtion. They may cause reduced growth rate. Sulfonamides commonly cause methemoglobinemia and carbonic anhydrase inhibition with resultant acidosis and diuresis. They reportedly cause agranulocytosis and hypoprothrombinemia. Sulfaquinoxaline causes increased clotting time, but small doses of sulfamethazine reportedly have improved the clotting time in pigs. Peripheral neuritis has been reported in chickens fed large quantities of sulfonamides. Sulfonamides may also cause reduced egg production in chickens, arrested fetal development in rats, and atrophy of the male genital tract when fed continuously at levels of 0.05 to 0.5 percent. Except for depression of growth and development, most of the latter miscellaneous toxic conditions are reversible. Short-term therapeutic doses and continuous use in rations at levels of 0.01 to 0.05 percent reportedly have not caused these types of toxicological problems.

Clinical Signs, Physiopathology, Diagnosis, and Treatment

Diagnosis of the acute "drug shock" phenomenon is based largely on history and symptomatology, and the cause usually is evident enough to warrant a diagnosis. The best treatment of any acute sulfonamide toxicosis is reduction of the dose or administration rate plus alleviation of the symptom.

Diagnosis of the "chronic" uremic form may be more difficult, especially if owners are treating animals or flocks covertly. History is nevertheless important, especially to ascertain the existence of sulfonamide therapy. It usually takes five to seven days to develop a lethal uremic toxicosis. Doses that cause toxicosis vary with the drug and the animals' states of hydration. In most cases, the traditional dosage of 70-100 mg/lb body weight or the dosing time limit of three to five days has been exceeded.

Symptomatology during the uremic form may reveal anorexia, depression, and collapse. Hematuria, albuminuria, and oliguria may be present; and frequently sulfonamide crystals may be observed on preputial or vulvar hairs. Antemortem chemical analyses of whole unclotted blood for BUN and sulfonamides are valuable. The presence of elevated BUN levels with total sulfonamide levels in excess of 15 mg/100 ml is diagnostic. Necropsy reveals few gross changes except the frequent presence of sulfonamide crystals in the renal tubules and pelvis. Histopathological specimens of kidneys should be fixed in a slightly acidified formalin solution or absolute ethanol to prevent dissolution of the crystals, which are readily noted in the tubules during microscopic examination of stained slides, especially with polarized lighting.

In cases involving forensic toxicology, chemical analyses of rations or tissues may be advisable. When chemically analyzing feeds for sulfonamides, it must be remembered that arsanilic acid and procaine penicillin give false positive reactions. Chemical analysis of tissues is difficult, but the drugs are stable and persist for several days after drug withdrawal. Levels in muscle, kidney, or liver above 20 ppm justify a positive diagnosis. Treatment involves drug withdrawal and reestablishment of renal function. Rehydration of the animal should be done by prudently administering isotonic mixed or alkalinizing solutions intravenously, plus oral administration of alkalinizing electrolytes and water.

Diagnosis of hypersensitive reactions is largely based on clinical signs and history, especially establishing the probability of previous sensitizing doses. In the case of intravenous medication, anaphylactoid asthmatic reactions may be mistaken for "drug shock," from which the animal usually recovers spontaneously. Treatment of hypersensitive reactions is symptomatic and should include immediate cessation of drug administration and injections of antihistamines. In the case of asthmatic reactions, epinephrine should be injected subcutaneously or intravenously.

Case History

An Iowa veterinary practitioner prescribed sulfaquinoxaline as the sodium salt to be administered in the drinking water of chicken broilers for the treatment of coccidiosis at the rate of 0.04 percent for three days. Five days later the flock owner returned with four dead birds and reported that several more were ataxic. Postmortem examination revealed swollen, light-colored kidneys that "grated" when cut due to the presence of crystals. The owner was questioned and it was revealed that he had administered the sulfaquinoxaline solution for five days plus a solution of 0.2 percent sulfamethazine for the past seven days and concurrently with the sulfaquinoxaline. The medicated water was replaced with clean, unmedicated water, and the flock recovered with a death loss of approximately 5 percent. This case exemplifies the importance of obtaining a complete and accurate history of each case, including the possibility of previous or concurrent medications. It also points out the dangers of overdosing of sulfonamides specifically. These principles should be considered in all cases involving suspected drug toxicoses.

REFERENCES

Goodman, L. S.; and Gilman, A. 1970. *The Pharmacological Basis of Therapeutics.* New York: The Macmillan Company.

Jones, L. M. 1965. *Veterinary Pharmacology and Therapeutics*. Ames, Iowa: Iowa State University Press.

Lloyd, W. E. 1971-72. Research data, Vet-A-Mis, Inc., Shenandoah, Iowa.

Righter, H. F.; Worthington, J. W.; and Mercer, H. D. 1971. Tissue-Residue Depletion of Sulfamethazine in Calves and Chickens. *Amer. J. Vet. Res.* 32(7):1003-06.

Schneller, G. H. *et al.* 1948. Sulfonamides in Veterinary Medicine. *Calco Technical Bull.* No. 723, American Cyanamid Company, Bound Brook, New Jersey.

Sodeman, W. A. 1968. *Pathologic Physiology, Mechanisms of Disease*. Philadelphia: W. B. Saunders Company.

Stowe, C. M.; Hartman, W.; and Pallesen, D. 1956. Studies with Sulfonamide Combinations in Dairy Cattle. *JAVMA* 129:384-87.

Fungicides

ORGANIC SYNTHETIC
FUNGICIDES

As a general class, fungicides are all those chemical agents used to prevent or eradicate fungal infections from plants and seeds. The types of fungicides used in agriculture and food processing range from those of relatively low toxicity to mammals to those which are highly lethal and tend to persist for long periods. The recommendations and restrictions concerning fungicides generally preclude poisoning in animals. Accidents and careless use constitute the major source of hazard to mammals.

The fungicides are used as seed protectants, foliage and blossom protectants, and fruit protectants. A few are used to eradicate established fungal infestations, and some are employed in soil fumigation. In general, those compounds designed to eradicate a fungus are inherently more toxic and thus more hazardous to plants and livestock than are the protectants.

There are at least 250 major brand names of fungicides. New brands or types are introduced each year. If problems of poisoning from fungicides are suspected, realization of the general type involved and its active ingredient will aid in diagnosis, prognosis, and treatment. Table 1 lists the major fungicides and their most probable usage classification.

In addition to problems arising from direct exposure to fungicides, these compounds are often combined with insecticides such as dieldrin or malathion. Thus, careful history gathering and examination may be necessary to obtain a proper diagnosis.

Many of the carriers or solvents for fungicides are in themselves toxic. Carbon disulfide, carbon tetrachloride, ethylene dibromide, formaldehyde, petroleum ethers, low molecular weight hydrocarbons, and sulfur dioxide may accompany or serve as a carrier for fungicides. Animals housed in close confinement near treated grain may suffer from the vapors of these volatile compounds.

Some of the fungicides are discussed on the following pages. Other fungicides are discussed under other headings. See the sections on **mercury, copper** and **pentachlorophenol.**

Benomyl

Benomyl is a new carbamate fungicide developed since 1968. It differs from the two older carbamate fungicides zineb and maneb in that benomyl does not contain a metal cation. The structural formula is shown in figure 1. It is a white crystalline solid that decomposes without melting above 300° C.

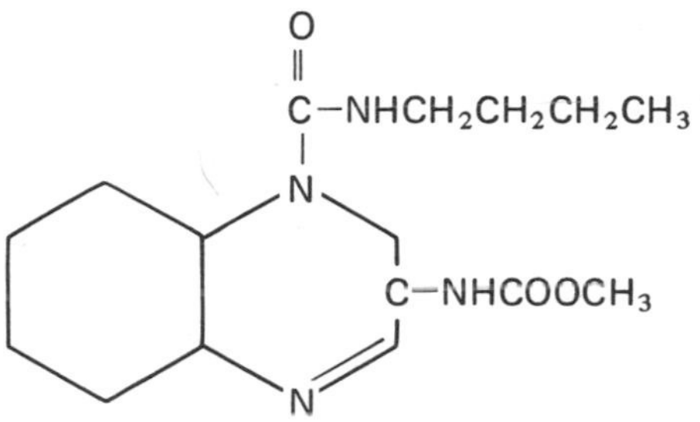

Figure 1. Structure of benomyl.

The oral LD_{50} in rats is greater than 10g/kg. Benomyl is excreted in the urine and feces with 99 percent of oral doses eliminated in seventy-two hours. Based on two-year feeding trials in dogs and rats, benomyl and its metabolites do not accumulate in animal tissues. The principal residues on crops are benomyl itself and methyl 2-benzimidazolecarbamate. (Baude *et al.,* 1973)

Feeding rats 0.25 percent benomyl in the diet in a three-generation reproduction study did not affect reproduction or lactation. No pathologic changes were found in tissues from weanling pups. No teratogenic effects were found when rats were fed up to 0.50 percent benomyl in the diet from days six to fifteen of gestation. Benomyl is rapidly metabolized to methyl 2- benzimidazolecarbamate in the rat. (Sherman *et al.,* 1975)

153

TABLE 1
Active Ingredients and Common Usage of Some Major Fungicides

Common Name	Chemical Name	Trade Names	Use
Benomyl	Methyl 1-(butylcarbamoyl)-2-benzimidazolecarbamate	Benlate	Foliage and soil, preventative and curative
Captan	N-Trichloromethylmercapto-4-Cyclohexene—1,2 dicarboximide	Orthocide 50-W Captan 50-W Orthocide 75	Seed, foliage and fruit protectants
Chloranil	Tetrachloroparabenzoquinone	Spergon	Seed protectant
Dichlone	2,3 Dichloro, 1,4-Naphthoquinone	Phygon XL Phygon 50-W	
Dodine	Dodecylguanidine acetate	Cyprex	
Ferbam	Ferric dimethyl dithiocarbamate	Fermate Ferradow	Foliage and blossom protectants
Glyodin	2—Heptadecyl-glyoxaladine		
HCB	Hexachlorobenzene-C_6Cl_6	No Bunt, Sanocide	Cereal grains
Maneb	Manganese ethylenebisdithiocarbamate	Manzate Dithane M 22	Fruit protectant
Metham sodium	Sodium N-methyldithiocarbamate	Vapam	
Nabam	Disodium ethylenebisdithiocarbamate	Dithane D-14 Parfate Liquid Thiodow	Fruit protectant
PCNB	Pentachloronitrobenzene	Teraclor	Soil
Terrazole	5-Ethoxy-3-trichloromethyl 1-1, 2, 4-thiadiazole	Terrazole	Soil
Tetrachloroisophthalonitrile	Tetrachloroisophthalonitrile	Daconil 2787 Exothermtermil Termil	Plants
Thiram	Tetramethyl-thiuram disulfide	Arasam Panoram Thylate	Seed and fruit protectant
Zineb	Zinc ethylenebisdithiocarbamate	Parzate Dithane Z-78	
Ziram	Zinc dimethyl dithiocarbamate	Corozate Karbam white	
Mercurials	Mercuric chloride Mercurous chloride	Corrosive sublimate Calogreem Calomel Subchloride of mercury	Eradicants Seed protectant
Organomercurials	Ethyl or Methyl mercury derivatives of various organic compounds	Argon Ceresan Chipcote Mersol Panogen Puratized Setrete	Seed protectants Fungal eradicants

Captan

Captan (N-trichloromethylmercapto-4-cyclohexene-1,2 dicarboxamide) is a widely used, organic nonmercurial fungicide. Its toxicity to mammals is quite low. The LD$_{50}$ for rats is approximately 480 mg/kg orally and 50 to 100 mg/kg intraperitoneally. The lowest lethal dose in the mouse is 9 mg/kg given intraperitoneally.

Acute poisoning may be caused by doses of 250 to 500 mg/kg in ruminants. Clinical signs are labored respiration, anorexia, depression, and death.

Necropsy examination reveals hydrothorax, ascites, petechial hemorrhage of the gall bladder, and inflammation of the gastrointestinal tract.

Repeated small doses of captan have no apparent adverse effect on weight gain.

Injecting captan into fertile eggs results in malformations of the head, wings, legs and lower body. However, captan is neither embryotoxic nor teratogenic in rabbits, albino rats, golden Syrian hamsters, or rhesus and stump-tailed monkeys.

Carbamate Fungicides

The carbamate fungicides are all derivatives of dithiocarbamic acid (NH_2CS_2H). There are three major derivatives of this basic structure as follows:

1. Thiuram disulfides—This is a combinatiom of two dithiocarbamic acid molecules joined in a disulfide linkage.
2. Metallic dithiocarbamates—Dithiocarbamic acid is complexed with a metal cation, usually iron or zinc.
3. Ethylenebisdithiocarbamates—Combination of two parallel metallic dithiocarbamates.

Two of the better known carbamate fungicides are maneb (manganous ethylene bisdithiocarbamate) and zineb (zinc ethylene bisdithiocarbamate). Both of these are used on vegetables, fruits and nuts, field crops and ornamentals. The rat oral LD_{50} for maneb is 6,700 mg/kg and 5,200 mg/kg for zineb. The acute toxicity is low with dosages of 500 mg/kg for fifteen days required to produce toxicosis in sheep (zineb). The clinical signs are nonspecific consisting of depression, anorexia and diarrhea.

Necropsy lesions include friable, hemorrhagic livers, degeneration and inflammation of kidneys and congestion of the lungs.

The metallic dithiocarbamates may have a chronic effect on the thyroid gland. Feeding rats or dogs for thirty days to two years resulted in thyroid hyperplasia and reduced iodine concentration rates. Some investigators suggest that the dithiocarbamates block the enzymatic organification of iodine.

The ethylenebisdithiocarbamate fungicides are degraded to several compounds including ethylenethiourea (ETU). ETU is a carcinogen in rats when fed at 125 ppm for twelve months. Thyroid weight is increased with thyroid nodular hyperplasia and adenocarcinoma. (Graham et al., 1973) ETU may be teratogenic in the rat (10-80 mg/kg) but not in the rabbit. (Klera, 1973)

Chloroneb

Chloroneb (Demosan 65W E.I. du Pont) 1,4-dichloro-2,5-dimethoxybenzene has been used to reduce seedling diseases of cotton, beans and soybeans when used in conjunction with a standard seed protective fungicide. Plants take up chloroneb into the roots and lower stems. The half-life in soil is three to six months when incorporated into the soil two to three inches below the surface. Residues in bean and cotton seed were 3-78 ppb.

A dog was fed 500 ppm for one year, rats were fed 2,500 ppm for two years, and two cows were fed 2 or 50 ppm for thirty days. Toxic effects, if any, were not discussed. The only metabolite found in the urine of the dog, rats, and cows was 2,5-dichloro-4-methoxyphenol (DCMP). At the 2 ppm feeding level no chloroneb or DCMP was found in the milk (0.02 ppm). At the 50 ppm feeding level 0.3-0.4 ppm DCMP was reported in the milk. The residue disappeared two days after feeding stopped.

Dinitroorthocresol

This compound is a by-product of the dye industry. It is used as a fungicide, insecticide, wood preservative, and herbicide.

Absorption may be either oral, respiratory, or percutaneous. Dinitro derivatives produce uncoupling of oxidative phosphorylation resulting in increased oxidative processes with energy converted to heat instead of ATP. Clinically, this is manifested as fever, acidosis, and parenchymatous damage to liver, kidneys, and myocardium. The toxic effects are potentiated by increased environmental temperature. The LD_{50} for dogs and swine is approximately 50 mg/kg.

All species exhibit similar clinical signs. Listlessness, anorexia, deep rapid respiration, thirst, oliguria, hyperpyrexia, weakness, and death are characteristic clinical signs. There is usually progressive respiratory distress until collapse or death. Abortion may occur. Recovery from acute exposure is usually within six to twelve hours. In animals dying of dinitrocresol or dinitrophenol poisoning, onset of rigor mortis is almost immediate.

Both dinitrocresol and dinitrophenol are persistent yellow dyes. External skin, hair and lips may be stained yellow. Yellowish or orange coloration of stomach contents and liver, and yellow-green tinged urine are suggestive of poisoning. The sclera may also be stained yellow.

Hyperpyrexia, dyspnea, early rigor mortis, and yellow discoloration of the organs should suggest dinitrocresol or dinitrophenol as possible etiologic agents. Whole blood levels in excess of 10 mg/100 ml dinitrocresol correlates with poisoning. Presence of β-carotene in blood may interfere with this test.

Administer gastric lavage for oral exposure, using 5 percent sodium bicarbonate and activated charcoal. Catharsis with sodium sulfate is also indicated. Paraffin oil (but not castor oil) may be used because the dinitrocresol is fat soluble, but the paraffin oil is not absorbed. Keeping the patient cool (*e.g.,* with ice packs) is helpful and administration of thiouracil to slow the metabolic rate may be indicated.

Dichlone

The LC_{50} in birds is greater than 5,000 ppm. The oral LD_{50} in rats is 1,300 mg/kg.

Ferbam

Approximately 40-70 percent of oral doses are absorbed from the gastrointestinal tract (rat). The compound is eliminated in the urine and to a small extent in bile. Urinary metabolites include inorganic sulfate, dimethylammonium ion and a glucuronide conjugate of dimethyl-dithiocarbamate.

Hexachlorobenzene (HCB)

Hexachlorobenzene is a crystalline substance (C_6Cl_6) that is insoluble in water. It is also used in organic synthesis. Residues have been found in predatory birds, fish and mussels. A mass poisoning occurred in Turkey involving 3,000 human cases with the main symptoms being photosensitization and porphyrinuria. (Cam and Nigogosyan, 1963)

The oral lethal dose in guinea pigs is greater than 3 g/kg. In Japanese quail 20 ppm killed two of fourteen birds in ninety days. The no-effect level is 1 ppm. Liver weights increase with some liver necrosis, bile duct proliferation and hypertrophy of nucleoli at 5 ppm. Tissue residues after ninety days feeding of 5 ppm were 7 ppm (liver) and 1 ppm (brain). (Vos *et al.,* 1971)

In rats the chronic oral LD_{50} is 640 ppm. Young rats are more susceptible with the LD_{50} less than 160 ppm. Doses of 120 mg/kg are embryotoxic. The oral LD_{50} values are: 3,500 mg/kg (rat), 1,700 mg/kg (cat) and 2,600 mg/kg (rabbit).

Maneb

Maneb is discussed under carbamate fungicides in this section.

Metham Sodium

The LC_{50} in birds is greater than 5,000 ppm. The oral LD_{50} values are 700 mg/kg (rat) and 50 mg/kg (mouse).

Methyl Bromide

Methyl bromide is a highly volatile, nonflammable, nonexplosive liquid with high penetrating power used as a fumigating agent. It no longer is used as a refrigerant and fire extinguisher because of its toxicity. The first fatal case of poisoning was reported in 1899. Lethal concentrations range from 300-6,425 ppm in the air.

Bromide residues were found in 232 food samples with a range of 0.5-84 ppm (total bromides) in the total diet survey for June 1968-April 1969. Other reports recorded natural bromide levels of 2.1 ppm (wheat), 2.3-3.9 ppm (oats), 1.5-1.9 ppm (corn), 5.6 ppm (barley), 2.1 ppm (peas), 10 ppm (lentils). Of 155 corn samples taken from ship holds 117 had residues less than 50 ppm. The samples were taken at the times of unloading. The residues are thought to decrease when the grain is aired or stored.

Chronic mild exposure leads to polyneuropathy. Acute exposure leads to headache, dizziness, nausea, vomiting, generalized weakness followed by mental excitement, focal or generalized seizures and tremors. In fatal cases coma, muscle spasms, seizure, fever and death compose the sequence of events. Convalescence may last eighteen months.

Nabam

The LC_{50} in birds is greater than 5,000 ppm. Eleven percent (11%) mortality occurred in Bobwhite at 5,000 ppm. The rat oral LD_{50} is 395 mg/kg.

Organotin Compounds

Organotin compounds, especially triphenyltin hydroxide and triphenyltinacetate, have been used commercially as fungicides since about 1954. In Britain about 25 percent of the potato acreage is treated with triphenyltin. Residues on harvested potatoes were only 1-6 ppb.

Acute toxicities of organotin compounds are listed in table 2.

Note that, as with mercury, the methyl, ethyl and propyl organic tin compounds are highly toxic and that toxicosis involves the nervous system.

PCNB

The no-effect level in a three-generation rat reproductive study was 500 ppm. In dogs the two-year no-effect level was 30 ppm. In dogs fed 180-1,080 ppm cholestatic hepatosis with secondary bile nephrosis occurred but was considered reversible. PCNB is not stored in the tissues of the rat, dog or cow. Traces of PCNB occur in cow's milk. The metabolites pentachloroaniline and methyl pentachlorophenyl sulfide are found in tissues at levels generally less than 1 ppm. The metabolites were not found in rat tissues when control diets were fed for sixty days after feeding the PCNB diet. (Borzelleca et al., 1971)

PCNB has produced renal agenesis in one strain of mice (C57BL/6) at doses of 215-464 mg/kg but not in a second strain of mice (AKR). (Courtney, 1973) PCNB at 125 mg/kg in rats was neither embryolethal or teratogenic. (Jordan et al., 1975)

Sulfur

Sulfur or lime sulfur is one of the oldest fungicides. Pure sulfur (flours of sulfur) or lime sulfur is not highly toxic. Approximately 250 mg/kg are required to poison cattle or horses. A ration containing 2 percent or more sulfur may be harmful to chickens.

The toxicity of sulfur is due to superpurgation and local irritation. Violent purgation, colic, dullness and "muddy" colored mucous membranes are seen. Dermal exposure may cause erythema, pruritis and pain.

Necropsy lesions are those of inflammatory gastroenteritis and congestion of liver and kidneys. There may be excess gas and a hydrogen sulfide odor from the gastrointestinal tract.

TABLE 2
Toxicity of Organic Tin Compounds

Compound	Species	Toxicity	Compound	Species	Toxicity
Di-n-octyl-tin-bis [2-ethyl-hexyl-mercaptoacetate]	Mouse	Oral LD_{50} = 2,010 mg/kg	Triethyl-tin	Rat	5 ppm in drinking water. Posterior paralysis in 15 days in adult female rat. Young rats were clinically normal but brains showed status spongiosus at 1, 3 and 4 months
Di-n-octyl-tin-bis [dodecyl-mercaptide]	Mouse	Oral LD_{50} = 4,000 mg/kg			
Di-n-octyl-tin-bis [butyl-mercapto-acetate]	Mouse	Oral LD_{50} = 1,140 mg/kg	Dimethyl dichloro tin	Rat	I.V. LD_{50} = 40 mg/kg
Mono-n-octyl-tin-tris-[2-ethyl-hexyl-mercapto-acetate]	Mouse	Oral LD_{50} = 1,500 mg/kg	Diethyl dichloro tin	Rat	I.V. LD_{50} = 25 mg/kg
			Di-n-propyl dichloro tin	Rat	I.V. LD_{50} = 7 mg/kg
Triethyl-tin	Rat	5 mg/kg for 3 days lead to 100% mortality in day old, 8 day and adult rats. Lesions included swollen brains, petechial hemorrhages of cerebrum and cerebellum, status spongiosus of myelinated tracts, cerebrum and cerebellum.	Diisopropyl dichloro tin	Rat	I.V. LD_{50} = 15 mg/kg
			Dibutyl dichloro tin	Rat	I.V. LD_{50} = 5 mg/kg
			Di-2-ethylhexyltin dichloride	Rat	I.V. LD_{50} = 5 mg/kg
			Bis (tri-n-butyltin) oxide	Rat	Oral LD_{50} = 194 mg/kg 32 or 10 ppm in food for 30 days—depressed growth but no deaths; 320 ppm for 30 days—some deaths.

Tetrachloroisophthalonitrile

Tetrachloroisophthalonitrile is a crystalline, white, tasteless compound with a slightly pungent odor.

The acute oral LD_{50} values are: rat = greater than 10 g/kg and dog = greater than 5 g/kg. The acute dermal LD_{50} in rabbits is greater than 10 g/kg. Mild to moderate skin irritation occurs at 500-1,000 mg/kg in rabbits. The acute oral LD_{50} in quail is 5,200 ppm. This compound is relatively toxic to fish with LD_{50} values of 250-432 ppb. At 1.5-3.0 percent of the diet, dogs showed anorexia and weight loss in a two-year feeding study. Liver, kidney and thyroid weights increased in dogs in the two-year exposure. The no-effect level in dogs is 120 ppm. The compound is not stored in tissues and is eliminated in the feces. (Eisler, 1970)

Terrazole®

The acute oral LD_{50} values are: rat = 1,077 mg/kg, rabbit = 779 mg/kg and dogs = more than 5 g/kg. The two-year oral no-effect level in rats is greater than 640 ppm. In dogs fed 1,000 ppm for two years there was decreased weight gain and increased serum cholinesterase, BSP retention and liver weights. Lesions included hepatosis with secondary bile nephrosis. No adverse effects were noted in dogs fed 10 or 100 ppm for two years. In a three-generation rat reproductive study no effects were found except for depressed weaning weights and adult weights in the 640 ppm group. (Borzelleca *et al.,* 1971)

Thiram

The LD_{50} in birds is greater than 5,000 ppm. Mallards fed 5,000 ppm had a 20 percent mortality. Oral LD_{50} values are: 560 mg/kg (rat) and 210 mg/kg (rabbit). The lowest lethal dose in the cat is 230 mg/kg.

Zineb

Zineb is discussed under carbamate fungicides in this section.

REFERENCES

Baude, F. J.; Gardiner, J. A.; and Han, J. C-Y. 1973. Characterization of Residues on Plants Following Foliar Spray Applications of Benomyl. *J. Agr. Food Chem.* 21:1084-90.

Borzelleca, J. F.; Larson, P. S.; Crawford, E. M.; Hennigar, G. R.; Kuchar, E. J.; and Klein, H. H. 1971. Toxicologic and Metabolic Studies on Pentachloronitrobenzene. *Toxicology and Applied Pharmacology* 18:522-34.

Borzelleca, J. F.; Larson, P. S.; and Kuchar, E. J. 1971. A Toxicologic Evaluation of 5-ethoxy-3-trichloromethyl 1-1,2,4-thiadiazole (Terrazole). *Toxicology and Applied Pharmacology* 19:400.

Cam, C., and Nigogosyan, G. 1963. Acquired Toxic Porphyria Cutanea Tarda Due to Hexachlorobenzene. *J. Amer. Med. Assn.* 183:88-91.

Courtney, D. 1973. The Effect of Pentachloronitrobenzene on Fetal Kidneys. *Toxicology and Applied Pharmacology* 24:455.

Eisler, M. 1970. The Toxicology and Biological Activity of Tetrachloroisophthalonitrile. Cleveland, Ohio: Diamond Shamrock Chemical Company.

Gerarde, H. W. 1964. Toxicology: Organic. *Ann. Rev. Pharm.* 4:223-46.

Graham, S. L.; Hansen, W. H.; Davis, K. J.; and Perry, C. H. 1973. Effects of One-year Administration of Ethylenethiourea Upon the Thyroid of the Rat. *J. Agr. Food Chem.* 21:324-29.

Greenberg, J. O. 1971. The Neurological Effects of Methyl Bromide Poisoning. *Ind. Med.* 40:27-29.

Heath, R. G.; Spann, J. W.; Hill, E. F.; and Kreitzer, J. F. 1972. Comparative Dietary Toxicities of Pesticides to Birds. Special Scientific Report. Wildlife No. 152. U.S. Department of the Interior, Fish and Wildlife Service, Washington, D.C.

Hodgson, J. R.; Hoch, J. C.; Castles, T. R.; Helton, D. O.; and Lee, C-C. 1975. Metabolism and Disposition of Ferbam in the Rat. *Toxicology and Applied Pharmacology* 33:505-13.

Ivanova-Chemishanska, I.; Markov, D. U.; and Dashev, G. 1971. Light and Electron Microscopic Observations on Rat Thyroid After Administration of Some Dithiocarbamates. *Environ. Res.* 4:201-12.

Jordan, R. L.; Sperling, F.; Klein, H. H.; and Borzelleca, J. F. 1975. A Study of the Potential Teratogenic Effects of Pentachloronitrobenzene in Rats. *Toxicology and Applied Pharmacology.* 33:222-30.

Klera, R. S. 1973. Ethylenethiourea: Teratogenicity Study in Rats and Rabbits. *Teratology.* 7:243-252.

Pelikan, Z., and Cerny, E. 1970. The Toxic Effects of Some Di- and Mono-N-octyl-Tin Compounds on White Mice. *Arch. Toxikol.* 26:196-202.

Sherman, H.; Culik, R.; and Jackson, R. A. 1975. Reproduction, Teratogenic and Mutagenic Studies with Benomyl. *Toxicology and Applied Pharmacology* 32:305-15.

Rhodes, R. C., and Pease, H. L. 1971. Fate of Chloroneb in Animals. *J. Agr. Food Chem.* 19:750-53.

Rhodes, R. C.; Pease, H. L.; and Brantley, R. K. 1971. Fate of C^{14}-Labelled Chloroneb in Plants and Soils. *J. Agr. Food Chem.* 19:745-49.

Truhaut, R.; Guerinot, F.; and Bohuvon, C. 1971. Biochemical Mechanism of the Toxicity of the Fungicides of Dithiocarbamates Series: Inhibitory Action upon Dopamine β-Hydroxylase Activity. *Annales Pharm. Franc.* 29:117-24.

Vondruska, J.; Fancher, O. E.; and Calandra, J. C. 1971. An Investigation into the Teratogenic Potential of Captan, Folpet and Difolatan in Nonhuman Primates. *Tox. Appl. Pharm.* 18:619-24.

Vos, J. G.; Van Der Mass, H. L.; Musch, A.; and Ram, E. 1971. Toxicity of Hexachlorobenzene in Japanese Quail with Special Reference to Porphyria, Liver Damage, Reproduction and Tissue Residues. *Toxicology and Applied Pharmacology* 18:944-57.

PENTACHLOROPHENOL

Pentachlorophenates have been used as herbicides, bactericides, fungicides, molluscacides, and insecticides. They resemble the dinitrophenols in increasing metabolism by uncoupling cellular oxidation and phosphorylation. Symptoms include weakness, loss of weight, dyspnea, and sweating.

Pentachlorophenol (PCP) compounds have been generally regarded as inert and causing few health problems. PCP residues in food products are infrequently found; and when detected, the levels are in the 5-40 ppb range.

Arthur Bevenue and Herman Beckman have written an excellent review, "Pentachlorophenol: A discussion of its properities and its occurrence as a residue in human and animal tissue," Residue Reviews 19:83-194, 1967. The reference list contains 150 citations. Portions of the review served as a basis in the following discussion.

Sources

Pentachlorophenol or its salts are used for the following applications.

1. Fungicide and/or bactericide in the processing of cellulose products, starches, adhesives, proteins, leather, oils, paints and rubber.
2. Rug shampoos and textiles to control mildew.
3. Food processing plants to control mold and slime.
4. Mothproofing of fabrics (pentachlorophenyl laurate).
5. Construction and lumber for mold and termite control; control powder post beetles and wood boring insects.
6. Herbicide and preharvest desiccant.
7. Fungicide on seeds and bulbs (SPERGON).
8. Molluscacide—snail intermediate hosts of human schistosomes.
9. Processing aid in manufacture of polyvinyl chloride emulsion polymers which are intended for use as articles that contact food at temperatures not to exceed room temperature.
10. Manufacture of closure-sealing gaskets for food containers (not to exceed 0.05 percent by weight).
11. Wood preservative in wooden crates for packaging raw agriculture products (not to exceed 50 ppm).

The chemical structure and physical properties are given below.

Molecular weight = 266.36
Melting pt = 190°C
Boiling pt = 293°C
Density = 1.85

PCP is decomposed by strong oxidizing agents. Sodium pentachlorophenate is decomposed by sunlight. The decomposition is increased by temperature and moisture. Decomposition products in aqueous solutions are chloranilic acid and chlorinated benzoquinones.

Toxicity and Clinical Signs

Rabbit Cutaneous—PCP in pine oil—lethal dose = 39 mg/kg
Rabbit Cutaneous—PCP in olive oil—lethal dose = 350 mg/kg
   Oral—257 mg/kg of Na-PCP
Rat No effect, oral feeding—3.9 mg/rat/day for 28 wks
Rat Sodium pentachlorophenate, LD_{50} = 100 mg/kg
Rat Pentachlorophenol, LD_{50} = 125-200 mg/kg

A cow was reported to have drunk a 5 percent PCP-kerosene solution with death occurring eight hours later. Two calves tolerated 500-600 mg/L in drinking water for five to seven weeks. A rhesus monkey (5 lb) tolerated 4 mg of PCP in water and a calf tolerated 3 gms in water over a four-day period. Swine (30 g) and sheep (23 g) were drenched with PCP solutions. The kidney, liver and spleen of the swine showed some changes but not severe enough to cause death. No harmful effects were noted in the kidney or liver of the adult sheep. The lambs suffered some liver damage. Pigs confined to farrowing pens treated with 4 percent PCP experienced high mortalities, with lesions in the kidney, liver, spleen, stomach and intestinal and respiratory tracts. Two sows placed in farrowing crates treated with large amounts of PCP died in twenty-four hours. A field case was reported where placing a sow and ten one-day-old pigs in a new farrowing house treated with PCP resulted in rapid death of the litter. The environmental temperature was about 100°F. The piglets were depressed, panting, ataxic, and exhibited fine muscle tremors. Necropsies revealed frothy blood in the nose, mouth and trachea; renal and cardiac petechia. Body temperatures were 107-108°F. The PCP had been applied in used crankcase oil at a level greater than manufacturers' recommendations.

Maximum nontoxic level for fish is 0.2-0.6 ppm. A level of 1 ppm is toxic with survival time related to pH and temperature. Depending on concentration of PCP salt the following enzymes were either stimulated or inhibited: aldolase, lactic dehydrogenase, glutamic-oxalacetic transaminase, glutamic-pyruvic transaminase and isocitric dehydrogenase. Levels of 10-20 ppm are lethal for snails.

Mechanism of Action

PCP is a powerful uncoupler of oxidative phosphorylation. PCP binds with actomyosin (muscle protein) and causes the muscle fibers to shorten. *In vitro* studies with mitochondria showed that PCP would uncouple oxidative phosphorylation, inhibit mitochondrial and myosin adenosine triphosphatase, inhibit glycolytic phosphorylation, inactivate respiratory enzymes and damage mitochondrial structure.

Clinical Signs

In mild cases there is muscular weakness, anorexia and lethargy. Moderate toxicosis involves accelerated respiration, hyperpyrexia, hyperglycemia, glycosuria, sweating, dehydration, irritation of skin (dermal exposure), irritation of respiratory tract, eyes, nose, and throat. Lethal exposures follow the symptoms described

above with the addition of cardiac and muscular collapse. There is rapid onset of rigor mortis.

Physiopathology

In the rabbit PCP is rapidly absorbed from the gut, and peak blood levels are reached in seven hours. In the rabbit 70 percent is eliminated in the urine in twenty-four hours. Traces of PCP persist in the blood for four days and in the urine for ten days.

In the rat 13 percent was excreted in the urine in the first twenty-four hours following oral ingestion.

In one species of shellfish studied (*Tapes philipinarum*) C^{14}-PCP was rapidly taken up from the water and distributed in all tissues with highest amounts in the Bojanus organ and the liver. The PCP was rapidly eliminated in either a free or bound form of unmetabolized PCP.

In mice given PCP excretion was via the kidneys and gastric and biliary secretion. Most of the PCP (72-83 percent) was excreted in the first four days, predominantly in the urine. About 50 percent was excreted in the first twenty-four hours. A metabolite tetrachlorohydroquinone (TCH) was found in the urine along with free and small amounts of conjugated (sulphuric or glucuronic acid) PCP. The PCP and TCH accounted for all the PCP and metabolites found in the urine (based on radio-tracer techniques). The PCP accounted for 30 percent and the TCH for 21 percent of the 51 percent PCP eliminated during the first twenty-four hours.

Diagnosis

Diagnosis in mild cases may be difficult to establish based on the relatively vague and general clinical symptoms.

Insufficient data is available to firmly establish a correlation between tissue residues, urinary excretion and severity of clinical signs.

PCP can be chemically identified in tissues and body fluids.

Treatment

No specific treatment has been reported. Once wood premises are contaminated it is very difficult to seal off the wood to prevent further vaporization.

Clinical Episode

A number of episodes have been reported, several of which are presented below. Of the fifty cases reported in the literature, thirty have resulted in death through 1967. A recent instance in the U.S. occurred in a small maternity hospital in St. Louis, Mo., in 1967. Nine infants were involved, of which two died. The infants were exposed via diapers, undershirts, sheets, blankets and other linens washed in an antimicrobial laundry neutralizer containing 22.9 percent Na pentachlorophenol (PCP) and 3.2 percent other chlorophenols. The PCP was used in the terminal rinse. The product was specifically *not recommended* for hospital laundries or for terminal rinses. Residues in the linens ranged from 11.50 ppm to 1,950 ppm. Residues in autopsy tissue of one infant were 20-34 ppm for kidney, adrenal, heart, fat and connective tissues. Serum levels in exposed but asymptomatic infants were 7-26 ppm and urine levels were < 1 ppm. Serum level in one ill infant was 118 ppm before exchange treatment and 31 ppm after. A urine level taken several days after blood exchange was 2.4 ppm. Serum levels in the nurses at the time of the episode were 1-12 ppm. Serum levels in infants sampled a year after PCP usage stopped were < 0.5 ppm and urine levels only 4-7 ppb. Reports related to this case include Armstrong *et al.,* (1969), Barthel *et al.,* (1969), and Robson *et al.,* (1969).

Bevenue, A. *et al.,* (1967b) reported a case of skin exposure resulting in a painful reddening of hands. Initial urine level was 236 ppb, which decreased to background levels in one month.

Bevenue *et al.,* (1967c) analyzed urine PCP levels in 541 people in Hawaii. In the occupationally exposed group (N = 130) the average urine PCP was 1.802 ppm with a range of 0.003-35.7 ppm. The nonoccupationally exposed individuals (N = 117) had a mean urine level of 0.040 ppm and a range of 0-1.84 ppm. Another group (N = 294) with mixed exposure had an average urine level of 0.217 ppm with a range of 3-38.6 ppm. The overall average for the three groups was 0.587 ppm.

Another report concerned the poisoning of a young girl following washing in contaminated water for thirteen days. The wooden water storage tank had been treated with PCP. (Chapman, 1965)

REFERENCES

Armstrong, R. W.; Eichner, E. R.; Klein, D. E.; Barthel, W. F.; Bennet, J. V.; Jonsson, V.; Bruce, H.; and Lovelass, L. E. 1969. Pentachlorophenol Poisoning in a Nursery for Newborn Infants. II. Epidemiologic and Toxicologic Studies. *J. Pediat.* 75:317-25.

Barthel, W. F.; Curley, A.; Thrasher, C. L.; and Sedlak, V. A. 1969. Determination of Pentachlorophenol in Blood, Urine, Tissue and Clothing. *JAOAC* 52:294-98.

Bevenue, A., and Beckman, H. 1967a. Pentachlorophenol: A Discussion of Its Properties and Its Occurrence as a Residue in Human and Animal Tissues. *Resid. Rev.* 19:83-134.

Bevenue, A.; Haley, T. J.; and Klemmer, H. W. 1967b. A Note on the Effects of a Temporary Exposure of an Individual to Pentachlorophenol. *Bull. Env. Cont. & Tox.* 2:293-96.

Bevenue, A.; Wilson, J.; Casarett, L. J.; and Klemmer, H. W. 1967c. A Survey of Pentachlorophenol Content in Human Urine. *Bull. Env. Cont. & Tox.* 2:319-32.

Blevins, D. 1965. Pentachlorophenol Poisoning in Swine. *Vet. Med.* 60:455.

Chapman, J. B., and Robson, P. 1965. Pentachlorophenol Poisoning from Bathwater. *Lancet.* 1:1266-67.

Jakobson, I., and Yllner, S. 1971. Metabolism of Pentachlorophenol in the Mouse. *Acta Pharm. et Toxic.* 29:513-24.

Kobayashi, K.; Akitake, H.; and Tomiyama, T. 1969. Studies on the Metabolism of Pentachlorophenate, Herbicide, in Aquatic Organisms. I. Turnover of Absorbed PCP in *Tapes philippinarum. Bull. Jap. Soc. Scientific Fisheries.* 35:1179-83.

Robson, A. M.; Kissane, J. M.; Elvick, N. H.; and Pundavela, L. 1969. Pentachlorophenol Poisoning in a Nursery for Newborn Infants. I. Clinical Features and Treatment. *J. Pediat.* 75:309-16.

Schipper, I. A. 1969. Toxicity of Wood Preservatives for Swine. *Am. J. Vet. Res.* 22:401-05.

Spencer, G. R. 1957. Poisoning of Cattle by Pentachlorophenol in Kerosene. *JAVMA* 130:299-300.

Herbicides

CHLORATES

Chlorate salts (usually as sodium or potassium chlorate) have been used for many years as herbicides and defoliants. In 1966, 900,000 pounds were used to defoliate cotton.

For weed control chlorate is used at 2-4 pounds per square rod, which is equivalent to 320-640 pounds per acre. Chlorate is used both as the dry salt and as a water spray. Chlorate is a strong oxidizing agent and is combustible.

Sodium chlorate should not be mixed with nor stored near organic compounds, oils, sulfur, sulfides, powdered metals, ammonium salts or phosphorous. Such mixtures may produce ignition or explosion.

Source

The major source is carelessly disposed chlorate salt or chlorate mistaken for sodium chloride and mixed in animal feeds. Animals deprived of access to NaCl are more likely to eat chlorate.

Sheep have safely grazed pastures treated with five pounds chlorate per square rod.

Chlorate decomposes in about seven days in warm moist soil.

Poisoning has occurred when lumps of chlorate are spread on the ground and animals allowed to graze.

Toxicity

The rat oral LD_{50} is 1.2 gm/kg. The toxicity for domestic animals is given in table 1.

Mechanism of Action

Chlorate in the blood converts hemoglobin to methemoglobin. The chlorate is not inactivated in the reaction and continues to form methemoglobin as long as it is present. Chlorate also irritates the intestinal tract resulting in diarrhea.

Clinical Signs and Physiopathology

Initially there is staggering, purging, evidence of abdominal pain, hematuria and hemoglobinuria.

As the hemoglobin becomes converted to methemoglobin there is dyspnea, increased respiratory effort and cyanosis. Death may occur without obvious symptoms. Animals which die suddenly may have "tarry" blood exuding from all body orifices.

On postmortem all the tissues will be brown.

Diagnosis

The history must include the presence of and access to chlorate on the farm. The extensive methemoglobinemia will be a valuable clue. *Care must be taken to differentiate chlorate poisoning from nitrate toxicosis.* The history may separate the two diseases. Additionally in

TABLE 1
Toxicity of Chlorate for Domestic Animals

Species	Dose	Effect
Horse	250 gm	Lethal
Cow	500 gm	Lethal
Calf	260 mg/kg	No effect
Calf	525 mg/kg	No effect
Cow	.1-.25 gm/kg for 5 days	Dark brown urine, methemoglobinemia
Cow	.06-.18 gm/kg for 3 days	Anorexia, watery feces, cow went down
Sheep	100 gm	Lethal
Sheep	10 gm or more	Produces methemoglobinemia
Chicken	5 gm/kg	Lethal
Dog	0.5-2.0 gm/kg	LD_{50} in 2-4 daily doses

chlorate poisoning the formation of methemoglobin is more severe and continues for a long period.

Treatment

The prognosis is unfavorable. The source should be found immediately to prevent further losses.

Gastric lavage with 1 percent sodium thiosulfate is recommended for monogastric animals. Milk or demulcents may be given to relieve gastric irritation.

Methylene blue at 10 mg/kg given I.V. in either a 2 or 4 percent solution is the treatment of choice for the cases that are recognized quickly enough. Several doses may have to be given at intervals during the several hours after exposure. Care should be exercised so that treatment is not stopped too soon. A suitable end point is when a blood sample no longer turns dark on standing.

REFERENCES

Arena, J. M. 1974. Poisoning. *Toxicology, Symptoms, Treatments*. 3rd ed. Springfield, Illinois: Charles C. Thomas, Publishers.

Dalgaard-Mikkelsen, S., and Paulsen, E. 1962. Toxicology of Herbicides. *Pharm. Rev.* 14:225.

McCulloch, F. C., and Murer, H. K. 1939. Sodium Chlorate Poisoning. *JAVMA* 95:675.

Moore, G. R. 1941. Sodium Chlorate Poisoning in Cattle. *JAVMA* 99:50.

ORGANIC SYNTHETIC HERBICIDES

Source

The control or elimination of noxious plants has long been a goal of the human race. The ideal situation would be to control or kill the harmful species and improve those which are beneficial without upsetting the delicate environmental balance in which we survive.

Early attempts at plant control were nonselective in nature. Such materials as arsenicals, chlorates, and phenols have been used to kill plants. Unfortunately, such compounds are not selective for plants and often are highly toxic to man and animals as well.

The advent of commercial farming and the decline of human labor in agriculture has prompted development of selective weed control chemicals. Thus, numerous mechanical passages over the several hundred acres under a producer's control are eliminated by herbicide usage. Both selective and nonselective herbicides, some highly toxic and some nearly nontoxic, remain with us today.

The herbicides are grouped chemically as inorganic and organic compounds. The inorganic herbicides are composed of various inorganic salts. Many are slowly removed from the soil or not at all. Compounds such as calcium cyanamide, cupric sulfate, mercurous chloride, potassium cyanate, sodium tetraborate, sodium and potassium chlorate, and arsenicals are available for use as herbicides. The arsenicals and chlorates are most frequently used. The characteristics of poisoning by these compounds have been treated elsewhere. A great variety of organic herbicides are used in agriculture and horticulture. The type of herbicide used is often dictated by the particular crop or conditions. For clinical and toxicologic purposes, the organic herbicides may be divided into several groups, since mode of action and toxicity are similar for compounds in that group.

Toxicity

Determination of the Hazard of Herbicide Use

Expressions of toxicity are usually given as mg/kg, mg/lb, or gm/kg. When dealing with herbicides, the direct ingestion of chemicals may come either from the concentrate or from the treated forage. The likelihood of poisoning (hazard) depends largely upon whether enough herbicide is applied to plants to allow sufficient intake for toxicosis to develop.

Several assumptions must be made in estimating the herbicide load on forages. A yield of 2 tons/acre (approximately 0.1 lb/sq ft) of air-dry forage can be used as a basis. It must also be assumed that an animal will consume approximately 3.0 percent of its body weight as forage daily, and that *all* chemicals applied adhere to the vegetation. With these limitations, applications of 1 lb of chemical/acre provides 10.4 mg/sq ft of area. This all simplifies to the single statement that 1 lb of actual herbicide/acre provides a dosage of 7 mg/kg of body weight.

As with other agricultural chemicals, the majority of problems are associated with human error or accident. Poisoning is not likely to result if proper application and withholding times are observed.

The toxicity of various selected herbicides by chemical class and their hazard at normal application rates are summarized in tables 1-10. (Palmer, 1963, 1964a, 1964b, 1964c, 1964d, and Palmer and Radeleff, 1969)

Phenoxy Derivatives of Fatty Acids

The toxicology of the phenoxy fatty acid herbicides deserves special mention for two reasons: (1) their ability to alter some aspects of plant toxicity and (2) their association with teratogenicity. This group is comprised of herbicides which are short chain fatty acids (*e.g.,* acetic, butyric, propionic) containing a phenoxy ring. The acid form of these compounds is not very soluble in water or oil. To increase solubility, an ester form of the herbicide is used. This form is also highly volatile.

The phenoxy acid derivatives are plant growth regulators. As such, they alter the metabolism of the plant. A side effect of this is that treated plants may build high levels of nitrates or cyanide prior to death. Also, many toxic weeds may become more palatable (*e. g.,* Jimsonweed, nightshade) and will be consumed for that reason. However, the inherent toxicity of poisonous plants apparently is not altered.

Concern was raised regarding the potential teratogenic effects of 2, 4, 5-T based on studies in laboratory animals and upon reports of increased congenital defects in South Vietnam as a result of warfare defoliation programs. (Clegg, 1971) In 1969, the use of 2, 4, 5-T in the United States was curtailed; and in 1970, reports supporting the teratogenic effects of 2, 4, 5-T were published, (Courtney *et. al.,* 1970) Changes reported included increased incidence of cleft palate, renal cysts, and skeletal malformations in mice.

The compounds known collectively as dioxins have been found as contaminants in several synthetic organic chemicals. In the phenoxy herbicides, 2, 4, 5-T has in the past been the major herbicide contaminated.

Several forms of dioxin exist and their toxicologic effects vary widely depending on the chemical structure. The highly toxic forms include hexachloro-dibenzo-p-dioxin (commonly abbreviated HCDD) and 2, 3, 7, 8, tetrachloro-dibenzo-p-dioxin (abbreviated as TCDD). Of the dioxins, the one of concern in herbicides has been TCDD. Contamination involved TCDD levels as high as 30 ppm (parts per million) in 2, 4, 5-T while present day production results in dioxin levels below 0.1 ppm.

Adverse effects from TCDD exposure in the past have been reported in workers in several industries producing synthetic organic chemicals. Other reports are available from research studies in laboratory animals used to evaluate TCDD hazards. A field case involving horses exposed to dioxin contaminated industrial waste oil used to control riding arena dust has recently been reported.

The effects of TCDD are both from direct toxicity and through production of birth defects (teratogenesis) or fetal death in laboratory animals. The effects of TCDD may be observed as separate and distinct from any effects due to 2, 4, 5-T or other phenoxy herbicides which do not contain TCDD.

The direct effects in TCDD administered to laboratory animals are skin damage, hepatic damage, hemorrhage, and suppression of the immune response. Wide variation in the effects of TCDD are seen among various animals. Furthermore, there is a great variation in the amount of TCDD to which animals are susceptible. For example, dogs are some 100 times more resistant to TCDD than are mice or guinea pigs.

Birth defects and fetal death can be produced by low doses of TCDD given to pregnant laboratory animals. This appears due to an effect on the fetus and not in the genetics of the pregnant animal.

Similar birth defects have been produced from dioxin-contaminated 2, 4, 5-T and from pure TCDD. When TCDD is present at less than 1 ppm in 2, 4, 5-T

herbicide, the number and severity of birth defects are markedly reduced. Furthermore, the changes induced by excessive levels of 2, 4, 5-T are of a less serious nature and in many respects are reversible. Such changes include reduced birth weight, hemorrhages, and delayed bone formation. While birth defects have been demonstrated in mice and hamsters from 2, 4, 5-T, studies in other animals (rats, dogs, and sheep) have been negative or inconclusive.

Detrimental effects in the rat fetus from contaminated 2, 4, 5-T vary with the amount of TCDD contamination in the herbicide. Levels of TCDD greater than 1 ppm are required to enhance the embryotoxic effect of 2, 4, 5-T. 2, 4, 5-T containing the currently accepted levels of less than 0.1 ppm TCDD or less would maintain a safety margin with regard to potentiation.

When TCDD itself is administered to rats, approximately 30 percent of the dose is passed through the digestive tract. Of the absorbed TCDD, the half-life is approximately seventeen days via urine and expired air. Most retained TCDD is in the liver and fat. Accumulation of TCDD in the body would not be expected unless high and continued doses were received.

Clinical Signs and Physiopathology

Chlorophenoxy Derivatives of Fatty Acids

Poisoning is almost entirely due to accidental ingestion of concentrates or sprays. Only occasionally would treated forages be hazardous to livestock. The toxicity, application rates, and hazard of various phenoxy derivatives of fatty acids are summarized in table 1.

Repeated and massive doses are required to produce poisoning in ruminants and dogs. In ruminants, there is anorexia, depression, rumen atony, muscle weakness, and sometimes diarrhea. There may be ulceration of oral mucosa from prolonged exposure. Animals gradually become emaciated and moribund. No struggle or convulsions are observed. Ruminants may bloat. In dogs, there is myotonia, ataxia, and posterior weakness. Periodic clonic spasms may occur. Vomiting and bloody feces may be evident.

Epicardial hemorrhage and hydropericardium may be found in phenoxy fatty acid-poisoned animals. A characteristic finding is rumen stasis with bright green, undigested feed. The liver is swollen and friable and kidneys are congested. There may be hyperemia and enlargement of the lymph nodes and mesenteric vessels.

In ruminants, generally ten days exposure is required to produce initial signs of poisoning from phenoxy herbicides. Calves, however, have been poisoned by single oral doses of 200 mg/kg body weight.

In swine, the minimum acutely toxic dose of 2, 4-D is approximately 100 mg/kg orally, and the fatal dose is of the order of 500 mg/kg. Effects in swine include diarrhea, stilted gait, and transitory depression. More severe poisoning causes vomiting, severe muscle weakness, and generalized depression. Acute lesions in swine were observed mainly in the digestive tract and the respiratory and excretory organs. Young pigs fed 500 ppm of 2, 4-D did not develop clinical signs of poisoning. The only adverse effect seen was an irregular or depressed growth rate during a twelve-month period. Histological examination of swine fed 500 ppm 2, 4-D in the feed reveals parenchymatous degeneration of the liver with variation in nuclear size of hepatic cells. Albuminuria may be observed but consistent renal changes are not found.

In chickens poisoned by 2, 4-D or other phenoxy herbicides the main lesion is a consistent enlargement of the kidneys, observable in dead as well as sacrificed animals.

Dogs appear somewhat more sensitive to phenoxy herbicides than do other classes of domestic animals. The approximate oral LD_{50} for 2, 4-D in the dog is 100 mg/kg. At this level death may not occur for from seven to ten days after administration of a single dose of the herbicide. The continued administration of 20 mg/kg 2, 4-D for two to three weeks in dogs has produced severe fatal poisoning. The clinical signs in dogs are characteristic and include an initial disinclination to move, and a passiveness which is gradually worsened as a pattern of myotonia develops. This rigidity of skeletal muscles is combined with ataxia, progressive apathy, depression, and muscular weakness particularly of the posterior limbs. Periodic clonic spasms, and finally coma are the typical sequelae of phenoxy herbicide poisoning in dogs. During the clinical course of poisoning there is a marked anorexia; there may be vomiting, and occasionally passage of blood-tinged feces. Postmortem reveals necrotic ulcers of the oral mucosa, signs of irritation in the gastrointestinal tract, and sometimes necrosis of the small intestine as well as focal necrosis in the liver and degeneration of renal tubules. Even at 20 mg/kg body weight it is not likely that dogs will be poisoned by exposure to properly treated lawns. More probable is the fact that discarded or excess spray which has been previously mixed or pools of spray which have collected in low spots or in containers may be the cause of hazards to dogs.

The phenoxy herbicides are generally short lived in the animal body. The half-life values for clearance from tissues range from five to ten hours in rats, up to ten to thirty hours in species such as swine, calves and chickens. The tissue half-life of 2, 4, 5-T in the dog may range as high as eighty-seven hours. At low levels of exposure most of the phenoxy compounds appear to be excreted largely unchanged in the urine and do not appear in appreciable amounts in milk or in body fat. However at conditions of high exposure in the dog there appear to be several metabolites of 2, 4, 5-T which may be a result of inability of body systems to handle excessive dosages in the normal manner. This could account for, in part, the increased susceptibility of dogs to phenoxy herbicides. Recent work with phenoxy herbicide residues in sheep and cattle has indicated that residues of the phenoxy compounds and their phenol metabolites are present at lowest levels in muscle and fat, and were found in greatest amounts in the liver and kidney. Maximum levels of phenoxy herbicides from feeding as much as 2,000 ppm herbicide in the diet amounted to 1 ppm in most cases in the kidney and liver tissues and less than .05 ppm herbicide or metabolites in the muscle or fat of experimental animals. Phenoxy herbicide residues are not likely to be greater than 300 ppm in or on forage immediately after treatment with these compounds at rates recommended for control of weeds and brush. Residues decline rapidly with a forage half-life generally of one to two weeks. Residues in meat are expected only when circumstances indicate extremely high exposure during continuous ingestion of freshly treated vegetation. Withdrawal of animals from treated forages for one to two weeks prior to slaughter would significantly reduce any residues present.

Herbicide treated forages appear not to alter rumen microbial functions nor development of the rumen. In addition, these herbicides are not readily degraded by rumen microorganisms.

The effect of 2, 4-D and other phenoxy herbicides on fertility, hatchability of eggs, and survival of various fowl has been studied. In general, exposure to phenoxy herbicide levels approximating or exceeding those equivalent to recommended field application rates do not alter the reproductive status of eggs from chickens, quail, and partridge. Evidence of the reproductive effects on pheasant eggs is somewhat in conflict, but generally indicates no adverse effect from rates of phenoxy herbicide application which are recommended for field weed control.

Amides

The amide herbicides are relatively toxic among the plant growth regulators. Anorexia is the initial and prominent sign of poisoning. Salivation, depression, and prostration follow.

Necropsy lesions are those of hemorrhage and congestion of the abomasal and intestinal mucosa and congestion of the lungs and tracheal mucosa. Kidneys of poisoned animals often are enlarged and congested.

At recommended levels of application, CDAA would be hazardous to livestock.

Residues of the amide herbicide Randox are not detected in the milk, urine or feces in dairy animals fed the herbicide at 5 ppm in the diet. The compound is stable to at least twenty-four hours of incubation in rumen content, but appears to disappear rapidly when incubated with beef liver. Under typical field conditions of use Randox would not be expected to result in residues in milk or meat.

Arsenicals

The organic arsenical herbicides act as trivalent arsenicals. Thus their clinical effects are similar to those described for inorganic arsenic poisoning and they should be treated accordingly (see Arsenic).

The persistence of arsenical compounds make their accumulation in soil and on plants a potential problem where repeated application is practical.

Dipyridyl Compounds

Diquat and Paraquat have several environmental assets including low application rates (2 oz/acre), rapid action on plants, inactivity when in contact with soil, and relatively rapid photodecomposition.

Acute effects from a single large exposure to dipyridyl herbicides (100-300 mg/kg) results in stomatitis, vomition, colic and diarrhea. If animals survive the acute phase, a second syndrome occurs from two to ten days after administration. This second phase is characterized by pulmonary congestion and edema, hyaline membrane formation and inflammatory infiltration. Animals surviving the subacute edema and inflammation often develop progressive diffuse pulmonary fibrosis with high mortality. It is noteworthy that the lesion develops long after the majority of the herbicide is eliminated from the body.

Substituted Urea Compounds

Diarrhea, anorexia, depression, incoordination, and prostration are caused by large doses of substituted urea compounds. Severe congestion of lungs, liver, spleen, and meninges is seen in animals receiving toxic doses of the substituted ureas.

The induction of hepatic microsomal enzymes by several substituted urea herbicides has been demonstrated. There occurs a dose related increase in the activities of three hepatic microsomal enzymes after exposure to this class of herbicides. The significance of this finding may be that a large number of environmentally available materials such as herbicides and other pesticides can influence not only their own toxicity but may also alter the effects expected when several compounds are combined in one animal.

Thiocarbamates

These compounds are of moderate toxicity on a mg/kg basis. However, their use is commonly at rather low concentrations and, when used as directed, should not cause problems.

Signs of poisoning in ruminants are muscle spasms, ataxia, depression, and prostration. Alopecia may be seen in chronically affected animals, often as long as sixty days after dosing. Congested, friable livers and congested kidneys are necropsy lesions observed in thiocarbamate herbicide poisoning.

The thiocarbamate herbicide diallate, in addition to causing anorexia and loss of body weight induces alopecia in sheep which are chronically affected. It also may cause muscular spasms, ataxia, and central nervous system depression. This generally is followed by prostration when large doses are administered. Continued exposure to dialate in the sheep results in development of tolerance to that herbicide over a period of twenty-one daily doses.

The thiocarbamate herbicide Pebulate is known to induce enlargement or congestion of the thyroid and kidneys. Yearling cattle dosed with 100 mg/kg body weight of Pebulate had marked decreases in the magnesium to calcium plasma ratio, acute toxic tubular nephritis, hepatic damage and mild congestion of the spleen. By contrast, sheep dosed with the same herbicide did not have significantly altered magnesium to calcium plasma ratios.

Triazines

Anorexia, depression, muscular spasms, and dyspnea are observed in triazine poisoning. Weakness and uncoordinated gait are commonly observed.

Necropsy lesions consist of pale friable livers, congested livers and kidneys, and petechia on the epicardium. These compounds would be a hazard to livestock if used at the higher application rates.

The triazine herbicides, atrazine and prometone when administered on forage at rates equivalent to or higher than recommended field applications cause no gross signs of adverse effects from consuming either herbicide. There were no significant changes in SGOT, SGPT, or LDH. Nor were changes in total protein, hemoglobin, packed cell volume and complete blood count observed.

Histopathologic changes attributable to ingestion of atrazine treated hay were not observed, although other workers have found that similar levels did cause adverse effects in cattle and sheep. The method of administration must be considered. In those cases where adverse effects occurred, dosage was by drench or capsule, whereas when no adverse effects were seen the dosage was as a result of spraying the herbicides on the forage consumed by animals, thus changing the rate and method of administration.

One of the authors has observed a field case of atrazine poisoning in which several dairy animals gained access to a bag of atrazine formulation prior to its being mixed for herbicidal use. The clinical signs observed by the attending clinician included hyperesthesia, moderate hypersalivation, muscle tremors, ataxia, recumbency, and death.

A limited amount of work on the metabolism and excretion of atrazine indicates that it is probably metabolized by dealkylation and then excreted primarily in the urine.

Benzoic Acid Derivatives

The benzoic acid herbicides are relatively nontoxic to animals. Their low application rates make poisoning quite unlikely at conditions of normal usage. Signs of poisoning are convulsions, tympanites, and prostration. Necropsy lesions are hemorrhages of the lymph nodes and epicardium and congestion of the liver and kidney.

Methyluracils

The methyluracil derivatives (bromacil, isocil) cause anorexia, depression, bloat, and incoordinated gait. Enlarged, hemorrhagic lymph nodes and congested lungs are features of the necropsy. These compounds are applied at rates up to 20 lbs actual/acre. Rates in excess of 5 lbs/acre could be hazardous to ruminants.

Polychlorobicyclopentadiene Isomers

Animals poisoned by this group of herbicides exhibit anorexia, depression, muscle tremors, and hyperexcitability. Uncoordinated gait and prostration follow. Hemorrhage along the brain stem and in the cerebrum is seen at necropsy. The liver is enlarged and friable, and kidneys are reduced in size.

Polychlorobicyclopentadiene isomers are applied to noncrop areas. They would be hazardous at 30-40 lbs/acre.

Picloram (4-amino-3, 5, 6-trichloropicolinic acid) Tordon®

Weakness, depression, and anorexia are prominent signs of poisoning. Necropsy examination reveals swol-

len cervical and cephalic lymph nodes, respiratory tract congestion, blood-tinged pericardial fluid, undigested rumen contents, and congestion of kidneys and intestinal mucosa. Picloram is a noncrop herbicide which would be hazardous used in excess of 25 lbs actual/acre.

Dinitroaniline Compounds

The dinitroaniline herbicide Planavin apparently disappears rapidly and is decomposed by fresh rumen fluids with production of several sulfur containing metabolites. At 5 ppm Planavin in the diet of dairy cows, no residues are detected in the urine or feces.

Diagnosis

The detection of adverse effects resulting from organic synthetic herbicides is difficult to define. Many of the clinical signs and lesions are nonspecific, and refer only to gastrointestinal irritation, poor growth rate, lowered feed efficiency, parenchymatous organ degeneration, and depression of normal activity. Evidence other than clinical signs and lesions must be considered. Establishment of exposure is of prime importance, without which a solid diagnosis can seldom be made. One must be prepared to estimate the degree of exposure of animals to various herbicides which may be in question; secondarily, to compare that exposure with known toxicity data to establish the hazards of poisoning. Analytical methods are available for most of the modern organic herbicides. Many of these methods involve costly and time consuming procedures and require a large investment in instrumentation and manpower. Suitable tissues for analysis would include the suspected forages or water, liver and kidney, urine, stomach contents, and feces. In the authors' experience, acute or subacute poisoning from the proper application and use of organic synthetic herbicides has not been proven. This would include observation of the proper application rates, as well as proper withholding times from consumption of treated forage. Further, there is no conclusive evidence of chronic effects including reproductive failure, teratogenesis, or carcinogenesis in domestic animals or wildlife as a result of low level long-term exposure to organic synthetic herbicides properly used.

Treatment

No specific antidotes for herbicide poisonings are available. Prompt removal of the gastrointestinal contents, intestinal protectants, forced diuresis, and hepatic and renal supportive therapy may aid in overcoming the clinical severity.

TABLE 1
Toxicity and Hazard of Phenoxy Derivatives of Fatty Acids and of Chlorinated Aliphatic Acids

Chemical Name	Common Name	Toxicity (mg/kg)	Application Rate (Actual lbs/Acre)	Hazard of Poisoning
2,4-Dichlorophenoxyacetic Acid, Ester	2,4-D	C 250[10] * S 250[9] P 250[10]	0.07-40.0	Yes @ 30+ lbs/acre
2,4,5-Trichlorophenoxy-acetic Acid	2,4,5-T	C 250[7] S 250[6] P 500[10]	0.5-4.5	No
2(2,4,5-Trichlorophenoxy) Propionic Acid	Silvex (2,4,5-TP)	C 100[29] S 100[11]	0.13-8.0	No
2-Methyl-4-Chlorophenoxy-acetic Acid	MCP Amine (MCPA, MCPB)	C 500[10] S 250[10] P 500[10]	0.13-2.1	No
2,2 Dichloropropionic Acid	Dalapon (Dowpon ®)	C 1,000** S 500[7] P 500**	1.1-14.8	No except for sheep @ 10+ lbs/acre

C = Cattle
S = Sheep
P = Chickens
 *Number of days to produce effects.
**No ill effects.

TABLE 2
Toxicity and Hazard of Amide Herbicides

Chemical Name	Common Name	Toxicity (mg/kg)	Application Rate (Actual lbs/Acre)	Hazard of Poisoning
N,N Dimethyl-2,2-Diphenyl-acetamide	Diphenamide	C 250[3] * S 250[7] P 500[10]	3-6	No
2-Chloro-N,N-diallyl-acetamide	CDAA (Randox ®)	C 25[10] C 50[1] S 50[1] P 50[10]	4-10	Yes
2-Chloro-N,N-diallyl-acetamide and Trichlorobenzyl chloride	Randox-T	C 50[2] C 100[1] S 25[10] S 50[2] P 250[1]	3.5-7	Yes for sheep and cattle

C = Cattle
S = Sheep
P = Chickens
*Number of days to produce effects.

TABLE 3
Toxicology of Substituted Urea Compounds

Chemical Name	Common Name	Toxicity (mg/kg)	Application Rate (Actual lbs/Acre)	Hazard of Poisoning
3-(p-Chlorophenyl)-1,1-Dimethyl Urea	Monuron (Telvar®)	C 500[1] * S 100[4] P 100[10]	1.2-6.4	Only to chickens @ 3+ lbs
3-(3,4-Dichlorophenyl)-1-Methoxymethyl Urea	Linuron (Lorox®)	C 50[10] S 50[8] P 100[8]	1-3	No
3-Phenyl-1,1-Dimethyl Urea	Fenuron (Dybar®)	C 500[2] S 100[8] S 500[3]	Spot treat 0.016	Yes if large area treated
3-(3,4-Dichlorophenyl)-1,1-Dimethyl Urea	Diuron (Karmex®)	C 100[10] S 100[2] P 50[10]	0.2-9.6	No except as noted**

C = Cattle
S = Sheep
P = Chickens
*Number of days to produce effects.
**May be used @ 80 lbs/acre actual in irrigation ditches; would be hazardous to all livestock at this level.

TABLE 4
Toxicology of Carbamate and Thiocarbamate Herbicides

Chemical Name	Common Name	Toxicity (mg/kg)	Application Rate (Actual lbs/Acre)	Hazard of Poisoning
3, 4-Dichlorobenzyl Methyl-carbamate	Dichlormate (Rowmate 4E)	C 10[10] * S 50[10] P 175[10]	1.0	@ 1 lb/acre, cattle
S-2, 3-Dichloroallyl Diiso-propylthiocarbamate	Diallate (Avadex®)	C 25[5] S 25[5] P 150[10]	1.25-2.0	No
S-2, 3, 3-Trichloroallyl Di-isopropylthiocarbamate	Triallate (Avadex BW®)	C 25[5] S 50[2] P 175[10]	1.0-1.25	
S-Ethyl-N, N-Propylthio-carbamate	EPTC (EPTAM®) (Knoxweed[R])	C 50[1] S 100[2] P 50[10]		Yes, for cattle and chickens
S-Propyl Dipropylthio-carbamate	Vernolate (Vernam®)	C 100[4] S 250[10] P 100[10]	2.0-3.0 Incorporated in soil	

C = Cattle
S = Sheep
P = Chicken
*Number of days to produce effects.

175

TABLE 4 (cont.)

Chemical Name	Common Name	Toxicity (mg/kg)	Application Rate (Actual lbs/Acre)	Hazard of Poisoning
Isopropyl M-Chlorocarbanilate	Chlorpropham	C 100^2 S 100^{10} P 100^{10}	2-10	Yes, 12+ all species
4-Chloro-2-Butynyl	Barban	C 25^1 S 10^2 P 50^{10}	0.38-1.00	Yes, sheep
2-Chloroallyl Diethyl Dithiocarbamate	CDEC	C 25^1 S 25^3 P 100^{10}	3-8	Yes, cattle and sheep
S-Propyl Butylethyl Thiocarbamate	Pebulate	C 50^3 S 175^3 P 100^{10}	4-6	Yes, cattle

C = Cattle

S = Sheep

P = Chicken

*Number of days to produce effects.

TABLE 5
Toxicology of Triazine and Benzoic Acid Herbicides

Chemical Name	Common Name	Toxicity (mg/kg)	Application Rate (Actual lbs/Acre)	Hazard of Poisoning
2-Chloro-4-Ethylamino-6-Isopropylamino-s-Triazine	Atrazine (Atrazine®)	C 25^{2*} S 5^{10} P 50^{10}	6-25	Yes sheep 1 lb/acre and cattle 3 lbs/acre
2-Chloro-4,6-Bis (Ethylamino)-s-Triazine	Simazine (Simazine®)	C 25^3 S 50^{17} P 50^{10}	1-9.6	Yes sheep 5 lbs/acre and cattle 3 lbs/acre
2-Chloro-4,6-Bis (Isopropylamino)-s-Triazine	Propazine (Propazine®)	C 25^3 S 25^5 P 100^{10}	2-4	Yes to sheep and cattle
2,4-Bis(Isopropylamino)-6-(Methylthio)-s-Triazine	(Prometryne®)	C 50^2 S 100^8 P 250^{10}	0.64-6	Maximum rate toxic for cattle

C = Cattle

S = Sheep

P = Chickens

*Number of days to produce effects.

**No ill effects.

TABLE 6
Substituted Dinitroanaline Herbicides

Chemical Name	Common Name	Toxicity (mg/kg)	Application Rate (Actual lbs/Acre)	Hazard of Poisoning
4-(Methylsulfonyl)-2,6-Dinitro-N,N-Dipropyl-aniline	Nitralin (Planavin®)	C 250[10]* S 375[2] P 500**	1.25-1.50	No
a,a,a-Trifluoro-2,6-Dinitro-N,N-Dipropyl-p-Toluidine	Trifluralin (Treflan®)	C 175[2] S 175[4] P 500[10]	0.5-2.0	Anorexia, diarrhea; reduced weight gain

C = Cattle
S = Sheep
P = Chickens
*Number of days to produce effects.
**No ill effects.

TABLE 7
Toxicology of Benzoic Acid Herbicides

Chemical Name	Common Name	Toxicity (mg/kg)	Application Rate (Actual lbs/Acre)	Hazard of Poisoning
2-Methoxy-3, 6-Dichlorobenzoic Acid, Dimethylamine Salts	Dicamba	C 250[2]* S 500[1] P 50[10]	0.125-1.000	No
2, 3, 6-Trichlorobenzoic Acid and Related Polychlorobenzoic Acids, Dimethylamine Salts	2, 3, 6-TBA	C 500[1] S 25[10] P 250[10]	(no reg.)	No
3-Amino-2, 5-Dichloro-benzoic acid	Chloramben	C 175[10] S 25[10] P 375[10]	2.0-4.1	No

C = Cattle
S = Sheep
P = Chickens
*Number of days to produce effects.

TABLE 8
Arsenical Herbicides

Chemical Name	Common Name	Toxicity (mg/kg)	Application Rate (Actual lbs/Acre)	Hazard of Poisoning
Monosodium Methanearsonate	MSMA (Ansar 170®)	C 10^2 S 50^3 P 100^{10}	2.0	Yes for cattle and sheep but not poultry
Disodium Methanearsonate	DSMA (Ansar 184®)	C 25^2 S 25^5 P 375^{10}	3.0	Yes for cattle and sheep but not poultry
Hydroxydimethylarsine	Cacodylic Acid (Phytar 560®)	C 25^8 S 25^{10} P 100^{10}	7.7-8.4	Yes for cattle and sheep but not poultry

C = Cattle
S = Sheep
P = Chickens
*Number of days to produce effects.

TABLE 9
Toxicology of Phthalmic Acid Herbicides

Chemical Name	Common Name	Toxicity (mg/kg)	Application Rate (Actual lbs/Acre)	Hazard of Poisoning
N-1-Naphthylphthalamic Acid, Sodium Salt	Naptalam	C 175^{6}* S 100^3 P 250^1	1.26-8.00	No
N-1-Naphthylphthalamic Acid and 2-Sec-butyl 4, 6-Dinitrophenol	Dinoseb	C 25^8 S 25^{10} P 25^2	2.25-3.00	Yes

C = Cattle
S = Sheep
P = Chickens
*Number of days to produce effects.

TABLE 10
Toxicology of Some Miscellaneous Herbicides

Chemical Name	Common Name	Toxicity (mg/kg)	Application Rate (Actual lbs/Acre)	Hazard of Poisoning
5-Bromo-3-Secbutyl-6-Methyluracil	Bromacil (Hyvar X®)	C 250[10]* S 50[8] P 500[10]	1.6-20	Yes for sheep @ 5 lbs/acre
5-Bromo-3-Isopropyl-6-Methyluracil	Isocil (Hyvar Isocil)	C 50[7] S 100[1] P 500[10]	1.6-26	Yes in excess of 5 lbs/acre
Polychlorobicyclopenta-diene Isomers	Bandane®	C 100[10] S 100[7] P 100[10]	30-40 on noncrop areas	Yes
2,6 Dichlorobenzonitrile	Dichlobenil (Casoron®)	C 50[1] S 25[10] P 25[10]	2-6	Yes for sheep @ 3 lbs/acre and cattle @ 6 lbs/acre
4-amino-3,5,6-Trichloro-picolinic Acid	Picloram (Tordon®)	C 500[8] S 250[9] P**	Use canceled for cropland	Yes for sheep @ 25 lbs/acre

C = Cattle
S = Sheep
P = Chickens
 *Number of days to produce effects.
**No ill effects.

TABLE 11

Clinical and Pathologic Effects of Organic Herbicides

Effect	Chlorophenoxy	Triazine*	Chlorinated Aliphatic*	Amide*	Phenyl Urea	Carbamate	Thiocarbamate	Arsenical*	Substituted Dinitroanaline	Dipyridyl*	Phthalamic Acid	Benzoic Acid
Depression		X					X	X	X			
Anorexia	X	X	X	X	X	X	X	X	X	X	X	
Rumen Stasis	X											
Vomition					X		X	X				
Diarrhea			X	X	X	X		X	X	X	X	
Salivation				X			X					
Bloat						X	X		X		X	X
Weakness	X							X				
Ataxia	X		X	X	X			X				
Muscle Spasms	X						X					X
Prostration				X					X			X
Dyspnea		X					X					
Urticaria					X							
Lung Congestion	X	X		X		X	X			X		
Liver Congestion		X	X	X			X					X
Kidney Congestion	X	X	X	X	X			X		X	X	X
Friable Liver	X	X					X	X	X	X		
G. I. Inflammation	X	X	X	X	X	X		X	X		X	X
Enlarged L. N.							X		X			X
Hemorrhage						X	X	X		X		X
Ascites							X					
Hydrothorax							X					

*Hazard at conditions of use.

REFERENCES

Audus, L. J. 1964. *The Physiology and Biochemistry of Herbicides.* New York: Academic Press.

Baily, G. W., and White, J. L. 1965. Herbicides: A Compilation of Their Physical, Chemical, and Biological Properties. *Residue Rev.* 10:97-122.

Clark, D. E., and Palmer, J. S. 1971. Residual Aspects of 2, 4, 5-T and an Ester in Sheep and Cattle with Observations on Concomitant Toxicological Effects. *J. Agr. Food Chem.* 19:761-64.

Clark, D. E.; Palmer, R. D.; Radeleff, H.; Crookshank, R.; and Farr, F. M. 1975. Residues of Chlorophenoxy Acid Herbicides and Their Phenolic Metabolites in Tissues of Sheep and Cattle. *J. Agric. Food Chem.* 23:573-78.

Clegg, D. J. 1971. Embryotoxicity of Chemical Contaminants of Foods. *Food Cosmet. Toxicol.* 9:195-205.

Council for Agricultural Science and Technology. 1975. The Phenoxy Herbicides. Cast. Report No. 39.

Courtney, K. D.; Gaylor, D. W.; Hogan, M. D.; Falk, H. L.; Bates, R. R.; and Mitchell, I. 1970. Teratogenic Evaluation of 2, 4, 5-T. *Science* 168:864.

Dalgaard-Mikkelson, S. V., and Poulson, E. 1962. The Toxicology of Herbicides. *Pharm. Rev.* 14:225-50.

Galston, A. W. 1971. Some Implications of the Widespread Use of Herbicides. *Bioscience* 21:891-92.

Gralleau, G.; de Lavaru, E.; and Siou, H. 1974. Effects of 2, 4-D on Reproduction of Quail and Partridge after Dusting onto Eggs. *Annals de Zoologie Ecologie Animale* 6:313-31.

Gutenmann, W. H., and Hardee, D. D. 1963. Residue Studies with 2-4-Dichlorophenoxyacetic Acid Herbicide in the Dairy Cow and in a Natural and Artificial Rumen. *J. Dairy Sci.* XLVI:1287-88.

Gutenmann, W. H., and Lisk, D. J. 1970. Metabolism of Planavin Herbicide in a Lactating Cow. *J. Dairy Sci.* 53:1289-91.

———. 1971. Metabolic Studies with Bexide (Herbisan) Herbicide in the Dairy Cow. *J. Agr. Food Chem.*

Ingham, B. 1975. Effect of Asulam in Wildlife Species. Acute Toxicity to Birds and Fish. *Bull. of Environ. Contam. and Toxi.* 13:194-99.

Johnson, E. A.; Van Kampen, K. R.; and Binns, W. 1972. Effects on Cattle and Sheep of Eating Hay Treated with Triazine Herbicides, Atrazine and Prometone. *Am. J. Vet. Res.* 33:1433-38.

Johnson, J. E. 1971. The Public Health Implications of Widespread Use of the Phenoxy Herbicides and Picloram. *Bioscience* 21:899-905.

Kenaga, E. E. 1974. Toxicological and Residue Data Useful to the Environmental Safety Evaluation of Dalapon. *Residue Reviews* 53:109-51.

Kinoshita, F. K., and DuBois, K. P. 1970. Induction of Hepatic Microsomal Enzymes by Herban, Diuron, and Other Substituted Urea Herbicides. *Tox. and Applied Pharm.* 17:406-17.

Klingman, G. C. 1961. *Weed Control As a Science.* New York: John Wiley & Sons, Inc.

Menzie, C. M. 1966. Metabolism of Pesticidies. Spec. Sci. Rep. 96. U.S. Dept. Interior, Fish and Wildlife Serv.

Newton, M. 1970. Herbicide Usage. *Science* 168:1605.

Palmer, J. S. 1963. Chronic Toxicity of 2, 4-D Alkanolamine Salt to Cattle. *JAVMA* 143:398-99.

———. 1964a. The Toxicologic Effects of Certain Fungicides and Herbicides on Sheep and Cattle. *Ann. N. Y. Acad. Sci.* 111:729-36.

———. 1964b. Toxicity of Carbamate, Triazine, Dichloropropionanilide, and Diallylacetamide Compounds to Sheep. *JAVMA* 145:917-20.

———. 1964c. Toxicity of Methyluracil and Substituted Urea and Phenol Compounds to Sheep. *JAVMA* 145:787-89.

———. 1964d. Toxicologic Effects of Silvex in Yearling Cattle. *JAVMA* 144:750-55.

Palmer, J. S.; Haufler, B. A.; Hunt, L. M.; Schlinke, J. C.; and Gatea, C. E. 1972. Chronic Toxicosis of Sheep from the Organic Herbicide Di-Allate. *Am. J. Vet. Res.* 33:543-46.

Palmer, J. S., and Radeleff, R. D. 1969. The Toxicity of Some Organic Herbicides to Cattle, Sheep, and Chickens. Prod. Res. Rep. No. 106. USDA-ARS.

Palmer, J. S., and Schlinke, J. C. 1973. Oral Toxicity of Tributyl Phosphorotrithioite, a Cotton Defoliant to Cattle and Sheep. *JAVMA* 163:1172-74.

Pinsent, P. J. N., and Lane, J.G. 1970. A Case of Possible 2, 4-D and 2, 4, 5-T Poisoning in the Horse. *Vet. Rec.* p.. 247.

Radeleff, R. D. 1964. *Veterinary Toxicology.* Philadelphia, Pennsylvania: Lea & Febiger.

Riper, W. N.; Rose, J. Q.; Leng, M. L.; and Gehring, P. J. 1973. The Fate of 2, 4, 5-Trichlorophenoxyacetic Acid (2, 4, 5-T) Following Oral Administration to Rats and Dogs. *Tox. and Applied Pharm.* 26:339-51.

Rogers, P. A.; Spillane, T. A.; Fenton, M.; and Henaghan, L. 1973. Short Communications. *The Veterinary Record* 92:44-45.

St. John, L. E. Jr.; Wagner, D. C.; and Lisk, D. J. 1964. The Fate of Atrazine, Kuron, Silvex, and 2,4,5-T in the Dairy Cow. *J. Dairy Sci.* 47:1267-70.

Smalley, H. E. 1973. Toxicity and Hazard of the Herbicide, Paraquat, in Turkeys. *Poultry Sci.* 52:1625-28.

Smalley, H. E., and Radeleff, R. D. 1970. Comparative Toxicity of the Herbicide Paraquat in Laboratory and Farm Animals. *Toxicol. Appl. Pharm.* 17:305.

Smith, A. E. 1973. Influence of 2, 4-D and 2, 4, 5-T on In Vitro Digestion of Forage Samples. *J. Range Management* 26:272-74.

Somers, J.; Morgan, E. T.; Reinhart, B. S. Jr.; and Stephenson, G. R. 1974. Effect of External Application of Pesticides to the Fertile Egg on Hatching Success and Early Chick Preformance. *Bull of Environ. Contam. and Tox.* II:33-38; 511-16.

Sparschu, G. L.; Dunn, F. L.; Lisowe, R. W.; and Rowe, V. K. 1971. Studies of the Effects of High Levels of 2, 4, 5-Trichlorophenoxyacetic Acid on Foetal Development in the Rat. *Food Cosmet. Toxicol.* 9:527-30.

Thomas, P., and Amor, O. F. 1968. A Case of Diquat Poisoning in Cattle. *The Vet. Rec.* 82:674-76.

United States Department of Agriculuture. 1967. *Suggested Guide for Weed Control.* Agr. Handbook 332.

Weed Science Society of America. 1974. *Herbicide Handbook.* 3rd ed. Geneva, New York: W. F. Humphrey Press.

Insecticides

NICOTINE

Source

Nicotine is an alkaloid extracted from the tobacco plant, *Nicotiana tabacum*. An aqueous solution containing 40 percent alkaloidal nicotine sulfate is available commercially as an insecticide. The generally used proprietary name is Black Leaf 40. Poisoning can result from the misuse of this preparation. Nicotine has also been combined with carbon tetrachloride, sodium arsenate and copper sulfate in an anthelmintic for use in cattle. Some problems including deaths occurred following the use of this combination. It was never determined whether the deaths were due to one of the active ingredients or to synergism of two or more components.

A death in a dog due to eating a package of cigarettes was reported by Kaplan (1968).

Nicotine solutions have also been used to spray plants for insect control.

Toxicity

Nicotine is highly toxic and should be handled with great care.

The LD_{50} in insects is 200-300 mg/kg. In laboratory rodents the oral LD_{50} is 24 mg/kg in the mouse and 55 mg/kg in the rat. The intravenous LD_{50} is 0.8 mg/kg in the mouse and 1 mg/kg in the rat.

The minimum lethal dose of nicotine for the dog and cat is 20-100 mg. If a cigarette contained 0.5-2 mg, then a package of twenty would contain 10-40 mg.

The lethal dose in the horse is 100-300 mg and for the sheep it is 100-200 mg.

Mechanism of Action

In small doses nicotine stimulates all autonomic ganglia and the central nervous system. The distribution of C^{14}-labelled nicotine in the mouse and cat brain has been described by Appelgren *et. al.,* (1962).

Large doses block the autonomic ganglia and the myoneural junction. Large doses cause a descending paralysis of the central nervous system.

Death is due to respiratory paralysis of the diaphragm and chest muscles.

Clinical Signs

A sequence of signs of excitement and stimulation followed by paralysis will be noted. There is excitement, rapid respiration, salivation, emesis and diarrhea. This is followed by depression, incoordination, rapid pulse, shallow and slow respiration, coma, flaccid paralysis and death.

Physiopathology and Diagnosis

There are no specific lesions. Signs of general anoxia will be present.

Treatment

The prognosis is poor. The first three to four hours after ingestion are critical. The effects of sublethal exposures should diminish in three hours.

Dermal exposures should be washed off.

Oral exposures are treated with gastric lavage with some recommending a 1:10,000 potassium permanganate solution.

Artificial respiration and oxygen should be used as indicated.

Variable success has followed the use of stimulants such as neosynephrine and amphetamine.

REFERENCES

Appelgren, L. E.; Hansson, E.; and Schmiterloew, C. G. 1962. The Accumulation and Metabolism of C- Labelled Nicotine in the Brain of Mice and Cats. *Acta. Physiol. Scand.* 56:249.

Kaplan, B. 1968. Acute Nicotine Poisoning in a Dog. *VM/SAC.* 63:1033.

Stowe, C. M. 1965. Ganglionic Blocking and Muscle Relaxant Drugs. L. M. Jones, ed. *Veterinary Pharmacology and Therapeutics.* Ames, Iowa: Iowa State University Press. pp. 334-35.

ORGANIC INSECTICIDES: GENERAL CONSIDERATIONS

Insects have always been a competitor of man and animals both for their food and as transmitters of disease-causing organisms. As population densities increased and as man turned to purposeful raising of crops and animals for his food supply, the battle lines were clearly drawn. A few insects and a small amount of insect damage could be tolerated; but when the productivity of crops and animals was threatened, then man was prepared to use whatever tools were available to protect his source of income and his food supply.

Marco Polo was reported to have brought pyrethrins back to Europe from his Asian trips. One can almost sense the awe the people must have expressed as they witnessed the quick knockdown of insects exposed to pyrethrins. By 1763 it was recognized that ground tobacco, a New World plant, killed insects. It was later recognized that this was due to the nicotine in tobacco. Also, in the eighteenth century various organic chemicals such as petroleum, kcroscnc, crcosotc, and turpentine were used to control mosquito larvae. These compounds were phytotoxic and, consequently, were of little value in protecting crops. Rotenone, another naturally occurring plant substance with insecticidal properties, was used in 1848.

Late in the nineteenth century highly refined oils with low toxicity to plants were developed as insecticides. Hydrogen cyanide (HCN) was used in 1886 to control the red scale insect, but by 1916 the insect was resistant to HCN. This is one of the earliest examples of insect resistance. Late in the 1800's a variety of metal salts of copper, zinc, thallium, lead, and chromium were used. Lead arsenate was used for gypsy moth control in 1892.

Synthetic organic compounds such as dinitrophenol, carbon disulfide, methyl bromide, thiocyanates, and cyclohexylamine were also introduced around 1892.

The insecticidal properties of DDT were recognized in 1939 and thc compound patented in 1942. DDT was used for public health purposes such as bedbug and body lice control during World War II. In 1945 DDT became available for general public use. The cyclodienes aldrin and dieldrin were developed in 1945. Another old chlorinated hydrocarbon insecticide is benzene hexachloride (hexachlorocyclohexane) which was developed in England and France in 1940.

The organophosphorus insecticides were also developed during World War II and are said to be, at least in part, a spin-off of research on organophosphorus nerve gases such as Tabun, Sarin, and Soman. The first organophosphorus insecticide was TEPP (tetraethylpyrophosphate), and the more widely known parathion and methyl parathion were introduced in 1944.

The carbamates are of more recent vintage with the exception of the pharmacologic carbamate, eserine or physostigmine, which was isolated from an African plant in 1864. Experimental work on carbamate insecticides began around 1947 with carbaryl (Sevin®) introduced in 1957.

During the late 1940's, Dr. R. D. Radeleff began studying the toxicity of the synthetic organic insecticides to livestock on a consulting basis with the Entomology Research Division of the Agricultural Research Service, Kerrville, Texas. Shortly thereafter Doctor Radeleff quit his private practice of veterinary medicine and became a full-time researcher with the U.S.D.A. laboratory at Kerrville. During the following twenty years, Doctor Radeleff and his colleagues continued to study the toxicity and metabolic effects of chemical compounds, many of which were later approved as insecticides. Much of the information obtained from studies with animals was eventually found to be also true in humans. Doctor Radeleff should be credited as a self-trained veterinary toxicologist whose contribution to our knowledge of the toxicity and metabolic effects of insecticides is yet to be equaled. His discussion of insecticides, acaricides, and anthelmintics is an excellent treatise on the toxicity of these compounds in domestic animals. (Radeleff, 1970)

Sources of Problems Resulting from Use of Insecticides

There are many classifications of insecticides. This discussion, however, will be limited primarily to the discussion of three major synthetic organic groups; namely, chlorinated hydrocarbon, organophosphorus, and carbamate compounds. We recognize that there are many other groups of insecticides such as activators or synergists, botanicals, nitrophenols, sulfonates, sulfides, sulfones, sulfonamides, sulfites, fumigants, attractants, and repellants. A summary of their toxicity to laboratory animals is presented by Kenaga and End (1974).

Poisoning in livestock and pet animals is usually accidental resulting from excessive or nonrecommended exposure to an insecticide. A common source of nonrecommended exposure to food-producing animals is the inadvertent mixing of granular or powdered pesticide formulations, mistaken for salt or mineral preparations, into animal feeds. Such formulations often appear physically similar to feed ingredients. Left-over portions of pesticides are often stored in feed bins along with other feed ingredients. At a later time during feed mixing operations, partially filled bags of insecticide may be misidentified as feed ingredients. Sometimes feed bins may be used for storing loose grain following their use for storage of insecticides resulting in contamination of the grain. Occasionally commercial grain elevators and feed manufacturers have stored pesticide formulations adjacent to feed ingredients resulting in the inadvertent mixing of pesticides in feed preparations. When livestock feeds are accidentally contaminated with such insecticide formulations, in addition to a possible high death loss, a chain reaction of insecticide exposure and contamination of food products may occur. The cadavers of animals killed by insecticide exposure may be used for the production of animal by-products used in swine and poultry feeds. Such cadavers may contain fifty to seventy-five or greater ppm insecticide in their fat. Although the carcasses may be diluted with other noncontaminated carcasses, a sufficient concentration may be present to result in low-level exposure to swine and poultry, resulting in contaminated meat and eggs. Also, animals and poultry which recover from accidental insecticide exposure in their feed have insecticide residues in their meat, milk, and eggs, especially if the pesticide was a chlorinated hydrocarbon such as DDT, aldrin, dieldrin, heptachlor, or chlordane, all of which have persistent residue characteristics.

Another source of low-level contamination of food-producing animals by insecticides is the use of persistent chlorinated hydrocarbon formulations such as DDT, aldrin, dieldrin, heptachlor, and endrin on crops which later may be used for animal feeds. These insecticides may persist in soil for several years. Thus, forage crops growing in soil treated with chlorinated hydrocarbon insecticides several years previously could be sufficiently contaminated to produce a residual level of insecticide in meat and milk from cows consuming the forage. One would not expect such exposure levels to be hazardous to the animals, but the public health significance of this problem is very apparent (see section on physiopathology, chapter on chlorinated hydrocarbon insecticides for more complete discussion of this problem). Table 1 summarizes the use of various insecticides on crops in the United States during a single year.

Another common source of insecticide poisoning in both large and small animals is the miscalculation of concentrations for spraying and dipping procedures and oral dosage preparations. A misplaced decimal point can result in a ten-, hundred-, or thousandfold increase in exposure, which may be disastrous for the treated animals or birds. A summary of the use of insecticides on livestock in the United States is given in table 2.

The use of insecticides not recommended for animals or formulations prepared for use on soils and crops are also common sources of poisoning. Relatively few of the chlorinated hydrocarbon insecticides are recommended for use on animals, some because they are highly toxic, others because of their persistence in animal tissues. Wettable powders and emulsifiable concentrates intended for spraying on plants are not suitable for dips or sprays for animals. This is because the wettable powder or emulsion particle for plant use is much larger than for animal use. (Radeleff, 1970) When a plant formulation is sprayed on an animal or used as a dip, there will be a tendency for the heavy particles to concentrate on the hair of the animal, resulting in excessive exposure and poisoning.

There are many other sources of insecticide poisoning in animals such as carelessness in leaving insecticides accessible to animals which will drink or eat them. Leaving insecticide preparations on sills of sheds and barns where they may be knocked down and trampled or eaten by animals is a common cause of poisoning in cattle, swine, and horses. Inadequate covers on backrubbers containing insecticide concentrates, using pesticide containers to water and feed animals without adequate decontamination, and treating animals under stress with certain insecticides are common causes of poisoning. It is unwise to expose an emaciated or sick animal to an insecticide. Also, castration, vaccination, and dehorning practices should not be done simultaneously with spraying or dipping with insecticides. It is important that the

TABLE 1

Use of Selected Insecticides[1] by U. S. Farmers on Certain Crops[2] in 1971

Insecticides—Pounds X 1000

Crop	DDT	Aldrin	Toxaphene	Disulfoton	Parathion	Diazinon	Phorate	Carbaryl
Corn	4	7,759	182	312	1,329	1,991	2,661	1,649
Cotton	13,158	—	28,112	225	2,560	—	100	1,214
Wheat	9	—	26	579	395	—	122	114
Soybeans	197	11	1,524	2	59	—	140	1,346
Tobacco	7	< 0.5	206	148	271	154	—	1,420
Alfalfa	—	1	18	227	247	151	22	104

[1] Other insecticides were used during 1971.

[2] Data available for other crops.

Source: See Table 2.

TABLE 2

Use of Selected Insecticides by U. S. Farmers on Livestock in 1971

Insecticides—Pounds X 1000

Animal	Lindane	DDT	Methoxy-chlor	Toxa-phene	Ruelene	Couma-phos	Ron-nel	Mala-thion	Cio-drin	Dichlor-vos	Car-baryl	Botan-icals
Dairy	14	55	872	200	2	18	33	142	693	2,109	18	78
Beef	226	158	1,011	3,483	215	147	384	357	176	153	196	38
Swine	164	27	58	843	< 0.5	2	44	88	26	26	52	6
Poultry	5	< 0.5	9	4	—	< 0.5	7	38	3	75	928	18
Sheep	4	3	18	39	—	1	1	3	1	2	< 0.5	2

Source: Quantities of Pesticides Used by Farmers in 1971, Agricultural Economics Report No. 252. Economic Research Service, USDA.

< = less than

insecticide applicator read the label on the container and observe any warning statements with regard to the insecticide's use.

Poisoning by systemic organophosphorus pesticides is usually associated with errors in administration for their systemic effect against cattle grubs, horse bots, flies, and other internal and external parasites. Some preparations are administered in the feed, others given orally in bolus or capsule form, while others are applied as a spray or dip. Sometimes an animal may suffer a reaction from a killed parasite within its body tissues. For example, cattle treated for grubs when the larval stage is in the esophagus may die of bloat because of the swelling and edema which occur in response to the killed larvae. Similarly, if the grub larvae are located in the spinal cord when the animal is treated, the killed grubs may cause a tissue reaction resulting in ataxia and paralysis. Although these reactions are not directly a toxicology problem, they frequently are encountered following the use of systemic organophosphorus compounds.

Toxicity

Toxicity data on the various chlorinated hydrocarbon, organophosphorus, and carbamate compounds are presented in their respective chapters. There are many factors which influence the toxicity of any particular insecticide. These include the species, breed, age, condition of the animal, state of lactation, accompanying stress, and weather conditions. Emaciated and lactating animals are several times more susceptible to such pesticides as benzene hexachloride and toxaphene than are nonlactating animals in good condition. Young animals generally are more susceptible to poisoning than are adults, although there are notable exceptions, such as ronnel, which is equally toxic to adult and young cattle. Certain breeds are more susceptible than others to specific insecticides. For example, Brahman cattle are highly susceptible to poisoning by the organophosphorus compound, Ciodrin® . It is generally considered that subjecting an animal to stress during or immediately following exposure to an insecticide may increase the likelihood of poisoning. Certain therapeutic agents may potentiate the toxicity of some insecticides. Examples of such potentiations that have been reported include phenothiazine compounds and high levels of vitamin A as possible potentiators of the organophosphorus insecticides coumaphos and trichlorfon. Efforts in our laboratory to substantiate this phenomenon, however, have not been successful.

Mechanism of Action

A large number of different compounds are used as insecticides which makes it difficult to present a comprehensive and coherent discussion of the biological effects of insecticides. The following discussions are not complete reviews of all that is known about insecticides since books have been written on individual or groups of chemical insecticides. What is presented are some of the major effects of insecticides that are of interest to the clinical toxicologist. The reader should keep in mind that insecticides were developed to control insects and not birds or mammals. Therefore, more is known about the mechanism of action of insecticides in insects than in birds or mammals.

Originally all that was required to be known was the actue toxicity of insecticides for birds and mammals, since the major problem in birds and mammals was considered to be overt poisoning due to accidental exposures. The history of insecticides since 1942, when DDT was patented and became available for public use in 1945, clearly shows that several types of unanticipated problems have developed which are distinctly different from acute toxicosis. Problems such as eggshell thinning, fish kills, enzyme induction, generalized low-level residues, and biological magnification of environmental residues have required more study of the mechanism(s) of action of insecticides, their metabolism and environmental impact.

The mechanism(s) of action of the three major classes of synthetic organic insecticides are discussed in their respective chapters.

BIBLIOGRAPHY

Buck, W. B. 1969. Pesticides and Economic Poisons in the Food Chain. Proc. 23rd An. Meet. U.S. Anim. Health Assn. pp. 221-26.

———. 1965. Diagnosis of Poisoning by Organic Pesticides. Proc. 69th An. Meet. U.S. Livestock Sanitary Assn. pp. 513-23.

———. 1969. Laboratory Toxicologic Tests and Their Interpretation. *JAVMA* 155:1938.

———. 1970. Diagnosis of Feed-Related Toxicoses. *JAVMA* 156:1440-41.

———. 1970. Lead and Organic Pesticide Poisoning in Cattle. *JAVMA* 156:1470-72.

Quantities of Pesticides Used by Farmers in 1971. Agricultural Economic Report No. 252. USDA.

Kenaga, E. E., and End, C. S. 1974. Commercial and Experimental Insecticides. Ent. Soc. Amer. Special Publication 74-1.

Radeleff, R. D. 1970. *Veterinary Toxicology.* Philadelphia, Pennsylvania: Lea & Febiger.

Report of the Secretary's Commission on Pesticides and Their Relationship to Environmental Health. 1969. E. M. Mrak, Chairman. U.S. Dept. HEW.

ORGANOCHLORINE INSECTICIDES

The organochlorine insecticides (chlorinated hydrocabons) include the diphenyl aliphatic (DDT), aryl and cyclodiene groups.

Toxicity

Toxicity data for certain organochlorine insecticides to domestic and laboratory animals and wildlife are presented in table 1.

Mechanism of Action

Although the use of some of the more persistent chlorinated hydrocarbon insecticides is either being discontinued or severely restricted, their history and the types of problems that developed serve as valuable models helping to define the relationship between the crop and livestock segments of modern agriculture.

The exact mechanism of action of the chlorinated hydrocarbon insecticides with the possible exception of DDT is unknown. Generally they are diffuse stimulants or depressants of the central nervous system. A discussion of other known biologic effects is given under *Physiopathology.*

As early as 1946 it was known that DDT increased the firing rate of nerve fibers. (Roeder and Weiant, 1946) DDT appeared to decrease the membrane threshold for an action potential to occur and once the nerve was stimulated a volley of action potentials occurred. This helps explain the generalized fine muscle tremors seen in DDT poisoning. More recent studies using voltage-clamp techniques in giant axons, have demonstrated that DDT slows down the turning off of the Na^+ membrane current and inhibits the turning on of the K^+ membrane current. (Narahashi, 1969) Recall that when a normal nerve membrane is stimulated there is an initial inward rush of Na^+ ions for 1-2 milliseconds followed by an outward flow of K^+ ions to restore the nerve membrane to its resting potential. Therefore, the net effect of DDT is to make the inside of the nerve membrane more positive and thus decrease the threshold (partially depolarized) for another action potential to occur. Of course, if the effect becomes severe enough then the nerve membrane would be permanently depolarized. Sensory nerves are more sensitive to DDT than are motor nerves.

The muscle tremors seen in DDT poisoning are the result of local effects on nerve fibers and stimulation of spinal reflexes, since the muscle tremors also occur in decerebrate and decerebellate animals. However, DDT also affects the brain in intact animals. Electroencephalographic (EEG) changes include a decrease in slow activity and a tendency for the EEG to become a diffuse pattern of low amplitude-fast frequency activity. After exposure has stopped, slow wave activity returns over a period of days to weeks. Spike activity that is in synchrony with the whole body muscle tremors can be recorded from the cerebellum. EEG changes occur in the cerebellum before they occur in the cerebrum.

Dieldrin affects the brain and causes high amplitude-slow frequency waves to appear in the cortical EEG. Convulsions are thought to be a result of ammonia buildup as a result of impairment of glutamine synthesis. (St. Omer, 1971)

Clinical Signs

The chlorinated hydrocarbon insecticides act as diffuse stimulants or depressants of the central nervous system. Clinical signs expressing stimulation or depression take many forms but usually are of a neuromuscular type. Although it is unlikely that a single poisoned animal will demonstrate all of the possible symptoms, there is sufficient similarity between animals to permit the recognition and identification of a definite syndrome. The onset of signs occurs within a few minutes or a few days after exposure, usually within twenty-four hours. The signs displayed may be progressively severe in nature or may be explosive and fulminating. At first, an animal may be apprehensive, hypersensitive, or belligerent. Fasciculations of the face and cervical muscles

TABLE 1
Toxicity of Some Common Organochlorine Insecticides to Livestock[1], Laboratory Animals[2], and Wildlife[3]

Chemical	Species	Age or Sex	Oral Maximum Non-Toxic Dose Tested mg/kg B. Wt.[4]	Oral Minimum Toxic Dose Found Mg/kg B. Wt.[5]	Dermal Maximum Non-Toxic Dose Tested	Dermal Minimum Toxic Dose Found[5]
Diphenyl Aliphatics—DDT Relatives						
DDT	Calves	1-2 wks.	100	250	8.0%	
1,1,1-trichloro-	Cattle	Adult	250	500	8.0%	
2,2-bis (p-chloro-	Sheep	Adult	250	500	8.0%	
phenyl) ethane	Goats	Adult	250		8.0%	
Chlorophenothene	Rat		CO 5 ppm	LD_{50} = 87		LD_{50} = 2000 mg/kg
	Mouse			LD_{50} = 150		
$C_{14}H_9Cl_5$	Rabbit			LD_{50} = 250		LD_{50} = 2820 mg/kg
	Dog		CO 400 ppm			
	Mallards	3 mos. F		LD_{50} > 2240		
	Pheasants	3 mos. F		LD_{50} = 1296		
	Coturnix	2 mos. M		LD_{50} = 841		
	Pigeons			LD_{50} > 4000		
	Lesser Sandhill Cranes	Adult		LD_{50} > 1200		
	Bullfrogs	F		LD_{50} > 2000		
Methoxychlor	Calves	1-2 wks.	250	500	8.0%	
1,1,1-trichloro-	Cattle	Adult			8.0%	
2,2-bis (p-methoxy-	Sheep	Adult	1000		8.0%	
phenyl) ethane	Rat		CO > 100	LD_{50} = 5000		LD_{50} > 3000 mg/kg
Marlate®	Mouse			LD_{50} = 1850		
	Rabbit			LD_{50} > 6000		
$C_{16}H_{15}Cl_3O_2$	Dog		CO > 4000			
	Mallards	3 mos. M		LD_{50} > 2000		
1,1-dichloro-2,2-	Calves	1-2 wks.	250	500	8.0%	
bis (p-ethylphenyl)	Sheep	Adult	1000			
ethane	Rat		CO 500	LD_{50} = 6600		
Perthane®	Mouse			LD_{50} = 9220		
$C_{18}H_{20}Cl_2$	Dog		CO 100			
Dicofol						
4,4-dichloro-						
2-(trichloro-						
methyl) benzhydrol						
Kelthane®						
$C_{14}H_9Cl_5O$	Rat		CO 20 ppm	LD_{50} = 575		LD_{50} = 1000 mg/kg
	Dog		CO 300 ppm	LD_{50} > 4000		
	Rabbit			LD_{50} = 1810		LD_{50} = 2100 mg/kg

1. Data adapted primarily from Radeleff (1970).

2. Data adapted primarily from Kenaga and End (1974).

3. Data adapted from Tucker and Crabtree (1970).

4. Maximum single dose which did not produce a toxic effect. CO = chronic oral exposure, 90 days or longer, in parts per million in diet which did not have toxic effects.

5. Minimum single dose which caused minimal toxic effects. Those levels given as LD_{50} are minimum values given that caused 50% death losses.

TABLE 1 (Cont.)

Chemical	Species	Age or Sex	Oral		Dermal	
			Maximum Non-Toxic Dose Tested	Minimum Toxic Dose Found	Maximum Non-Toxic Dose Tested	Minimum Toxic Dose Found
			mg/kg B. Wt.	mg/kg B. Wt.		
Aryl and Cyclodiene Organochlorines						
Aldrin	Calves	1-2 wks.	2.5	5.0	0.1%	0.25%
1,2,3,4,10,10-hexachloro-1,4,4a,5,8,8a-hexahydro-1,4-endo-exo-5,8-dimethanonaphthalene	Cattle	Adult	10	25		
	Sheep	3 wks.	10	15	4.0%	
	Goats	3 wks.			4.0%	
	Rat		CO 0.5 ppm	$LD_{50} = 39$		$LD_{50} = 80$ mg/kg
	Mouse			$LD_{50} = 44$		
Octalene	Dog		CO 1 ppm	$LD_{50} = 65$		
	Rabbit			$LD_{50} = 50$		$LD_{50} < 150$ mg/kg
$C_{12}H_8Cl_6$	Mallards	3-4 mos. F		$LD_{50} = 520$		
	Pheasants	3-4 mos. F		$LD_{50} = 17$		
	Quail	3-4 mos. F		$LD_{50} = 7$		
	Fulvous Tree Duck	3-6 mos. M		$LD_{50} = 29$		
Chlordane	Calves	1-2 wks.	10	25	1.0%	1.5%
1,2,4,5,6,7,8,8-octachloro-3a,4,7,7a-tetrahydro-4,7-methanoindane	Cattle	Adult	75	90	2.0%	
	Lambs	3 wks.			1.5%	2.0%
	Sheep	Adult	35	50	3.0%	4.0%
Octachlor®	Goats	Adult			3.0%	4.0%
	Horses	Adult			1.5%	
	Pigs	Adult			1.5%	
$C_{10}H_6Cl_8$	Rat		CO > 25	$LD_{50} = 283$		$LD_{50} = 580$ mg/kg
	Rabbit					$LD_{50} < 780$ mg/kg
	Mallard	4-5 mos. F		$LD_{50} = 1200$		
Dieldrin	Calves	1-2 wks.	5	10	0.1%	0.25%
1,2,3,4,10,10-hexachloro-6,7-epoxy-1,4,4a,5,6,7,8,8a-octahydro-1,4-endo-exo-5,8-dimethanonaphthalene	Cattle	Adult	10	25	1.0%	2.0%
	Lambs	2 wks.			2.0%	3.0%
	Sheep	Adult	10	25		4.0%
	Goats	Adult		$LD_{50} = 100$		4.0%
	Horses	Adult		25	1.0%	
Octalox	Pigs	8 wks.	25	50	4.0%	
HEOD	Rat		CO 0.5	$LD_{50} = 40$		$LD_{50} = 52$ mg/kg
	Mouse			$LD_{50} = 38$		
	Rabbit			$LD_{50} = 45$		$LD_{50} = 250$ mg/kg
	Dog			$LD_{50} = 65$		
$C_{12}H_8Cl_6O$	Mallard	6-7 mos. F		$LD_{50} = 381$		
	Pheasant	10-23 mos. M		$LD_{50} = 79$		
	Chukar	8-11 mos.		$LD_{50} = 23$		
	Coturnix	2 mos. M		$LD_{50} = 70$		
	Pigeon			$LD_{50} = 27$		

TABLE 1 (Cont.)

| Chemical | Species | Age or Sex | Oral | | Dermal | |
			Maximum Non-Toxic Dose Tested mg/kg B. Wt.	Minimum Toxic Dose Found mg/kg B. Wt.	Maximum Non-Toxic Dose Tested	Minimum Toxic Dose Found
	Sparrow	F		LD_{50} = 48		
	Canada Geese	Adult		LD_{50} = 50		
	Fulvous Tree Duck	F		LD_{50} = 100		
	Partridges	3-10 mos. F		LD_{50} = 9		
	Mule Deer	8-18 mos. M		LD_{50} = 75		
Endrin	Goats	Adult		LD_{50} = 25		
1,2,3,4,10,10-hex-achloro-6,7-epoxy-1,4,4a,5,6,7,8,8a-octahydro-1,4-endo-endo-5,8-di-methanonaphthalene	Rat			LD_{50} = 3		LD_{50} = 12 mg/kg
	Mouse		CO >1 – <25			
	Rabbit			LD_{50} = 7		LD_{50} = 60 mg/kg
	Mallard	10-13 mos. F		LD_{50} = 6		
	Pheasant	3-4 mos. F		LD_{50} = 2		
$C_{12}H_8Cl_6O$	Pigeon			LD_{50} = 2		
	Grouse	4 yrs. F		LD_{50} = 1		
Heptachlor	Calves	1-2 wks.	15	20	0.25%	0.5%
1,4,5,6,7,8,8-hep-tachloro-3a,4,7,7a-tetrahydro-4,7-methanoindene	Cattle	Adult			0.5%	
	Sheep	Adult	25	50	4.0%	
	Rat		CO 0.5	LD_{50} = 40		LD_{50} = 119 mg/kg
Velsicol 104®	Mouse			LD_{50} = 68		
	Rabbit					LD_{50} = 2000 mg/kg
$C_{10}H_5Cl_7$	Dog		CO 4			
	Mallard	3 mos. M		LD_{50} = 2000		
Lindane	Calves	1-2 wks.	2.5	5.0	0.025%	0.05%
1,2,3,4,5,6-hex-achlorocyclohex-ane, gamma isomer	Cattle	6-8 mos.			0.1%	
	Cattle	Adult	10	25	0.1%	0.25%
gamma BHC	Lambs	3 wks.				0.15%
	Sheep	Adult	10	25	0.15%	
$C_6H_6Cl_6$	Horses	Adult			0.15%	
	Pigs	3 mos.			1.0%	
	Rat		CO 50	LD_{50} = 76		LD_{50} = 500 mg/kg
	Mouse			LD_{50} = 86		
	Rabbit			LD_{50} = 60		LD_{50} = 300 mg/kg
	Dog		CO >15	LD_{50} = 40		
	Mallards	3-4 mos. M		LD_{50} > 2000		
Mirex	Rat			LD_{50} = 235		
Dodecachloro-octahydro-1,3,4-metheno-1H-cyclo-buta[cd] pentalene	Rabbit					LD_{50} = 800 mg/kg
	Mallard	3-4 mos. M		LD_{50} > 2400		
Dechlorane®						
$C_{10}Cl_{12}$						

TABLE 1 (Cont.)

Chemical	Species	Age or Sex	Oral Maximum Non-Toxic Dose Tested mg/kg B. Wt.	Oral Minimum Toxic Dose Found mg/kg B. Wt.	Dermal Maximum Non-Toxic Dose Tested	Dermal Minimum Toxic Dose Found
Toxaphene	Calves	1-2 wks.	5	10	0.5%	0.75%
Chlorinated Camphene Containing 67-69% Chlorine Camphechlor	Cattle	4 mos.			1.0%	
	Cattle	Adult	25	35	2.0%	4.0%
	Sheep	Adult	10	25	1.5%	4.0%
	Goats			25	1.5%	4.0%
	Goats			$LD_{50} > 160$		
	Horses				1.5%	
	Pigs	Adult			1.5%	
	Rat		CO 10	$LD_{50} = 40$		$LD_{50} = 600$ mg/kg
	Mouse			$LD_{50} = 112$		
	Rabbit			$LD_{50} < 780$		$LD_{50} = 780$ mg/kg
	Dog		CO 400	$LD_{50} = 15$		
	Mallard	1 wk.		$LD_{50} = 31$		
	Mallard	3-5 mos. F		$LD_{50} = 71$		
	Pheasant	3 mos. F		$LD_{50} = 40$		
	Quail	3 mos. M		$LD_{50} = 85$		
	Grouse	Adult M		$LD_{50} = 10$		
	Fulvous Tree Duck	3-6 mos. M		$LD_{50} = 99$		
	Lesser Sandhill Crane	F		$LD_{50} = 100$		
	Mule Deer	Adult M		$LD_{50} = 139$		

soon follow. Spasms of the eyelids, muscles of the forequarters, and finally the hindquarters may occur continuously or intermittently. Clonic-tonic seizures often follow, which may progress to death or be repeated intermittently, interrupted by periods of CNS depression. Some animals may become increasingly agitated, often frenzied, and lose coordination. They may stumble while walking, jump imaginary objects, walk aimlessly about, or move in circles. Abnormal posturing may be assumed such as resting the sternum on the ground while the hind legs remain in the standing position. Others persist in keeping the head between the forelegs. There may be continuous chewing movements accompanied by an increased flow of saliva. Some animals may continue to chew for hours and even days. Poisoned animals may become comatose and remain so for several hours prior to death, or they may regain consciousness and fully recover. Sometimes animals will suffer a convulsive seizure while standing. They may raise their head in the air as if having been stung on the nose and then go backwards in a circle, often falling down in a convulsive seizure. When an entire herd has been in convulsive seizures, this will be evident by the mud and debris on the animals' bodies. All animals including poultry exhibit similar signs of poisoning by the chlorinated hydrocarbon insecticides. Animals with a simple stomach will usually vomit following oral consumption of insecticides. This may result in increased salivation and frothy accumulation at the mouth.

Physiopathology

Pathologic changes associated with acute poisoning by chlorinated hydrocarbon insecticides are usually minimal and nonspecific. If convulsive activity has preceded death, accompanied by high body temperature (as is often the case with chlorinated hydrocarbon compounds), cloudy swelling of the viscera and blanching of the intestines is often present. Small hemorrhages occur at random throughout the body, especially the heart. There may be diffuse endocardial and epicardial hemorrhages. Generally there is pulmonary congestion, hemorrhages and edema. The brain and spinal cord are frequently congested and edematous. Excess cerebrospinal fluid causing increased pressure frequently occurs.

Chronic exposure to chlorinated insecticides can cause liver cell changes, including increased deposition of fat, margination of cytoplasmic granules, hypertrophy of hepatic cells, formation of lipoid cytoplasmic bodies and an increased amount of smooth endoplasmic reticulum. The rat seems to be more susceptible to these changes than other animals. The no-effect level for DDT in the rat is about 5 ppm while in the rhesus monkey levels of 5,000 ppm are required. Liver function tests are altered at DDT feeding levels of 400 ppm in the rat and liver necrosis occurs at feeding levels of 1,000 ppm in the rat.

The dog adrenal gland is susceptible to DDD (TDE). Adrenal cortical atrophy occurs without any effect on the medulla and the atrophy does not involve the pituitary gland. The o,p'-DDD isomer is effective and appears to block the ACTH regulated mitochondrial conversion of cholesterol to pregnenolone. (Hart and Straw, 1971) Because of this effect, o,p'-DDD has been used to treat Cushing's syndrome.

The no-effect level of aldrin, dieldrin, and endrin is approximately 0.05 mg/kg or 1 ppm in the dog, rat and monkey. At 2 ppm there is increased metabolism of steroids in birds. The chlorinated insecticides cross both the placental and blood-brain barriers.

Biological Magnification

The chlorinated hydrocarbon insecticides have pointed out the relationships within the food web. In one example DDD was applied to a lake at a concentration of 0.02 ppm. About a year later DDD levels in the plankton were 10 ppm, in small fish 900 ppm and in large fish and fish-eating birds over 2,000 ppm. (Hunt and Bischoff, 1960) This is an example of biological magnification where relatively low background levels become concentrated in different levels of the food chain. Similar phenomena may occur with other persistent fat soluble chemicals. This process is of interest to veterinarians for several reasons. The dairy cow is located near the top of the food chain and is known to concentrate chlorinated hydrocarbon insecticide in the milk. The situation is similar for the chicken that is fed a diet of plant and animal origin. Residues present in the feed are eliminated in the egg.

Enzyme Induction

Dieldrin and heptachlor are the best enzyme inducers in the rat. Levels of 1 ppm in the diet will induce aldrin epoxidase activity. DDT is also a good inducer with a level of 2— 2.5 ppm required to induce hexobarbital oxidase. Most of the other insecticides must be present at levels greater than 5 ppm for enzyme induction to occur. Enzyme induction results in an increased breakdown of both exogenous and endogenous chemicals. The medical concern is whether the levels of pesticide residues occurring in man and animals are sufficient to increase the metabolism of endogenous hormones and whether this results in altered health or decreased production.

Eggshell Thinning

The relationship between DDT and its metabolites and the thin eggshell problem in certain wild birds is beginning to be understood. Neither DDT nor DDE have much influence on eggshell thickness in gallinaceous birds such as chickens, pheasants, or Japanese quail if there is sufficient calcium in the diet, although it is possible to produce some decrease in eggshell thickness and reductions in shell calcium if high doses of DDT are fed. The same is true for mallards and kestrels. However, if DDE is fed rather than DDT then eggshell thinning has been demonstrated in sparrow hawks, mallards and black ducks even in the presence of adequate dietary calcium. DDE levels of 10-30 ppm reduce eggshell thickness by 15-25 percent. DDE residues in the eggs from the experimentally fed birds are similar to those found in wild birds that were producing thin eggshells. In addition to the decrease in shell thickness there is an increase in shell magnesium and decreases in shell barium, strontium and calcium.

The mechanism of action is not understood. Originally it was hypothesized that DDE inhibited carbonic anhydrase as do acetazolamide and sulfanilamide which also cause thin eggshells. However, both *in vivo* and *in vitro* carbonic anhydrase measurements have failed to produce convincing evidence that the degree of inhibition is sufficient to account for the observed effects. Other theories suggest that since o,p'-DDT is estrogenic that it might be serving in the biofeedback mechanism to the hypothalamus and thus upsetting the hormonal mechanisms involved in production of the egg. Still others suggest that liver microsomal enzymes are induced and there is a faster breakdown of endogenous hormones.

Some evidence suggests that DDT acts by inhibiting ATPase and thus limits the amount of energy available for the active transport of calcium into the shell gland.

Environmental Residues

Environmental contamination is a result of translocation of insecticides from the soil to plants, drift of sprays onto forage or soil dust precipitating onto forage. A survey of animal feed grains and forages in Pennsylvania found 54 percent of the forages and 62 percent of the grain and commercial feed supplements containing detectable residues of DDT ranging from 0.003 ppm to 0.33 ppm. (Cole *et al.*, 1966) A Canadian study found dieldrin residues in sixteen of twenty sweet clover and alfalfa samples. (Saha, 1969) The available data can be criticized for being fragmentary.

Unfortunately for the veterinarian, more is known about the uptake of soil insecticides by potatoes, beets, and rutabagas than alfalfa and corn.

Residues found in corn grain and soybeans are shown in table 2. Generally residues are lower in the seed (grain) than in the roughage portion of the plant. A limited amount of work has been reported on the translocation of DDT from soil to forage in crops, but some recent work suggests that the DDT vaporizes from the soil and reaches the plant through the air or on dust particles rather than via translocation from the roots. The direct application of DDT to forage crops results in residues of a few to over 100 ppm depending on the elapsed time.

TABLE 2
Average Chlorinated Hydrocarbon Insecticide Residues (PPM) in Corn Grain and Soybeans—1964-66*

Insecticide	Corn	Soybeans	Soybean Oil	Soybean Meal
DDT	0.007	0.006	0.015	0.005
TDE	0.003	t	0.006	t
DDE	t*	t	0.002	0.001
Dieldrin	0.001	0.002	0.013	t
Toxaphene		0.004	0.024	

t = trace

*Adapted from Duggan, 1968.

Heptachlor residues in alfalfa, sudan grass, birdsfoot trefoil and corn ranged from 4 to 30 ppb when grown in soil treated with 1 pound heptachlor/acre. Table 3 shows the slow decline in heptachlor residues in alfalfa grown up to three years after the ground was last treated with heptachlor.

Alfalfa growing in soil treated with aldrin at 1.3 to 1.5 pounds/acre resulted in residues of 9 ppb. Dieldrin applied at 3 to 5 pounds/acre resulted in 10 to 90 ppb dieldrin in alfalfa thirty-two months after application. A report on translocation of dieldrin by corn is summarized in table 4.

TABLE 3
Heptachlor Persistence in the Alfalfa Production Environment*

Time Since Last Treatment (years)	N	Heptachlor Residue (ppm)
3	56	0.017
2	528	0.050
1	934	0.181
0.5	45	0.416

*Adapted from Engel *et al.*, 1965.

TABLE 4
Translocation of Dieldrin by Corn*

Soil** Dieldrin Level	1 ppm	5 ppm
Plant part	Plant Residue (ppb)	
Leaves—Top 1/2 of plant	20-30	30-180
Stalk—Top 1/2 of plant	10-160	30-220
Ear	10-30	30-110
Lower Leaves	10-500	110-1200
Lower Stalk	100-3920	520-10,910
Subdivision of ear		
Ear Leaf	10-40	30-90
Cob	40-80	130-270
Kernels	4-10	20-40

*Adapted from Beestman *et al.*, 1969.

**Part of variation in residues is due to difference in soil types studied.

Uptake and Excretion in Domestic Animals

In order to adequately understand and be able to derive reasonable recommendations, rules, and regulations for insecticide usage, we must know how efficient domestic animals are in accumulating insecticides and how much time is required for their elimination.

First, it can be stated that, based on available evidence, the concentration of an insecticide in milk will rise rapidly within a few hours or days following the initial feeding of contaminated feed and will level off at a plateau characteristic for each concentration in the diet and for each insecticide. The data in table 5 shows the average milk/diet ratios for various insecticides.

Stated another way, cows can consume a diet containing 800 ppm methoxychlor and will have milk levels of 0.13 ppm methoxychlor; while cows consuming 0.3 ppm heptachlor epoxide will secrete milk containing 0.140 ppm heptachlor epoxide. Thus, not only the level in the diet but also the specific insecticide involved must be considered. Therefore, trace amounts of aldrin, dieldrin, and heptachlor epoxide represent a much

TABLE 5

Relative Efficiency of Dairy Cows in the Oral Uptake and Secretion in Milk of Chlorinated Hydrocarbon Insecticides*

Insecticide	Range of Feeding Levels (ppm)	Average Milk/Diet Ratio
Heptachlor Epoxide	0.05-0.30	.90-.37
Heptachlor Epoxide	0.005-0.020	.56-.21
Telodrin	0.005-0.020	.4-.5
Aldrin	1-40	0.39
Dieldrin	0.05-0.30	0.39
Endrin	0.05-0.30	0.07
DDT — direct feeding	0.05-0.30	0.030
DDT + weathered DDT	0.023-4	1.08-.15
Kelthane	2	0.15
Gamma BHC	0.05-0.30	0.04
Heptachlor	50-200	0.020
Chlordane	50-5000	0.0016
Toxaphene	20-140	0.014
Methoxychlor	800-7000	0.00023

*Adapted from Saha, 1969.

greater threat to the marketability of a food product of animal origin than do trace amounts of methoxychlor.

Based on feeding trials in dairy cattle, a dietary level of more than 1.3 ppm DDT will likely result in milk residues above 0.05 ppm (actionable level). However, DDT is broken-down under field conditions so that residues in plants will consist of DDT, DDE, and DDD. Administration of 4 ppm DDT dissolved in oil results in 0.87 ppm DDT and metabolites in milk. Therefore, rather than a milk/feed ratio of 0.03 (table 5) based on direct feeding of DDT, weathered DDT residues on crops result in milk/feed ratios of 0.15 to 0.5 when the dietary level is greater than 1 ppm. One study demonstraed that a feed level of 0.023 ppm (weathered DDT residues, no extraneous DDT was added) resulted in milk residues of 0.025 ppm or a milk/feed ratio of 1.08, which is thirty-six times the milk/feed ratio based on direct DDT feeding trials. Thus, "weathered" DDT residues in excess of 0.05 ppm may result in actionable residue levels. It is this rather fragmentary information on very low-level feeding studies (*i.e.,* levels at or near "naturally" occurring environmental levels) that brings into focus the importance of translocation and surface contamination of plants used for animal feed. (Saha, 1969)

Both plants and animals readily convert aldrin to dieldrin. The ratio of dieldrin in milk to aldrin in feed is 0.39 which is the same as the ratio of dieldrin in milk to dieldrin in feed (table 5). Thus, residues of aldrin and dieldrin in excess of 0.03 ppm in fresh plants will lead to more than 0.01 ppm dieldrin in milk.

Even less data is available on the rate of excretion than on the uptake of chlorinated hydrocarbon insecticides by domestic animals. Based on available data, the biological half-life for several insecticides is given in table 6. The data is limited by few observations and in most instances by lack of experimental design which would allow for adequate determination of excretion rates.

Some information is available to describe the toxicodynamics of DDE and dieldrin in cows milk. Recent work (Fries *et. al.,* 1969) has suggested a two component first-order model to describe the elimination of DDE from cows milk. The normalized equation was of the form $C = .41e^{-0.31t} + .59e^{-0.013t}$* which suggests

*C = Concentration; e = base of natural logarithm; t = time in days. (See chapter on *Toxicokinetics*)

TABLE 6

Estimated Biologic Half-Life of Chlorinated Hydrocarbon Insecticides in Domestic Animals

Insecticide	Animal	Tissue	Half-Life (days)	Reference
Dieldrin	Heifer	Fat	85	Hironaka, 1968
	Steer	Fat	245	Hironaka, 1968
	Hens	Fat	49	Liska and Stadelman, 1969
	Swine	Fat	28	Dobson *et al.,* 1971
	Cow	Milk Fat	22	Liska and Stadelman, 1969
	Cow	Milk Fat	30	Moubry *et al.,* 1968
DDT	Cow	Milk Fat	14-20	Moubry *et al.,* 1968
	Hen	Fat	49	Liska and Stadelman, 1969
	Hen	Fat	56	Liska and Stadelman, 1969
DDE	Cow	Milk Fat	52	Fries *et al.,* 1969

a rapid loss of approximately 41 percent of the residue followed by a much slower elimination of the remaining 59 percent. The biological half-life of the first part is 2.2 days and 53 days for the second part. A similar equation with different constants can also be used to describe the elimination of dieldrin in milk fat. The following normalized equation closely fits the milk excretion curves published for dieldrin. The normalized equation is $C = .52e^{-.2t} + .48e^{-.012t}$. The half-life of the first component is 3.46 days and 57 days for the second component. This suggests that for both DDE and dieldrin there is a rapid elimination of about 40-50 percent of the residue during the first 3 to 4 days following contamination. Dieldrin would seem to be eliminated slightly slower than DDE but in both cases the time is quite lengthy for the elimination of the second half of the initial residue.

These equations can be of some use in estimating the time required to maintain animals on clean diets before residues decline to acceptable levels. However, a word of caution is needed. The two component equation assumes that you have milk residue data immediately after exposure has occurred. If the data you are working with was obtained from samples taken more than a few days after exposure occurred then only the second component of the equation is valid, since the rapid elimination phase would have already occurred. In the case of DDE you would assume a half-life of 53 days and for dieldrin a half-life of 57 days.

Diagnosis

A history that animals have been exposed to an insecticide coupled with clinical signs, manifested primarily by convulsive seizures and neuromuscular involvement would warrant a tentative diagnosis of chlorinated hydrocarbon insecticide poisoning.

The absence of definitive lesions upon necropsy except for pulmonary congestion and edema and occasional ecchymotic hemorrhages in the cardiac and digestive tract are also compatible with synthetic organic insecticide poisoning. If an animal has been in prolonged convulsive seizures and suffered an extremely high body temperature, the intestines may have a blanched appearance.

Chemical analysis of liver, kidney, stomach contents, fat and hair will usually confirm exposure to a specific insecticide. The presence of an insecticide in the tissues, however, does not necessarily substantiate a diagnosis. Since the chlorinated hydrocarbon insecticides are cumulative in the tissues substantial levels may accumulate in normal animals exposed to recommended levels of insecticide. However, the presence of excessive levels of insecticide in the liver and kidney in addition to stomach contents or hair may enable a diagnostician to confirm a diagnosis of poisoning. Recent studies have indicated that brain levels may have more consistent diagnostic value. Furr (1974) found that 4-5 ppm or more dieldrin in whole macerated swine brain and 3-4 ppm in chicken brain were associated with aldrin poisoning and death. Clinical signs without death were associated with 2 ppm or less. Similar data was obtained with toxaphene.

Chlorinated hydrocarbon insecticide poisoning must be differentiated from several other infectious and non-infectious conditions in animals. In cattle, polioencephalomalacia (polio) and lead poisoning often produce central nervous system disturbances similar to those produced by chlorinated hydrocarbon insecticides. Blood and tissue analyses for lead can be confirmatory and growth and histopathologic changes in the brain can be used for diagnosis of polio. Infectious thromboembolic meningoencephalitis, rabies, nervous forms of coccidiosis and ketosis, and brain abscesses all may produce clinical signs similar to those produced by the chlorinated hydrocarbon insecticides. In swine, water deprivation-sodium ion toxicity and pseudorabies are manifested by clinical signs similar to those produced by chlorinated hydrocarbon insecticides. These conditions can be differentiated by histopathologic examination of the brain and suitable tissue isolation and innoculation techniques. In dogs and cats, strychnine, and in dogs fluoroacetate (1080) produce signs very similar to the chlorinated hydrocarbon insecticides. These toxicants can be differentiated only by chemical analysis. Rabies and some forms of acute food poisoning may also be manifested by central nervous system disturbances.

Treatment

Since the precise mechanism by which chlorinated hydrocarbon insecticides produce poisoning in animals is not yet known, no specific antidote is available. Poisoned animals manifesting convulsive seizures or other neuromuscular hyperactivity should be lightly anesthetized with chloral hydrate or a long-acting barbiturate. If exposure was by the dermal route, the animal should be washed thoroughly with soap and water. If exposure was oral, a saline cathartic, activated charcoal (about 900 gm per adult cow), or a gastric lavage may be indicated. Usually animals need not be anesthetized for longer than twenty-four hours; and in some instances recovery may be complete after three to six hours. Some affected animals are dull, listless, and generally unreactive. The administration of stimulants may be indicated in such cases. Several practicing veterinarians have reported that various tranquilizing agents are useful in controlling the more violent neuromuscular activity.

Decontamination of Domestic Animals

Several methods have been tested to increase the excretion rate of insecticide residues in domestic animals. The first consideration is obviously to remove the source of contamination. However, this is not always as easy as it may appear since the attending veterinarian must first identify the source. This may require extensive laboratory analysis, and may not always be conclusive. In cases where dermal application is involved, the animals should be washed immediately with a warm water, soap solution in order to limit dermal absorption.

If feed is suspected then the various feed constituents such as grain, roughages, protein supplement and mineral must be analyzed for the offending insecticide. The laboratory costs incurred can range from fifteen to fifty dollars per sample. The costs may or may not be charged directly to the livestock owner.

Once the source is identified, the problem becomes one of either allowing time and clean feed to solve the problem or of using an experimental drug treatment. Currently, the most commonly used treatment is the simultaneous feeding of phenobarbital and activated charcoal. It has been demonstrated in ruminants that dieldrin is recycled from the blood to the gastrointestinal tract. The feeding of charcoal as an adsorbent will tend to trap the insecticide in the gut and render it unavailable for further recycling. Phenobarbital (5 gm/ cow/day for 3-4 weeks; off 3-4 weeks, repeated for 3-4 weeks) has been shown to stimulate liver microsomal enzymes which increase the rate of detoxification of chlorinated insecticides. The varied results following use of this method can be seen in table 7. Our experiences in attempting to increase the rate of dieldrin excretion from dairy and beef cattle indicate that phenobarbital alone is as effective as phenobarbital plus charcoal. Our tests were performed, however, on herds of animals in which the time of exposure was unknown. Undoubtedly charcoal would be beneficial if given shortly after the insecticide is consumed.

The use of phenobarbital in dairy cattle has not always been successful in reducing DDE and dieldrin milk residues. In some cases the response has been transient. One experimenter has reported both no effect and some effect from two separate experiments. It is difficult to completely assess the feasibility of using the phenobarbital treatment. It is possible that the effect is related to the time elapsed since contamination and to the duration of phenobarbital feeding. Most of the experiments completed in dairy cows do not include data past the time when phenobarbital feeding was stopped. This makes it impossible to determine if there was a rebound effect. Milk production and feed consumption are not affected by the daily feeding of 5 grams of phenobarbital per cow. It appears that most of the effect on accelerating elimination of DDT, DDE and dieldrin is due to the phenobarbital and not the activated charcoal.

Other treatment procedures have been tried. Placing hens on a high protein diet and in a forced molt increased depletion of DDT. Conflicting reports have been published on the effect of thyroprotein in speeding

TABLE 7
Application of Charcoal and Phenobarbital Feeding to Increase Excretion
of Chlorinated Hydrocarbon Residues in Domestic Animals

Insecticide	Animal	Treatment	Effect	Reference
Dieldrin	Swine	125 grams phenobarbital per ton of feed + 0.5 pounds charcoal briquets/ head/day.	Shorten time 50%	Dobson et al., 1971
Dieldrin	Dairy Cow	10 mg phenobarbital/kg body weight + 0.91 kg activated carbon/head/day.	Shorten time 50%	Braund et al., 1971
Dieldrin, DDT, DDE	Dairy Cow	1 kg activated carbon/head/day.	No effect	Fries et al., 1970
Dieldrin, DDE	Dairy Cow	5 grams phenobarbital/head/day.	Shorten time for DDE —25%, for dieldrin— 50%	Fries et al., 1971
DDT	Dairy Cow	5 mg phenobarbital/kg/day.	Transient response	Alary et al., 1971
Dieldrin, DDT	Dairy Cow	5 grams phenobarbital/cow/day for 14 days.	No effect	Fries et al., 1971

up removal of DDT in milk. Intramuscular administration of vitamins A (1,000,000 IU), D$_2$ (100,000 IU), and E (100 IU) resulted in a trend (not statistically significant, also only 7 animals tested) toward an increased excretion of dieldrin by heifers and steers.

Case History 1

An Iowa farmer had 95 head of 550-pound steers in a feedlot. He purchased feed from the local elevator, which included corn cobs, cracked corn, alfalfa, soybean oil meal, molasses, urea, mineral and vitamins. On the afternoon of February 24, the feed elevator delivered a load of the mixed feed and placed it in two self-feeders, as had been the custom for the past three months. The next morning nearly all of the 95 animals were exhibiting convulsive seizures, central nervous system depression, abnormal posturing, or other forms of aberrant central nervous system behavior. About 9 a.m. on February 25, or approximately sixteen hours after delivery of the feed, 30 animals were dead. The remainder were exhibiting the various clinical signs described above. The seizures were intermittent; an animal would start jerking his head upwards and circling backwards, falling down in a series of clonic-tonic convulsions. Some lasted only a few seconds; others several minutes. In some instances, the animals continued in convulsive seizures until death. Because of the muddy conditions in the lot, many of the animals actually drowned in the mud during convulsive seizures. Postmortem examinations were conducted on three of the animals. No lesions were apparent except for congestion of the blood vessels of the gastrointestinal tract and the meninges. The livers were severely congested with apparent centrilobular hemorrhages. The rumens were full of feed. Specimens of rumen contents from several animals and feed from the self-feeders; plus brain, omental fat, liver, and kidney were obtained for insecticide analysis.

An investigation of the procedure followed in the mixing the feed by the elevator was conducted. It was found that corn cobs were being stored in a large warehouse and that a partition used to hold the cobs in place consisted of a large stack of 50 pound bags of 20 percent aldrin granules. In the process of scooping the corn cobs with the tractor loader, it was apparent that the workmen had ripped open the bags of aldrin, spilling out the granules into the corn cobs. Samples of the granules were obtained and it was considered that this was the source of insecticide exposure.

Thirty-six of the 95 animals died acutely. The remaining 59 recovered and were fed out for slaughter. The results of laboratory analysis of tissues and feed samples for insecticide levels are presented in table 8.

TABLE 8

Specimen	Insecticide	Concentration (ppm)
Samples obtained from an animal that died of poisoning on February 25		
Brain	Dieldrin	6.3
Omental Fat	Dieldrin	57.0
	Aldrin	1.00
	Heptachlor epoxide	0.17
	Endrin	0.35
	p,p'—DDD	0.10
	p,p'—DDT	0.66
Liver	Dieldrin	25.8
	Aldrin	0.21
Kidney	Dieldrin	3.82
	Aldrin	0.14
Rumen Contents	Aldrin	611
Contaminated Feed	Aldrin	1200
Samples obtained from an animal slaughtered August 6		
Omental Fat	Dieldrin	2.77
	Heptachlor epoxide	0.088
	Lindane	0.66
	p,p'—DDE	0.074
	p,p'—DDT	0.210
Liver	Dieldrin	0.047
	Lindane	0.08
Kidney	Dieldrin	0.140
	Lindane	0.160
Skeletal Muscle	Dieldrin	0.057
	Lindane	0.032

Case History 2

This is a case of dieldrin contamination in a dairy herd. An Iowa dairy farmer was notified that excessive dieldrin residues had been detected in the milk from his herd of 18 Holstein cows. At this time the residue level was 670 ppb (milk fat). Samples taken some months earlier were also above the 300 ppb actionable level. The milk fat also had been found to contain 28 ppb BHC, 11 ppb lindane, 120 ppb heptachlor epoxide, and 112 ppb DDT and metabolites.

Although the dairyman had known for six to eight months that he had a potential residue problem, outside assistance was not requested until the milk was no longer allowed on the market. The Toxicology Section of the Iowa Veterinary Diagnostic Laboratory was contacted by the dairyman's veterinarian and a field investigation was made. The veterinarian had made arrangements for obtaining a supply of activated charcoal and phenobarbital. Also, on the farm were heifers that were pastured the same as the cows, drank from the same source, and were fed hay from the same fields. The cows were fed pelleted commercial dairy supplement. The heifers were fed the supplement only during severe winter weather. The heifers also gleaned the cornfield and were not fed hay at this time. All of the corn fed was grown on the farm. The alfalfa hay came from two fields; one field had been in corn four years previously and the other five years previously. The hay lost its field identity in the barn and loafing shed. The heifers and cows were fed a commercial mineral mixture.

Aldrin had been used for corn soil insect control at the rate of 2 lb/acre. Corn used for silage was treated with one pound of aldrin/acre. Heptachlor, DDT, and BHC had not been used on the farm according to the farmer. Part of the herd had been fed silage from November 1969 until April 1970. First calf heifers (raised on the farm) were added to the herd in September, 1970. Blood samples for dieldrin analysis were obtained from all the animals on December 23, 1970 (designated Day 0) and 57 days later. Blood samples were collected from the cows after 25 days. Beginning on December 24, 1970, the cows (not the heifers) were fed two pounds of charcoal and five grams phenobarbital/head/day for 57 days. Milk samples from individual cows and herd composites were also obtained. In addition a herd composite milk sample was taken 75 days after treatment began. The results of the blood and milk analyses are presented in table 9. The results of the insecticide analysis on the

TABLE 9
Results of Dieldrin Analysis
on Blood and Milk Samples
from a Contaminated Herd

Residue Level (ppb) Mean ± Standard Deviation			
	Day 0	Day 25	Day 57	Day 75
Blood				
Cows	1.33 ± 0.17 ppb	0.49 ± 0.13	0.26 ± 0.03	
Heifers	0.85 ± .09 ppb		0.54 ± 0.07	
Milk fat (herd average)	661 ppb	335	317	471

feed and other materials are shown in table 10. A milk sample obtained July, 1971, contained 244 ppb dieldrin (fat basis). Fecal samples from two cows were found to contain 6-7 ppb dieldrin. The milk samples were also found to contain approximately 100 ppb heptachlor epoxide and 20-30 ppb DDT and metabolites. In April and May of 1971 soil samples from the farm were analyzed and found to contain 14-159 ppb dieldrin and

TABLE 10
Results of Dieldrin Analysis
on Feed and Other Materials
Related to Contaminated Herd

Sample	Residue Level (ppb)
Dairy Supplement	1.77
Hay (average of 8 hay samples)	12.4
Oats	negative
Corn (grain)	2.51
Corn cobs	3.0
Mineral Supplement	2.06
Salt	6.0
Water (300 ft. drilled well)	negative
Methoxychlor Insecticide	no dieldrin
Milk filter pad	negative
Dairy detergent used to clean milk equipment	negative

2-497 ppb aldrin in soil from the hayfields. Water runoff from neighboring farms that traveled through the pasture contained approximately 50 ppb dieldrin in late May, 1971. Heptachlor epoxide (10 ppb) was also found in the runoff.

Several comparisons were made on the data set. The average blood dieldrin level in the 10 cows fed the corn silage was 1.25 ppb in the samples collected on December 23, 1970. The level in the eight first calf heifers that had not been fed silage was 1.50 ppb dieldrin. It was concluded that whatever effect the corn silage may have had, it was not a factor at this time. An analysis of variance was done on the blood residue data collected on Day 0 and 57 in the cows and the heifers in order to determine the effectiveness of the charcoal-phenobarbital treatment. On Day 0 and Day 57 the levels in the cows and heifers were significantly different ($P < 0.01$). Inspection of table 9 shows that the cows (treated group) started with a higher blood dieldrin level and after treatment had a lower blood level than the heifers (control group), which indicates that the treatment had some effect in the cows. Unfortunately the treatment was not sufficiently effective to reduce milk residues below actionable levels (300 ppb).

Williams et. al., (1964) fed cows 50 ppb dieldrin and obtained milk residues of 21 ppb, or a milk/feed ratio of 0.4. Based on this, the theoretical level in the feed should be approximately 30 ppb when the milk residue is 12 ppb whole milk, or 300 ppb fat basis, (4% butter fat), yet the analyses conducted in this case did not detect these levels.

In this case it was concluded that either an unknown source of dieldrin existed in this herd or the cow is very efficient in the uptake and excretion in milk of trace levels of dieldrin.

BIBLIOGRAPHY

Alary, Jean-Gy; Guay, P.; and Brodeur, J. 1971. Effect of Phenobarbital Pretreatment on the Metabolism of DDT in the Rat and the Bovine. *Tox. Appl. Pharm.* 18:456-68.

Alexander, M. 1965. Presistence and Biological Reactions of Pesticides in Soil. *Proc. Soil Sci. Am.* 29:1-7.

Beestman, G. B.; Keeny, D. R.; and Chesters, G. 1969. Dieldrin Translocation and Accumulation in Corn. *Agron. J.* 61:390-92.

Braund, D. G.; Brown, L. D.; Huber, J. T.; Leeling, N. C.; and Zabik, M. J. 1969. Excretion and Storage of Dieldrin in Dairy Cows Fed Thyroprotein and Different Levels of Energy. *J. Dairy Sci.* 52:1-11.

Braund, D. G.; Langlois, B. E.; Conner, D. J.; and Moore, E. E. 1971. Feeding Phenobarbital and Activated Carbon to Accelerate Dieldrin Residue Removal in a Contaminated Dairy Herd. *J. Dairy Sci.* 54:435-38.

Brown, W. H.; Witt, J. M.; Whiting, F. M.; and Stull, J. W. 1966. Secretion of DDT in Milk by Fresh Cows. *Bull. Env. Cont. and Tox.* 1:21

Buck, W. B., and Van Note, W. 1968. Aldrin Poisoning Resulting in Dieldrin Residues in Meat and Milk. *JAVMA* 153:1472-75.

Cole, H.; Barry, D.; and Frear, D. E. H. 1966. DDT Contamination of Feed Grains and Forages in Pennsylvania. *Bull. Env. Cont. Tox.* 1:212-18.

Cook, R. M. 1969. Pesticide Removal from Dairy Cows. Extension Bulletin E-668. Michigan State University.

——. 1970. Metabolism of Xenobiotics in Ruminants. *J. Ag. Food Chem.* 18:434-36.

Cummings, J. G.; Zee, K. T.; Turner, V.; and Quinn, F. 1966. Residues in Eggs from Low-Level Feeding of Five Chlorinated Hydrocarbon Insecticides in Hens. *JAOAC* 49:354-64.

Dobson, R. C.; Fahey, J. E.; Ballee, D. L.; and Baugh, E. R. 1971. Reduction of Chlorinated Hydrocarbon Residues in Swine. *Bull. Env. Con. Tox.* 6:189-92.

Duggan, R. E. 1968. Residues in Food and Feed: Pesticide Residues in Vegetable Oil Seeds, Oils and By-Products. *Pest. Mon. J.* 1:2-7.

Edwards, C. A. 1970. Persistent Pesticides in the Environment. Cleveland, Ohio: CRC Press, Chemical Rubber Co.

Engel, R. W.; Young, R. W.; Samuels, B. L.; and Midyette, Jr.J. W. 1965. Heptachlor Persistence in the Alfalfa-Production Environment. *J. Dairy Sci.* 48:110105.

Furr, A. A. 1974. Correlation of Body Tissue Levels with Aldrin and Dieldrin Exposure and Onset of Toxicity. M.S. Thesis. Ames, Iowa 50010: Iowa State University Library.

Fries, G. F.; Flatt, W. P.; and Moore, L. A. 1969. Energy Balance and Excretion of DDT into Milk. *J. Dairy Sci.* 52:684-86.

Fries, G. F.; Marrow, Jr. G. S.; and Gordon, C. H. 1969. Comparative Excretion and Retention for DDT Analogs by Dairy Cows. *J. Dairy Sci.* 52:1800-05.

Fries, G. F.; Marrow, Jr. G. S.; Gordon, C. H.; Dryden, L. P.; and Hartman, A. M. 1970. Effect of Activated Carbon on Elimination of Organochlorine Pesticides from Rats and Cows. *J. Dairy Sci.* 53:1632-37.

Fries, G. F.; Marrow, Jr. G. S.; Lester, J. W.; and Gordon, C. H. 1971. Effect of Microsomal Enzyme Inducing Drugs on DDT and Dieldrin Elimination from Cows. *J. Dairy Sci.* 54:364-68.

Gannon, N.; Link, R. P.; and Decker, G. G. 1959. Insecticide Residue in the Milk of Dairy Cows Fed Insecticides in Their Daily Ration. *J. Ag. Food Chem.* 7:829-32.

Hart, M. M., and Straw, J. A. 1971. Studies on the Site of Action of o,p'-DDD in the Dog Adrenal Cortex. I. Inhibition of ACTH-Mediated Pregnenolone Synthesis. *Steroids* 17:559-74.

Hironaka, R. 1968. Elimination of Dieldrin from Beef Cattle. *Can. Vet. J.* 9:167-69.

Hunt, E. G., and Bischoff, A. I. 1960. Inimical Effects on Wildlife of Periodic DDD Applications to Clear Lake. *California Fish and Game.* 46:91-106.

Jager, K. W. 1970. *Aldrin, Dieldrin, Endrin and Telodrin.* New York: Elsevier Publishing Co.

Kenaga, E. E., and End, C. S. 1974. Commercial and Experimental Insecticides Ent. Soc. Amer. Special Publication 74-1.

Lichtenstein, E. P.; Schulz, K. R.; Fuhremann, T. W.; and Liang, T. T. 1970. Degradation of Aldrin and Heptachlor in Field Soils During a Ten-Year Period. *Ag. and Food Chem.* 18:100-106.

Liska, J., and Stadelman, W. J. 1969. Accelerated Removal of Pesticides from Domestic Animals. *Res. Rev.* 29:51-60.

Moubry, R. J.; Myrdal G. R.; and Sturges, A. 1968. Residues in Food and Feed: Rate of Decline of Chlorinated Hydrocarbon Pesticides in Dairy Milk. *Pest. Mon. J.* 2:72-79.

Narahashi, T. 1969. Mode of Action of DDT and Allethrin on Nerve: Cellular and Molecular Mechanisms. *Res. Rev.* 25:275-88.

Radeleff, R. D. 1970. *Veterinary Toxicology.* 2nd ed. Philadelphia, Pennsylvania: Lea & Febiger. pp. 197-263.

Roeder, K. D., and Weiant, E. A. 1946. The Site of Action of DDT in the Cockroach. *Science* 103:304-06.

Saha, J. G. 1969. Significance of Organochlorine Insecticide Residues in Fresh Plants as Possible Contaminants of Milk and Beef Products. *Res. Rev.* 26:89-126.

St. Omer, V. 1971. Investigation into Mechanisms Responsible for Seizures Induced by Chlorinated Hydrocarbon Insecticides: The Role of Brain Ammonia and Glutamine in Convulsions in the Rat and Cockerel. *J. Neurochem.* 18:365-74.

Tucker, R. K., and Grabtree, D. G. 1970. Handbook of Toxicity of Pesticides to Wildlife. Resource Pub. No. 84. Bureau of Sport Fisheries and Wildlife, Denver Wildlife Research Center, USDI; 131 pages.

Williams, S. P.; Mills, P. A.; and McDowell, R. E. 1964. Residues in Milk of Cows Fed Rations Containing Low Concentrations of Five Chlorinated Hydrocarbon Pesticides. *JAOAC* 47:1124.

Zweig, G.; Smith, L. M.; Peoples, S. A.; and Cox, R. 1961. DDT Residues in Milk from Dairy Cows Fed Low Levels of DDT in Their Daily Food Rations. *J. Ag. Food Chem.* 9:481-84.

ORGANOPHOSPHORUS AND CARBAMATE INSECTICIDES

The organophosphorus insecticides consist of aliphatic derivatives of phosphorus compounds, carbon cyclic (phenyl, etc.) derivatives, and heterocyclic derivatives. Certain of these compounds have systemic action: absorbed by plants or animals (by way of roots, leaves, stems, skin, digestive tract, mucous membranes and otherwise) and translocated generally throughout the treated plant or animal in sufficient amounts to kill insects, ticks, mites or other pests feeding on tissues or fluids.

The carbamate insecticides consist of cyclic or aliphatic derivatives of carbamic acid. Kenaga and End,

(1974) have described a total of ninety-four organophosphorus insecticides (thirty-one aliphatic, thirty-nine cyclic, twenty-four heterocyclic) and twenty carbamate insecticides.

Toxicity

Toxicity data for certain of the organophosphorus and carbamate insecticides to domestic and laboratory animals and wildlife are presented in table 1.

TABLE 1

Toxicity of Some Common Organophorus and Carbamate Insecticides to Livestock[1], Laboratory Animals[2], and Wildlife[3]

Chemical	Species	Age or Sex	Oral Maximum Non-Toxic Dose Tested mg/kg B. Wt.[4]	Oral Minimum Toxic Dose Found mg/kg B. Wt.[5]	Dermal Maximum Non-Toxic Dose Tested	Dermal Minimum Toxic Dose Found
ORGANOPHOSPHATES						
ABATE®	Rat		CO 2	LD_{50} = 1000		$LD_{50} > 4000$ mg/kg
O,O-dimethyl phosphorothioate O,O-diester with 4,4'-thiodiphenol	Mouse			LD_{50} = 4000		
BITHION®	Rabbit					LD_{50} = 1024 mg/kg
Temephos						
$C_{16}H_{20}O_6P_2S_3$						
Azinphosmethyl	Calves	1-2 wks.	0.1	0.5		
O,O-dimethyl S(4-oxo-1,2,3-benzotriazin-3(4H)-ylmethyl) phosphorodithioate	Sheep	Adult	12	25		
	Rat		CO 5	LD_{50} = 13		LD_{50} = 220 mg/kg
	Mouse			LD_{50} = 8		
Guthion®	Dog		CO 5			
Gusathion®	Mallard	3-4 mos. M		LD_{50} = 136		
	Pheasant	3-5 mos. M		LD_{50} = 75		
$C_{10}H_{12}N_3O_3PS_2$	Chukar	3-4 mos. M		LD_{50} = 84		
Carbophenothion	Calves	1-2 wks.				0.05%
S-[(p-chlorophenylthio) methyl] O,O-diethyl phosphorodithioate	Cattle	Adult			0.1%	1.0%
	Sheep	Adult	10	25		
	Rat		CO 5	LD_{50} = 6		LD_{50} = 22 mg/kg
Trithion®	Mouse			LD_{50} = 218		
	Rabbit			LD_{50} = 1250		
	Dog		CO 0.8			
$C_{11}H_{16}ClO_2PS_3$	Mallard	3-4 mos. M		LD_{50} = 121		
Chlorfenvinphos	Cattle	All ages		20		0.15%
2-chloro-1-(2,4-dichlorophenyl) vinyl diethyl phosphate	Rat			LD_{50} = 12		LD_{50} = 31 mg/kg
	Mouse			LD_{50} = 117		
	Rabbit					LD_{50} = 420 mg/kg
Compound 4072	Dog			$LD_{50} > 12,000$		
SUPONA®						
BIRLANE®						
$C_{12}H_{14}Cl_3O_4P$						

1. Data adapted primarily from Radeleff (1970).

2. Data adapted primarily from Kenaga and End (1974).

3. Data adapted from Tucker and Crabtree (1970).

4. Maximum single dose which did not produce a toxic effect. CO = chronic oral exposure, 90 days or longer, in parts per million in diet which did not have toxic effects.

5. Minimum single dose which caused minimal toxic effects. Those levels given as LD_{50} are minimum values given that caused 50% death losses.

TABLE 1 (Cont.)

Chemical	Species	Age or Sex	Oral Maximum Non-Toxic Dose Tested mg/kg B. Wt.	Oral Minimum Toxic Dose Found mg/kg B. Wt.	Dermal Maximum Non-Toxic Dose Tested	Dermal Minimum Toxic Dose Found
Chlorpyrifos						
Dursban®	Goats	F		LD_{50} = 500		
O,O-diethyl O-(3, 5,6-trichloro-2-py-ridyl) phosphoro-thioate	Rat			LD_{50} = 97		
	Rabbit			LD_{50} = 1000		LD_{50} = 2000 mg/kg
	Mallard			LD_{50} = 75		
Dowco®179	Pheasant	3-5 mos. M		LD_{50} = 8.4		
	Pheasant	3-5 mos. F		LD_{50} = 18		
$C_9H_{11}Cl_3NO_3PS$	Chukar	3-5 mos. F		LD_{50} = 61		
	Coturnix	2-3 mos. M		LD_{50} = 16		
	Pigeon			LD_{50} = 27		
	Sparrow	M		LD_{50} = 21		
	Canada Geese			LD_{50} = 80		
	Lesser Sandhill Crane	M		LD_{50} = 25		
	Bullfrog	M		$LD_{50} > 400$		
Coumaphos	Calves	under 3 mos.			0.25%	0.5%
O-(3-chloro-4-methyl-2-oxo-2H-1-benzopyran-7-y1) O,O-diethyl phosphor-othioate	Cattle	over 3 mos.	20	25	0.5%	1.0%
	Sheep	Adult		8	0.25%	0.5%
	Goats	Adult			0.25%	0.5%
	Horses	Adult		25 (severe)	0.5%	
CO-RAL®	Swine	Adult			0.5%	
ASUNTOL®	Rat		CO 5	LD_{50} = 13		LD_{50} = 860 mg/kg
MUSCATOX®	Dog		CO 2			
$C_{14}H_{16}Cl_5PS$	Mallard	3-4 mos. M		LD_{50} = 30		
Counter®	Sheep*	Adult	1.5	3.0		
S [(tert-butylthio) methyl] O,O-diethyl phosphorodithioate	Cattle*	Yearling	—	1.5		
$C_9H_{21}O_2PS_3$						
Crufomate						
Ruelene®	Calves	1-2 wks.	25	50	1.5%	2.0%
4-tert-butyl-2-chlorophenyl methyl methylphosphorami-date	Cattle	Adult		100	0.5%	1.5%
	Sheep	Adult	150	200		5.0%
	Goats	Adult		100		2.5%
	Pigs	Adult		15		
$C_{12}H_{19}Cl NO_3P$	Horses	Adult	25	50		
	Rat		CO 10	LD_{50} = 660		
	Rabbit			LD_{50} = 490		
	Dog			$LD_{50} > 1000$		LD_{50} = 2000 mg/kg

*Furr and Carson (1975a).

TABLE 1 (Cont.)

Chemical	Species	Age or Sex	Oral Maximum Non-Toxic Dose Tested mg/kg B. Wt.	Oral Minimum Toxic Dose Found mg/kg B. Wt.	Dermal Maximum Non-Toxic Dose Tested	Dermal Minimum Toxic Dose Found
Crotoxyphos						
Ciodrin®	Calves	1-2 wks.			0.5%	2.0%
α-methylbenzyl	Cattle	Adult			2.0%	
3-hydroxycrotonate	Goats	Adult			1.0%	
dimethyl phosphate	Sheep	Adult			1.0%	
$C_{14}H_{19}O_6P$	Swine	3 mos.			2.0%	
	Rat		CO 7	$LD_{50} = 125$		
	Mouse			$LD_{50} = 90$		
	Rabbit					$LD_{50} = 385$ mg/kg
	Mallard	3-4 mos. M		$LD_{50} = 790$		
Demeton	Goats			$LD_{50} = 8$		
Mixture of O,O-	Rat		CO 1	$LD_{50} = 2$		$LD_{50} = 8$ mg/kg
diethyl S-(and O)	Rabbit					$LD_{50} = 24$ mg/kg
-2-[(ethylthio)	Dog		CO 1			
ethyl] phosphoro-	Mallard	3 mos. M		$LD_{50} = 7.2$		
thioates	Pheasant	2 mos. F		$LD_{50} = 8.2$		
Systox®	Chukar	3 mos.		$LD_{50} = 15$		
$C_8H_{19}O_3PS_2$	Coturnix	2 mos. F		$LD_{50} = 8.5$		
	Pigeon	Adult		$LD_{50} = 8.5$		
	Grouse	Adult		$LD_{50} = 4.8$		
	Sparrow	F		$LD_{50} = 9.5$		
	Finch			$LD_{50} = 2.4$		
	Bullfrog	M		$LD_{50} = 562$		
Diazinon	Calves	1-2 wks.	0.5	2.5	0.05%	0.1%
O,O-diethyl O-(2-	Cattle	6-12 mos.	10	25	0.25%	
isopropyl-4-methyl-	Sheep	Adult	20	30		
6-pyrimidyl) phos-	Goats	Adult	20	30		
phorothioate	Horses	Adult	20			
$C_{12}H_{21}N_2O_3PS$	Chicken	Adult		2		
	Rat		CO 1	$LD_{50} = 66$		$LD_{50} = 379$ mg/kg
	Mouse			$LD_{50} = 80$		
	Rabbit			$LD_{50} = 130$		$LD_{50} = 4000$ mg/kg
	Dog		CO 0.8			
	Mallard	3-4 mos. M		$LD_{50} = 3.5$		
	Pheasant	3-4 mos. M		$LD_{50} = 3.3$		
	Bullfrog	F		$LD_{50} > 2000$		
Dichlofenthion	Calves	1-2 wks.			0.25%	0.5%
O-2,4-dichloro-	Cattle	Adult			2.0%	3.0%
phenyl O,O-diethyl	Sheep	Adult			2.0%	3.0%
phosphorothioate	Goats	Adult			0.25%	0.5%
V-C 13®	Rat			$LD_{50} = 270$		
	Rabbit					$LD_{50} = 6000$ mg/kg
$C_{10}H_{13}Cl_2O_3PS$	Dog		CO 0.8			

TABLE 1 (Cont.)

Chemical	Species	Age or Sex	Oral Maximum Non-Toxic Dose Tested mg/kg B. Wt.	Oral Minimum Toxic Dose Found mg/kg B. Wt.	Dermal Maximum Non-Toxic Dose Tested	Dermal Minimum Toxic Dose Found
Dichlorvos	Calves	1-2 wks.		10		
2,2-dichloro-vinyl dimethyl phosphate	Cattle	Adult			1% dust—2 oz. (cattle) total	
	Horses	Adult		25	2% mist—200 ml (cattle) total	
Vapona®	Sheep	Adult		25		
DDVP	Rat		CO < 250	LD_{50} = 25		LD_{50} = 59 mg/kg
$C_4H_7Cl_2O_4P$	Rabbit					LD_{50} = 107 mg/kg
	Mallard	5-7 mos. M		LD_{50} = 7.8		
	Pheasant	3 mos. M		LD_{50} = 9.0		
Dicrotophos						
Bidrin®	Rat		CO 1.5	LD_{50} = 22		
3-hydroxy-N,N-dimethyl-cis-crotonamide, dimethyl phosphate	Mouse			LD_{50} = 15		
	Rabbit					LD_{50} = 225 mg/kg
	Mallard	3 mos. M		LD_{50} = 4.2		
	Pheasant	2 mos. M		LD_{50} = 3.2		
$C_8H_{16}NO_5P$	Chukar	Adult		LD_{50} = 9.6		
	Coturnix	2 mos. M		LD_{50} = 4.3		
	Pigeon	Adult		LD_{50} = 2		
	Grouse	Adult		LD_{50} = 2.3		
	Sparrow	M		LD_{50} = 3		
	Finch	Adult		LD_{50} = 2.8		
	Canada Geese	Adult		LD_{50} = 2.3		
	Bullfrog	Adult M		LD_{50} = 2000		
Dimethoate	Calves	1-2 wks.		5	1.0%	
O,O-dimethyl S-(N-methylcarbamoyl-methyl) phosphoro-dithioate	Cattle	1 yr.	10	15	1.0%	
	Sheep	Adult		50	1.0%	
	Horse	Adult	50	60		
CYGON®	Rat		CO 5	LD_{50} = 250		LD_{50} = 150 mg/kg
	Mouse			LD_{50} = 200		
$C_5H_{12}NO_3PS_2$	Rabbit			LD_{50} = 300		
	Dog			LD_{50} = 400		
	Mallard	3-4 mos. M		LD_{50} = 42		
	Mule Deer			LD_{50} = 200		
Dioxathion	Calves	1-2 wks.		5		0.1%
S,S'-p-dioxane-2,3-diyl O,O-diethyl phosphorodithioate	Cattle	Adult			0.5%	
	Sheep	Adult			0.5%	
	Goats	Adult			0.25%	
Delnav®	Swine	Adult			0.25%	
$C_{12}H_{26}O_6P_2S_4$	Rat		CO 4	LD_{50} = 19		LD_{50} = 53 mg/kg
	Mouse			LD_{50} = 50		
	Rabbit					LD_{50} = 107 mg/kg
	Dog		CO 1	LD_{50} = 10		
Disulfoton	Goats	Adult M		LD_{50} < 15		

TABLE 1 (Cont.)

Chemical	Species	Age or Sex	Oral Maximum Non-Toxic Dose Tested mg/kg B. Wt.	Oral Minimum Toxic Dose Found mg/kg B. Wt.	Dermal Maximum Non-Toxic Dose Tested	Dermal Minimum Toxic Dose Found
O,O-diethyl S-2-[(ethylthio) ethyl] phosphorodithioate Di-Syston® Dithiodemeton $C_8H_{19}O_2PS_3$	Rat			$LD_{50} = 2$		$LD_{50} = 20$ mg/kg
	Mouse		CO 2			
	Dog		CO 1			
	Mallard	3-4 mos. M		$LD_{50} = 6.5$		
EPN O-ethyl O-p-nitrophenyl phenylphosphonothioate $C_{14}H_{14}NO_4PS$	Rat		CO $>$ 5	$LD_{50} = 7$		$LD_{50} = 22$ mg/kg
	Mouse			$LD_{50} = 42$		
	Rabbit					$LD_{50} = 30$ mg/kg
	Dog		CO 80	$LD_{50} > 100$		
	Mallard	3 mos. F		$LD_{50} = 3.1$		
	Pheasant	3-5 mos. F		$LD_{50} = 53$		
	Chukar	3 mos. F		$LD_{50} = 14$		
	Coturnix	2 mos. F		$LD_{50} = 5.3$		
	Pigeon			$LD_{50} = 5.9$		
	Sparrow			$LD_{50} = 1.3$		
Ethion O,O,O',O'-tetraethyl S,S'-methylene bisphosphorodithioate $C_9H_{22}O_4P_2S_4$	Calves	1-2 wks.			0.25%	0.5%
	Cattle	Adult			0.25%	0.5%
	Sheep	Adult		25	0.5%	1.0% (lethal)
	Goats	Adult			0.25%	0.5%
	Rat		CO 6	$LD_{50} = 27$		$LD_{50} = 62$ mg/kg
	Rabbit					$LD_{50} = 915$ mg/kg
	Dog		CO 2			
MOCAP® O-ethyl S,S-dipropyl phosphorodithioate $C_8H_{19}O_2PS_2$	Pig	2 mos.		65 (lethal)		
	Rat	Adult		$LD_{50} = 61$		
	Rabbit					$LD_{50} = 26$ mg/kg
Famphur O-[p-(dimethylsulfamoyl) phenyl] O,O-dimethyl phosphorothioate WARBEX® Famophos $C_{10}H_{16}NO_5PS_2$	Calves	1-2 wks.	10	$>$10		
	Cattle	Adult	50	$>$50	2000 mg/kg	
	Sheep	Adult	50	100		
	Horse	Adult	50			
	Rat		CO 1	$LD_{50} = 35$		
	Mouse			$LD_{50} = 30$		
	Rabbit					$LD_{50} = 1460$ mg/kg
	Dog		CO 4			
	Mallard	3-4 mos. M		$LD_{50} = 9.9$		
Fensulfothion Dasanit® O,O-diethyl O-[p-(methylsulfinyl) phenyl] phosphorothioate $C_{11}H_{17}O_4PS_2$	Pig	2 mos.		15 (lethal)		
	Rat		CO 1	$LD_{50} = 2$		$LD_{50} = 3$ mg/kg
	Mallard	5-7 mos. F		$LD_{50} = 0.7$		

TABLE 1 (Cont.)

Chemical	Species	Age or Sex	Oral Maximum Non-Toxic Dose Tested mg/kg B. Wt.	Oral Minimum Toxic Dose Found mg/kg B. Wt.	Dermal Maximum Non-Toxic Dose Tested	Dermal Minimum Toxic Dose Found
Fenthion	Calves	1-2 wks.			0.25%	
O,O-dimethyl O-	Cattle	Adult	20	25		
[4-(methylthio)-m-	Sheep	Adult	25	50 (lethal)	0.5%	
tolyl] phosphorothi-	Goats	Adult				0.25%
oate	Horses	Adult	20			
BAYTEX®	Rat		CO 2	LD_{50} = 178		LD_{50} = 275 mg/kg
TIGUVON®	Dog		CO 2			
$C_{10}H_{15}O_3PS_2$	Mallard	4 mos. F		LD_{50} = 5.9		
	Pheasant	Adult F		LD_{50} = 18		
	Chukar	3 mos.		LD_{50} = 26		
	Coturnix	3 mos. F		LD_{50} = 11		
	Pigeon			LD_{50} = 4.6		
	Dove			LD_{50} = 2.7		
	Sparrow	F		LD_{50} = 23		
	Finch			LD_{50} = 10		
	Canada Geese			LD_{50} = 12		
Fonofos						
Dyfonate®	Pig			50 (lethal)		
O-ethyl S-phenyl	Rat			LD_{50} = 8		
ethylphosphonodi-	Rabbit					LD_{50} – 147 mg/kg
thioate						
$C_{10}H_{15}OPS_2$						
Malathion	Calves	1-2 wks.	10	20	0.5%	1.0%
Diethyl mercapto-	Cattle	Adult	50	100	2.0%	
succinate, S-ester	Sheep	Adult	50	100	1.0%	
with O,O-dimethyl	Goats	Adult	50	100	1.0%	
phosphorodithioate	Dogs	Adult	CO 100		2.0%	
CYTHION®	Rat		CO 100	LD_{50} = 885		LD_{50} > 4000 mg/kg
$C_{10}H_{19}O_6PS_2$	Mouse			LD_{50} = 720		
	Rabbit					LD_{50} = 4100 mg/kg
	Mallard	3-4 mos. F		LD_{50} < 485		
Methyl Parathion	Rat		CO 5	LD_{50} = 9		LD_{50} = 63 mg/kg
O,O-dimethyl O-ρ-	Mouse			LD_{50} = 32		
nitrophenyl phos-	Rabbit					LD_{50} = 1270 mg/kg
phorothioate	Mallard	3 mos. M		LD_{50} = 10		
$C_8H_{10}NO_5PS$	Pheasant	2 mos. F		LD_{50} = 8.2		
Methyl Trithion®	Calves	1-2 wks.			0.5%	
S-[(ρ-chlorophenyl-	Cattle	Adult			0.5%	
thio)methyl] O,O-	Sheep	Adult	25			
dimethyl phosphoro-	Goats	Adult			0.1%	
dithioate	Rat			LD_{50} = 98		LD_{50} = 198 mg/kg
$C_9H_{12}ClO_2PS_3$	Mouse			LD_{50} = 390		
	Rabbit					LD_{50} = 2420 mg/kg

TABLE 1 (Cont.)

Chemical	Species	Age or Sex	Oral Maximum Non-Toxic Dose Tested mg/kg B. Wt.	Oral Minimum Toxic Dose Found mg/kg B. Wt.	Dermal Maximum Non-Toxic Dose Tested	Dermal Minimum Toxic Dose Found
Mevinphos	Rat		CO = 0.8	LD_{50} = 3		LD_{50} = 3 mg/kg
Methyl 3-hydroxy-	Mouse			LD_{50} = 8		
alpha-crotonate,	Rabbit					LD_{50} = 13 mg/kg
dimethyl phosphate	Dog		CO = 1			
Phosdrin[®]	Mallard	6-7 mos. F		LD_{50} = 4.6		
	Pheasant	3-4 mos. M		LD_{50} = 1.4		
$C_7H_{13}O_6P$	Grouse	Adult M		LD_{50} = 1		
Monocrotophos						
Azodrin[®]	Goats	1 yr.		LD_{50} = 20		
3-hydroxy-N-	Mule Deer	Adult		LD_{50} = 25		
methyl-cis-croton-	Rat		CO = 1.5	LD_{50} = 21		
amide dimethyl	Rabbit					LD_{50} = 354 mg/kg
phosphate	Mallard	4-10 mos. M		LD_{50} = 4.8		LD_{50} = 30 mg/kg
Nuvacron[®]	Pheasant	7-8 mos. F		LD_{50} = 2.8		
	Chukar	4 mos. F		LD_{50} = 6.5		
	Quail	Adult M		LD_{50} = 0.94		
	Pigeon	Adult		LD_{50} = 2.8		
	Sparrow	Adult		LD_{50} = 1.6		
	Canada Geese			LD_{50} = 1.6		
	Turkey	Adult		LD_{50} = 1		
	Golden Eagle	M		LD_{50} < 0.8		
Naled	Mule Deer			LD_{50} = 200		
1,2-dibromo-2,2-	Rat			LD_{50} = 430		
dichloroethyl di-	Rabbit					LD_{50} = 1100 mg/kg
methyl phosphate	Dog		CO 7.5			
DIBROM[®]	Mallard	M		LD_{50} = 52		
	Grouse	M		LD_{50} = 65		
$C_4H_7Br_2Cl_2O_4P$	Canada Geese			LD_{50} = 37		
Parathion	Calves	1-2 wks.		0.5		0.01%
O,O-diethyl O-ρ-	Cattle	Adult		50		1.0%
nitrophenyl phos-	Sheep	Adult		20 (lethal)		1.0%
phorothioate	Goats	Adult		20 (lethal)		
BLADAN[®]	Swine	Adult		25 (severe)		
Niram[®]	Rat		CO 1	LD_{50} = 3		LD_{50} = 4 mg/kg
Alkron[®]	Mouse			LD_{50} = 6		
$C_{10}H_{14}NO_5PS$	Rabbit			LD_{50} = 10		LD_{50} = 40 mg/kg
	Dog		CO 1	LD_{50} = 3		
	Mallard	3-4 mos. M		LD_{50} = 2.1		
	Pheasant	2-3 mos. M		LD_{50} = 12		
	Chukar	3-12 mos.		LD_{50} = 24		
	Coturnix	2 mos. F		LD_{50} = 5.6		
	Pigeon			LD_{50} = 2.5		
	Grouse	Adult		LD_{50} = 4.0		
	Sparrow	F		LD_{50} = 3.4		

TABLE 1 (Cont.)

Chemical	Species	Age or Sex	Oral Maximum Non-Toxic Dose Tested mg/kg B. Wt.	Oral Minimum Toxic Dose Found mg/kg B. Wt.	Dermal Maximum Non-Toxic Dose Tested	Dermal Minimum Toxic Dose Found
	Fulvous Tree Duck			$LD_{50} = 0.2$		
	Partridge	3-10 mos. M		$LD_{50} = 16$		
	Mule Deer	10 mos. M		$LD_{50} = 22$		
Phorate	Calves	1-2 wks.	0.1	0.25		
O,O-diethyl-S-[(ethylthio) methyl] phosphorodithioate	Cattle	Adult	0.5	1.0		
	Cattle*	Yearling	0.75	1.5		
	Sheep*	Adult	0.75	0.75		
Thimet®	Rat			$LD_{50} = 1$		$LD_{50} = 2$ mg/kg
$C_7H_{17}O_2PS_3$	Mallard	3-4 mos. F		$LD_{50} = 0.6$		
	Pheasant	3-4 mos. F		$LD_{50} = 7.1$		
	Chukar	3 mos. F		$LD_{50} = 12.8$		
	Bullfrog	F		$LD_{50} = 85$		
Phosmet						
Imidan®	Calves	1-2 wks.		25		
O,O-dimethyl S-phthalimidomethyl phosphorodithioate	Cattle	Adult	10	25	0.5%	1.0%
	Sheep	Adult		50		
	Goats	Adult				0.5%
Prolate®	Rat		CO 40	$LD_{50} = 147$		
Phosmet	Rabbit					$LD_{50} > 3160$ mg/kg
$C_{11}H_{12}NO_4PS_2$	Dog		CO 40			
	Mallard	3-4 mos. M		$LD_{50} = 1830$		
Phosphamidon	Calves	1-2 wks.		5		
2-chloro-N,N-diethyl-3-hydroxy-crotonamide, dimethyl phosphate	Cattle	Adult		5	0.25%	0.5%
	Sheep	Adult	5		0.25%	
	Rat		CO 2.5	$LD_{50} = 15$		$LD_{50} = 125$ mg/kg
Dimecron®	Mouse			$LD_{50} = 6$		
	Rabbit					$LD_{50} = 267$ mg/kg
$C_{10}H_{19}ClNO_5P$	Mallard	3 mos. F		$LD_{50} = 3$		
	Chukar	3-5 mos.		$LD_{50} = 9.7$		
	Pigeon	Adult		$LD_{50} = 2$		
	Doves	Adult		$LD_{50} = 2$		
Stirofos						
RABON®	Swine	2 mos.	50	100		
2-chloro-1-(2,4,5-trichlorophenyl) vinyl dimethyl phosphate	Rat			$LD_{50} = 4000$		
	Mouse			$LD_{50} > 5000$		
	Rabbit					$LD_{50} > 5000$ mg/kg
GARDONA®	Mallard	1 yr.		$LD_{50} > 2000$		
	Pheasant	2-4 mos.		$LD_{50} = 2000$		
$C_{10}H_9Cl_4O_4P$	Chukar	1 yr.		$LD_{50} > 2000$		
Ronnel	Calves	1-2 wks.	100	125		
O,O-dimethyl O-2,4,5-Ronnel	Cattle	Adult	100	125	2.5%	

*Furr and Carson (1975a).

TABLE 1 (Cont.)

Chemical	Species	Age or Sex	Oral		Dermal	
			Maximum Non-Toxic Dose Tested	Minimum Toxic Dose Found	Maximum Non-Toxic Dose Tested	Minimum Toxic Dose Found
			mg/kg B. Wt.	mg/kg B. Wt.		
trichlorophenyl phos-phorothioate	Sheep	Adult		400	2.5%	
Korlan®	Horse	Adult	110			
Trolene®	Rat		CO 10	$LD_{50} = 906$		
Nankor®	Mouse			$LD_{50} = 2000$		
Viozene®	Dog		CO 100	$LD_{50} > 500$		
	Rabbit			$LD_{50} = 640$		$LD_{50} = 1000$ mg/kg
Fenchlorphos						
$C_8H_8Cl_3O_3PS$						
tepp	Rat			$LD_{50} = 0.5$		$LD_{50} = 2$ mg/kg
	Mouse			$LD_{50} = 1.0$		
Tetraethyl pyro-phosphate	Rabbit					$LD_{50} = 5$ mg/kg
	Mallard	3-4 mos. M		$LD_{50} = 3.5$		
Tetron®	Pheasant	3-4 mos. M		$LD_{50} = 4.2$		
	Chukar	3-4 mos.		$LD_{50} = 10$		
$C_8H_{20}O_7P_2$	Bullfrog	F		$LD_{50} = 89$		
Trichlorfon	Calves	1-2 wks.	5	10	1.0%	
Dimethyl (2,2,2-trichloro-1-hydroxy-ethyl) phosphonate	Cattle	Adult	50	75	2.0%	
	Sheep	Adult		100		
	Horse	Adult		100		
Dipterex®	Rat		CO 500	$LD_{50} = 450$		$LD_{50} > 2800$ mg/kg
Dylox®	Mouse			$LD_{50} = 300$		
Neguvon®	Rabbit					$LD_{50} = 5000$ mg/kg
$C_4H_8Cl_3O_4P$						
CARBAMATES						
Carbaryl	Calves	1-2 wks.			2.0%	4.0%
1-naphthyl methylcarbamate	Cattle	Adult			4.0%	
	Sheep	Adult			2.0%	
SEVIN®	Goats	Adult			1.0%	
Carpolin	Rat		CO 200	$LD_{50} = 307$		$LD_{50} > 500$ mg/kg
$C_{12}H_{11}NO_2$	Rabbit			$LD_{50} = 710$		
	Dog		CO 200	$LD_{50} = 759$		$LD_{50} > 2000$ mg/kg
	Mallard	3 mos. F		$LD_{50} > 2179$		
	Pheasant	3 mos. M		$LD_{50} > 2000$		
	Pheasant	3 mos. F		$LD_{50} = 707$		
	Coturnix	2 mos. M		$LD_{50} = 2990$		
	Pigeon			$LD_{50} = 1000$		
	Grouse	3-12 mos.		$LD_{50} > 80$		
	Canada Geese			$LD_{50} = 1790$		
	Mule Deer	11 mos. F		$LD_{50} = 200$		
	Bullfrog	M		$LD_{50} > 4000$		

TABLE 1 (Cont.)

Chemical	Species	Age or Sex	Oral Maximum Non-Toxic Dose Tested mg/kg B. Wt.	Oral Minimum Toxic Dose Found mg/kg B. Wt.	Dermal Maximum Non-Toxic Dose Tested	Dermal Minimum Toxic Dose Found
Carbofuran	Cattle*	Yearling	3.0	4.5		
				18 = death		
	Sheep*	Adult	—	4.5		
				9 = death		
	Rat		CO 25	LD_{50} = 8		
	Dog		CO 20	LD_{50} = 19		
2,3-dihydro-2,2-dimethyl-7-benzo-furanyl methylcarbamate	Rabbit					LD_{50} = 10200 mg/kg
	Mallard	3-4 mos. F		LD_{50} = 0.4		
	Pheasant	3 mos. F		LD_{50} = 4.2		
Furadan®	Quail	3 mos. F		LD_{50} = 5.0		
CURATERR®	Fulvous Tree Duck	3-6 mos. F		LD_{50} = 0.2		
$C_{12}H_{15}NO_3$						
LANDRIN	Cattle	8-10 mos.		50		
3,4,5-trimethyl-phenyl methylcarbamate, 75%; 2,3,5,-trimethyl-phenyl methylcarbamate, 18%	Goat	Adult		LD_{50} = 210		
	Rat			LD_{50} = 178		
	Mouse			LD_{50} = 103		
	Rabbit					LD_{50} > 2500 mg/kg
$C_{11}H_{15}NO_2$	Mallard	4 mos. F		LD_{50} = 17		
	Pheasant	3 mos. M		LD_{50} = 52		
	Chukar	7-11 mos.		LD_{50} = 60		
	Coturnix	2 mos. M		LD_{50} = 71		
	Pigeon			LD_{50} = 168		
	Sparrow			LD_{50} = 46		
	Mule Deer	5-11 mos. M		LD_{50} = 50		
Metalkamate						
BUX®	Swine	2 mos.	100	212 (severe)		
m-(1-ethylpropyl) phenyl methylcarbam-ate mixture (1-4) with m-(1-methyl-butyl)phenyl methyl-carbamate	Rat			LD_{50} = 87		
	Rabbit					LD_{50} = 400 mg/kg
	Dog					LD_{50} = 1400 mg/kg
Bufencarb						
$C_{13}H_{19}NO_2$						
Methomyl						
Methyl N-[(methyl = carbamoyl)oxy] thioacetimidate	Rat		CO > 100	LD_{50} = 17		
	Rabbit					LD_{50} = 1000 mg/kg
Lannate®	Dog		CO > 100			
Nudrin®	Mallards	8 mos.		LD_{50} = 12-20		
	Pheasants	3-4 mos.		LD_{50} = 9-27		
$C_5H_{10}N_2O_2S$	Mule deer	Yearling		LD_{50} = 11-22		

*Data from Furr and Carson (1975a).

TABLE 1 (Cont.)

Chemical	Species	Age or Sex	Oral		Dermal	
			Maximum Non-Toxic Dose Tested	Minimum Toxic Dose Found	Maximum Non-Toxic Dose Tested	Minimum Toxic Dose Found
			mg/kg B. Wt.	mg/kg B. Wt.		
Propoxur						
Baygon®	Goats	1 yr. M		$LD_{50} > 800$		
o-isopropoxyphenyl methylcarbamate	Rat		CO 800	$LD_{50} = 95$		$LD_{50} > 1000$ mg/kg
UNDEN®	Mallard	4-6 mos. F		$LD_{50} = 12$		
Blattanex®	Pheasant	3-5 mos. M		$LD_{50} = 20$		
	Chukar	4-6 mos.		$LD_{50} = 24$		
Arprocarb	Coturnix	20 mos. F		$LD_{50} = 28$		
SLINCIDE®	California Quail	Adult M		$LD_{50} > 30$		
$C_{11}H_{15}NO_3$	Pigeon			$LD_{50} = 60$		
	Dove			$LD_{50} = 4.2$		
	Sparrow	F		$LD_{50} = 13$		
	Finch	Adult		$LD_{50} = 3.6$		
	Lesser Canada Geese			$LD_{50} = 6.0$		
	Lesser Sandhill Crane			$LD_{50} = 40$		
	Mule Deer	11 mos. F		$LD_{50} = 100$		
	Bullfrog	M		$LD_{50} = 595$		

Mechanism of Action

Acetylcholinesterase (AChE) is the enzyme present at cholinergic nerve endings, myoneural junctions and in red blood cells that is responsible for the nearly instantaneous hydrolysis of acetylcholine. The function of acetylcholinesterase in the red blood cell is unknown, but it does not appear to participate in functioning of the nervous system.

There are other esterases in the body capable of hydrolyzing acetylcholine. These are found in the brain and blood plasma and are referred to as pseudocholinesterases (PChE).

Organophosphorus and carbamate compounds are inhibitors of both true and pseudo-ChE. The inhibition involves removal of a hydroxyl ion from serine at the active site on the enzyme. Other compounds that have limited anticholinesterase activity include quaternary ammonium bases, and phenothiazines.

The organophosphorus insecticides share fundamental characteristics: structurally all contain a phosphorous radical in a combination which permits the compound to competitively inhibit acetylcholinesterase and other cholinesterases. The carbamate compounds characteristically contain carbamic acid and produce parasympathomimetic action by inhibiting acetylcholinesterase, allowing acetylcholine to accumulate. In general inhibition by the organophosphates tends to be irreversible whereas inhibition by the carbamates is reversible. (Murphy, 1975)

Spontaneous reversal of enzyme inhibition by organophosphates and carbamates can occur at various rates depending on the compound. The reversal involves hydrolysis of the phosphorylated cholinesterase. With some compounds a phenomenon known as "aging" takes place. A chemical change occurs that makes the phosphorylated enzyme very stable. Recovery of cholinesterase activity occurs through the synthesis of new enzyme. Agents such as 2-PAM accelerate the hydrolysis of the phosphorylated enzyme and consequently the regeneration of active cholinesterase. Phosphorylated enzyme that has "aged" is not reversible by the oximes. Consequently, the earlier treatment is initiated the more likely are positive results.

True AChE is inhibited by an excess of acetylcholine, while PChE is not inhibited by an excess of acetylcholine. Both true AChE and PChE will hydrolyze acetylthiocholine and propionylcholine. Substrates which are specific for each type of ChE and thus can be used to distinguish true and pseudo ChE activity are acetyl-B-methylthiocholine for true AChE and either butyrylcholine or butyrylthiocholine for PChE.

Both the absolute amount of ChE activity and the proportion of true AChE and plasma PChE vary with species. In the rabbit, pig, man and rat there is more RBC ChE than plasma activity. In terms of absolute amounts of blood ChE activity the ranking from most to least activity is man, horse and monkey, cattle, sheep, goat, turkey, dog, rat, duck, cat, goose, mouse and rabbit. The ranking is only a relative indicator since the position of individual species is influenced by the analytical method used.

Plasma ChE is replaced more rapidly than RBC AChE. Plasma ChE is replaced more slowly in animals with liver disease. AChE is bound to the surface membrane of the RBC, therefore, the RBC ChE activity of blood is proportional to the packed cell volume. RBC AChE activity is lower in the newborn.

Blood ChE is stable for several weeks if the sample is stored at 0-5° C. Plasma samples can be frozen for several months. It is also possible to place the blood sample on a filter paper, dry it and then store at 0-5° C for several months. However, when later measuring the ChE activity the reaction must take place in the presence of filter paper since 80 percent of the enzyme stays on the paper if one tries to wash it off.

Certain organophosphorus compounds, such as the triester, triorthocresyl phosphate (TOCP) inhibit carboxylesterases (aliesterases) and this may account for delayed neurotoxic effects characterized by peripheral nerve demyelination preceded by axonal degeneration. Malathion and dimethoate are apparantely hydrolyzed by the carboxylesterases. Thus, an excess of these compounds at the tissue level may deplete carboxylesterase activities resulting in delayed neurotoxicity, especially if the exposure is continuous for a long period of time. (Murphy, 1975)

Clinical Signs

In general, signs of organophosphorus and carbamate poisoning are those of overstimulation of the parasympathetic nervous system. They may be grouped into three different categories: muscarinic, nicotinic, and central nervous system effects. Those signs included in the *muscarinic* group are profuse salivation; gastrointestinal hypermotility resulting in severe pain, abdominal cramps, vomiting, diarrhea, excessive lacrimation, sweating, dyspnea, miosis, pallor, cyanosis, and incontinence of urine and feces. The clinical signs included in the *nicotinic* group reflect excessive stimulation of the skeletal muscles manifested by twitching of the muscles of the face, eyelids, tongue, and ultimately the general musculature. Often, there is generalized tetany causing the animal to walk in a sawhorse, stifflegged fashion. This hyperactivity often is followed by weakness and paralysis of the skeletal muscles as acetylcholine accumulation increases at the myoneural junctions. The *central nervous system* effects vary with the class of animal involved. Domestic food- producing animals may exhibit hyperactivity reflecting excessive stimulation of the CNS but rarely, if ever, exhibit convulsive seizures. More commonly, severe CNS depression occurs. In small animals such as dogs and cats hyperstimulation of the central nervous system may progress to convulsive seizures. Extreme CNS depression, however, commonly occurs in those animals poisoned by the cholinesterase inhibitors. It is important to realize that not every animal will exhibit all the clinical signs when poisoned by an organophosphorus or carbamate compound. If several animals are poisoned, however, most of the reported clinical signs will be present in some of the animals. Often, poisoned animals will cough frequently, probably due to excessive secretion in the respiratory tract thereby eliciting the cough reflex. The clinical signs of organophosphorus and carbamate poisoning are similar in all species of animals. Usually, death results from hypoxia due to bronchoconstriction; excessive respiratory secretions in the bronchial tree; and erratic, slowed heartbeat. Constriction of the pupils or miosis is a characteristic muscarinic sign.

The clinical signs of poisoning by the systemic organophosphorus insecticides reflect the complexity of their chemical structure; and in many instances, a combination of signs similar to those produced by chlorinated hydrocarbon and organophosphorus compounds probably are produced because many are, in fact, combined chlorinated hydrocarbons and organophosphates. There are several differences between poisoning by the systemic, coumaphos, and other organophosphates. First, the onset of signs may not occur until eighteen to thirty hours have elapsed after exposure; and in some instances, the time lapse may be a week to ten days, depending on the degree of exposure. Signs usually occur sooner in young animals than adults, and also the time of onset is shortened with massive doses. The coumaphos-poisoned animal may initially exhibit excessive salivation, dyspnea, stiff movements, and diarrhea typical of the other O-P compounds. However, later in the poisoning syndrome, the clinical signs more nearly approach those produced by the chlorinated hydrocarbon insecticides. Animals may show extreme muscle rigidity resulting in abnormal posturing and ataxia. They may progress into tetany and in some cases convulsive seizures. The convulsive seizures usually occur during the terminal stages prior to death. Coumaphos and most of the other systemic insecticides almost always produce a gastrointestinal upset. A diarrhea often flecked with blood is usually present during some stage of the poisoning syndrome. When poisoning occurs as a result of Ruelene® exposure, the clinical signs are usually in the reverse to those produced by coumaphos; that is, the muscle rigidity, abnormal posturing, and ataxia, probably reflecting the presence of the chlorinated phenyl moiety, occur early in the syndrome which may be from twelve to thirty-six hours after exposure. If the poisoned animal survives, the syndrome may progress into one of central nervous system depression, excessive salivation, weakness, dehydration, diarrhea, and other signs typical of O-P poisoning. As with many of the other systemic compounds, the poisoning syndrome may be prolonged for several days to a week. Animals may lie on their sides paddling. Often, eye movements are not coordinated. A characteristic swaying of the head and neck from side to side with an awkward movement has been described as an abnormal labyrinth effect.

Poisoning by the systemic organophosphorus compounds in the horse almost invariably is manifested by severe gastrointestinal disturbances. Slobbering, abdominal distress, tucked abdomen, and severe diarrhea are characteristic. The diarrhea may be very fluid and will often result in dehydration.

Physiopathology

Pathologic changes associated with acute poisoning by organophosphorus and carbamate insecticides are usually minimal and nonspecific. The effects of overstimulation of the parasympathetic nervous system are readily apparent. The continuous stimulation of secretory glands leads to excessive salivary fluids in the mouth and bronchial secretions in the respiratory tract. Extensive pulmonary edema may occur. Digestive tract secretions may increase and result in fluid accumulation. There may be diffuse endocardial and ectocardial hemorrhages and petechial and ecchymotic hemorrhages in the serosa and mucosa of the GI tract.

Activation and Inactivation

Certain of the organophosphorus insecticides are not inhibitors of ChE unless they undergo microsomal oxidation. Parathion, a thionophosphate, must be oxidized to paraoxon before it can phosphorylate ChE, and this phenomonen is apparently necessary for all thionophosphates. In addition to the thionophosphate→ phosphate activating metabolic reaction, there are other metabolic reactions known to occur with certain organophosphates. They include alkyloxidation, sulfide oxidation, dealkylation, dearylation and carboxyesterase—catalyzed hydrolysis. (Norton, 1975)

There is evidence that animals and man develop tolerance to repeated sublethal doses of organophosphates. The cholinergic receptor sites become refractory to repeated exposures. (Murphy, 1975)

Serum and liver esterases participate in the detoxification of organophosphorus compounds. These esterases are also inhibited by some of the organophosphorus insecticides and in some instances are inhibited before there is significant depression of either RBC or brain acetylcholinesterase. (Su et al., 1971) This may be the mechanism that accounts for the potentiation of one organophosphate by another. The plasma esterases also metabolize drugs such as succinylcholine. Therefore if a horse has been exposed to an organophosphorus insecticide, there may be inhibition of plasma esterases and subsequent potentiation of a therapeutic dose of succinylcholine. (Short et al., 1971) Evidence has also been presented which shows that at least some organophosphorus compound also inhibit certain enzymes involved in cellular metabolism.

Toxic Interactions

There are also interactions between other drugs and organophosphorus insecticides. The tranquilizer chloropromazine increases the toxicity of parathion six hours after administration. But twenty-four hours later the toxicity is decreased and there is less inhibition of brain cholinesterase and the inhibition of RBC cholinesterase is unchanged. At the same time the conversion of parathion to paraoxon is increased. (Vukovich et al., 1971)

Insecticide "synergists" such as piperonyl butoxide have been shown to inhibit or induce microsomal drug—metabolizing enzymes and to potentiate or antagonize phosphorothioate insecticides, depending upon the dose and time of pretreatment with the "synergist". (Murphy, 1975)

Delayed Neurotoxicity

In the 1930s it was found that tri-ortho-cresyl phosphate (TOCP) caused peripheral nerve damage that resulted in weakness and ataxia. (Smith et al., 1930) The early episodes in man resulted from drinking ginger liquor contaminated with TOCP and resulted primarily in leg weakness, ataxis and paralysis, hence the syndrome was called "ginger jake paralysis".

The paralysis is a delayed neurotoxic reaction occurring several days or weeks after exposure. (Johnson, 1969) The monkey, dog and rat are more resistant to organophosphorus delayed neurotoxicity, while man, chicken, calf, cat, lamb and rabbit are more sensitive. The chicken has been the most commonly used experimental animal for studying the physiopathology of this syndrome. (Cavanagh, 1954) There appears to be a critical age factor since delayed neurotoxicity does not occur in chickens until they are fifty-five to seventy days old. This most likely involves the maturation of the nervous system and some suggest that it involves development of myelination. In chickens at least nine months old, ataxia and weakness develop eight to fourteen days after exposure and there is little to no recovery in two months. The dosage required is as little as 70 micrograms/kg or 4 or 5 doses of 20 micrograms/kg. (Davis *et. al.,* 1966) This suggests the presence of a very specific and extremely sensitive site of action.

Several esters of phosphoric acid have been shown to produce a similar clinical syndrome. The three most widely studied compounds are di-isopropylphosphorofluoridate (DFP), bis-mono-isoprophylphosphorodiamide fluoride (Mipafox®) and TOCP. All of the compounds are inhibitors or are converted to inhibitors of esterases. But the delayed neurotoxic reaction is not a result of acute cholinergic effects.

The delayed onset has led some investigators to postulate that the biochemical lesion involves the permanent blocking of a vital synthesis pathway so that no additional "essential substance" can be formed and as soon as the existing intracellular supply is exhausted in the eight to fourteen days following exposure then clinical signs appear. The "essential substance" is unknown. The clinical picture resembles thiamine and nicotinic acid deficiency, but administration of these vitamins does not delay the onset of the syndrome.

The lesions involve a dying back of long axons in the sciatic nerve and in the spinal cord particularly in the spino-cerebellar and vestibulo-spinal tracts. There is myelin disintegration secondary to the axonal destruction. In some cases myelin disruptions are not observed until fourteen days after clinical signs have developed. Changes have not been observed in the brain. Some suggest that the lesion starts at the annulospinal endings of nerves to the muscle spindle and that the motor nerves are relatively unaffected. Large osmiophilic multi-lamellated inclusions and smaller membrane-bound bodies occurring between myofibrils in the foot muscles of TOCP poisoned cats have recently been reported. (Prineas, 1969)

Biochemical studies have concentrated on the effects of TOCP on nerve lipids. (Morazain and Rosenberg, 1970) Phospholipids of sciatic nerve but not brain in a TOCP poisoned chicken are more readily hydrolyzable by phospholipase. There is also an increase in sciatic nerve cholesterol and a decrease in triglyceride content following TOCP exposure in chickens. The mechanism of organophosphorus induced delayed neurotoxicity remains a mystery. But there is considerable interest in finding out how a single exposure to a small amount of TOCP is capable of causing such a profound change in the nervous system of susceptible species. There are also similarities between the pathology of TOCP neurotoxicity and several other types of degenerating nerve diseases that increase the importance of discovering the

mechanism of TOCP neurotoxicity. Because a variety of organophosphorus compounds can cause the delayed neurotoxicity there is constant concern that new organophosphorus materials are not released that might produce these effects. Present drug testing procedures would likely detect these effects, but at the same time the investigators conducting the studies must be careful not to expose themselves to chemicals that produce such drastic and prolonged effects.

Carbaryl, a carbamate insecticide, causes ataxia and incoordination in swine following continuous exposure at high levels. (Smalley, 1970) Feeding 150-300 mg/kg body weight daily for eight to twelve weeks resulted in a functional neuromuscular dissociation starting with relaxation of suspensory ligaments in the rear legs and incoordination followed by stringhalt gait and partial paralysis. Animals recovered when carbaryl exposure was discontinued. Pathologic changes included a discrete myodegeneration of traumatic or ischemic type, acute hyaline and vacuolar myodegeneration, dystrophic calcification, and edema of myelinated tracts of the cerebellum, brain stem, and upper spinal cord associated with vascular degenerative changes. (Smalley et al.,1969)

Environmental Residues

In general residue problems with organophosphorus insecticides are of considerably less significance than are similar problems with the chlorinated hydrocarbon insecticides. Table 2 shows the decline in methyl and ethyl parathion residues on treated alfalfa.

TABLE 2
Decline in Parathion Residues on Alfalfa*

| Treatment | Days Post-Treatment | | |
| | 0 | 10 | 15 |
	Residue—ppm		
Methyl Parathion			
0.5 lb/A	36	0.8	0.3
1.0 lb/A	55	1.5	1.0
Ethyl Parathion			
0.5 lb/A	33	1.5	3.0
1.0 lb/A	80	4.0	5.0

*Adapted from Waldron and Goleman, 1969.

Some of the organophosphorus insecticides used for control of soil insects do persist for some period of time. The persistence of four organophosphates in soil is shown in table 3.

Residues are also minimal in milk from cows treated with organophosphorus insecticides. (Table 4)

TABLE 3

Residues of Four Organophosphorus Insecticides
in Two Types of Soil Seven Months
after Treatment at 1.9 Pounds Per Acre*

Compound	Percent of Original Residue	
	Sandy Soil	Loam Soil
Chlorfenvinphos (Birlane®)	25%	45%
Diazinon	1%	10%
Fonofos (Dyfonate)	25%	45%
Phorate (Thimet®)	25%	35%

*Adapted from Suett, 1971.

TABLE 4

Residues (PPM) in Milk of Dairy Cows
Sprayed or Dusted with Insecticide*

Insecticide	ppm—Whole Milk Time—Post-Treatment			
	12 hrs.	1 day	3 days	7 days
0.2% Methoxychlor[a]	0.2	0.1	0.05	———
0.06% Diazinon[b]	0.35	0.14	0.02	0.02
.25% Coumaphos[b]	0.03	0.02	<0.01	<0.01
.03% Ciodrin®[b]	0.007	0.004	0.001	———

[a] = chlorinated hydrocarbon

[b] = organophosphate

*Adapted from Matthysse and Lisk, 1968.

Dimethoate [O,O-dimethyl-S-(N-methylcarbamoyl-methyl) phosphorodithioate] residues in sheep were approximately 0.02 ppm in heart and muscle two to four weeks after intramuscular injections (20 mg/kg). (Chamberlain et. al., 1961) Dimethoate residues in milk were < 0.2 ppm after the second milking and were not detected in milk from the fourth milking. (Fechner et al., 1970)

Ronnel [O,O-dimethyl O-(2, 4, 5-trichlorophenyl) phosphorothioate] at 100 mg/kg resulted in residues of 20-40 ppm in omental fat of sheep one to seven days after dosing. Ronnel residues were not detected twenty-one days after treatment. (Crookshank and Smalley, 1970)

Tissues from pigs sprayed with one quart of 0.5% Rabon® [2-chloro-1-(2, 4, 5-trichlorophenyl) vinyl dimethyl phosphate] were free of residues within seven days. (Ivey et al., 1970)

Dursban® (O,O-diethyl 0-3, 5, 6-trichloro-2-pyridyl phosphorothioate) was used at 4 pounds/acre to control chiggers in turkeys. Residues in turkeys housed on the treated ground were primarily limited to the skin and fat. Residues were not detected after six to eight weeks. Residues were very low in the muscle and liver after seven to twenty-eight days. (Claborn et al., 1970)

Cows fed up to 3 grams of carbofuran (2, 3-dihydro-2, 2-dimethyl-7-benzofuranyl methylcarbamate, FURADAN) for five days excreted small amounts (< .3 ppm) of 3-hydroxycarbofuran in the milk. (Miles et al., 1971)

Diagnosis

A history of possible excessive exposure within the past forty-eight hours, coupled with characteristic parasympathomimetic signs could warrant a tentative diagnosis of organophosphate or carbamate poisoning.

Chemical analyses of body tissues for organophosphorus and carbamate compounds usually yield disappointing results, probably because of the rapid metabolism of these insecticides. If a sample of feed, stomach contents or suspected insecticide formulation is available in sufficient quantities to chemically analyze, feed or apply to a laboratory animal to determine its toxicity, positive results may be significant. If negative results are obtained from biologic testings however, one cannot always be assured that the field conditions were duplicated.

The single-most important aid in determining if an animal has experienced excessive exposure to the cholinesterase inhibitors is a test for cholinesterase activity in blood and tissue. If the acetylcholinesterase has been phosphorylated its activity will be drastically reduced from normal. It is important to keep in mind, however, that depletion of cholinesterase activity in blood is not directly involved with the appearance of signs of poisoning. This is because depletion of blood cholinesterase may not correlate with depletion of cholinesterase activity at the myoneural junction. If the depletion in blood cholinesterase activity happens to reflect the depletion of true cholinesterase at the nerve endings, as is the case with some organophosphorus and carbamate compounds, it then has diagnostic significance (see subsequent paragraph on cholinesterase measurement and significance). Brain ChE activity (cerebrum) may have more diagnostic value than does blood. (Furr and Carson, 1975)

Signs of organophosphorus and carbamate poisoning may be confused with urea toxicosis and acute grain overload in cattle. Nitrate and cyanide poisoning and bloat in cattle also occur rapidly and could be confused with acute poisoning by the cholinesterase inhibitors. Many diseases and toxicoses which produce labored breathing, excessive salivation, muscle stiffness or paralysis and, in general, parasympathomimetic effects may be confused with organophosphorus and carbamate poisoning.

Diagnosis of poisoning by the systemic organophosphorus compounds is much more difficult than diagnosis of poisoning by the chlorinated hydrocarbon and pure organophosphates. This is especially true concerning coumaphos and Ruelene® because the clinical signs are not typical of either organophosphorus or chlorinated hydrocabon insecticides. Since the syndrome produced by these compounds may last for several days or even weeks, they may be confused with infectious and nutritional disorders. Certain types of calf pneumonia and infectious diarrheas may result in dehydration and central nervous system depression causing syndromes very similar to those produced by both Ruelene® and coumaphos. Other systemics such as trichlorfon, dichlorvos, famphur and dimethoate often produce clinical signs typical of organophosphates, but frequently the gastrointestinal and central nervous system effects are more pronounced. Although ronnel has a relatively low order of toxicity in the sense of producing systemic signs of poisoning, animals often exhibit weakness in the rear limbs for as long as six or eight weeks after exposure. This weakness may be manifested by dragging of the hind feet while walking. Diarrhea, muscular weakness, loss of hair luster and general unthriftiness may be evident for several months after initial poisoning. If one keeps the limitations of the blood cholinesterase test in mind, it can be used as a diagnostic aid. One can assume that if blood cholinesterase activity is reduced to 25 percent of the normal range, the animal has been excessively exposed to a cholinesterase inhibiting agent (see paragraph below). Many infectious, parasitic and nutritional diseases of both large and small animals can be confused with the syndromes produced by the systemic organophosphorus compounds. One should make every attempt to rule out such possibilities before concluding his diagnostic effort.

Measurement of Cholinesterase

All of the commonly used methods for measuring cholinesterase activity are based on the hydrolysis of acetylcholine or a suitable synthetic ester. (Wills, 1972) It is assumed that the rate of hydrolysis is proportional to the amount of enzyme present and that the substrate is being hydrolyzed by a cholinesterase. But since esterases other than cholinesterase can hydrolyze acetylcholine special methods have been developed to separate nonspecific esterase activity from cholinesterase activity. Most of the methods utilize the change in pH that occurs when acetylcholine or similar substrate is hydrolyzed. Older methods depended on color changes of pH sensitive chemicals. For a long time the Michel method (1949) was used which recorded the change in pH occurring in the sample following incubation for a fixed period using standardized test concentrations and volumes. Results with the Michel method

were then reported as change (Δ) in pH with a large change indicating cholinesterase activity and zero pH change meaning complete inhibition of cholinesterase. Normal values for most species have been reported.

Recently more rapid and automated methods have been developed which utilize somewhat expensive and sophisticated equipment. These are referred to as titrimetric or pH Stat methods. These methods neutralize the acid as it is formed by the automatic injection of a base solution of known strength into the reaction vessel. This serves to hold the pH of the reaction at a constant and the amount of base used is then directly related to the amount of cholinesterase activity. In addition the amount of base titrated is often plotted against time to establish the kinetics of the reaction. Samples can be analyzed in two to ten minutes once the measuring system is calibrated.

Cholinesterase Determination in Domestic Animals

For a number of years clinical veterinary toxicologists used a modified Michel method for whole blood cholinesterase determinations. The Michel method was originally developed for analyzing human blood where approximately 50 percent of the total cholinesterase activity is in each of the red blood cells and plasma fractions. Since only true acetylcholinesterase activity is found in the RBC's, they were separated from the plasma, resuspended and the ChE activity measured. Work with animal blood demonstrated that in most species 80 percent or more of the total blood ChE activity was in the RBC (table 5) and, therefore, whole blood could be used in a modified

TABLE 5
Percent of Total Blood Cholinesterase Found in Red Blood Cells of Animals[*]

Species	Percent of Total ChE in RBC
Rabbit	81
Pig	67-88
Rat	71
Monkey	80
Dog	61
Goat	89
Cow	90 (estimated)
Horse	90 (estimated)
Sheep	90 (estimated)

[*]Adapted from Wills, 1972.

Michel procedure. (Radeleff and Woodward, 1956) The range and median values using the modified Michel method are given in table 6. The Michel method requires less equipment and is, therefore, more widely used in routine diagnostic veterinary laboratories at the present time.

TABLE 6
Whole Blood Cholinesterase Activity in
Domestic Animals Using the Modified Michel Method*

Species	Range**	Median or Mean
Horse	0.20-0.65	0.39
Cattle	0.30-0.75	0.40-0.55
Sheep	0.10-0.30	0.15-0.20
Goat	0.04-0.24	0.14
Dog	———	0.43

*Adapted from Wills, 1972; Radeleff and Woodard, 1956.
**Units are ΔpH.

Special Consideration with Carbamate Inhibited Cholinesterase

The inactivation of ChE by carbamates involves a much weaker and less stable binding than with organophosphates. For this reason in cases of carbamate toxicosis blood samples should not be diluted and they should be refrigerated immediately and analyzed as soon as possible.

The method used to analyze the samples should produce results within minutes and should not involve periods of standing of the diluted sample. As soon as the sample is diluted it is possible that the carbamate-ChE complex reverses and active ChE is released. If this occurs then the results of the ChE determination would indicate normal or near normal ChE activity and the diagnosis could be missed. This point is supported by the data in table 7. Rats were fed one of three carbamate

TABLE 7
Effect of Analytical Method on Measuring
Carbamate Cholinesterase Inhibition in
Rat Red Blood Cells*

Group	Michel Method ΔpH	% of Cont.	Titrimetric μmoles acid/ ml/min	% of Cont.
Control	0.54	———	3.01	———
Banol	0.57	105%	1.54	51%
Mobam	0.51	94%	0.60	20%
Carzol	0.55	101%	1.19	40%

*Adapted from Williams and Casterline, 1969.

insecticides and RBC ChE determined by both the Michel and titrimetric methods. In the Michel method the sample is diluted and incubated for thirty to sixty minutes and the pre- and postincubation pH values compared. In the titrimetric method the results are obtained two minutes after the sample is placed in the reaction vessel. Both the absolute values and the percent inhibition are given.

Treatment

Atropine sulfate is the pharmacologic antidote for organophosphorus and carbamate poisoning. Although atropine is highly effective as an antidote, it is important to realize that it has no effect on the fundamental biochemical lesion. Atropine acts only to block or counteract some of the more important effects of acetylcholine accumulation. Animals poisoned by cholinesterase inhibitors have an increased tolerance to atropine and the dosage should be greater than is usually recommended. For ruminants, an average of 0.5 mg/kg body weight, a total of 65 mg for an average horse, or 2 mg for an average dog should be given. About one fourth of the dosage should be given intravenously and the remainder subcutaneously or intramuscularly. Improvement in the animal's condition should be seen within a few minutes. It may be necessary to repeat the dosage every three to four hours for one to two days, depending upon the response of the animal. With each successive treatment, however, the response becomes less and less apparent.

The development of specific antidotes for organophosphorus poisoning shows promise in the hydroximic acids and oximes. Compounds such as 2-PAM (pralidoxime) and TMB-4 act competitively breaking down the phosphorylated enzyme complex, freeing acetylcholinesterase and at the same time tying up the organophosphate, making it available for hydrolysis and excretion. Dosages of approximately 20 mg/kg body weight have been effectively used in animals. The oximes may not be effective in the treatment of carbamate poisoning because the anionic site of the acetylcholinesterase is not available for complexing. In those cases of massive oral exposure, especially in ruminants, the use of both atropine and the oximes may be ineffective because of the continued absorption of the insecticide from the rumen. Animals may make a transient recovery only to relapse into more severe poisoning than was initially observed. Therefore, based on recent clinical trials by Furr and Carson, (1975) we recommend that activated charcoal be given orally, along with atropine and oxime treatment. The charcoal should be of a very fine mesh and activated. Dosages of 1/4-1/2 pound (100-250 gm) in sheep to 2 pounds (900 gm) in large cattle should be given.

A number of drugs should be avoided in treating poisoning by organophosphorus compounds. These include morphine, succinylcholine, and phenothiazine tranquilizers.

Poisoning by some of the systemic organophosphorus compounds is readily alleviated with atropine sulfate. Trichlorfon, dichlorvos and famphur are in this category. Atropine has much less therapeutic benefit with poisoning by coumaphos, ronnel, Ruelene® and dimethoate. Good therapeutc results have been obtained, however, by using atropine in combination with the oximes such as TMB-4 and 2-PAM. The atropine should be given every six to twelve hours at a rate of approximately 0.5 mg/kg body weight and the oximes should be given twice each day at a rate of approximately 20 mg/kg body weight. The atropine should be given to effect, the criteria being the alleviation of excessive salivation and central nervous system effects. Thus one should expect to observe gradual recovery in a poisoned animal treated with a combination of atropine and oximes over a period of twenty-four to forty-eight hours. One should not expect the results to be immediate and dramatic, rather there should be a gradual, but steady recovery during this type of treatment regime. Atropine does not alleviate the neuromuscular effects.

Case History

An Iowa farmer used 15% Thimet® (phorate) granules as a soil insecticide treatment for corn. He placed the insecticide granules in a corn planter, hooked it on a tractor and traveled through the pig lot to the cornfield. Unfortunately, a small trail of granules was left behind the corn planter as it went through the pig lot. There were 77 pigs weighing 30-50 pounds in the lot. Shortly thereafter the pigs were noticed rooting in the ground along the area where the corn planter had traveled. They apparently were eating the granules. About six hours later the farmer noticed ten pigs salivating excessively, vomiting, sweating and exhibiting dyspnea, tensed muscles, twitching and moist rales. He called his veterinarian and by the time he arrived, approximately 20 pigs were affected, some having already died. Several were treated with atropine and promptly recovered. A total of ten died, of the twenty that were affected. Several of the pigs that died were laid aside by the farmer. Shortly thereafter three dogs and seven cats were noticed eating on the carcasses of the dead pigs. Over a period of the next twelve hours the dogs were noticed salivating, vomiting, twitching, with stiffened muscles and difficult breathing. Several cats were observed quivering, kicking, with dyspnea and some had a severe diarrhea. All seven cats died and two of the three dogs died. One dog was treated with atropine and recovered.

Liver and kidney tissues from a pig, dog and cat were analyzed and found to be negative for phorate and other insecticides. The stomach contents of the pig contained approximately 20 ppm phorate. A blood sample from the recovered dog was taken one week after the episode and the cholinesterase determination was done by the modified Michel method and found to have 0.25 Δ pH per hour.

BIBLIOGRAPHY

Cavanagh, J. B. 1954. The Toxic Effects of Tri-Ortho-Cresylphosphate on the Nervous System. An Experimental Study in Hens. *J. Neurol. Neurosurg. Psychiat.* 17:163-72.

Chamberlain, W. F.; Gatterdam, P. E.; and Hopkins, D. E. 1961. The Metabolism of p³²-Labelled Dimethoate in Sheep. *J. Econ. Ent.* 54:733-40.

Claborn, H. V.; Kunz, S. E.; and Mann, H. D. 1970. Residues of Dursban in the Body Tissues of Turkeys Confined in Pens Containing Treated Soil. *J. Econ. Ent.* 63:422-24.

Crookshank, H. R., and Smalley, H. E. 1970. Ronnel Residues in Adult Sheep. *Ag. Food Chem.* 18:326.

Davies, D. R.; Holland, P.; and Rumens, M. J. 1966. The Delayed Neurotoxicity of Phosphorodiamidic Fluorides. *Biochem. Pharm.* 15:1783-89.

Fechner, G.; Berger, H.; Hoernicke, E.; and Ackermann, H. 1970. Rueckstandsbildung in der Milch nach der Pour- on-Applikation des systeminsektizids Dimethoat bei laktierenden Rindern. *Arch. Exp. Vet.* 24:1137-40.

Furr, A. A., and Carson, T. L. 1975a. Comparative Results of Therapeutic Measures Used in the Treatment of Thimet® 15G, Counter® 15G, and Furdan® Toxicosis in Sheep and Cattle. Unpublished Data.

Furr, A. A., and Carson, T. L. 1975. Therapeutic Measures Used in the Treatment of Organophosphorus Insecticide Toxicosis in Sheep. *Vet. Tox.* 17:(4)121-22.

Ivey, M. C.; Eschle, J. E.; and Hogan, B. F. 1971. Residues of Rabon in Body Tissues of Pigs Treated for Control of Hog Lice. *J. Econ. Ent.* 64:320-21.

Johnson, M. K. 1969. Delayed Neurotoxic Action of Some Organophosphorus Compounds. *Brit. Med. Bull.* 25:231-35.

Kenaga, E. E., and End, C. S. 1974. Commercial and Experimental Insecticides. Ent. Soc. Amer. Special Publication. 74-1.

Matthysse, J. G., and Lisk, D. 1969. Residues of Diazinon, Coumaphos, Ciodrin, Methoxychlor, and Rotenone in Cows Milk from Treatments Similar to Those Used for Ectoparasite and Fly Control on Dairy Cattle, with Notes on Safety of Diazinon and Ciodrin for Calves. *J. Econ. Ent.* 61:1394-8.

Michel, H. O. 1949. An Electronic Method for the Determination of Red Blood Cell and Plasma Cholinesterase Activity. *J. Lab. Clin. Med.* 34:1564-68.

Miles, J. T.; Demott, B. J.; Hinton, S. A.; and Montgomery, M. J. 1971. Effect of Feeding Carbofuran on the Physicology of the Dairy Cow and on Pesticide Residues in Milk. *J. Dairy Sci.* 54:478-80.

Morazain, R., and Rosenberg, P. 1970. Lipid Changes in Tri-o-Cresylphosphate-Induced Neuropathy. *Tox. Appl. Pharm.* 16:461-74.

Murphy, S. D. 1975. Pesticides in *Toxicology, the Basic Science of Poisons.* Casarett, L. J., and Doull, J. eds. New York pp. 408-37. Macmillan Publishing Co.

Norton, T. R. 1975. Metabolism of Toxic Substances in *Toxicology, the Basic Science of Poisons.* Casarett, L. J., and Doull, J. eds. New York: Macmillan Publishing Co., pp. 45-132.

Prineas, J. 1969. Triorthocresylphosphate Myopathy. *Arch. Neur.* 21:150-56.

Radeleff, R. D. 1970. *Veterinary Toxicology.* 2nd ed. Philadelphia, Pennsylvania : Lea & Febiger pp. 197-263.

Radeleff, R. D., and Woodard, G. T. 1956. Cholinesterase Activity of Normal Blood of Cattle and Sheep. *Vet. Med.* 51:512-14.

Short, C. E.; Cuneio, J.; and Cupp, D. 1971. Organophosphate-Induced Complications During Anesthetic Management in the Horse. *JAVMA.* 159:1319-27.

Smalley, H. E. 1970. Diagnosis and Treatment of Carbaryl Poisoning in Swine. *JAVMA.* 156:339-44.

Smalley, H. E.; O'Hara, P. J.; Bridges, C. H.; and Radeleff, R. D. 1969. The Effects of Chronic Carbaryl Administration on the Neuromuscular System of Swine. *Tox. Appl. Pharm.* 14:409-19.

Smith, M. I.; Elvove, E.; and Frazier, W. H. 1930. The Pharmacological Action of Certain Phenol Esters, with Special Reference to the Etiology of So-Called Ginger Paralysis. *Pub. Health Rep.* 45:2509-24.

Suett, D. L. 1971. Persistence and Degradation of Chlorfenvinphos, Diazinon, Fonofos and Phorate in Soils and Their Uptake by Carrots. *Pest. Sci.* 2:105-12.

Su, Mei-Quey; Kinoshita, F. K.; Frawley, J. P.; and DuBois, K. P. 1971. Comparative Inhibition of Aliesterases and Cholinesterase in Rats Fed Eighteen Organophosphorus Insecticides. *Tox. Appl. Pharm.* 20:241-49.

Tucker, R. K., and Crabtree, D. G. 1970. Handbook of Toxicity of Pesticides to Wildlife. Resource Pub. No. 84. Bureau of Sport Fisheries and Wildlife, Denver Wildlife Research Center, USDI pp. 131.

Vukovich, R. A.; Triolo, A. J.; and Coon, J. M. 1971. The Effect of Chloropromazine on the Toxicity and Biotransformation of Parathion in Mice. *J. Pharm. and Exp. Ther.* 178:395-401.

Waldron, A. C., and Goleman, D. L. 1969. Ethyl and Methyl Parathion Residues in Green and Cured Alfalfa. *J. Ag. Food Chem.* 17:1066-69.

Williams, C. H., and Casterline, J. L. Jr. 1969. A Comparison of Two Methods for the Measurement of Erythrocyte Cholinesterase Inhibition after Carbamate Administration to Rats. *Food & Cos. Tox.* 7:149-51.

Wills, J. H. 1972. The Measurement and Significance of Changes in the Cholinesterase Activites of Erythrocytes and Plasma in Man and Animals. *Crit. Rev. Tox.* 1:153-202.

Molluscacides

METALDEHYDE

Metaldehyde is used as a molluscicide and is the active component of many proprietary slug and snail killers. It may be marketed as a liquid preparation or in the form of pellets containing from 3 to 3.5 percent metaldehyde. Unfortunately, dogs and other domestic animals may be attracted to the pelleted bait and consume large quantities. There are reports in the literature of metaldehyde poisoning in dogs, cats, sheep and children.

Source

A common source of pelleted metaldehyde is called Snarol® which looks and apparently tastes very much like dog or cat food. It is a meal preparation containing 3.15 percent metaldehyde and 5 percent tricalcium arsenate. Although many of the commercially available preparations contain arsenic, the clinical signs and course of poisoning indicate that most of the problem from these products come from the metaldehyde content of the material. Metaldehyde molluscicides are used primarily in the coastal areas of the United States and the southern lowlands where snails and slugs are prominent pests. In areas where the pelleted material is used, incidents of poisoning in dogs are very common.

Toxicity

In dogs, dosages of approximately 400 mg/kg have produced toxicoses. Thus, 3-4 ounces of Snarol® would be sufficient to poison a 20-50 pound dog. Sheep have been poisoned after consuming 3-4 ounces per head of a commercial preparation. (Simmons and Scott, 1974)

Clinical Signs

Metaldehyde gives rise to incoordination, polypnea, tachycardia, loss of consciousness and cyanosis. Animals may exhibit hyperaesthesia and muscle tremors leading to opisthotonus and continuous convulsions. Nystagmus is almost a characteristic sign in the cat. In man, a depressed cardiac and respiratory rate often occur and barbiturates are contraindicated. Elevated body temperatures have been reported in sheep (102-107° F) and may occur in dogs poisoned on metaldehyde.

Physiopathology

Lesions include hyperemia of the liver and kidneys and degeneration of liver cells and of ganglion cells in the brain. The lungs may be hyperemic and contain interstitial hemorrhages. In sheep, the liver was pale and friable and the trachea and bronchi were full of froth. (Simmons and Scott, 1974) The stomach contents may have a distinct odor of acetaldehyde, which is less pungent than formaldehyde. Ecchymotic and petechial hemorrhages may be present in the mucosa of the gastrointestinal tract.

Diagnosis

The occurrence of clinical signs as described above, together with a history of use of a molluscicide to which the animal had opportunity for consumption are sufficient evidence to warrant a tentative diagnosis of metaldehyde poisoning. Stomach contents can be analyzed for acetaldehyde, a breakdown product of metaldehyde, and its presence can be considered confirmatory.

Treatment

There is no specific antidote. Treatment should be directed toward (1) sedating the animal to a point of general anesthesia to control the muscle spasms, (2) removal of the compound from the stomach with an emetic or gastric lavage, and (3) fluid therapy to maintain hydration and to correct the acidosis that is frequently associated with metaldehyde poisoning.

If the dog is still ambulatory, apomorphine can be

given to produce vomition. Depending upon the degree of muscle tremor, a variety of depressants may be used, such as methocarbamol (Robaxin®) or xylazine (Ropun®), given intravenously to effect. Diazepam (Valium®) given intravenously to effect is good for relatively early or mild cases which may completely recover within three to twelve hours. (Custer, 1974)

If the animal is presented while unable to stand or if there are worsening tremors following emesis, a general anesthetic should be used to maintain light anesthesia for twelve to seventy-two hours. Thiamylal (Surital®) can be used repetitively or as a continuous drip or can be followed by an inhalation anesthetic (Metofane®). An endotracheal tube should be inserted to prevent accidental aspiration of fluids.

The patient should be monitored, as done with any surgical anesthesia case. The stomach should be lavaged immediately after anesthetization. After thoroughly lavaging, a tablespoonful of pectin-bismuth in water should be introduced into the stomach before withdrawing the gastroscope.

The acidosis associated with metaldehyde poisoning can be controlled by the intravenous administration of 1.6 M-Na lactate. The dosage should be 22 ml/kg body weight, administered by continuous infusion during each twelve hours that the patient is anesthetized. (Custer, 1974)

BIBLIOGRAPHY

Custer, M A. 1974. In *Current Veterinary Therapy Small Animal Practice* Vol. 5, Kirk, R. W. ed. Philadelphia, Pennsylvania: W. B. Saunders Company. pp. 129-30.

Simmons, J. R., and Scott, W. A. 1974. An Outbreak of Metaldehyde Poisoning in Sheep. *Vet. Rec.* 95:211-12.

Udall, N. D. 1973. The Toxicity of the Molluscdies Metaldehyde and Methiocarb to Dogs. *Vet. Rec.* 93:420-22.

Rodenticides

ALPHA-NAPHTHYL THIOUREA (ANTU)

Source

ANTU (alpha-naphthyl thiourea) is used exclusively as a rodenticide. It is a gray powder, free from the bitter taste characteristic of most thioureas. It is insoluble in water and is usually prepared in sausage or bread as a bait containing 1 to 3 percent ANTU.

Toxicity

Rodents, especially rats, are very susceptible to ANTU toxicity. The Norway or brown rat is the most susceptible, others being more resistant. Dogs, cats, and swine are the most susceptible domestic animals and are most likely to eat baits containing ANTU. Mature and aged dogs are more susceptible than young ones. Since the advent of more effective rodenticides' ANTU poisoning in dogs has declined to the point of being a rarity.

ANTU rates very high in its speed of action as a toxicant, just under that of sodium fluoroacetate. Its toxicity varies with many factors:

1. The particle size affects absorption and, therefore, toxicity. Apparently, the larger particle size (50-100 microns in diameter) is more toxic than smaller particles (5 microns in diameter).
2. Mature animals are more susceptible than younger ones.
3. Animals with partially filled stomachs are less likely to vomit and thus are more susceptible than animals with empty stomachs.

The single oral lethal dose in the mature dog is recorded to be between 10 and 50 mg/kg body weight. In young dogs the single lethal dose is 85-100 mg/kg.

Mechanism of Action

ANTU causes an increase in permeability of the pulmonary capillaries. Pulmonary edema develops, and the animal actually drowns in its own fluid. In acute cases, pulmonary edema and pleural effusions may be the only effects observed. ANTU is also a strong emetic. This property undoubtedly has protected animals that can vomit. This is why rodents are more susceptible to ANTU—they are unable to vomit and expel the poison. The emetic effect is apparently mediated centrally as well as locally.

Clinical Signs

Vomition, salivation, and other evidence of gastric irritation may be the first signs of ANTU poisoning. They appear within a few minutes to a few hours after ingestion, and the course lasts twelve hours or less. Survival for as long as twelve hours suggests a more favorable prognosis. Other signs include dyspnea, coughing, increased heart rate, heart sounds which are often muted because of pericardial effusion, hypothermia which develops as the animal approaches coma, and diarrhea. The cause of death is anoxia resulting from the accumulation of fluid in and around the lungs and heart. Many animals try to relieve the increased intrathoracic pressure by sitting; they rapidly become cyanotic and too weak to do anything except lie in a sternal position.

Physiopathology

There is cyanosis on postmortem examination. Pleural effusions and pulmonary edema resulting in hydrothorax are characteristic. The trachea, bronchi, and gastrointestinal mucosa may be inflamed. Hyperemia of the kidneys and liver is usually found.

Diagnosis

One must rely upon history, signs, and characteristic postmortem changes of lung edema and hydrothorax for a tentative diagnosis. Chemical tests for thiourea are usually inconclusive. Gastric contents or vomitus are the most suitable specimens for analysis. Tissues and blood may be used for chemical analysis, but the tests must be conducted within twenty-four hours after exposure. Animals surviving longer than twenty-four hours after ingestion usually give negative tests for ANTU. ANTU poisoning should be differentiated from urea poisoning, which is not commonly encountered in dogs. Organophosphorus insecticide poisoning may result in edema of the lungs, but pleural effusions are almost never found.

Treatment

There is no satisfactory specific treatment for ANTU poisoning. Silicone aerosol may help prevent foaming in the bronchioles. N-amylmercaptan or other substances providing thiol (—SH) groups may reduce mortality. Emetics such as apomorphine may be indicated if treatment can be accomplished early but are of no value once pulmonary edema has developed.

REFERENCES

Clarke, E. G. C., and Clarke, M. L. 1967. *Garner's Veterinary Toxicology*. 3rd ed. Baltimore: The Williams & Wilkins Co.

Radeleff, R. D. 1964. *Veterinary Toxicology*. Philadelphia: Lea & Febiger.

FLUOROACETATE AND FLUOROACETAMIDE

Source

Sodium monofluoroacetate (1080) and fluoroacetamide were developed for insecticidal and rodent control purposes. They are colorless, odorless, tasteless, and quite water soluble. For these reasons, some countries have investigated them as a possible chemical warfare agent for addition to water supplies. Presently, the primary commercial use of fluoroacetate is in rodent control. The compound is commonly mixed with bread, carrots, bran, or other baits. In the United States, fluoroacetate compounds are mixed with a black dye and are available only to licensed exterminators. Some countries (*e.g.*, Great Britain) restrict the use of these compounds to areas such as sewers and ship holds.

Compound 1080 is commonly used at a concentration of 0.6 percent in grain baits, and approximately 2,500 pounds are produced annually. The manufacturer (of which there are two in the United States) requires the following of purchasers:

1. Purchaser assumes full responsibility for use and agrees to use only for rodents.
2. Purchaser must be covered by public liability insurance for exterminator operations.
3. Purchaser agrees that chemical purchased will not be given away or resold in any form.
4. Purchaser agrees that fluoroacetate will be used only by trained and experienced personnel.
5. Purchaser agrees to deliver to the manufacturer any unused 1080 if required liability insurance is cancelled or if his use of 1080 is discontinued.

As an exterminating agent, 1080 is quite effective. It is highly toxic and not detectable to the sense organs. In addition, the characteristic lag period after ingestion minimizes bait shyness in rodents and other pests. Unfortunately, 1080 is not selective and is even more toxic to pet animals and livestock than to rodents. A further disadvantage is that biological chain reactions can occur, and animals may be poisoned by eating rodents or birds killed by 1080.

Monofluoroacetic acid is recognized as the naturally occurring toxicant in a number of plants from several countries (see table 1).

TABLE 1
Plants Which Contain Monofluoroacetic Acid as the Toxic Principle

Plant	Geographic Location
Dichapetalum cymosum	South Africa
Dichapetalum toxicarum	West Africa
Acacia georginae	Australia
Gastrolobium grandiflorum	Australia
Oxylobium parviflorum	Australia
Palicourea margravii	Brazil

Several investigators (Lovelace, *et al.,* 1968; and Cheng, *et al.,* 1968) have found accumulation of fluoroacetate in forage and grain crops grown in areas of high atmospheric fluorides. The toxicologic significance of these findings have not been assessed.

Toxicity

1080 is highly toxic. Nonprimate mammals may be killed by dosages of 0.1 to 5.0 mg/kg. Dogs are quite susceptible, and as little as 0.05mg/kg may be lethal. Primates and man are less susceptible. Rats and mice are more resistant than dogs, cats, or livestock; and 5.0 to 8.0 mg/kg is required to produce poisoning. Dogs are most likely to be poisoned by the oral route. Both dogs and swine have been killed by ingestion of birds or rodents poisoned on 1080.

The acute toxicity of 1080 for various mammals and birds is summarized in table 2.

Fluoroacetate may be absorbed through the gastrointestinal tract, respiratory tract, and abraded skin, but not via the intact skin.

TABLE 2
Acute LD_{50} Values in Some Animals Susceptible
to Sodium Fluoroacetate

Species	LD_{50} (mg/kg)	Route
Man	0.7-2.1[1]	Oral
Rhesus monkey	4.0	IV
Cattle (adult)	.39	Oral
Cattle (calves)	.22	Oral
Horse	0.35-0.55	Oral
Sheep	0.25-0.50	Oral
Swine	0.4-1.0	Oral
Bear	0.5-1.0	Oral
Domestic cat	0.20	IV
Coyote	0.10	IV
Norway rat	2.1-3.0	Oral
House mouse	8.0	Oral
Dog	0.05-1.0	Oral
Domestic pigeon	4.24	Oral
Mallard	10.0	Oral
Golden eagle	1.25-5.00	Oral
Great horned owl	~ 10.0	Oral

[1] estimated

Mechanism of Action

Fluoroacetate is not particularly toxic. However, fluoroacetate can replace acetyl CoA, combining with oxalacetic acid in the Krebs cycle to form fluorocitric acid. Fluorocitric acid then acts to inhibit the enzyme aconitase in the Krebs cycle. There is a blockage of the Krebs cycle with a buildup of citric acid. The net result is that the animal suffers a loss of cellular respiration (fig. 1).

The metabolic involvement of fluoroacetate makes it a powerful tool for research in carbohydrate metabolism, and particularly in brain research on the mechanisms of convulsions. Peters and Shorthouse (1975) have recently found that conversion of fluoroacetate to fluorocitrate in rat and dog brain mitochrondria does not occur *in vitro,* but is dependent in some way on an *in vivo* association.

There is generally a short delay between ingestion of 1080 and appearance of clinical signs. This is because fluoroacetate must be converted to the more toxic fluorocitrate, which then must accumulate to toxic levels.

Other halogenated acetates (e.g., monochloroacetate and monoiodoacetate) do not cause inhibition of aconitase as does 1080.

Clinical Signs

There is a characteristic latent period of from one-half to two hours after ingestion of sodium fluoroacetate. When signs commence, the onset is acute and the course rapid and usually violent. The physiologic and clinical effects are different depending on the species affected. In general, herbivores exhibit cardiac failure while carnivores have marked CNS disturbance, convulsions, and gastrointestinal hypermotility.

In 1080 poisoned dogs there is an initial period of restlessness and hyperirritability. Aimless wandering progresses to wild, frenzied running and barking. Often affected dogs will run a straight course until a building or fence is encountered. There appears to be hallucination and pain (barking, anxious appearance). Vomition is observed early in the course, and repeated defecation and urination are characteristic. The tenesmus continues even after the bowels and bladder are evacuated. The stools passed are usually soft and formed, not watery. Wild running and barking are interrupted by tonic-clonic seizures, opisthotonus, and paddling. Body temperature may be elevated in the range of 105-108° F in affected dogs during convulsive seizures. After such a siezure the dog lies for a time in a state of apparent exhaustion. As the disease progresses, convulsions become weaker and more frequent. Terminally, the animal is semicomatose and gasps for breath. Death from respiratory failure ensues within two to twelve hours after onset of signs.

Cats may exhibit signs similar to the dog, but generally do not display the marked excitement characteristic of the dog. Cardiac arrhythmia, hyperesthesia, and vocalization may be quite pronounced.

In ruminants and other herbivores, cardiac signs predominate. There is marked cardiac arrhythmia, a rapid, weak pulse, and finally ventricular fibrillation. Animals may be found dead with no signs of struggle. Live animals may stagger, tremble, and fall. There may or may not be urination and defecation. Moaning and grinding of teeth attest to extreme pain. Terminal convulsive seizures occur, but they are generally not the violent type seen in carnivores. Horses are observed to tremble and sweat profusely. They may be somewhat hypersensitive but not to the extreme degree seen in strychnine poisoning. Swine may display both cardiac and nervous signs of about equal magnitude.

Animals which die of 1080 poisoning experience rapid onset of rigor mortis with the limbs fixed in extensor rigidity.

Secondary intoxication occurs in highly susceptible animals such as carnivores (especially dogs) consuming rodents or birds which have died of 1080 poisoning. The hazard of secondary poisoning will depend, in part, on the amount of bait consumed by the primary species, the portions of that species consumed (alimentary tract versus carcass) and the susceptibility of the consuming species. When 1080 is used in an area, all dead rodents and birds should be promptly collected and safely disposed of.

Physiopathology

Interference with the Krebs cycle results in accumulation of citrate especially in the kidney. Secondarily, glucose is poorly utilized so there is hyperglycemia as well as lactic acidemia and resultant depression of blood pH. Some investigators have reported elevations in brain ammonia, but this effect generally occurs after convulsions are initiated. (St. Omer, 1975) Fluoroacetate effects on central nervous function are not well defined. Various theories include involvement of citrate, ammonia, and glutamate. This aspect of 1080 intoxication is presently an area of active research.

There is general cyanosis of mucous membranes and other tissues. The liver and kidney are dark and extremely congested. The heart is usually in diastole and may have subepicardial hemorrhages. Dogs and cats almost invariably have an empty stomach, colon, and urinary bladder. Diffuse visceral hemorrhage has been described, especially in cattle.

Histologic lesions may be absent, although cerebral edema and lymphocytic infiltration of the Virchow-Robin Space have been described.

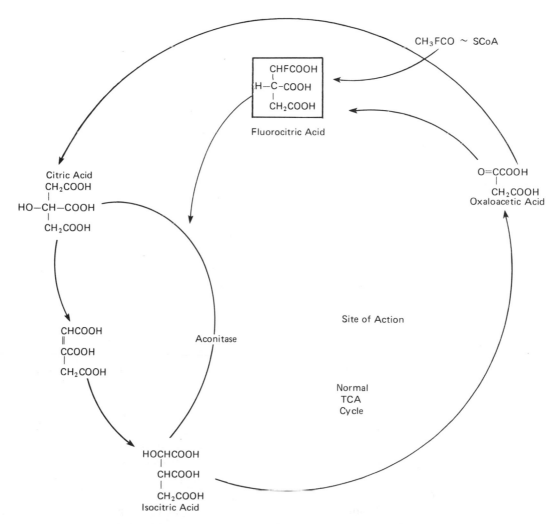

Figure 1. Scheme of the mechanism of fluoroacetate inhibition of the TCA cycle.

Diagnosis

Heavy reliance is placed on history, clinical signs, and necropsy findings as well as negative analyses for other convulsant poisons. Methods currently utilized to chemically confirm 1080 poisoning include gas-liquid chromatography as well as use of the fluoride-ion specific electrode.

Samples for submission to the chemistry laboratory should include suspected baits, vomitus, stomach contents, liver and kidney.

There is hyperglycemia in affected animals, and this may be a rapid clinical laboratory aid. Citric acid accumulates to high levels in the kidneys of poisoned animals, and chemical analysis revealing markedly elevated citrate is suggestive when correlated with the clinical history.

Many compounds produce convulsions or CNS aberrations in animals. Strychnine causes extreme hyperesthesia resulting in tetanic seizures in response to external stimuli. Strychnine-poisoned dogs usually do not vomit or void urine and feces, nor is there the extreme running and yelping which characterizes 1080 intoxication. Chlorinated hydrocarbon insecticides (*e.g.,* toxaphene, chlordane) produce intermittent epileptiform convulsions, fine muscle tremors, and mild hypersensitivity. Vomiting and defecation are not common. Elevated temperature may occur during or after chlorinated hydrocarbon convulsions. Lead poisoning is characterized by tremors, convulsions, and vomiting or colic. These are usually intermittent and follow a much longer course. A differential blood smear with nucleated erythrocytes and basophilic stippling is tentative confirmation of lead poisoning in dogs. Garbage intoxication in dogs may cause weakness, mild convulsions, vomiting, and diarrhea. Extreme agitation and excitability are not associated with garbage poisoning, however.

Plant alkaloids such as nicotine and taxine (Japanese yew), or cicutoxin (water hemlock) may cause violent seizures and/or sudden death, especially in large animals.

Hypocalcemia in bitches, hypomagnesemia, acute pancreatic necrosis, acute massive liver necrosis, and brain injury can cause various degrees of CNS stimulation and vomiting.

A careful history, clinical examination, and necropsy will help to establish or rule out 1080 as a possible toxicant. Citrate levels in kidney tissue may aid in confirmation of the clinical diagnosis.

Treatment

There is no specific antidote. Control of the violent convulsions is of first importance. Barbiturates should be used with caution since they may further depress the respiratory center. The dosage of barbiturate should be just enough to control the more violent convulsions, but complete anesthesia should not be attempted. Calcium gluconate (4 to 10 cc of a 10 to 20 percent solution) may be used as an additional means of controlling convulsions and combating possible hypocalcemia. Gastric lavage with milk or limewater is recommended.

Glycerol monoacetate (Monacetin) may be given intramuscularly at 0.55 gm/kg. This may help to overcome the acetate to citrate change believed responsible for the toxicity of 1080. Oral administration of 8.8 ml/kg each of 50 percent alcohol and 5 percent acetic acid may be substituted for Monacetin. In advanced or severe cases, prognosis is always grave and treatment is often unrewarding.

REFERENCES

Anon. 1964. Fluoroacetamide Poisoning. *J. Sm. Animal Pract.* 5:209-11.

Artyushkova, V. A; Kirzon, M. V.; and Chernova, G. G. 1968. Change of External Respiration in White Rats Following Sodium Fluoroacetate Poisoning. *Biol. Nauk.* 11:29-33.

Atzert, S. P. 1971. A Review of Sodium Monofluoroacetate (Compound 1080). It's Properties, Toxicology, and Use in Predator and Rodent Control. United States Department of the Interior, Fish and Wildlife Service. Wildlife No. 146: 1-34.

Cheng, J. Y.; Yu, M. H.; Miller, W.; and Welkie, H. W. 1968. Fluoroorganic Acids in Soy Bean Leaves Exposed to Fluoride. *Environmental Sci. & Tech.* 2:367-70.

Cheng, S. C.; Kumar, S.; and Casella, G. A. 1972. Effects of Fluoracetate and Fluorocitrate on the Metabolic Compartmentation of Tricarboxylic Acid Cycle in Rat Brain Slices. *Brain Res.* 42:117-28.

Chenoweth, M. B. 1967. Fluoroacetate: Still a Portal to Comparative Toxicology. *Fed. Amer. Soc. Ex. Bio.* 16:1074.

Fanshier, D. W.; Gottwald, L. K.; and Kun, E. 1964. Studies on Specific Enzyme Inhibitors VI. Characterization and Mechanism of Action of the Enzyme Inhibitory Isomer of Monofluorocitrate. *Jour. Biol. Chem.* 239:425-34.

Godoy, H. M.; Cignolig, E. V.; and Castro, J. 1968. Effect of Fluoroacetate Poisoning on the Glycogen Content of Rat Heart and Skeletal Muscle. *Life Sci. Biochem. Gen. Molec. Biol.* 7:847-54.

Guarda, F., and Dotta, U. 1964. Experimental Poisoning with Sodium Fluoroacetate in Dogs: Symptoms and Lesions. *Annal. Fac. Med. Vet. Torino.* 12:241-70.

Harris, W. F. 1964. Clinical Syndromes of Three Common Convulsants. *Southwest. Vet.* 17:214-17.

Haynes, F. D.; Short, R. D.; and Hibson, J. E. 1973. Differential Toxicity of Monochloroacetate, Monofluoroacetate and Monoiodoacetate in Rats. *Toxicology and Applied Pharmacology* 26:93-102.

Jensen, R.; Tobiska, J. W.; and Ward, J. C. 1948. Sodium Fluoroacetate (Compound 1080) Poisoning in Sheep. *Am. J. Vet. Res.* 8-9: 370-72.

Lahiri, S., and Quastel, J. H. 1963. Fluoroacetate and the Metabolism of Ammonia in Brain. *Biochem. J.* 89:157-63.

Lovelace, J.; Miller, G. W.; and Welkie, G. W. 1968. Short Communication. The Accumulation of Fluoroacetate and Fluorocitrate in Forage Crops Collected Near a Phosphate Plant. *Atmospheric Environment* 2:187-90.

Matsumura, F., and O'Brien, R. D. 1963. A Comparative Study of the Modes of Action of Fluoroacetamide and Fluoroacetate in the Mouse and American Cockroach. *Biochem. Pharmacol.* 12:1201-05.

Peters, R. A., and Morselli, P. L. 1965. Observations on the Use and Action of Monacetin in Fluoroacetate Poisoning. *Biochem. Pharmacol.* 14:1891-93.

Peters, R. A. 1963. Organo-Fluorine Compounds Present in Certain Plants and Their Effect on Animals. Proceedings of the Biochemical Society. 49th Annual Meeting: 8-9.

————. 1970. Lethal Synthesis. *Biol. Nutr. Dieta.* 15:19-28.

Powell, G. L., and Beevers, H. 1968. Fluoroacetyle CoA as a Substrate for Malate Synthase (Fluoroacetate Toxicity, Mammals). *Biochem. Biophys. Acta.* 151:708-10.

Robinson, W. H. 1970. Acute Toxicity of Sodium Monofluoroacetate to Cattle. *J. Wildlife Management* 34:647-48.

Roszkowski, A. P. 1967. Comparative Toxicity of Rodenticides. *Fed. Proc.* 126:1082-88.

St. Omer, V. V. E. 1975. Personal Communication. University of Missouri: College of Veterinary Medicine.

Spencer, A. F., and Lowenstein, J. M. 1967. Citrate Content of Liver and Kidney of Rat in Various Metabolic States and in Fluoroacetate Poisoning. *Biochem. J.* 103:342-48.

Vickery, B., and Vickery, M. L. 1973. Toxicity for Livestock of Organofluorine Compounds Present in Dichapetalum Plant Species. *The Vet. Bul.* 43:537-42.

MISCELLANEOUS RODENTICIDES

Numerous compounds have been used by man in an attempt to control unwanted populations of rodents and other undesirable mammals. In the United States, control of rats and mice constitutes the major use of such materials. Table 1 enumerates the toxicants commercially available for rat and mouse control. Of those listed, arsenic, coumarins, indane-diones, phosphorous, strychnine, thallium, zinc phosphide and sodium flouroacetate are treated under appropriate separate chapter headings.

This chapter will deal primarily with those specialized rodenticides of less toxicity to other mammals. These include alpha-chloralose, castrix, norbormide, red squill, and vacor.

TABLE 1
Toxicants Used in Control
of Rats and Mice

Alpha chloralose
Arsenic
Barium salts
Coumarin anticoagulants
Crimidine® (castrix)
Indane-dione anticoagulants
Alpha-napthyl thio urea (ANTU)
Norbormide
Phosphorous
Red squill
Sodium fluoroacetate
Strychnine
Sulfaquinoxaline
Thallium
Warfarin
Zinc phosphide
Vacor®

Alpha-Chloralose

Source

Alpha-chloralose is a condensation of chloral (CCl_3CHO) with various pentose or hexose sugars. It is a centrally active drug with both stimulant and depressant properties on the central nervous system.

Three principal uses of alpha-chloralose are recognized. They are (1) a general rodenticide primarily for indoor use, (2) a general anesthetic in laboratory animals, and (3) an activating agent in electroencephalography in man.

Toxicity

The toxicity of alpha-chloralose in several species is given as follows:

mouse (oral LD_{50})	300mg/kg
rat (oral LD_{50})	400 mg/kg
cat (oral LD_{50})	400 mg/kg
dog (oral LD_{50})	600 mg/kg

Mechanism of Action and Clinical Signs

Alpha-chloralose selectively depresses the neurons of the ascending reticular formation, suppressing the normal arousal response. The EEG of anesthetized animals, however, suggests that cortical neurons are in a "subconvulsive state." Small doses of the drug increase motor activity and there are myoclonic movements which may progress eventually to deep anesthesia as dosage increases. Moderate to marked hypothermia may also occur.

Alpha-chloralose is metabolized to chloral which is converted to trichloroethanol, a CNS depressant. Hepatic formation of a glucuronide then occurs to form pharmacologically inactive urochloralic acid which is excreted in the urine. (Lees and Pharm, 1972)

Early clinical effects are mild ataxia followed by hyperexcitability. Some cats may become quite aggressive. In severe poisoning the early signs rapidly give way to posterior weakness, prostration, increased salivation, shallow respiration, weak pulse and hypothermia.

A sort of "psychic blindness" is described in dogs (Lees and Pharm, 1972) in which affected animals do not respond to normal stimuli or familiar surroundings.

Physiopathology

Under clinical circumstances fatalities are rarely described. No reports of clinicopathologic changes or pathologic lesions have been found.

Treatment

Treatment recommended includes restraint to prevent injury, maintenance of normal body temperature, and evacuation of the gastrointestinal tract by appropriate means (see therapy). In severe cases, analeptics are recommended, but their duration is much shorter than that of alpha-chloralose. Artificial ventilation in combination with other general toxicologic management is also advised for severe intoxications.

CASTRIX (CRIMIDINE)

Castrix (2, chloro-4-dimethylamino-6- methylpyrimidine) is a rapidly-acting convulsant chemical with no reported age or sex differences in toxicity.

Toxicity values include the following:

Species	Oral LD_{50}
mice	1.2 mg/kg
rats	1.5 mg/kg
chicks	22.5 mg/kg

The drug is apparently an antagonist of vitamin B_6 and clinical signs are reflected in the CNS as convulsant activity.

Twenty lethal doses of Castrix can be eliminated within twenty-four hours in the urine of poisoned dogs, provided convulsions are controlled by barbiturates. (Jones, 1965)

NORBORMIDE

Norbormide 5-(α-hydroxy-α-2-pyridylbenzyl)-7-(- 2-pyridylbenzylidene)-5-norbornene-2, 3-dicarboxamide, is a modern rodenticide which approaches the ideal of a target specific toxicant. It kills Norway rats in from fifteen minutes to four hours and has an approximate LD_{50} for rats of 5 mg/kg. The compound is non-cumulative, tolerance does not develop, and it kills rats in one feeding.

Toxicity

The toxicity of norbormide in several species of animals is given as follows:

Species	Oral LD_{50}
rat	5.3 mg/kg
mouse	2,250 mg/kg
guinea pig	620 mg/kg
hamster	140 mg/kg
cat	no deaths at 1,000 mg/kg
dog	no deaths at 1,000 mg/kg
swine	no deaths at 1,000 mg/kg

Mechanism of Action

Norbormide causes peripheral vasoconstriction in the rat. There is blanching of the extremities and widespread ischemia. The norbormide sensitive receptor is apparently different from those of vascular smooth muscle responsive to norepinephrine.

Clinical Signs, Physiopathology

The clinical signs described in rats include restlessness ataxia, posterior weakness, labored breathing, paleness of the extremities and death preceded by mild convulsions.

Treatment

None is described.

RED SQUILL

Source

Red squill is a red powder obtained from *Urginea maritima* (Fam. Liliacae) and is native to several mediterranean countries. It is considered the oldest rodenticidal material known.

Toxicity

The acute oral toxicity of red squill is given as follows:

Species	LD_{50} (mg/kg)
rat	490
bovine (adult)	250
bovine (young)	100
sheep	250
swine	200
dog	145
cat	100

Mechanism of Action

As is characteristic of many of the lily family, red squill contains glycosides of the digitalis type. Rats appear quite sensitive to the glycoside and in addition to any cardiac effect convulsions and paralysis are produced in rats.

Clinical Signs

Vomiting is an early and characteristic sign in animals other than the rat and ruminants. There is development of convulsions, hyperesthesia, incoordination, and in ruminants alternating periods of depression. Diarrhea may occur approximately one day after emesis and early signs. Death usually occurs within one to three days after initial ingestion, but recovery is common.

Physiopathology

Pathologic changes of gastritis, enteritis and alimentary mucosal ulceration may be seen, as well as congestion of abdominal and thoracic organs.

Diagnosis

No good chemical test is available. Diagnosis is based on history of exposure correlated with compatible signs and lesions.

Treatment

Specific therapy is not described. General detoxication and supportive therapy should be of value however.

VACOR

Vacor (N-3-pyridylmethyl N¹-p-nitrophenyl urea) is a newly developed rodenticide with high toxicity to rats as compared to other animals. It is available as a 10 percent tracking powder or a 2 percent bait. (Whitmoyer Laboratories, Myerstown, PA)

Toxicity

Available toxicity data are as follows:

Species	Oral LD_{50} (mg/kg)
rat	12
rabbit	300
dog	500-1,000
cat	62-200
chicken	700
swine	300
sheep	300
rhesus monkey	2,000

From available data, only the cat would appear to be under hazard from potential field exposure. Trials for secondary toxicity in dogs and cats consuming poisoned rats have been negative. (Mock, 1975)

Mechanism of Action

Vacor appears to be a vitamin B antagonist (Mock, 1975), specifically against nicotinamide. Experimentally, large doses of nicotinamide counter the effects of the toxicant. Response to nicotinamide is best if administered soon after exposure to Vacor.

Clinical Signs

Rats are killed in four to eight hours in a non-convulsive depressive manner.

Diagnosis

Poisoning under field conditions is not likely. Diagnosis would be based on determination of quantitative exposure to Vacor. Chemical analysis is on a research basis and at present diagnostic analyses are not utilized.

BIBLIOGRAPHY

Fitzpatrick, R. J.; McGirr, J. L.; and Papworth, D. S. 1955. The Toxicity of Rodenticides II. Red Squill and Zinc Phosphide. *Vet. Rec.* 67:142.

Hammond, P. B. 1965. Drugs Having Special Lethal Effects. *Veterinary Pharmacology and Therapeutics.* L. M. Jones, ed. Ames, Iowa: I.S.U. Press.

Lees, P., and Pharm, V. 1972. Pharmacology and Toxicology of Alpha-Chloralose: A Review. *Vet. Rec.* 91:330.

Lisella, F. S.; Long, K. R.; and Scott, H. G. 1970. Toxicity of Rodenticides and Their Relation to Human Health. *J.E.H.* 33:231.

McGirr, J. L., and Papworth, D. S. 1955. The Toxicity of Rodenticides I. Sodium Fluoroacetate, ANTU and Warfarin. *Vet Rec.* 67:124.

Mock, J. F. 1975. Personal Communication. Whitmoyer Laboratories. Meyerstown, PA.

Peregrine, D. J. 1973. Toxic Baits for the Control of Pest Animals. *PANS* 19:523.

Roszowski, S. P. 1965. The Pharmacologic Properties of Norbormide, a Selective Rat Toxicant. *J. Pharm. Exp. Therap. 149:288-99.*

PHOSPHORUS

Occasionally, white or yellow phosphorus is used as a rodenticide. Dogs may rarely be poisoned by the consumption of baits containing this material. Red phosphorus and most other phosphorus compounds are relatively nontoxic; however, dogs are quite susceptible to white phosphorus poisoning with 50-100 mg often producing lethal effects. Initial signs of toxicity are related to abdominal irritation and vomition. The vomitus may be luminous in the dark and may have a garlic like odor.

Signs commence very soon after ingestion of phosphorus. Animals may then appear to recover for a few hours or a few days only to relapse into vomiting, abdominal pain accompanied by icterus, nervous signs, convulsions, coma, and death. The secondary phase of this condition is the result of severe hepatic and renal degeneration. Necropsy reveals acute gastroenteritis. Fatty degeneration of the liver, muscles, and blood vessels may be seen. There may be extravasation of blood into subcutaneous and muscular tissue. Icterus is quite evident in dogs which have been ill for more than a few days.

Diagnosis of the condition is dependent upon the detection of phosphorus in the gastrointestinal tract, vomitus, or feces. Treatment should be initiated immediately after exposure, if possible. Vomiting should be induced or a gastric lavage should be performed. Oral administration of 0.1-0.2 percent potassium permanganate helps to neutralize the phosphorus. This chemical may be incorporated into the lavage solution. Also, rinsing the stomach with a 0.2 percent copper sulfate solution may be beneficial. The administration of 100-200 ml of mineral oil has been recommended, since it dissolves phosphorus and renders it unavailable for absorption. Avoid the use of castor oil or milk because phosphorus is highly fat soluble, and absorption would be promoted. Cardiac stimulants and 5 percent glucose intravenously may be indicated.

REFERENCES

Clarke, E. G. C., and Clarke, M. L., 1967. *Garner's Veterinary Toxicology*. 3rd ed. Baltimore: The Williams & Wilkins Co.

STRYCHNINE

Source

Strychnine is an indole alkaloid. The following formula for strychnine has been established:

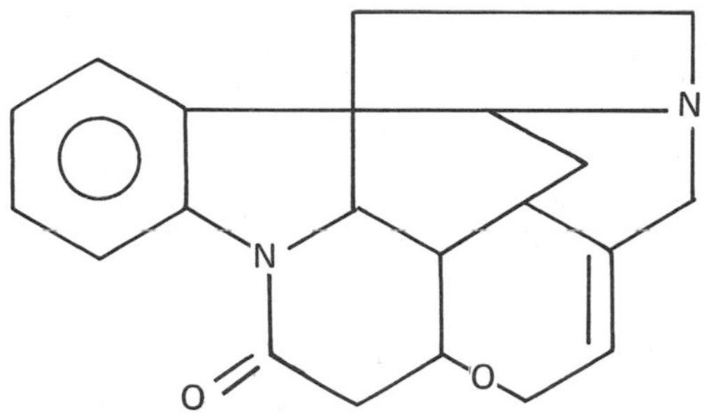

Brucine is a structurally close relative of strychnine, and has similar physiologic effects (although less potent) as strychnine.

The morphine alkaloids thebaine, morphine and codeine are structurally similar to strychnine in many respects, but have obvious depressant activity rather than the excitatory properties of strychnine.

The commercial sources of strychnine are primarily from Southeast Asia, being derived from seeds of the plants *Strychnos nux-vomica* and *Strychnos ignatii*. It was first used in medicine about 1540 and has been used in Europe as an animal poison since the sixteenth century.

Present day usage of strychnine is primarily as a ruminatoric (tartar emetic), stimulant, and pesticide. However, there is no modern rational basis for the use of strychnine in therapy.

Its principal pesticidal applications are for rat, gopher, mole, and coyote control. Many commercial forms are pelleted and are dyed either bright green or red. Strychnine is available to the public through many retail outlets.

Toxicity

Strychnine is a highly toxic compound to most domestic animals. The approximate oral lethal toxicity to various animals is as follows:

Bovine	0.5 mg/kg
Equine	0.5 mg/kg
Porcine	0.5-1.0 mg/kg
Canine	0.75 mg/kg
Feline	2.0 mg/kg
Fowl	5.0 mg/kg
Rat	3.0 mg/kg

Injected strychnine is some two to ten times more toxic than oral strychnine.

Mechanism of Action

As alkaloids characteristically do, strychnine appears to directly affect the central nervous system by selectively antagonizing certain types of spinal inhibition. It interferes with postsynaptic inhibition in the spinal cord and medulla. Thus, the moderating and controlling effects in the reflex are eliminated. Chief examples of postsynaptic inhibition are the inhibitory influences between motoneurons of antagonistic muscle groups, and the recurrent spinal inhibition mediated by Renshaw cells. Renshaw cells are those which mediate inhibition from collaterals of lower motoneurons to adjacent motoneurons. The purpose of such inhibitions is to allow discrete and controlled activity mediated through anterior motoneurons.

The amino acid glycine is an accepted inhibitory transmitter in the spinal cord and medulla. Strychnine reversibly and selectively antagonizes glycine in the spinal cord and medulla, possibly by a competitive type of antagonism. Postsynaptic membrane permeability is changed and the net effect is that strychnine reduces the inhibitory postsynaptic potential normally controlled by glycine.

The physiologic effect of strychnine, then, is to allow uncontrolled and relatively diffuse reflex activity to proceed basically unchecked. All striated muscle groups are affected, but the relatively more powerful extensors predominate to produce symmetrical and generalized rigidity and tonic seizures.

Gross or microscopic changes in the neurons, axons, or myelin sheath have not been observed.

Clinical Signs

Clinical signs of strychnine poisoning appear within ten minutes to two hours after ingestion of the poison. Early signs are apprehension, nervousness, tenseness, and stiffness. Palpation in early stages reveals tense abdomen and rigid cervical musculature. Violent tetanic seizures may appear spontaneously or be initiated by stimuli such as touch, sound, or a sudden bright light. There is extreme and overpowering extensor rigidity causing the animal to assume a "saw horse" stance. The strength of the tetanic spasm may throw an animal off its feet. The legs and body are stiff, the neck arched, ears erect, and the lips are pulled back from the teeth. Breathing may cease momentarily. Duration of a tetanic convulsion may vary from a few seconds to a minute or more. Intermittent periods of relaxation are observed but become less frequent as the clinical course progresses. During convulsions the pupils are dilated, and cyanotic mucous membranes are evidence of anoxia. Convulsive seizures become more frequent and death eventually occurs from exhaustion or anoxia during a tetanic seizure. The entire syndrome, if untreated, is often less than one to two hours.

Physiopathology

Rigor mortis occurs rapidly after death from strychnine poisoning. Relaxation of body musculature also follows in more rapid than normal succession. No gross or microscopic lesions characteristic of strychnine poisoning can be consistently detected. Cyanosis, petechial or ecchymotic hemorrhages, and traumatic lesions are evidence of a violent and hypoxic state. Characteristically, the stomach of strychnine-poisoned animals is filled with food or bait which has not been completely digested.

Absorbed strychnine is transported in the blood by both plasma and erythrocytes, but rapidly passed from blood to tissues. It does not appear to concentrate in nervous tissue.

Excretion is accomplished in urine and via secretion into the stomach. The ionization of strychnine, a basic drug, is influenced by pH. Thus ion trapping of strychnine occurs in the acid conditions of the stomach and urinary excretion may be enhanced by acidification of the urine.

Diagnosis

Tentative diagnosis is usually based on history of ingestion, characteristic clinical signs, and lack of lesions. Similar clinical signs may be caused by chlorinated hydrocarbons, zinc phosphide, metaldehyde, lead, hypocalcemia, and acute massive hepatic necrosis.

Samples for analysis should include stomach contents, liver, kidney, urine, and central nervous system. In addition, baits or vomitus should be kept for analysis. Most chemical confirmations of strychnine poisoning are from stomach contents or liver. In many cases, animals die so rapidly that urinary excretion has been insignificant.

In some field cases suspected to be strychnine poisoning, pentobarbital is administered to control the convulsions. Since pentobarbital is metabolized in the liver and has amine properties like alkaloids, it may react with iodoplatinate to give a spot on thin-layer chromatography (TLC) which might be confused with strychnine. The condition of the TLC plate is critical for insuring against the above. If the plate is inactive, both pentobarbital and strychnine will travel at the solvent front and upon spraying will have the same Rf. In screening for strychnine, it would be possible to neglect to notice that strychnine is at solvent front and interpret the pentobarbital as strychnine.

Cases where pentobarbital might occur and give false positives are those which give negative results for stomach contents but positive results for the liver. This problem can be avoided by making sure the TLC plates are active.

Biologic verification of strychnine poisoning may be accomplished by the following procedure:

1. Extract stomach contents or urine by mixing with equal volume of acid.
2. Centrifuge or filter the acid extract.
3. Neutralize the supernate with ammonium hydroxide to a range of pH 7.0 to 8.0.
4. Inject 0.5 ml in the dorsal sac of a frog or intraperitoneally in a mouse.
5. Typical strychnine convulsive seizures usually occur within 2 to 4 minutes.

Treatment

Of prime concern in strychnine poisoning is the maintenance of relaxation and prevention of asphyxia. In emergency situations, pentobarbital in doses just sufficient to maintain relaxation are acceptable. However, far more prolonged maintenance of relaxation may best be accomplished by inhalation anesthesia or by administration of methocarbamol (150 mg/kg) and continued maintenance as needed.

Other successful therapeutic regimens for strychnine toxicosis have included use of diazepam or glyceryl guiacolate ether, both of which have central muscle relaxant properties. Glyceryl guiacolate has been employed at 110 mg/kg intravenously with repeated maintenance doses as needed. In man, 10 mg of diazepam has been utilized intravenously and repeated as needed. The animal dosage for diazepam is 2.5 to 20 mg intravenously or orally.

The advantage of combination therapy is primarily the reduction of exposure to high levels of barbiturates for prolonged periods.

Early induction of vomiting is recommended using apomorphine. Rapid recovery from strychnine toxicosis may be enhanced by prompt application of the entero-gastric lavage technique.

If anesthesia must be maintained, gastric lavage can be employed using 1 to 2 percent tannic acid or 1:2,000 potassium permanganate. Following this, activated charcoal and sodium sulfate may be left in the stomach to aid adsorption and more rapid elimination of the alkaloid.

Forced diuresis with 5 percent mannitol in 0.9 percent sodium chloride administered at the rate of 6.6 ml/kg/hour and acidification of the urine with 132 mg/kg of body weight of ammonium chloride orally will enhance excretion of strychnine. This must be subsequent to establishment of adequate urine flow.

Toxic doses of strychnine will be depleted from the body within twenty-four to forty-eight hours. One must expect to continue maintenance of relaxation and sedation for twelve to forty-eight hours. It should be emphasized that the sedation time can be considerably shortened if prompt and aggressive action is taken to clear the gastrointestinal tract, inactivate unabsorbed strychnine, and hasten elimination of alkaloid via diuresis.

Facilities for positive pressure pulmonary ventilation, oxygen administration, and warm quiet conditions should be readily available. When prompt and thorough action is taken, recovery of a high proportion of strychnine poisoning cases can be expected.

REFERENCES

Bailey, E. M., and Szabuniewicz, M. 1975. The Use of Glyceryl Guiacolate Ether in the Treatment of Strychnine Poisoning in the Dog. *Vet. Med. Sm. An. Cl.* 70:170-74

Clarke, E. G. C., and Clarke, M. L.1967. *Garner's Veterinary Toxicology.* 3rd ed. Baltimore: The Williams & Wilkins Co.

Curtis, D. R., and Johnston, G. A. R. 1974. *Convulsant Alkaloids In Neuropoisons.* Vol. 2. L. L. Simpson and D. R. Curtis, eds. New York: Plenum Press.

Franz, D. 1975. *Central Nervous System Stimulants In The Pharmacologic Basis of Therapeutics.* 5th ed. L. S. Goodman and A. Gilman, eds. New York: Macmillan Company Publishers.

Frye, F. L. 1974. Enterogastric Lavage in Small Animal Practice. *Vet. Med. Sm. An. Cl.* 69:835-36.

Kirk, R. W. 1971. *Current Veterinary Therapy.* 4th ed. Philadelphia: W. B. Saunders Company.

Lloyd, T. S. 1973. Accidental Poisoning in Birds. *Vet. Rec.* (May 5) 92:489.

McConnell, E. E.; van Rensburg, I. B. S.; and Minne, J. A. 1971. A Rapid Test for the diagnosis of Strychnine Poisoning. *J. S. Afr. Vet. Med. Assoc.* 42(1):81-84.

MacKinnon, J.; Waite, P. R .; and Hilbery, A. D. R. 1973. Accidental Poisoning of Animals. *Vet. Rec.* (May 5) 92:489.

Maron, B. J.; Krupp, J. R.; and Tune, B. 1971. Strychnine Poisoning Successfully Treated with Diazepam. *J. Ped.* (April) 78:697-99.

Osweiler, G. D. 1973. *Strychnine Poisoning* In *Current Veterinary Therapy* V. R. W. Kirk, ed. Philadelphia: W. B. Saunders' Company.

THALLIUM

Thallium (atomic number 81) is a heavy metal which occurs in the periodic chart of the elements between mercury (atomic number 80) and lead (atomic number 82). Thallium was discovered in 1861, and its toxic effects on animals were first described in 1863. During the years thallium was used as a treatment for infectious diseases prior to the development of antibiotics and later found use as a depilatory agent for human usage. More recently, in the early part of the 20th century, thallium (as thallous acetate or sulfate) came to be used as a rodenticide.

Thallium is a general cellular poison that is absorbed through the skin and from the digestive tract. All animals are susceptible, however, due to eating habits and access thallium toxicosis is more frequently seen in cats and dogs.

Source

Thallium has been largely replaced by other rodenticides. However cases are still occasionally reported indicating that there is some continued usage.

Toxicity

The lethal dosage for most species is of the order of 20-25 mg/kg. The LD_{50} for most species is in the range of 10-15 mg/kg. Thallium will accumulate in the body and repeated small doses will accumulate to produce toxicosis.

Mechanism of Action

Thallium is rapidly absorbed from the gastrointestinal tract with peak blood levels occurring two to four hours after ingestion. Thallium is excreted both in the urine and in the feces but is only slowly removed from the body. Approximate excretion rates are 4percent the first day, 37 percent in seven days and 60 percent after twenty-eight days.

Thallium is thought, similar to lead and arsenic, to combine with mitochondrial sulphydryl enzymes, thereby interfering with oxidative phosphorylation. *In vitro* tests demonstrated that thallium will inhibit aerobic respiration in the skin, brain and kidney. In addition, recent evidence indicates that thallium exchanges for potassium in excitable tissues, primarily muscle and nerve. Thallium will cause granules to appear in the mitochondria. It is felt that these granules represent deposits of thallium which have been exchanged for other cations, probably potassium.

Thallium is fairly evenly distributed in all tissues, being found in muscle, liver, kidney, brain, lung and skin. Of considerable importance is the necrotizing effect of thallium upon the intestinal tract, the kidney, and in some cases, the brain.

Clinical Signs

Thallium ingestion can result in acute, subacute or chronic toxicosis. An individual case of thallium poisoning may progress through all three stages.

Acute Form

In the acute form of intoxication the symptoms usually appear within one to four days of ingestion. The first signs observed are severe gastric distress. In the dog this is usually manifested by vomition within one to three days of exposure. This is followed by a severe hemorrhagic diarrhea, abdominal pain and anorexia. Lingual ulcers have been reported in cats. One of the first subtle signs observed experimentally is a labored breathing or dyspnea. In the acute form the dog or cat may die from the severe gastritis, depression and renal damage within three to six days. In the acute form motor paralysis and trembling may occur.

Subacute Form

In the subacute form of intoxication symptoms appear three to seven days after ingestion. In this form the gastric distress and motor disturbance are similar to but more mild and of longer duration than in the acute form. In the subacute form the skin changes are more prominent and may become apparent after four to seven days. There is a reddening of the skin and early pustular formation. This usually begins on the ears and nose and then will proceed to involve the axillary region, ventral abdomen and torso in general.

A very pronounced lesion is the marked reddening of the oral membranes and to a lesser extent the skin seen approximately four to six days after ingestion. Once he has had the opportunity to observe this very marked and severe reddening of the oral mucous membranes, the veterinarian will not mistake this for any other toxic or infectious disease process. The eyes are involved with a conjunctivitis and injection of the sclera. The eyes frequently become matted with a mucopurulent discharge quite similar to that seen in distemper in a young dog. Pneumonia or bronchitis may develop, and with the secondary infections body temperature is frequently elevated. In approximately seven to ten days loss of hair begins and the skin becomes encrusted. The dog may die at this stage.

Chronic Form

In the chronic form symptoms may take seven to ten days to appear. The digestive and nervous system are only mildly involved. The loss of hair and the drying and scaling of the skin after one to three weeks is pronounced. Depending on the exposure, there may be a nearly complete loss of body hair. If exposure was not too severe, hair follicles will not be permanently damaged and the hair will slowly reappear.

Physiopathology

Postmortem lesions will vary with the level of exposure and the duration of the illness. In the acute cases there will be a very severe hemorrhagic gastroenteritis and occasionally an inflammation of the respiratory mucosa. In subacute cases the gastritis is usually not as severe, but degeneration of cardiac muscle, nephrosis, a fatty degeneration and necrosis of the liver, and congestion and hemorrhage of the spleen, heart and kidneys may be observed. Thallium will cause cast formation in the proximal and distal renal tubules in approximately twenty-four hours after acute exposures. In less severe exposures albumin appears in the urine in approximate-

ly four days. In chronic cases the only lesion is severe loss of hair and drying and cracking of the skin.

The histopathology of thallium poisoning is not diagnostic, but the skin changes are marked, consisting of hyperkeratosis, parakeratosis, hyperemia and some hyalinization. Other histologic lesions include necrosis and hyalinization of skeletal muscle, and centrolobular necrosis of the liver. In the brain, cyton degeneration, demyelination and perivascular cuffing in the basal ganglia, pons and temporal cortex is seen.

Diagnosis

A history of the dog having had gastrointestinal upset with episodes of vomiting and diarrhea a few days prior to onset of signs such as dyspnea, reddening of the oral mucosa, injected scleral vessels, anorexia, and general debilitation should lead one to suspect thallium toxicosis.

Often the course of poisoning has passed through the acute and subacute stages and has reached the stage of early skin lesions by the time the dog is presented for treatment.

The detection of thallium in the urine of a dog suspected of poisoning is quite significant. The following rapid test is available.

Reagents

1. Bromine and water: saturate distilled water with bromine in a glass-stoppered amber bottle. Allow to stand for 12 hours before use. (Caution: very corrosive poison. Neutralize with sodium thiosulfate solution if it comes in contact with the skin.)
2. Sulfosalicylic acid: 10% solution in distilled water.
3. Concentrated hydrochloric acid.
4. Rodamine B: disolve 0.05 grams of Rodamine B in 100 ml concentrated hydrochloric acid.
5. Standard thallium: dissolve thallium acetate or sulfate in distilled water.
6. Benzene.

Procedure

1. Label three tubes: blank, standard, and unknown.
2. In the respective tubes place four drops each of water, standard, and the test urine.
3. To each tube add bromine water until a yellow color remains.
4. Add sulfosalicylic acid to each tube drop-wise until the bromine color is just removed.

5. To all tubes add one drop hydrochloric acid and 1-2 drops Rodamine B.
6. Add about 1/2 ml benzene to each tube; allow the two layers to separate.
7. Observe the upper layer: a positive test is indicated by a reddish to purple color. Disregard color of the lower layer.
8. If possible, observe under UV light; positive test will show yellow green fluorescence in upper layer.

This test rarely gives false-positives but may give false-negative results: therefore, a negative urine thallium does not necessarily mean thallium is not present. One should analyze repeated samples of urine from a suspected case.

The finding of any amount of thallium in tissues is of diagnostic significance. Kidney and liver levels may be 80 ppm or more with other tissues containing lesser amounts. Postmortem changes such as hemorrhagic gastroenteritis, injected sclera, skin erythema, pustulation, denudation, and hyperkeratosis are all important in making the diagnosis.

Thallium toxicosis in dogs may be confused with distemper in the early stage because of the increased body temperature, reddening and mattering of the eyes, nasal discharge, and inspiratory dyspnea. Other conditions that may be confused with thallium toxicosis include severe heart worm infestation, other heavy metal toxicoses, especially arsenic and lead, and skin conditions resulting in denudation and pustular formation. Occasionally corneal lesions develop in thallium poisoning which may be confused with the hepatitis complex.

Treatment

If it is known that the dog has recently consumed thallium, it is important to remove it from the gastrointestinal tract by giving emetics such as apomorphine or equal parts of mustard and table salt. Because of the rapid absorption of thallium from the gut, it is doubtful whether emetics are of much use if given three to four hours after exposure.

Diphenylthiocarbazone (dithizone) has been beneficial in acute thallium poisoning in dogs when accompanied with supportive therapy. In cases of *acute thallium poisoning* 70 mg/kg dithizone given orally three times per day has been recommended. The drug is not currently recommended for use in cats poisoned on thallium, and if further attempts are made to use this drug, it should be used at much lower dosages. The few cases reported where cats were treated with diphenylthiocarbazone are not encouraging. Although the cats were in reasonably good condition prior to treatment,

they developed a severe depression, jaundice and died within four days of initiation of treatment. It is possible that the cat reacts adversely to this drug or that the dosage used was too high.

The major beneficial treatment is good supportive medicine consisting of one or more of the following: the concurrent administration of potassium chloride (2-6 grams daily in divided doses) may aid in the elimination of thallium. However, potassium chloride should not be given unless renal function has been firmly established.

If the animal develops acidosis, sodium bicarbonate should be given at the rate of 0.3-3.0 grams daily.

Supportive therapy should accompany the specific treatment. Parenteral fluids, vitamin B complex and antibiotics may be beneficial.

Since thallium-poisoned dogs are usually dehydrated because of the vomiting, diarrhea and skin denudation a solution of 5 percent glucose and normal saline containing water soluble vitamins should be given parenterally. If the skin lesions are particularly prominent, antibiotics should be given to control secondary infection.

The thallium-poisoned dog is generally anorectic and should be fed easily digestable, palatable, and nutritious foods such as boiled meat, cottage cheese and boiled eggs with cooked cereal.

In chronic poisoning our experience indicates that a much lower dosage level of dithizone should be used. It appears that thallium is stored in tissues during the chronic form of the syndrome and administering large doses of the chelating agent, dithizone, may result in a rapid transfer of thallium into the blood vascular system leading to acute thallium poisoning.

REFERENCES

Buck, W. B.; Ramsey, F. K.; and Duncan, J. R. 1968. *Canine Medicine.* Disease Caused by Physical and Chemical Agents. Santa Barbara: Amer. Vet. Pub., pp. 229-51.

Gabriel, K. L., and Dubin, S. 1963. A Method for the Detection of Thallium in Canine Urine. *JAVMA* 143:722.

Garner, R. J. 1961. *Veterinary Toxicology.* Baltimore: The Williams & Wilkins Co., pp. 124-214.

Mather, G. W., and Low, D. G. 1960. Thallium Intoxication in Dogs. *JAVMA* 137-544.

Radeleff, R. D. 1964. *Veterinary Toxicology.* Philadelphia: Lea & Febiger, pp. 161-62.

Schwartzman, R. M., and Kerschbaum, J. O. 1962. The Cutaneous Histopathology of Thallium Poisioning. *J. Inv. Derm.* 39:169.

Skelly, J. R., and Gabriel, K. L. 1964. Thallium Intoxication in the Dog. *An. N. Y. Ac. Sci.* 3:612.

Wilson, J. R. 1961. Thallotoxicosis. *JAVMA* 139:116.

Zook, B. C.; Holzworth,J.; and Thornton, G. W. 1968. Thallium Poisoning in Cats. *JAVMA* 153:285-99.

WARFARIN AND OTHER ANTICOAGULANT RODENTICIDES

In the early 1920s, a hemorrhagic syndrome of cattle was observed in North Dakota and Canada. Observation of field cases established that the disease was associated with consumption of improperly cured or moldy sweet clover hay. Some ten years later, the bleeding was found to be due to a prothrombin deficiency caused by a breakdown product of coumarin in moldy sweet clover. During the early 1940s, the Wisconsin Agricultural Experimental Station synthesized an active and anticoagulant principle called dicoumarol or bishydroxycoumarin.

Following the synthesis of bishydroxycoumarin, the compound was rapidly adapted for use in thrombotic disorders, coronary disease, and rodent control. Coumarins or related compounds are the most frequently used class of rodenticides today.

Source

The anticoagulant rodenticides are structurally related to coumarin. All have the basic coumarin or indandione nucleus.

4-Hydroxycoumarin

Indane-1,3-dione

Three common rodenticides used extensively by professional exterminators and the layman are the following:

Warfarin, 3 (alpha-phenyl-beta-acetylethyl)-4- hydroxycoumarin, D-Con®

Pindone, 2-pivalyl-1, 3-indandione, Pival®

Diphacinone, 2-diphenylacetyl-1, 3-indandione, Diphacin®

Various other products are available. They vary in their side chains, solubility, and toxicity but contain the same basic nucleus. Many anticoagulant rodenticides incorporate sulfonamides in the bait to inhibit synthesis of vitamin K by intestinal flora.

Toxicity

The anticoagulant rodenticides are a potential hazard to all mammals and birds. Dogs and cats appear to be more frequently affected, and swine are occasionally poisoned by warfarin. The toxicity of these compounds varies widely from one to another. Susceptibility also varies among species. Massive single exposure or repeated low dosages may cause poisoning. Some values for warfarin toxicity in various species are listed as follows:

Species	Single Dose	Repeated Doses
Rats	50-100 mg/kg	1mg/kg for five days
Dogs	50 mg/kg	5 mg/kg for 5-15 days
Cats	5-50 mg/kg	1 mg/kg for 5 days
Swine	3 mg/kg	0.05 mg/kg for 7 days
Ruminants		200 mg/kg for 12 days
Poultry	50% of body wt. of feed containing 0.1 mg/kg	

The toxicity of the indandione products varies among compounds, but toxicity generally ranges from 50-100 mg/kg in dogs.

Several factors may influence the toxicity of coumarin and indandione compounds as follows:

1. The bioavailability of vitamin K may vary as in decreased bacterial synthesis of vitamin K.
2. The metabolic fate of coumarins may be modified by such things as absorption, protein binding, biotransformation, and excretion.
3. Prothrombin complex synthesis or catabolism may be altered.
4. The receptor affinity for coumarins at their site of action may be influenced.
5. Nonprothrombin-dependent hemostatic mechanisms may be changed.

Vitamin K deficiency resulting from high dietary fat intake or prolonged oral antibiotic therapy may increase the susceptibility of animals to warfarin. Likewise, liver disease makes animals more sensitive to a loss of prothrombin production.

Deykin (1970b) reviewed the literature concerning therapy with the anticoagulant drug warfarin and concluded that drugs can influence the response of patients to warfarin. Concomitant administration of a second drug can alter the absorption of an anticoagulant, if intestinal pH, motility, or drug solubility are changed.

The binding of coumarin drugs to plasma proteins may be a significant factor in the response of animals to anticoagulant coumarin drugs. Coumarins are bound to plasma proteins and become pharmacologically inactive, protected from biotransformation and excretion, and excreted only when the unbound drug is available in the plasma in equilibrium with its site of action. Albumin binding is readily reversible, and the total plasma bound reservoir is gradually released as biotransformation lowers the concentration of free drug. Drugs known to increase the displacement of warfarin from plasma binding sites include phenyl butazone, sulfonamides, and adrenocorticosteroids.

Mechanism of Action

The anticoagulant rodenticides interfere with the normal synthesis of clotting factors by the liver. Their major effect is due to inhibition of the prothrombin complex as a result of interference with the action of vitamin K.

In animals deficient in vitamin K or receiving coumarin anticoagulants, a protein is formed which has chemical and immunological properties similar to prothrombin. This protein is designated as "abnormal prothrombin" and is not converted to thrombin *in vivo*. (Anon. 1974, 1975) The coumarin anticoagulants competitively inhibit vitamin K in the synthesis of active prothrombin.

Warfarin resistant rats have been discovered. It is noteworthy that such rats while susceptible only to high doses of warfarin also have an abnormally high requirement for vitamin K. Thus, these rats are evidence for a common receptor for vitamin K and warfarin.

The coumarins do not destroy prothrombin, although they may interfere with the conversion of prothrombin to thrombin. Depending on the species of animal involved and the respective half-life of the clotting factors inhibited, defects in blood coagulation occur from two to five days after initial exposure to coumarin anticoagulants. Even massive exposure to coumarin anticoagulants require a latent period prior to clinical effects. There is also a definite depression of factors VII, IX, and X in the serum of warfarin-poisoned animals. Platelet adhesiveness may be slightly decreased, but platelet counts are not depressed.

There does not appear to be any direct hepatotoxic action from warfarin. Hypoxia and anemia, as a result of hemorrhage, may cause liver necrosis as a sequel to the basic lesion.

Absorption of warfarin from the intestine is rather complete but occurs slowly at enteric pH. Warfarin may be detected in circulating blood within one hour after ingestion, but peak levels are not reached for six to twelve hours. Most of the warfarin present is bound to plasma protein. High concentrations are also found in liver, spleen, and kidney. Warfarin is metabolized slowly, two to four days being required for degradation of the compound.

Coumarins are hydroxylated by hepatic microsomal mixed-function oxidases. Several ring-hydroxylated pharmacologically inactive metabolites of warfarin may be found in urine. Warfarin and bishydroxycoumarin are subject to the same major biotransformation pathways and the half-life varies widely among species. Warfarin concentrations in plasma decline exponentially with time in each species. The acute toxicity of warfarin and bishydroxycoumarin in animals is reduced when phenobarbital is used as an enzyme inducing drug. Administration of vitamin K does not enhance the rate of disappearance of warfarin.

Clinical Signs

The clinical signs of coumarin or indandione poisoning reflect some manifestations of hemorrhage. Onset may be acute, and occasionally animals are found dead with no previous signs of illness. This is especially true when hemorrhage in the cerebral vasculature, pericardial sac, mediastinum, or thorax occurs. In subacute cases, animals are anemic and weak; and pale mucous membranes, dyspnea, hematemesis, epistaxis, and bloody feces are common signs. Scleral, conjunctival, and intraocular hemorrhage may be seen. With severe blood loss, weakness and staggering or ataxia are observed. Blood loss and pulmonary hemorrhage are reflected in dyspnea with moist rales and blood-tinged froth around the nose or mouth. Cardiac rate is irregular and heartbeat is weak. Extensive external hematomata may occur, especially in areas of trauma. Swollen, tender joints are commonly seen. If hemorrhage involves the brain, spinal cord, or subdural space, CNS signs will be manifest as paresis, ataxia, convulsions, or acute death. When the course of poisoning is prolonged, autolysis of impounded blood can cause icterus.

Warfarin has caused abortions in cattle, both in natural cases and under experimental conditions.

Physiopathology

There is generalized hemorrhage; areas commonly affected are the thoracic cavity, mediastinal space, periarticular tissues, subcutaneous tissues, cerebral subdural space, and the spinal canal. Gastric, intestinal, and intraabdominal hemorrhage may be present. The heart is rounded and flaccid with subepicardial and subendocardial hemorrhages. Centrilobular hepatic necrosis, a result of anemia and hypoxia, may be observed. In prolonged cases, the tissues are icteric due to absorption of blood pigments.

Diagnosis

Warfarin poisoning should be differentiated from other hemorrhagic disorders. Some of these are aflatoxicosis, thrombocytopenia, radiation injury, infectious canine hepatitis, and vitamin K deficiency (especially in poultry and swine). Clinical pathology utilizing clotting time, prothrombin time, hematocrit, differential leucocyte count, and clot retraction may be employed if doubt exists. Clinical coumarin anticoagulant toxicosis would be expected to result in the following:

bleeding time	-variable
clotting time	-elevated
one stage prothrombin time	-elevated
activated partial thromboplastim time	-elevated
thrombocyte count	-normal
clot retraction	-normal
packed cell volume	-low
leucocyte count	-normal
differential leucocytes	-normal

One stage prothrombin time (OSPT) measures changes in fibrinogen, Factor II, V, VII, and X. These factors are part of the extrinsic system of blood coagulation.

Activated partial thromboplastin time (APTT) is recommended to measure the intrinsic system of the coagulation scheme. APTT measures deficiencies in Factors II, V, VIII, IX, X, XI, and XII. It is less sensitive to abnormalities occurring at early stages of coagulation leading up to prothrombin activation.

Plasma warfarin levels from live animals or liver warfarin levels in necropsy specimens can aid in confirming the diagnosis.

Treatment

Warfarin-poisoned animals should be handled to minimize trauma. Sedation or light anesthesia can aid in gentle manipulation. If respiratory difficulty or severe anemia is encountered, oxygen therapy may prolong life until treatment can be continued. In acute cases, whole blood should be administered to supply prothrombin and factors VII, IX, and X. Give 20 ml/kg of fresh, citrated whole blood intravenously. Half the dose should be given rapidly and the remainder at about 20 drops per minute.

Stored blood or plasma will retain a significant level of coagulation factors for up to two weeks and may be used if fresh blood is unavailable.

If dyspnea continues to be a problem, a thoracic radiograph is indicated. Thoracentesis to remove excess blood may save an animal's life and make further therapy possible.

Vitamin K_1 should be administered intravenously (15-75 mg) as a 5 percent suspension in 5 percent dextrose. Keep fluids to a minimum. Poisoned animals need blood more than extracellular fluid. Vitamin K_1 begins to reverse the hypoprothrombinemia in about thirty minutes, but several hours are required for full clinical response. Synthetic vitamin K (menadione) is less effective than vitamin K_1.

Animals should be kept warm and free of physical trauma for at least twenty-four hours. Convalescent animals may be given oral vitamin K_1 for four to six days to allow for complete degradation of the circulating warfarin.

REFERENCES

Anderson, G. F. 1967. Distribution of Warfarin (Coumarin) in Rat. *Thromb. Diat.* 18:754.

Anonymous. 1974. Vitamin K and Prothrombin Structure. *Nutrition Reviews* 32:279.

————. 1975. Vitamin K and the Carboxylation of Glutamyl Residues in the Formation of Prothrombin. *Nutrition Reviews* 33:25.

Blood, D. C., and Henderson, J. A. 1963. *Veterinary Medicine*. 2nd ed. Baltimore, Md.: The Williams & Wilkins Co.

Clarke, E. G. C., and Clark, M. L. 1967. *Garner's Veterinary Toxicology*. 3rd ed. Baltimore, Md.: The Williams & Wilkins Co. 1967.

Dakin, G. W. 1968. Postmortem Toxicological Findings in a Case of Warfarin Poisoning. *Vet. Rec.* 83:664.

Goodman, L S., and Gilman, A. 1966. *The Pharmacological Basis of Therapeutics*. 3rd ed. New York: The Macmillan Company.

Hunningh, D. B., and Azarnoff, D. L. 1968. Drug Interactions with Warfarin. *Arch. In. Med.* 121:349.

Jones, L. M., 1965. ed. *Veterinary Pharmacology and Therapeutics*. 3rd ed. Ames, Iowa: Iowa State University Press

Kirk, R. W. 1968. ed. *Current Veterinary Therapy III*. 3rd ed. Philadelphia, Pa.: W. B. Saunders Company.

Koch-Weser, J., and Sellers, E. M. 1971a. Drug Interactions with Coumarin Anticoagulants. *New Eng. J. Med.* 285:487-98.

———. 1971b. Drug Interactions with Coumarin Anticoagulants. *New Eng. J. Med.* 285:547-58.

Langdell, R. D. 1969. Coagulation and Hemostasis, Chapter 7. In I. Davidson and J. Henry, eds. *Clinical Diagnosis by Laboratory Methods*. Philadelphia, Pa.: W. B. Saunders Company.

Lawson, J., and Doncaster, R. A. 1965. A Treatment for Warfarin Poisoning in the Dog. *Vet. Rec.* 77:1183.

Nagashim, R.; O'Reilly, R. A.; and Levy, G. 1969. Kinetics of Pharmacologic Effects in Man— Anticoagulant Action of Warfarin. *Clin. Pharm.* 10:22.

O'Reilly, R. A. *et al.* 1962. The Metabolism of Warfarin. *J. Clin. Invest. 41:1390*

Osweiler, G. D. 1973. The Influence of an Antibiotic Combination on the Toxicity of Warfarin to Swine. Ph.D. Thesis. Iowa State University, Ames, Ia.

Pugh, D. M. 1968. Abortifacient Action of Warfarin in Cattle. *Br. J. Pharm.* 33:210.

Quick, A. J. 1966. Hemorrhagic Diseases and Thrombosis. Philadelphia, Pa.: Lea & Febiger.

Radeleff, R. D. 1964. *Veterinary Toxicology*. Philadelphia, Pa.: Lea & Febiger.

Schalm, O. W. 1965. *Veterinary Hematology*. 2nd ed. Philadelphia, Pa.: Lea & Febiger.

Sher, S. P. 1971. Drug Enzyme Induction and Drug Interactions: Literature and Tabulations. *Toxicol. App. Pharm.* 18:780-834.

Suttie, J. W. 1973. Vitamin K and Prothrombin Synthesis. *Nutrition Reviews* 31:105.

Walker, R. G. 1968. Pulmonary Complications in Cases of Suspected Warfarin Poisoning in the Dog. *Vet. Rec.* 83:148.

Welch, R. M.; Harrison, Y. E.; Conney, A. H.; and Burns, J. J. 1969. An Experimental Model in Dogs for Studying Interactions of Drugs and Bishydroxycoumarin. *Clinical Pharmacol. and Therap.* 10:817.

Welling, P. A.; Lee, K. P.; Khanna, U.; and Wagner, J. G. 1970. Comparison of Plasma Concentrations of Warfarin Measured by Both Simple Extraction and TLC Methods. *J. Pharm. Sci.* 59:1621.

ZINC PHOSPHIDE

Source

Zinc phosphide has been available commercially for rodent control since 1930. The cessation of importation of red squill during World War II resulted in a great increase in the use of zinc phosphide. It has found favor as an exterminating agent because rats tend to die in open areas and the effect is psychologically rewarding. (Chitty, 1954) Zinc phosphide, or occasionally aluminum phosphide, is employed in baits of bread, bran mash, soaked wheat, damp rolled oats, or sugar at concentrations of from 2 to 5 percent. The compound is a dull, grayish black powder, insoluble in water and having a faint phosphine or acetylene odor in atmospheric air.

Thomson (1975) lists preparations available in the United States under the names, Zinc Phosphide, Mous-Con, KilRat, and Rumetan.

Zinc phosphide is stable for long periods when kept dry but deteriorates rapidly under damp or acid conditions. Toxic activity persists for approximately two weeks under average atmosphere exposure.

Toxicity

The toxicity of zinc phosphide varies, depending on the species exposed and the acidity of the bait or the gastric contents. Most animals and poultry can be poisoned by 40 mg/kg, depending upon the pH in the stomach. (Blaxland and Gordon, 1945; Ingram, 1945; Fitzpatrick *et al.,* 1955; Roszkowski, 1967) Dogs fed zinc phosphide in amounts of 300 mg/kg can survive if the toxicant is given on an empty stomach. Feeding dogs a normal ration stimulates gastric HCl secretion and greatly increases their susceptibility to zinc phosphide. Thus, an empty stomach makes animals more resistant to zinc phosphide poisoning. (Johnson and Voss, 1962)

Some commercial products contain tartar emetic in order to stimulate vomiting as a protective measure in nontarget species. Zinc phosphide itself has a strong tendency to induce emesis in nonrodent animals, and it does not consistently cause fatal poisoning when accidentally ingested.

A dose of 40 mg/kg zinc phosphide administered to a dog by gelatin capsule induced sudden onset of convulsive seizures seven hours after administration, and the animal expired within thirty minutes after the onset of convulsions. The same dosage given repeatedly by mixing with food caused vomiting within a few minutes after consumption, but toxicosis was not produced. (Buck, *et al.,* 1971)

Mechanism of Action

The toxicity of zinc phosphide ($Zn_3 P_2$) is due to the release of phosphine gas (PH_3) in the presence of acid pH. (Buck, 1968) Both phosphine and intact zinc phosphide are absorbed from the GI tract. The phosphine is believed to cause the majority of acute signs, while the intact phosphide may cause hepatic and renal damage later.

Clinical Signs

The onset of poisoning is rapid, usually within fifteen minutes to four hours after ingestion of a toxic amount of zinc phosphide. Death from large doses is usually within three to five hours, and animals rarely survive longer than twenty-four to forty-eight hours. In some instances onset of clinical signs may be delayed as long as twelve to eighteen hours after ingestion. Commercially available zinc phosphide appears to contain two fractions. One is rapidly attacked, probably by direct release of phosphine when the toxicant mixes with gastric acids. The other appears to be slowly acted upon at some point in the gastrointestinal tract. This biphasic action may explain, in part, the variability in toxicity and onset of clinical signs observed in animals exposed to zinc phosphide.

Clinical signs are not characteristic but do suggest toxemia. An early sign is anorexia and lethargy. This is followed by rapid, deep respiration which often becomes wheezy or stertorous. Vomiting is common in the early stages, and gastric contents often contain dark blood. Abdominal pain, colic in horses, and ruminal tympany in cattle are observed. Ataxia, weakness, and recumbency follow. There may be terminal hypoxia, gasping for breath, and struggling. Also, hyperesthesia or convulsions can be seen. In some dogs, zinc phosphide signs may closely resemble strychnine poisoning. (Buck *et al.,* 1971) Careful attention to history, other signs such as GI upset, and a possible phosphine or acetylene odor of the breath may help.

Physiopathology

There is marked congestion of the lungs and interlobular edema in some cases. Pleural effusion and subpleural hemorrhages may be seen. The liver and kidney are extremely congested in acute cases. Subacute cases may show pale yellow mottling of the liver. Gastritis may be present and is most consistent in the pig. (Fitzpatrick *et al.,* 1955; Clarke and Clarke, 1967) The freshly opened stomach has a characteristic odor of acetylene. (Stephenson, 1967)

Histologic lesions of hepatic cloudy swelling, fatty change, and congestion of the liver and kidney are seen. Renal tubular degeneration, hyaline change, and necrosis may occur.

Diagnosis

A history of exposure to zinc phosphide, accompanied by rapid death characterized by dyspnea, vomiting, pulmonary edema, and visceral congestion are suggestive of zinc phosphide poisoning. Chemical detection of zinc phosphide in stomach contents or gastric lavage is possible. Zinc levels in blood, liver, and kidney may be elevated. A portion of zinc phosphide may be absorbed intact and detected in liver or kidney. (Stephenson, 1967)

Treatment

There is no specific treatment. However, indications from human literature are that therapy should be directed against acidosis, hypocalcemia, and liver damage. (Moeschlin, 1965; Stephenson, 1967) If detected early, the breakdown of zinc phosphide to phosphine may be retarded by gastric lavage with 5 percent sodium bicarbonate. Zinc phosphide should be cleared from the entire gastrointestinal tract to prevent additional poisoning from the delayed onset described earlier. Calcium gluconate and 1/6 M sodium lactate may aid in counteracting the acidosis present. Sodium thiosulfate (10 percent solution), lipotropic agents, and dextrose are rational therapy for possible liver injury.

REFERENCES

Blaxland, J. D., and Gordon, R. F. 1945. Zinc Phosphide Poisoning in Poultry. *Vet. J.* 101:108-10

Buck, W. B.; Osweiler, G. D.; and Van Gelder, G. A. 1971. Unpublished data, Iowa State University, Ames, Iowa.

Buck, W. B. 1968. Catcott, E. J., ed. *Canine Medicine,* Wheaton, Illinois: American Veterinary Publications.

Chitty, D. 1954. *Control of Rats and Mice.* Vol. I. New York: Oxford University Press.

Clarke, E. G. D., and Clarke, M. L. 1967. *Garner's Veterinary Toxicology.* 3rd ed. Baltimore: The Williams & Wilkins Co.

Fitzpatrick, R. J.; McGirr, J. L.; and Papworth, D. S. 1955. The Toxicity of Rodenticides. II. Red Squill and Zinc Phosphide. *Vet. Rec.* 67:142-45.

Ingram, P. L. 1945. Zinc Phosphide Poisoning in a Colt. *Vet. Rec.* 57:103-104.

Johnson, H. D., and Voss, E. 1952. Toxicologic Studies of Zinc Phosphide. *J. Amer. Pharm. Ass.* 16:468-72.

Moeschlin, S. 1965. *Poisoning, Diagnosis and Treatment.* New York: Grune and Stratton.

Roszkowski, A. P. 1967. Comparative Toxicity of Rodenticides. *Fed. Proc.* 26:1082-88.

Stephenson, J. B. P. 1967. Zinc Phosphide Poisoning. *Arch. Environ. Health.* 15:83-88

Thomson, W. 1975. *Agricultural Chemicals III.* Indianapolis, Indiana: Thomson Publications.

Biotoxins

MYCOTOXICOSES

Source

A mycotoxin is defined as a secondary toxic metabolite produced by mold. (Lillehoj *et al.,* 1970)

In a mycotoxicosis, mold growth is not directly involved in the host animal, while mycoses generally involve invasion of living tissue by actively growing microorganisms.

The earliest recognized mycotoxicosis in recorded history was ergotism. Outbreaks of convulsive and gangrenous ergotism were associated in the sixteenth century with fungal invasion of cereals. (Radeleff, 1970) Little scientific interest in the biochemical and biological effects of mycotoxins occured until the 1960s when studies were stimulated by turkey X disease in England in which 100,000 turkey poults were lost from toxic peanut meal. (Sargeant *et al.,* 1961) Prior veterinary reports (Forgacs and Carll, 1962) on moldy corn toxicosis, hepatitis X of the dog, and leucoencephalomalacia of horses were available; but potential problems in man had not been compared.

The historic attitude that animals have some innate ability to detect and reject toxigenic molds is not true. Toxin producers cannot be recognized visually, and processing may grossly mask mold growth.

Investigation of a number of field outbreaks has resulted in a listing of some principles that characterize mycotoxicosis (Feuell, 1969):

1. Frequently arise as veterinary problems whose true cause is not readily identified.
2. The disorders are not transmissible from animal to animal (neither infectious or contagious).
3. Treatment with drugs or antibiotics usually has little effect on the course of the disease, and antigenic stimulation is minimal or absent.
4. Field outbreaks are often seasonal and associated with particular climatic sequences.
5. Careful study indicates association with a particular feedstuff.
6. Examination of the suspected foodstuff reveals signs of fungal activity.

Conditions Allowing Fungal Growth and Spoilage of Feeds

The spoilage of foods and feeds by fungi depends upon the qualities of both the environment and the substrate. As much as 1 percent of the world supply of grain and oilseed is rendered unfit by fungal invasion. Moisture content of the seed, its viability and physical state, and stored product insect activity are factors in the initiation and extent of mold growth. (Golumbic and Kulik, 1969)

Fungal invasion may produce either toxic or nontoxic effects. Both field fungi such as *Alternaria, Helminthosporium, Fusarium,* and *Rhizopus* and the storage fungi which include *Aspergillus, Fusarium,* and *Penicillium* are associated with grain storage.

Under present-day harvest methods, storage fungi are the greatest problem and are associated with most of the livestock poisoning problems reported. The notable exception to this are the *Claviceps spp.* which invade rye, Dallis grass, and other grasses.

Storage fungi require the following for adequate growth:

1. A proper *substrate* (carbohydrate) in a readily available form.
2. *Moisture* in the grain (10.0 to 18%) and relative humidity (greater than 70%) in the storage atmosphere.
3. Adequate *temperature* for growth. This varies with fungi; but as an example, *Aspergillus flavus* can elaborate toxin from 12-47° C and some *Fusaria* may be active at or near freezing temperatures.
4. A supply of oxygen. Under usual storage conditions this is not a limiting factor.
5. Acidity. Organic acids, favoring low pH inhibit mold growth and spore formation.

In general, the toxigenic molds are extremely common potential contaminants and may grow under a wide range of conditions on a variety of substrates.

Numerous toxigenic fungi and their metabolites have been identified from a variety of substrates. A majority of these are produced by genera of *Aspergilli,* *Penicillia,* and *Fusaria* and are most often isolated from cereal grains or corn. Table 1 summarizes some of the major mycotoxins and data pertinent to those compounds.

Effects of Mycotoxins

Mycotoxins may cause acute to chronic effects in a variety of species and in almost every organ system of animals. Heavy mold growth may also lower the palatability and energy level of feeds, quite aside from any toxic effects.

The major toxic effects of mycotoxins in veterinary medicine may be classified as follows:

1. Hepatotoxins. There is degeneration, fatty change, hemorrhage, and necrosis of hepatic parenchyma. In some instances there may be abnormal size of hepatocytes and their nuclei. Bile duct hyperplasia can occur and some mycotoxins may induce hepatoma. Acute toxicosis results in icterus, hemolytic anemia, and elevated serum levels of liver enzymes. Chronic toxicosis results in poor performance, impaired protein synthesis, hypoproteinemia, hypoprothrombinemia, hepatic fibrosis, and cirrhosis. Photosensitization may be a secondary effect.
2. Nephrotoxins. Oxalic acid and other nephrotoxic agents may be produced by *Aspergillus sp.* and *Penicillium sp.* Renal tubular damage results in signs and lesions characteristic of toxic tubular nephrosis.
3. Changes in bone marrow, erythrocytes, and the vascular bed. Clinical effects seen include widespread hemorrhages, hematomata, weakness, anemia, granulocytopenia, and increased susceptibility to infection.
4. Direct Irritation. Dermonecrotic effects, oral ulceration and necrosis, gastroenteritis and intestinal bleeding are characteristic signs. Most of the toxins are produced by *Fusarium spp.*
5. Reproductive and/or Endocrine Disturbances. This is primarily seen as hyperestrinism in female swine and decreased fertility and libido in male swine. The effects are very similar to stimulation by exogenous estrogen.
6. Respiratory Function. Mold damaged sweet potatoes produce a toxin, ipomearone, which has been associated with hyaline membrane formation and production of "pulmonary adenomatosis in cattle".
7. Central Nervous System. Acute effects of ergot as well as several *Penicillium spp* produce toxins which affect the nervous system. Acute ergotism is the result of a lysergic acid related principle. Other "tremorigens" reported may induce hyperexcitability, incoordination, hypermetria and tremors. In addition equine "moldy corn poisoning" or leukenoencephalomelacia is a destructive lesion resulting in somnolence and death.
8. Immune System. Aflatoxins and rubratoxin have been shown to impair the efficacy of the immune system. Affected animals have lowered antibody production and increased susceptibility to infectious disease.

Table 5 lists the major organ systems affected by mycotoxins. For additional information, either the text or table 1 may be consulted, using the toxin name for cross-reference.

Diagnosis of Mycotoxicoses

The use of all available evidence is of utmost importance when dealing with mycotoxicoses. Certain facts and limitations must be kept in mind when confirmation of a mycotoxicosis is desired.

1. Samples of feed or forage for analysis or feeding trials should reflect all the sources of feed available *at the time the problem occurred.* The effects of a low-level contamination may not be apparent until weeks or months after the offending feed was consumed. The course and type of lesions and signs *must be correlated* with the class of mycotoxin and its availability to the animals. Representative sampling is important since contamination can vary widely within the same storage unit, or even among kernels on the same ear of corn.
2. A major effect from moldy feeds is refusal of the animal to eat it, and further the reduction in feed value of heavily infested feeds. This may be the true cause of poor performance in many cases.
3. Heat, chemicals, and sunlight all have the potential for altering the mold metabolites from their original structure and activity. Destruction of either the toxin or the fungus could occur, especially if time lapse and environmental changes have taken place.
4. Any laboratory is dependent on submission of a well-perserved, representative sample and an accurate and thorough clinical history. If specific toxins are suspected, these should be requested. A laboratory may be able to suggest other appropriate tests if the history is well presented.
5. Many more toxins exist than do tests to measure them. Probably no more than four to six good, practical, economical procedures are available for the mycotoxins most often implicated in veterinary medicine.

TABLE 1
Some Mycotoxicoses of Importance in Veterinary Medicine

Toxins[1]	Fungus	Common Substrate	Animal Species Involved	Disease Produced
Aflatoxins	*Aspergillus flavus*	Cottonseed, corn, peanuts, sorghum	Duck, dog, turkey, cattle, swine	Aflatoxicosis; hepatotoxicosis and hepatic carcinogenesis; cholangio-hepatitis, hemorrhage, slow growth
Butenolide	*Fusarium tricinctum*	Fescue hay	Cattle	Fescue foot; gangrene of the extremities
Citrinin	*Penicillium viridicatum*	Barley, corn, commercial feed	Swine, horses, sheep	Renal tubular necrosis, perirenal edema, hepatic damage
Diacetoxyscirpenol	*Fusarium tricinctum*	Corn	Cattle	Diarrhea, milk reduction, weight loss; possible dermonecrosis, gangrene
Emetic factor	*Fusarium sp.*	Corn, wheat	Swine	Emesis
Ergot alkaloids	*Claviceps purpurea*	Ovary of rye and cereal grains	Swine, cattle, poultry	Dry gangrene of extremities; hypogalactia in lactating sows; may be convulsions, ataxia, tremors
Ergot, lysergic acid	*Claviceps paspali*	Dallis grass	Cattle, sheep, horses	Paspalum staggers; ataxia, tremors, nervousness, convulsions; recovery in 5-10 days
Ipomearone	*Fusarium solani*	Sweet potatoe	Cattle	Pulmonary hyperplasia
Ochratoxin A	*Aspergillus ochraceus*	Corn barley, legumes	Swine, rats, mice,	Renal tubular necrosis,
	Penicillium viridicatum	Legumes	Guinea pigs	Hepatosis
Oxalic acid	*Aspergillus niger*	Hay, cereal, grain	Swine, others	Nephritis, prolonged clotting time
Rubratoxin	*Penicillium rubrum*	Corn	Cattle, swine	Hepatotoxicity, gen'l. hemorrhage
Slaframine	*Rhizoctonia leguminicola*	Clover hay and pasture	Cattle, sheep	Slobber factor; histamine-like disease, excessive salivation, lacrimation, diarrhea, bloat
Trichothecene T-2 toxin	*Fusarium tricinctum*	Corn, hay	Cattle, swine, poultry	Gastroenteritis, widespread hemorrhage, hematopoeitic depression
Sporodesmin	*Pythomyces chartarum*	Perennial rye grass	Sheep, cattle	Facial eczema; cholangiohepatitis; photosensitivity
Tremorigen Penitrem A	*Penicillium cyclopium and P. palitans*	Corn, silage, feed	Sheep, swine, cattle	Tremors, convulsions, ataxia; possible smooth muscle stimulation
Unknown	*Fusarium moniliforme*	Corn	Horses	Leucoencephalomalacia; ataxia, blindness, impaired mastication, coma, death
Stachybotrys toxin	*Stachybotrys atra*	Straw fodder	Horses	Stachybotryotoxicosis; hemato-poietic depression, stomatitis, epithelial ulceration, dermatitis; death
Zearalenone (F-2)	*Fusarium graminearum*	Corn	Swine	Vulvovaginitis; prolonged estrus; spontaneous estrus, vulvar swelling mammary enlargement, preputial enlargement; abortion

[1] Sources utilized in this table are marked by * in the reference list for this chapter.

6. Mold activity (even molds known to produce toxins) is no sure indicator of mycotoxicosis. Variables such as temperature variations, type of substrate, moisture, and number of contaminating molds all have a bearing on toxin production.

7. Some natural components of feeds or forages may cause false positive results for certain mycotoxin procedures.

8. Mixed feeds (meals, pellets) are complex and difficult to "clean up" for analysis. If individual components cannot be supplied, a complete listing of ingredients should be made available.

9. Extrapolation of feeding studies from one species to another is often not applicable, and feeding cattle and swine is expensive, even though feeding trials with similar species are best. Chronic (2-3 months) effects may occur and are most difficult to predict.

Specific Mycotoxicoses in Veterinary Medicine

Numerous mycotoxicoses are reported to affect domestic livestock. Of those reported, the most important in our experience appear to be (1) gangrenous ergotism caused by *Claviceps purpurea,* (2) vulvovaginitis of swine caused by *Fusarium graminearum,* (3) aflatoxicosis from *Aspergillus flavus* toxins, and (4) actual or potential toxicosis from the trichothecene metabolites of various *Fusarium spp.* These four mycotoxins will be discussed separately because of their individual characteristics and importance. Brief descriptions of other mycotoxicoses are also included.

The major characteristics of other mycotoxicoses are presented in table form with appropriate references for the interested reader. If a clinical problem is suspected from one of the toxins listed, contact with an appropriate laboratory or specialist is usually essential to diagnosis.

Aflatoxin

Toxicity

Variations in extent of aflatoxin contamination occur from year to year as well as in aflatoxin content of individual kernels or seeds. Furthermore, areas of excessive moisture in storage bins may result in foci of high aflatoxin production. Thus, in field situations only portions of a herd may receive a toxic feed; and then the exposure may be sporadic in nature. Toxicity data from experimental trials have generally been based on continuous exposure at a given level in feed. Wogan (1968) has summarized data on dietary levels toxic to cattle, swine, and poultry (see table 2).

TABLE 2
Dietary Aflatoxin Levels
Causing Toxicity in Domestic Animals*

Animal	Aflatoxin Level, ppm	Feeding Time	Toxicity Symptoms
Calves (weanling)	2.2	16 wks	Death
	0.22-0.44	16 wks	Growth suppression, liver damage
Steers (2 yrs old)	0.22-0.66	20 wks	Liver damage
Cows (heifers)	2.4	7 mo	Liver damage, clinical illness
Pigs (4-6 wks old)	0.41-0.69	3-6 mo	Growth suppression, liver damage
Chickens (1 wk old)	0.84	10 wks	Growth suppression, liver damage
Ducklings	0.30	6 wks	Death, liver damage

*From Wogan (1968).

The toxic effects of aflatoxin are both dose dependent and time dependent. Furthermore, species and breed specificity plays a significant role both in susceptibility and manifestation of aflatoxicosis. Established acute LD_{50} values for ducklings and dogs are approximately 1 mg/kg.

In general, poultry appear more sensitive to aflatoxins than do mammals. Within poultry the susceptibility ranges from ducklings > turkey poults > chickens. Among the mammals, the order is dogs > young swine > pregnant sows > calves > fattening pigs > mature cattle > sheep. There is no explanation given for the relative resistance (ca. 500 mg/kg) of the sheep. A summarization of the comparative susceptibility of various animals to aflatoxin is presented in table 3.

Mechanism of Action

Aflatoxin refers to a closely related group of metabolites of *Aspergillus flavus.* Those toxins generally recognized are B_1, B_2, G_1, G_2, M_1 M_2, B_{2a}, and G_{2a}. The letters B and G refer to blue and green fluorescence on chromatographic plates, while M refers to "milk" as the original source of M toxin. The most abundant member of the group present under natural contamination is aflatoxin B_1, the structure of which is shown in figure 1.

Other forms of aflatoxin have similar structure, varying primarily in location of double bonds or oxygen. (Goldblatt, 1969) All are highly substituted coumarins with a furocoumarin configuration characteristic of a large group of naturally occurring compounds with pharmacologic activities. (Wogan, 1966)

The bulk of information to date indicates that aflatoxin suppresses messenger-RNA synthesis. A further effect on DNA synthesis has also been shown. (Lillehoj *et al.,* 1970; Wogan 1975) The site of the RNA

TABLE 3
Detrimental Dietary Concentrations of Aflatoxin*

Class of Animal	Dietary Aflatoxin Content PPM (mg/kg)	Period of Feeding	Toxic Effects	
			Liver Lesions	Performance (Weight Gain and Feed Efficiency)
Pigs				
Growing (40-140 lb)	0.14	12 weeks	Mild	Normal
	0.28	12 weeks	Moderate	Reduced
	0.41	12 weeks		
Growing and finishing (40-200 lb)	0.28 & 0.41	20 weeks	Moderate	Reduced
Finishing stage (140-200 lb)	0.69	7 weeks	Mild	Normal
Sows (pregnant)	0.3-0.5	4 weeks	Marked	Anorexia and some deaths
Cattle				
Calves (initial age 4 days)	0.2	16 weeks	Mild	Reduced over 0-3 months
Fattening cattle (2-2½ yrs. old)	0.66	20 weeks	Mild	Normal
Milk cows	1.5	4 weeks	No information	Decreased milk production
				Excretion of aflatoxin M_1 in milk
Poultry				
Turkey poults (day old)	0.25	4 weeks	Marked	Reduced growth
Broiler chicks (day old)	0.21	7 weeks	Moderate	Normal growth
	0.42	7 weeks	Moderate	Weight loss in last 3 weeks
Ducklings (7 days old)	0.03	4 weeks	Characteristic of aflatoxicosis	Weight loss and death in 16 of 37 birds

*Adapted from Allcroft (1969).

effect is primarily in the nucleus via inhibition of precursor incorporation into RNA. There is also inhibition of DNA-dependent RNA polymerase activity. As a result of nuclear RNA inhibition, it is suspected that cytoplasmic RNA is altered as well. There is a probable inhibition of protein synthesis via the depression of messenger-RNA synthesis.

The impairment of protein synthesis and related ability to mobilize fats apparently relates to the early lesions seen primarily in the liver of affected animals. Hepatic necrosis and fatty change are early lesions of aflatoxicosis, and many of the clinical signs and other lesions stem from this effect. (Wogan, 1975)

Aflatoxin affects resistance to infection and development of acquired immunity. At low concentrations (0.25-0.5 ppm) there is a demonstrated reduction in resistance of poultry to some bacterial and protozoal diseases. (Pier, 1973) There is reduced resistance of turkeys to *P. multocida* when vaccinated for fowl cholera, and it apparently is not an antibody deficit, but

may be related to other nonspecific humoral mechanisms. The timing of aflatoxin exposure may be important in that acquired immunity to *P. multocida* is depressed only when aflatoxin is present simultaneously with or prior to immunization for fowl cholera. However, if aflatoxin is discontinued prior to vaccination, no reduction in resistance is seen.

The immunologic effects of aflatoxin appear due in part to depression of nonspecific humoral substances (e.g., complement) and in part to altered interaction between immunogen and aflatoxin-influenced host tissues.

In guinea pigs, aflatoxin produces an increase in γ-globulin, a decrease in α_2-globulin and usually a decrease in total protein concentration. (Richard, *et al.,* 1974)

The induction of hepatoma or hepatic carcinoma in rats and trout is a well-known effect of low-level exposure to aflatoxin, and other species are probably susceptible.

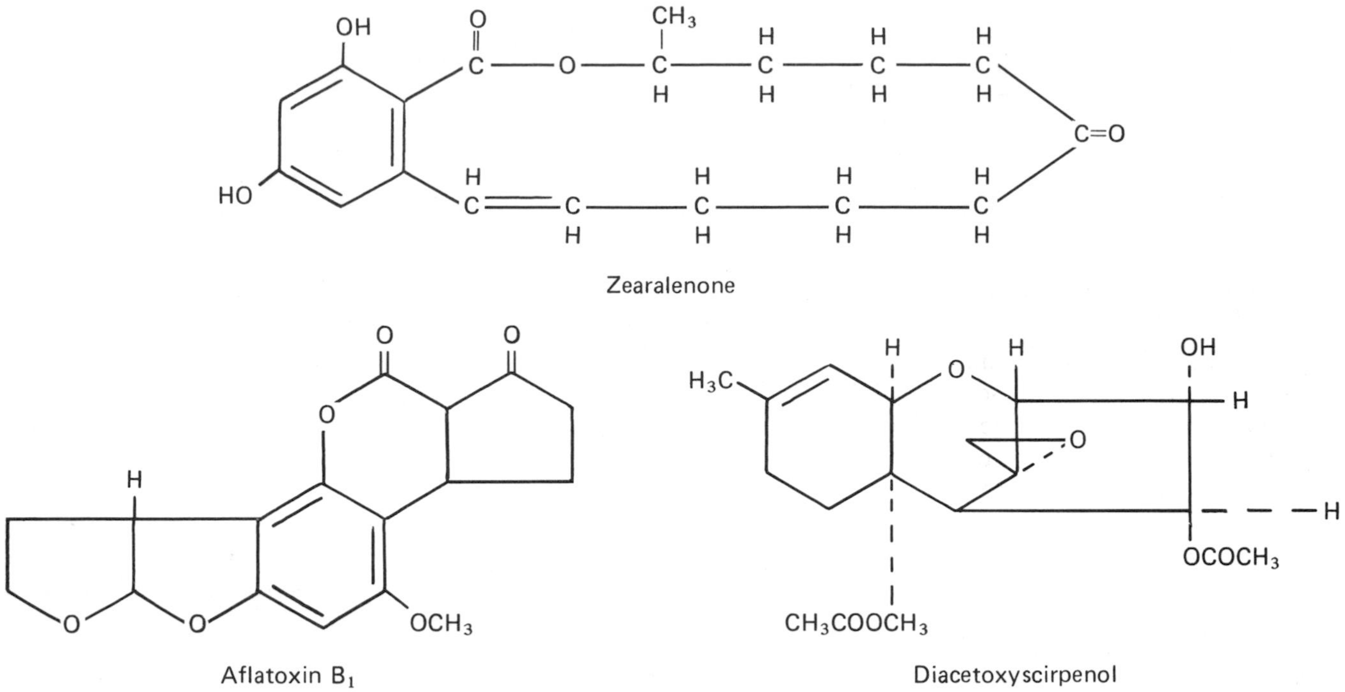

Figure 1. Chemical structures of some representative mycotoxins.

Recent work (Shalkop and Armbrecht, 1974) indicates that long-term low-level feeding of aflatoxin in swine can initiate hepatoma formation. Other mycotoxins implicated as tumorigens or carcinogens are included in table 5.

Clinical Signs

Animals may be affected acutely, subacutely, or chronically with aflatoxicosis. Acute signs can include death with no observed clinical signs. Other animals may be anorectic, depressed, ataxic, dyspneic, and anemic. Expistaxis and blood stained feces are observed. Occasionally, convulsions are present. In subacute cases, animals live longer and may develop icterus, hypoprothrombinemia, hematomata, and hemorrhagic enteritis.

Chronic aflatoxicosis probably poses a greater threat to the economics of livestock production than do the acute cases. The onset of chronic aflatoxicosis is insidious. There may be a reduction of feed efficiency, reduced daily gain, rough hair coat, anemia, enlarged abdomen, mild icterus, and eventually depression and anorexia. This stage of the disease is most difficult to recognize and confirm clinically. Animals on marginal or protein-deficient diets appear more severely affected.

Chronic aflatoxin poisoning causes icterus and cirrhosis of the liver. Hepatic cell necrosis may be minimal while bile duct proliferation and periportal fibrosis are pronounced. Continued feeding of low levels of aflatoxin may cause development of benign hepatoma, cholangiocarcinoma or hepatocellular carcinoma. Other signals of chronic toxicosis are reduced weight gain, reduced production, and increased susceptibility to various infectious diseases.

In swine, decreased feed conversion and failure to gain weight at a normal rate may be a major economic factor even at low concentrations of aflatoxin in feed.

Dogs are quite susceptible to aflatoxins, and the liver is the main target organ. Acute poisoning causes severe gastrointestinal disturbance, ascites, and hemorrhage into the lumen of the intestine. Subserosal hemorrhages are common. Chronic toxicosis may result in loss of thriftiness, decreased appetite, and soft feces. As the disease advances, there is clinical evidence of hepatic insufficiency.

While sheep are considered the most resistant of the domestic species, animals given less than 2 ppm aflatoxin for several years developed hepatic carcinomas and nasal tumors. Intermittent larger doses may be effective in causing chronic toxicosis or carcinogenesis in sheep.

Poultry, particularly chickens, may be poisoned by from 1 to 1.5 ppm aflatoxin B_1. The effects in chickens are similar to those in mammals, with fibrosis, regeneration of parenchymal cells in the liver, and bile duct proliferation being the main features. In addition, poultry may suffer significant increases in prothrombin time, clotting time, and recalcification time.

Physiopathology

Affected animals are anemic and often have low serum protein values which may reflect decreased protein synthesis and/or blood loss. Increases in serum transaminases and alkaline phosphatase, elevated icterus index, and decreased BSP excretion are evidence of the acute to chronic liver disease involved.

Gross pathologic changes include icterus, widespread petechial to ecchymotic hemorrhages, hemorrhagic gastroenteritis, focal hemorrhagic necrosis and fatty change in the liver, hepatomegaly (acute), fibrosis (chronic), and cirrhosis, ascites, hydrothorax, and edema of the wall of the gallbladder (table 4).

Microscopic alterations are centered in the liver. Hepatic necrosis occurs with or without hemorrhage. Fatty change is common in all but acute cases, and bile duct hyperplasia is characteristic of the subacute to chronic disease. In prolonged cases, there may be extensive interlobular fibrosis and this can progress to true cirrhosis. (Newberne, 1970)

Diagnosis

A diagnosis of aflatoxicosis in livestock must include many factors. A history of mold-contaminated feed may be helpful, but fungal growth may be masked by grinding or pelleting processes. Furthermore, the current feed source may not be contaminated, since observed chronic effects stem from prior low-level contamination. Evidence of characteristic lesions and clinical-pathologic changes is helpful. In addition, recent exposure can result in detectable levels of M toxin in the urine. Bioassay of feed supplies with ducklings or chemical analysis of the feed will indicate low levels of aflatoxin. A simple screening procedure for fluorescence of the feed under UV light is presumptive but not confirmatory. Elimination of alternative diagnoses such as leptospirosis, coal tar poisoning, copper intoxication, and crotalaria poisoning should be attempted. (Newberne, 1970)

Treatment

There is no specific treatment for aflatoxicosis. Easily digested low-fat diets, lipotropic agents, and avoidance of stress should be helpful in cases where aflatoxin-induced liver damage has occurred. Adequate dietary protein will aid in resistance to aflatoxins.

No practical way of destroying aflatoxin in contaminated feeds is presently available. Contaminated feeds are not allowed to move in grain trade channels.

Fusarium graminearum Toxin
(Porcine Vulvovaginitis)

Source

Fusarium graminearum appears to be the major fungal invader of stored corn associated with vulvovaginitis in swine. The early report by McNutt *et al.,* (1928) associated estrogenic effects in swine with moldy feed.

Wet corn (above 25 percent moisture) appears susceptible to mold invasion. A period of warm temperature followed by constant or intermittent lower temperature is needed for toxin production.

Mechanism of Action

A toxin, zearalenone, produced by *F. graminearum* has apparent estrogenic activity causing increases in uterine activity and weight in virgin rats.

TABLE 4
Comparative Pathology in Animals Fed Aflatoxin-Contaminated Feed

Liver Lesions	Calves	Cattle	Swine	Sheep	Duckling	Adult Duck	Turkey Poult	Chick
Acute necrosis and hemorrhage	−	−	+	−	+	−	+	−
Chronic fibrosis	+	+	+	0	−	+	−	−
Regeneration nodules	−	+	+	0	±	+	+	−
Bile duct hyperplasia	+	+	+	0	+	+	+	±
Veno-occlusive disease	+	+	−	0	−	−	−	
Enlarged hepatic cells	+	+	+	0	+	+	+	−
Liver tumors	0	0	0	0	−	+	0	0

*Data from Wogan (1966).

TABLE 5
Organ Systems Affected by Mycotoxins

Organ System Primarily Affected	Secondary Effects	Toxin Responsible
Liver	Immune System	Aflatoxin
Liver	Skin (photosensitization)	Sporidesmin
Liver	Kidney hemorrhage	Rubratoxin
Kidney	Liver	Ochratoxin A
Kidney		Citrinin
Hematopoeisis	Stomatitis	Stachybotyrs toxin
Hematopoeisis	Alimentary tract	Fusariotoxin T-2
Blood coagulation		Aflatoxin
Blood coagulation		Rubratoxin
Blood coagulation		Dicoumarol
Blood coagulation		Fusariotoxin T-2
Immune suppression		Aflatoxin
Immune suppression		Rubratoxin
Alimentary irritation		Fusariotoxin T-2
Alimentary irritation		Diacetyoxyscirpenol
Alimentary irritation		Stachybotrys toxin
Alimentary irritation		Slaframine
Emesis		Fusariotoxins
Pulmonary hyperplasia		Ipomearone
Reproductive system		Zearalenone (F-2)
Nervous system	Gangrene	Ergot alkaloids
Nervous system		Penitrem A
Nervous system		Patulin
Nervous system		Puberulum toxin
Nervous system		Fusarium moniliforme
Vascular system		Ergot alkaloids
Carcinogenesis, liver		Aflatoxin
Carcinogenesis, liver		Luteoskyrin
Carcinogenesis, liver		Sterigmatocystin
Carcinogenesis, adenoma		Streptozotocin
Carcinogenesis, adenocarcinoma		Elaiomycin
Carcinogenesis, sarcoma		Patulin
Teratogenesis		Aflatoxin
Teratogenesis		Ochratoxin
Teratogenesis		Cytochalasin B

Clinical Signs

Initially there is enlargement or swelling of the vulva similar to that seen during estrus. This continues to an extreme degree so that the mucosa of the vaginal vault begins to evert. There is obvious edema and hyperemia of the vaginal mucosa. The swelling may cause congestion and increased edema. Vaginal prolapse often results. Affected animals strain repeatedly, and rectal prolapse is a common sequel. In males, there is preputial enlargement, and gilts may have precocious mammary development. Gilts from one to four months are commonly affected. (Sippel, 1970) Reproductive performance after recovery does not appear affected. Access of pregnant swine to a contaminated ration may cause abortion or a reduction in numbers of viable pigs delivered. (Nelson *et al.*, 1971)

Physiopathology

Lesions are confined to the reproductive tract. Edema and hyperplasia of the uterus are observed with endometrial thickening and mammary gland duct proliferation. (Nelson *et al.,* 1971) There also may be squamous metaplasia of the cervix.

Diagnosis

A history of consumption of contaminated grain correlated with characteristic clinical signs usually is sufficient for a diagnosis. Chemical and bioassay methods are available for detection of F-2 toxin or zearalenone in feeds.

Treatment

Removal of swine from the contaminated feed will result in recovery from estrogenic signs in seven to ten days. Replacement of rectal or vaginal prolapses, local treatment of lacerations or abrasions, and suppression of secondary bacterial invasion are helpful.

Trichothecene Mycotoxins

Source

These mycotoxins are a group of naturally occurring sesquiterpenes with an epoxy group at positions 12 and 13 and a double bond at 9 and 10 of the cyclic structure. (Wilson, 1973) The basic structure for the group is as indicated in figure 1. These toxins are stable for long periods of storage and are not destroyed by normal cooking procedures.

The trichothecenes of greatest potential veterinary importance are produced by mainly *Fusarium spp,* particularly *F. tricinctum.* See table 1 for a listing of the toxins and their fungal sources. The source fungi are ubiquitous and can grow and elaborate toxins under a wide variety of conditions. For example, many trichothecene producing fungi will grow at low temperatures, and T-2 toxin may be produced well at temperatures of 8 to 15 °C, and in some cases production has occurred at temperatures below freezing. The *Fusaria* are common contaminants both as storage and field fungi. In the middle and northern temperate regions of the world *Fusaria* are more common toxicogenic contaminants than are the *Aspergilli.* Thus, along with zearalenone (cause of hyperestrinism) the trichothecenes have a widespread potential for harm.

Of the trichothecenes, fusariotoxin T-2 has probably been implicated most often in field outbreaks of trichothecene mycotoxicosis. Therefore, the following discussion is oriented specifically toward T-2 toxin. Other trichothecenes will be found in table 1.

Toxicity

The acute oral LD_{50} in swine and rats given T-2 toxin is approximately 4 mg/kg body weight, while for rainbow trout 6.5 mg/kg is an acute-oral LD_{50}.

Dietary levels of 16 ppm T-2 toxin caused reduction in growth of broiler chicks, production of oral lesions, and prolongation of prothrombin time. Albino rats were severely stunted by dietary T-2 at concentrations of 5 to 15 ppm. Dairy cattle exposed under field conditions to feed shown to contain 2 ppm T-2 toxin suffered chronic to subacute toxicosis with an eventual 20 percent death loss. It must be noted in this instance that total exposure could have been considerably higher. (Hsu, *et al.,* 1972) Other data in cattle have supported the high toxicity of T-2 toxin for cattle with 0.1 mg/kg body weight daily being lethal within sixty-five days.

While data on the chronic effects of T-2 are fragmented and incomplete, there appears to be little doubt that T-2 toxin is highly toxic to domestic and laboratory animals. In addition, although highly toxic, T-2 has not been found associated with carcinogenesis in either field or experimental studies.

Mechanism of Action

The biochemical mechanisms for T-2 or other trichothecene toxicoses remain obscur. Available evidence suggests that there is inhibition of amino acid incorporation into protein. There may also be inhibition of thymidine incorporation into DNA and marked disaggregation of polysomes.

Direct pathologic effects are similar in many species. There is direct dermal toxicosis characterized by inflammation and necrosis. Severe effects are commonly manifest in the alimentary tract and include vomiting, oral ulceration and necrosis, diarrhea, and intestinal hemorrhages. A radiomimetic effect is also reported, with granulocytopenia, anemia, and impaired immune response. The radiomimetic effect appears selective for dividing cells both *in vivo* and in cell culture.

Clinical Signs

Clinical effects are variable, but usually include prominent effects in the alimentary tract and vascular or coagulation systems. Acutely affected animals are depressed and may vomit. The epithelionecrotic effects of T-2 toxin result in salivation, stomatitis and oral and esophageal ulceration or necrosis. Early acute episodes of emesis may progress to diarrhea, which in many cases is hemorrhagic. Elevated prothrombin time and potential vascular damage result in widespread hemorrhaging. This may range from hematemesis to melena to subcutaneous bruising with formation of hematomata and hemarthroses.

Fever, anemia, and increased infectious disease may result from the radiomimetic effects of T-2 and other trichothecenes. The chronic effects of T-2 and other trichothecenes are less well-known. Growth inhibition and poor feed efficiency are known experimentally. Chronic effects on blood coagulation and the immune system are not well documented, but are probably present to some degree.

Although some few instances of infertility and abortion have been associated with field exposure to T-2, reproductive problems are not well defined.

Physiopathology

The lesions of T-2 toxicosis are a reflection of the actions of the toxin described earlier. Direct application of toxin results in inflammation, transudation of fluids, and eventually necrosis. Oral necrotic plaques and ulcers are found in poultry consuming T-2 contaminated feed. There may be gastric, enteritis, bloody intestinal contents, subserosal intestinal hemorrhages, and dark tarry feces.

Hemorrhages can be found in various organs and locations including lungs, heart, urinary bladder, kidneys, subcutis, and articular cavities.

Laboratory examination may include elevations in prothrombin time, blood lactic acid, sulfobromophthalein (BSP) retention, and lactic dehydrogenase (LDH) isoenzyme.

At present, clinicopathologic examination in T-2 or trichothecene toxicosis is not well characterized and would be utilized to assess prognosis rather than confirm a diagnosis.

Diagnosis

Trichothecene toxicosis may appear similar to many naturally occurring diseases. Similarities exist with bovine virus diarrhea, bracken fern poisoning, and dicoumarol toxicosis in cattle. In swine anticoagulant poisoning, crotalaria toxicosis, swine erysipelas, and acute salmonellosis could appear similar. The oral and hematologic lesions in poultry might suggest *Candidiasis,* fowl pox, Newcastle disease, or sulfaquinoxaline hemorrhagic disease. Diagnosis of trichothecene toxicosis is subject to the same limitations as for other mycotoxins as described earlier in this chapter. Careful attention to clinical history, sequence and duration of signs, gross and microscopic findings, and the quality of feed are essential.

Chemical analyses for trichothecenes are possible, but often limited to certain laboratories. Both thin-layer chromatography and gas-liquid chromatography have been used for chemical detection.

A bioassay has been developed which is quite sensitive to as little as $0.05 \mu g$ T-2 toxin. (Wer, *et al.,* 1972) Feed is extracted with ethyl acetate and applied to the shaved skin of an albino rat. The dermal reaction may be graded, but ranges from erythema through necrosis depending on the concentration of T-2 toxin.

Treatment

Removal of the source of toxin and supportive therapy are the only recourse. Attention to hypoprothrombinemia, anemia, hemorrhage, local ulcerations and infections is most important.

Ergot

Source

Ergot is a parasitic fungus which attacks the developing ovary of the grass flower. Rye is most commonly infected, but other cereal grains and grasses may be affected. (Hulbert and Oehme, 1968) The fungus replaces or invades the grass ovary with the resultant structure called a sclerotium. The sclerotium is a dark brown to purple body considerably larger than the ovary.

Growth of the ergot fungus is promoted by warm, moist conditions. Ascospores are spread by wind and serve as the primary infective source. Secondary spread of asexual conidia is accomplished by insects attracted to the sclerotia by its secretion of a yellow nectarlike material known as "honeydew." (Wilson, 1966)

Two important species of fungi parasitize the cereal grains. *Claviceps purpurea* commonly invades rye, oats, wheat, and Kentucky bluegrass; it is most often associated with outbreaks of gangrenous ergotism. *Claviceps paspali* parasitizes species of *Paspalum* or Dallis grass and may cause nervous dysfunction known as paspalum staggers.

Toxicity

The major toxic alkaloids in ergot have been divided into three groups: ergotamine, ergotoxine, and ergometrine. Ergotamine and ergotoxine are polypeptide derivatives of lysergic acid. The varied physiologic effects of ergot (*e.g.,* smooth muscle contraction gangrene, and CNS derangement) result primarily from mixtures of *levo*-isomers of ergotamine along with smaller amounts of histamine, tyramine, and acetylcholine.

The total concentration and proportions of alkaloids of ergot may vary among species and according to environmental conditions. As little as 1 percent ergot in rye has been associated with classical gangrenous ergotism in man (Feuell, 1969), while the tolerance limit set for grain by the USDA Grain Division is 0.30 percent on a crude weight basis. (Wilson, 1966) Such "ergoty" grain is seldom encountered in grain inspection. Data on animal toxicity are scarce. Sows fed 0.5-1.0 percent barley ergot for twenty-five to eighty-seven days delivered weak pigs and failed to lactate properly. (Hulbert and Oehme, 1968) Rats fed 0.1 percent ergot during the first twelve days of pregnancy produced no young.

In cattle, 0.02 percent of body weight as ergot fed for eleven days produced gangrenous ergotism. (Kingsbury, 1964) Because of variations in alkaloid content, individual animal response, and intermittent ingestion, a toxic level of ergot based on field conditions and/or scant experimental evidence is difficult to establish.

Mechanism of Action

Ergotamine, given in high doses, produces an initial stimulation of the central nervous system followed by depression. There is also a direct effect upon adrenergic nerves supplying arteriolar musculature, causing vasoconstriction and a rise in blood pressure. (Clarke and Clarke, 1967) Chronic administration of ergotamine can cause development of local anoxia, especially to extremities poorly supplied with blood. This effect is combined with injury to capillary endothelium resulting in blockage of capillary flow, vascular thrombosis and stasis, and dry gangrene. The tone of uterine and other smooth musculature is increased by ergotamine, and this effect may be exacerbated or influenced by other impurities present in crude ergot (*e.g.*, histamine, acetylcholine).

Clinical Signs

Two forms of ergotism, convulsive and gangrenous, are recognized. Of these gangrenous ergotism is apparently more economically important.

Gangrenous ergotism affects all classes of livestock. The extremities are involved, including nose, ears, tail, and limbs. Early signs generally occur in the hind limbs first. There may be lameness, evidence of pain, stamping of the feet, and coolness of the affected areas. A constricted, sharply demarcated band encircles the limb between the affected and gangrenous areas. As the disease progresses, dry gangrene develops, and the affected portion sloughs leaving a clean, readily healing surface. Sometimes serum exudation and secondary infection may occur.

Crude ergot may affect the digestive system, and gangrenous signs may be preceded by vomition, colic, and constipation or diarrhea.

Several days to a week of consumption of ergot is required for gangrenous lesions to appear. Abortion may occur in pregnant animals. Sows may deliver live pigs but are affected with a noninflammatory afebrile agalactia when fed ergot-infected grain. The authors have observed this phenomena in swine fed oats containing 0.30 percent ergot sclerotia by weight. Swine usually need seven to ten days to recover.

Convulsive ergotism in cattle appears to result from higher daily doses of ergot. While *Claviceps purpurea* may cause convulsive ergotism, the most common organism involved is *Claviceps paspali*. Clinical signs, which appear from two to seven days after ingestion of *C. paspali* forage, include hyperexcitability, belligerency, exaggerated appendicular flexure, ataxia, recumbency, convulsions, and opisthotonus. Excitement and handling tend to exacerbate the condition. Early removal of cattle from the source will sometimes allow recovery in from three to ten days.

Physiopathology

Dry gangrene of the effected extremities is the primary lesion. (Hulbert and Oehme, 1968) Increased cerebrospinal fluid volume has been reported in convulsive ergotism. (Blood and Henderson, 1970)

Treatment

Removal of the contaminated grain is the only primary treatment. Supportive treatment, *e.g.*, supplemental feeding, antibiotics, and pain control, may be indicated.

Ochratoxin A

At low levels ochratoxin A is primarily nephrotoxic. The renal changes include accelerated hyaline degeneration, principally in the proximal convoluted tubules. Desquamation of tubular cells may occur and clinical proteinuria develops. Persistent liver glycogen depletion occurs and hepatic degeneration or necrosis may develop.

Limited evidence indicates that ochratoxin A may be

embryotoxic, and abortions in dairy cattle and experimental rats have been noted.

Ochratoxin A is excreted by both feces and urine; concentrations are maximal at six to eighteen hours after oral exposure and decline to low concentrations by seventy-two hours.

Rubratoxin

The fungi *Penicillium rubrum* and *P. purpurogenum* produce a hepatotoxic and hemorrhage-inducing metabolite called rubratoxin. While much experimental evidence has accumulated concerning the effects of rubratoxin, the substance has not been implicated in naturally occurring diseases, although it has been suspected. Hepatotoxic effects of rubratoxins are quite similar to those described for aflatoxins. However, in contrast to aflatoxin, rubratoxin has not been shown to be carcinogenic.

Rubratoxin may decrease the resistance of animals and poultry to infectious diseases. In addition, combinations of rubratoxin with aflatoxin have been shown to be extremely potent in interfering with development of acquired immunity in poultry and guinea pigs.

Tremorgen Toxicosis

The toxins Tremortin A and Penitrem A are produced by several species of fungi in the genus *Penicillium*. Animals susceptible to these toxins include calves, mice, rats, chickens, rabbits, guinea pigs, and hamsters. The toxin is active by either oral or parenteral routes. In cattle, early signs of intoxication begin with a fine tremor which increases in severity when animals are forced to move or are excited. As consumption continues, animals may stand with their limbs stiff and spread wide apart while swaying rhythmically from side to side. When forced to move, such animals' gait is stiff, stilted and often ataxic. Paddling, extensor rigidity, opisthotonos and nystagmus can be seen. There are increases in plasma lactic acid, pyruvic acid, creatine phosphokinase and transaminase enzymes.

Diagnosis of tremorgen intoxication must be based on clinical signs as well as the demonstration of toxin in feed. The tremors may be reversed with mephenesin or diazepam as well as chlorpromazine.

REFERENCES

Alfin-Slater, R. B.; Aftergood. L.; and Wells, P. 1975. Dietary Factors and Aflatoxin Toxicity: I. Comparison of the Effect of Two Diets Supplemented With Aflatoxin B₁ upon Two Different Strains of Rats. *J. Am. Oil Chemists Society* 52:266.

Allcroft, R. 1969. Aflatoxicosis in Farm Animals. In *Aflatoxin*. L. A. Goldblatt, ed. New York: Academic Press.

Badiali, L.; Abou-Youssef M.; Radwan,A.; Hamdy, G.; and Hildebrandt, P. 1968. Moldy Corn Poisoning as the Major Cause of an Encephalomalacia Syndrome in Egyptian Equidal. *Am. J. Vet. Res.* 29:2029-35.

Blood, D. C., and Henderson, J. A. 1970. *Veterinary Medicine*. 3rd ed. Baltimore: The Williams & Wilkins Co.

Bristol, F. M., and Djurickovic, S. 1971. Hyperestrogenism in Female Swine as the result of Feeding Moldy Corn. *Can. Vet. J.* 12:132.

Brook, P. J. 1966. Fungus Toxins Affecting Mammals. *Ann. Rev. Phytopathol.* 4:171-94.

Burmeister, H. R.; Ellis, J. J.; and Hesseltine, C. W. 1972. Survey for Fusaria that Elaborate T-2 Toxin. *Applied Micro.* 23:1165.

Burnside, J. E.; Sippel, W. L.; Forgacs, J.; Carll, W. T.; Atwood, M. B.; and Doll, E. R. 1957. A Disease of Swine and Cattle Caused by Eating Moldy Corn. II. Experimental Production with Pure Cultures of Molds. *Am. J. Vet. Res.* 18:817-24.

Carr, S. B., and Jacobson, D. R. 1972. Bovine Physiological Responses to Toxic Fescue and Related Conditions for Application in a Bioassay. *J. Dairy Sci.* 52:1792-99.

Chaffee, V. W.; Edds, G. T.; Himes, J. A.; and Neal, F. C. 1969. Aflatoxicosis in dogs. *Am. J. Vet. Res.* 30:1737-49.

Clarke, E. G. C., and Clarke, M. L. 1967. *Garner's Veterinary Toxicology*. 3rd ed. Baltimore: The Williams & Wilkins Co.

Crump, M. H.; Smalley, E. G.; Nichols, R. E.; and Rainey, D. R. 1967. Pharmacologic Properties of a Slobber-Inducing Mycotoxin from *Rhizoctonia leguminicola*. *Am. J. Vet. Res.* 28:865-74

Cysewski, S. J.; Pier, A. C.; Engstrom, G. W.; Richard, J. L.; Dougherty, R. W.; and Thurston, J. R. 1968. Clinical Pathologic Features of Acute Aflatoxicosis of Swine. *Am. J. Vet. Res.* 29:1577.

Doerr, J. A.; Huff, W. E.; Tung, H. T.; Wyatt, R. D.; and Hamilton, P. B. 1974. A Survey of T-2 Toxin, Ochratoxin, and Aflatoxin for Their Effects on the Coagulation of Blood in Young Broiler Chickens. *Poultry Sci.* 53:1728.

Edds, G. T. 1973. Acute Aflatoxicosis: A Review. *JAVMA* 162:304-09.

Feuell, A. J. 1969. Types of Mycotoxins in Foods and Feeds. In *Aflatoxin*. L. A. Goldblatt, ed. New York: Academic Press, pp. 187-221.

Forgacs, J. 1965. Stachybotryotoxicosis and Moldy Corn Toxicosis. In *Mycotoxins in Foodstuffs*. G. N. Wogan, ed. Cambridge, Mass: M. I. T. Press, pp. 87-144.

Forgacs, J., and Carll, W. T. 1962. Mycotoxicoses. *Adv. Vet. Sci.* 7:277.

Gardner, S. 1974. Aflatoxin in Milk. *JAVMA* 165-85.

Goldblatt, L. A. 1969. *Aflatoxin.* New York: Academic Press.

Golumbic, C., and Kulik, M. M. 1969. Fungal Spoilage in Stored Crops and Its Control. In *Aflatoxin.* L. A. Goldblatt, ed. New York: Academic Press

Gumberman, M. R., and Williams, S. N. 1969. Biochemical Effects of Aflatoxin in Pigs. *Tox. Appl. Pharm.* 15:393-404.

Hesseltine, C. W. 1969. Mycotoxins. *Mycopathalogia et Mycologia Applicata.* 39:371-83.

Hsu, I. C.; Smalley, E. B.; Strong, F. M.; and Ribelin, W. E. 1972. Identification of T-2 Toxin in Moldy Corn Associated with a Lethal Toxicosis in Dairy Cattle. *Applied Micro.* 24:684.

Hulbert, L. C.; and Oehme, F. W. 1968. *Plants Poisonous to Livestock.* 3rd ed. Manhattan, Kansas: Kansas State University Printing Service

Kellerman, T. S.; Marasas, W. F. O.; Pienaar, J. G.; and Naude, T. W. 1972. A Mycotoxicosis of Equidae Caused by *Fusarium Moniliforme* Sheldon. A preliminary communication. *Onderstepoort J. Vet. Res.* 39:205.

Kingsbury, J. M. 1964. *Poisonous Plants of the United States and Canada.* Englewood Cliffs, New Jersey: Prentice-Hall, Inc.

Kosuri, N. R.; Grave, M. D.; Yates, S. G.; Tallent, W. H.; Ellis, J. J; Wolf, I. A.; and Nichols, R. E. 1970. Response of Cattle to Mycotoxins of *Fusarium tricinctum* Isolated from Corn and Fescue. *JAVMA* 157:938.

Kosuri, N. R.; Smalley, E. B.; and Nichols, R. E. 1971. Toxicologic Studies of *Fusarium tricinctum* (Corda) Snyder et Hans, from Moldy Corn. *Am. J. Vet. Res.* 32:1843.

Krogh, P.; and Hasselager, E. 1968. *Studies on Fungal Nephrotoxicity.* Copenhagen, Denmark: Royal Vet. Coll. Agr. College Yearbook.

Kurtz, H. J.; Nairn, M. E.; Nelson, G. H.; Christensen, C. M.; and Mirocha, C. J. 1969. Histologic Changes in the Genital Tracts of Swine Fed Estrogenic Mycotoxin. *Am. J. Vet. Res.* 30:551.

Leach, C. M., and Tulloch, M. 1971. *Pithomyces chartarum,* a Mycotoxin-Producing Fungus, Isolated from Seed and Fruit in Oregon. *Mycologia.* 63:1086-89

Lillehoj, E. B; Ciegler, A.; and Detroy, R. W. 1970. Fungal Toxins. In *Essays in Toxicology.* F. R. Blood, ed. New York: Academic Press.

Lynch, G. P.; Todd, G. C.; Shalkop, W. T.; and Moore, L. A. 1970. Responses of Dairy Calves to Aflatoxin Contaminated Feed. *J. Dairy Sci.* 53:63-71.

McNutt, S. H.; Purwin, P.; and Murray, C. 1928. Vulvovaginitis in Swine. *JAVMA* 73:484.

Marasas, W. F. O.; Bamburg, J. R.; Smalley, E. B.; Strong, F. M.; Ragland, W. L; and Degurse, P. E. 1969. Toxic Effects on Trout, Rats and Mice of T-2 Toxin Produced by the Fungus *Fusarium tricinctum* (Cd.) Synd. et Hans. *Toxicol. Appl. Pharm.* 15:471.

Miller, J. K.; Hacking, A.; and Gross, V. J. 1973. Stillbirths, Neonatal Mortality, and Small Litters in Pigs Associated with the Ingestion of *Fusarium* Toxin by Pregnant Sows. *Vet. Rec.* 93:559.

Mirocha, C. J.; Christensen, C. M.; and Nelson, G. H. 1968. Physiologic Activity of Some Fungal Estrogens Produced by *Fusarium. Cancer Res.* 28:2319-22.

Mirocha, C. J.; Harrison, J.; Nichols, A. A.; and McClintock, M. 1968. Detection of a Fungal Estrogen (F-2) in Hay Associated with Infertility in Dairy Cattle. *Appl. Microbiol.* 16:797-98.

Nelson, G. H.; Bornes, D. M.; Christensen, C. M.; and Mirocha, C. J. 1971. Effect of Mycotoxins on Reproduction . Paper 1379, Miscellaneous Journal Series, Institute of Agriculture, University of Minnesota.

Newberne, P. M. 1970. Aflatoxins In *Diseases of Swine.* H. W. Dunne, ed. Ames, Iowa: I.S.U. Press

Prentice, N., and Dickson, A. D. 1968. Emetic Material Associated with *Fusarium sp.* in Cereal Grains and Artificial Media. *Biotechnol. Bioeng.* 10:413-27.

Radeleff, R. D. 1970. *Veterinary Toxicology.* 2nd ed. Philadelphia, Pa.: Lea & Febiger.

Rutquist, L., and Persson, P. A. 1966. Studies on *Aspergillus fumigatus,* Experimental Mycotoxicosis in Mice, Chicks and Pigs with the Appearance in Pigs of Perirenal Edema. *Acta Vet. Scand.* 7:21-34.

Sargeant, K.; Sheridan, A.; O'Kelly, J.; and Carnaghan, R. B. A. 1961. Toxicity Associated with Certain Samples of Groundnuts. *Nature* 192:1096-97.

Shalkop, W. T., and Ambrecht, B. H. 1974. Carcinogenic Response of Brood Sows Fed Aflatoxin for 28 to 30 Months. *Am. J. Vet. Res.* 35:623.

Shreeve, B. J., and Patterson, D. S. P. 1975. Mycotoxicosis. *Vet. Rec.* 97:279.

Shreeve, B. J.; Patterson, D. S. P.; and Roberts, B. A. 1975. Investigation of Suspected Cases of Mycotoxicosis in Farm Animals. *Vet. Rec.* 97:275.

Sippel, W. L. 1970. Moldy Corn Poisoning. Vulvovaginitis, and Ergotism. In *Diseases of Swine.* H. W. Dunn, ed. Ames, Iowa: I.S.U. Press

Speers, G. M.; Meronuck, R. A.; Barnes, D. M.; and Mirocha, C.J. 1971. Effect of Feeding *Fusarium Roseum F. Sp. Graminearum* Contaminated Corn and the Mycotoxin F-2 on the Growing Chick, and Laying Hen. *Poultry Sci.* 50:627.

Tatsuno, T. 1968. Toxicological Research on Substances from *Fusarium nivale. Cancer Res.* 28:2393-96.

Todd, G. C.; Shalkop, W. T.; Dooley, K. L.; and Wiseman, H. G. 1968. Effects of Ration Modifications on Aflatoxicosis in the Rat. *Am. J. Vet. Res.* 29:1855.

Tookey, H. L.; Yates, S. G.; Ellis, J. J. Grove, M. D.; and Nichols, R. E. 1972. Toxic Effects of a Butenolide Mycotoxin and of *Fusarium tricinctum* Cultures in Cattle. *JAVMA* 160:1522.

Ueno, Y.; Sato, N.; Ishu, K.; Sakai, K.; Tsunoda, H.; and Enomoto, M. 1973. Biological and Chemical Detection of Trichothecene Mycotoxins of *Fusarium* Species. *Applied Micro.* 25:699.

Wei, R. D.; Smalley, E. B.; and Strong, F. M. 1972. Improved Skin Test for Detection of T-2 Toxin. *Applied Micro.* 23:1029.

Wilson, B. J. 1966. Fungal Toxins. In *Toxicants Occurring Naturally in Foods.* Publ. 1354, Washington D. C.: National Academy of Sciences

Wilson, B. J.; Wilson, C. H.; and Hayes, A. W. 1968. Tremorigenic Toxin from *Penicillium cyclopium* Grown on Food Materials. *Nature* 220:77-78.

Wilson, B. J. 1973. Toxicity of Mold-Damaged Sweet Potatoes. *Nutrition Reviews* 31:73.

Wilson, B. J. 1973. 12, 13-Epoxytrichothecenes: Potential Toxic Contaminants of Food. *Nutritional Reviews* 31:169.

Wogan, G. N. 1966. Chemical Nature and Biological Effects of the Aflatoxins. *Bact. Rev.* 30:460-70.

———. 1968. Aflatoxin Risks and Control Measures. *Federation Proc.* 27:932-38.

———. 1975. Mycotoxins. *Annual Rev. Pharmacol.* 15:437.

Wyatt, R. D.; Weeks, B. A.; Hamilton, P. B.; and Burmeister, H. R. 1972. Severe Oral Lesions in Chickens Caused by Ingestion of Dietary Fusariotoxin T-2[1]. *Applied Micro.* 24:251.

Yang, C. Y. 1972. Comparative Studies on the Detoxification of Aflatoxins by Sodium Hypochlorite and Commercial Bleaches. *Applied Micro.* 24:885.

Yates, S. G.; Tookey, H. L.; Ellis, J. J.; and Burkhardt, H. J. 1968. Mycotoxins Produced by *Fusarium nivale* Isolated from Tall Fescue (*Festuca arundinacea*). *Phytochem.* 7:139-46.

Yates, S. G.; Tookey, H. L.; Ellis, J. J.; Tallent, W. H.; and Wolff, I. A. 1969. Mycotoxins as a Possible Cause of Fescue Toxicity. *Ag. and Food Chem.* 17:437-42.

FOOD POISONING

Source

Adverse reactions and poisonings from foods or their decomposition products are a major cause of the toxicologic problems encountered in small animals. Dogs, by virtue of their voracious appetites and scavenging habits, are most prone to indiscriminate ingestion of potentially toxic foods. Animals may experience adverse reactions to foods in several ways:

1. Naturally occurring toxins which are components of certain food products (*e.g.,* cyanogenetic glycosides, nitrates, goitrogens).
2. Allergies to ingested foods.
3. Toxicity from ingestion of foods which contain preformed toxins.
4. Bacterial infection from grossly contaminated foods.

The scope of this discussion will be limited to the latter two categories, involving those foods which are normally wholesome but are rendered unfit or dangerous by virtue of contamination or spoilage. The chief offenders to be considered in this group are the *Salmonella spp.,* the *Clostridium spp., Escherichia coli, Staphylococcus spp.,* and certain polypeptides or amines which may result from protein decomposition.

Sources of the organisms listed include the skin, abscesses, soil, and alimentary tract. Contamination of high protein and readily usable food products results in proliferation of microorganisms with elaboration of their toxic metabolites. Enzymatic and microbial processes may also result in formation of polypeptide or amine fractions.

Salmonella

The primary reservoir of salmonella is the vertebrate intestine, with as many as 10^9 organisms/gm of feces in infected animals. In general, the salmonellae are excreted from carrier animals long after clinical disease has passed. Infected viscera consumed directly, food contaminated during butchering, and poor hygenic practices of persons preparing foods can account for sources of contamination.

Clostridium

Clostridium perfringens, a spore-forming, anaerobic bacillus, is widespread in soil and is found in the alimentary tract of nearly all warm-blooded species. It is a frequent postmortem invader in the tissues of man and animals. (Bruner and Gillespie, 1966) In man, most outbreaks are reported due to heat-resistant strains of *C. perfringens..* (Hobbs, 1969) Ideal medium is a high-meat food usually cooked at 100° C or less for two to three hours and allowed to cool slowly.

Clostridium botulinum may be found in almost any food material with pH above 4.5. Chief offending foods reported in man include canned string beans, beans, corn, and asparagus. Home canning or low-temperature cooking ($\leq$100° C) may not kill all *C. botulinum* organisms or spores. Fish and seafoods are also subject to *C. botulinum* invasion. Once formed, botulinus toxin is stable, even under acid conditions.

Staphylococcus

Staphylococcus aureus lives in close association with man and animals with a relatively stable host-parasite relationship. The enterotoxic staphylococci do not differ measurably in other respects from other members of the species. The staphylococci are ubiquitously distributed in the environment in air, dust, water, milk, food, feces, and sewage. Except for dairy products from mastitis-infected cows, man is the single most important source of *S. aureus* in foods.

Escherichia coli

This organism is a normal inhabitant of the lower intestinal tract and colon of all warm-blooded animals. Carnivora and omnivora usually harbor greater numbers of the organism than do herbivora. Other sources of food contamination may be soil and water. Strains containing K antigen appear most often associated with toxic reactions and infections.

Polypeptides and Amines

During putrefaction and decomposition of protein-aceous foods, polypeptides and amines may be formed. Some of these could have structural and biologic properties similar to known agents with CNS, cardiovascular, or histamine activity.

Toxicity

Salmonella

Certain types of salmonellae appear more pathogenic for dogs. These include *Salmonella typhimurium, S. anatum, S. cholerasuis, S. newport,* and *S. enteriditis.* Some endotoxin reactions could occur to massive *Salmonella* exposure, but most salmonella problems are the result of proliferation after ingestion and not of preformed exotoxin ingestion.

Clostridium

Clostridium perfringens, types B, C, and D, have been reported to cause acute enterotoxemia in lambs, calves, and small pigs. Experimental production of irreversible shock and rapid progression to death has been accomplished in dogs.

Clostridiun botulinum toxin is the most toxic material known. There are approximately 32×10^9 mouse LD_{50}/gm of toxin. Animal species differ in their susceptibility from the extremely sensitive guinea pig to the relatively resistant turkey buzzard. Dogs, cats, and pigs are relatively resistant. While dogs are susceptible to injected botulinum toxin types A and B, no verified natural cases have been reported. (Riemann, 1969) Mink, poultry, and horses are most commonly affected.

Staphylococcus

Several toxins are produced by *Staphylococcus aureus.* Under certain conditions, toxins are hemolytic, leukocytic, dermonecrotic, and lethal to mice and rabbits. In addition, a potent exotoxin known as enterotoxin is produced by certain strains. The primary toxin of clinical importance in man and animals is enterotoxin. Dogs have been poisoned mildly by 20-40 ml of toxin

filtrate. The enterotoxin of *S. aureus* is heat resistant and water soluble.

Escherichia coli

Some strains of *E. coli* appear to be harmless parasites while others are routinely associated with disease of the alimentary tract. All of the *E. coli* appear capable of releasing endotoxin upon lysis or death of their cells. This endotoxin has experimentally caused signs and lesions of irreversible shock in dogs. The presence of high numbers of *E. coli* in spoiled or contaminated foods may conceivably be a situation that could lead to endotoxic shock in animals consuming such foods.

Mechanism of Action

Certain factors other than exposure to specific agents may predispose small animals to enterotoxemic or food poisoning disease. Thus, exposure to bacteria, excessive proliferation of those organisms, a decrease in body resistance to the organism, or conditions promoting the absorption of toxin may precondition an animal to food poisoning.

Normally, five primary bacterial types inhabit the canine intestine: *E. coli, Clostridium perfringens, Lactobacillus acidophilus, Enterococcus,* and *Bacteroides.* They characteristically are fermentative and putrefactive. (Sudduth, 1971) These bacteria grow and elaborate toxin in alkaline or near-alkaline media, but production generally stops below pH 6.

Stasis of the intestine may allow excess proliferation of bacteria in the small intestine. The stasis also allows increased absorption of toxin from intrinsic or extrinsic sources. High protein meals, achlorhydria, and inflammation contribute to destruction of the intestinal barrier to bacteria and toxins. Enterotoxemialike conditions in dogs commonly result from: (1) eating garbage, spoiled food or feces; (2) ingestion of bones or foreign matter; (3) eating low-grade poor quality foods; (4) lack of exercise; (5) intestinal parasites; (6) nervous and psychologic problems; and (7) achlorhydria.

Salmonella

Salmonella food poisoning is the result of ingestion of these microorganisms and their multiplication in the intestine. (Taylor and McCoy, 1969) In this manner, salmonellosis is not a poisoning but a bacteriologic infection. Further details regarding salmonella infectious mechanisms can be obtained from appropriate bacteriology texts.

Clostridium

Clostridium perfringens food poisoning has generally been ascribed to presence of actively sporulating organisms ingested in contaminated meat products. The lecithin in food may be hydrolyzed by the clostridial enzyme phospholipase C to form phosphorylcholine. Experimental production of diarrhea eight to ten hours after phosphorylcholine administration has verified this. (Hobbs, 1969)

Clostridium botulinum acts as a preformed neurotoxin. It is adsorbed to nervous tissue and acts to prevent the release of acetylcholine or to inactivate it at synaptic sites. The clinical effect is flaccid motor paralysis.

Staphylococcus

Specific mechanisms for the action of staphylococcal enterotoxin remain unclear. At least three specific, weakly antigenic enterotoxins, A, B, and C, are known. Except that most enterotoxigenic strains of *S. aureus* are coagulase positive, no correlation has been shown between enterotoxigenicity and production of other toxins. (Angelotti, 1969)

Escherichia coli

Pathogenic *E. coli* may cause intestinal disease by bacterial infection. In addition, ingestion of large numbers of gram-negative bacteria may be followed by bacterial lysis and release of endotoxin. Experimental evidence (Hardaway *et al.,* 1961) has supported the possibility that endotoxin may account for acute illness and death in dogs. Potential cases of endotoxin shock from ingestion of garbage or spoiled food should be investigated more thoroughly.

Polypeptides and Amines

Protein degradation can result in formation of polypeptides and amines at various stages of autolysis. It is conceivable that these compounds could contain potent principles affecting the cardiovascular or nervous system. Further research in this area is needed.

Clinical Signs

Clinical disease from garbage or food poisoning is characterized by two major syndromes—gastrointestinal and clinical shock.

The gastrointestinal form of food poisoning or enterotoxemia includes a history of ingestion of spoiled foods, over-consumption on rich or unusual foods, or intake of dead animals or parts thereof. Such ingestion may occur from several hours to a week or more prior to the appearance of clinical signs.

Acute signs of food poisoning include vomition, colic, mucoid to watery diarrhea, weakness, stiffness, ataxia, nervousness, prostration, dehydration, and occasionally death.

Less severe cases of food poisoning or enterotoxemia may give evidence of anorexia, dull hair coat, drowsiness, and abnormal stools.

In those cases where endotoxic shock or clostridial exotoxin shock is suspected, there is dyspnea, depression, weakness, rapid pulse, cold extremeties, prostration, and circulatory collapse. Occasionally, a hemorrhagic diarrhea may be observed. Some animals may be found dead with no premonitory signs.

Specific agents induce certain clinical differences in food poisoning in the dog. Botulism causes a flaccid ascending paralysis, respiratory difficulty, and excess salivation. Salmonella infections cause vomiting, diarrhea, and fever after a period of twelve to twenty-four hours from the time of ingestion. Staphylococcal food poisoning results in clinical signs in from one to six hours after consumption of contaminated foods. Death is rare.

Physiopathology

Staphylococcal enterotoxin is associated with dehydration and related electrolyte disturbances. Postmortem examination of the relatively few fatal cases reveals serosanguineous exudate in the body cavities, petechial hemorrhages in the viscera, and hyperemia of the stomach and intestines. The stomach is often empty, while foul-smelling, fluid feces are present in the terminal alimentary tract.

Salmonella infections cause lesions of hyperemic gastritis and hemorrhagic to fibrinonecrotic enteritis. There may be hemorrhages in the viscera and subserosal areas indicative of septicemia. Leukocytosis and neutrophilia are commonly observed.

Clostridial and endotoxic shock syndromes cause a rapid drop in blood pressure, intravascular stasis and thrombosis, elevated packed cell volume, hemorrhagic necrosis of the intestine, acute congestion of the liver and kidney, and tubular degeneration in the kidney. (Lillehei and MacLean, 1959)

In cases where putrefactive changes have occurred *in vivo* or large amounts of high-protein spoiled foods have been eaten, urinary indican is elevated and urine pH is commonly alkaline.

Diagnosis

After careful examination of the history, clinical signs, and clinical pathologic data, confirmation of the specific agent may be attempted.

Culture of the GI tract, suspected foods, and other organs should be attempted. Serologic identification of staphylococcal and clostridial toxins, as well as injection and protection tests using laboratory animals, may be utilized. Filtrates of suspected material rendered harmless by specific antitoxin is evidence for a specific food poisoning agent.

Treatment

Therapy should be directed toward alleviating acute signs of shock and electrolyte imbalance, elimination of the offending agent or toxin, and promotion of normal gastrointestinal status.

Broad spectrum antibiotics and enteric sulfonamides will aid in elimination of pathogenic organisms and control of bacterial putrefaction. Administration of phthalysulfathiazole (100-200 mg/kg) and tetracycline (6-10 mg/kg) for three to five days is recommended. (Sudduth, 1971) Kaolin may be used as an adjunct in removal of bacteria, acidification of fecal flora, and elimination of gas-forming bacilli.

Appropriate intravenous therapy with fluids and electrolytes is reconmended to correct dehydration, acid-base imbalance, and shock. Laboratory determination of packed cell volume, blood urea nitrogen, electrolytes, and blood pH, pCO_2, and bicarbonate are valuable in assessing specific electrolyte and fluid needs. Maintenance of low intestinal pH with glutamic acid hydrochloride, 0.3 gram, before meals is useful in patients with gastric hypochlorhydria or alkaline urine. *Lactobacillus acidophilus* preparations may also aid in promoting the aciduric and competitive flora helpful in prophylaxis or convalescence of enterotoxemic conditions.

REFERENCES

Angelotti, R. 1969. *Food-Borne Infections and Intoxications.* Hans Riemann, ed. New York: Academic Press

Bruner, D. W.; and Gillespie, J. H. 1966. *Hagans Infectious Diseases of Domestic Animals.* Ithaca, New York: Cornell University Press

Crosby, D. G. 1969. Natural Toxic Background in the Food of Man and His Animals. *J. Agr. Food Chem.* 17:532-38.

Hardaway, R. M.; Husni, E. A.;. Geever, E. F.; Noyes, H. E.; and Burns, J. W. 1961. Endotoxin Shock. *Ann. of Surg.* 154:791-802.

Hobbs, B. C. 1969. *Clostridium perfringens and Bacillus cereus* Infections. In *Food-Borne Infections and Intoxications.* Hans Riemann, ed. New York: Academic Press

Lillehei, R. C.; and MacLean, L. D. 1959. Physiological Approach to Successful Treatment of Endotoxin Shock in the Experimental Animal. *AMA Arch of Surg.* 78:464-71.

McNeil, E. 1968. Food Poisonings. In *Canine Medicine.* E. J. Catcott, ed. Wheaton, Ill.: American Veterinary Publications

Reimann, H. 1969. Botulism-Types A, B, and F. In *Food-Borne Infections and Intoxications.* Hans Riemann, ed. New York: Academic Press

Sudduth, W. H. 1971. Enterotoxemia. In *Current Veterinary Therapy.* R. W. Kirk, ed. Philadelphia: W. B. Saunders Company

Taylor, J.; and McCoy, J. H. 1969. Salmonella and Arizona Infections. In *Food-Borne Infections and Intoxications.* Hans Riemann, ed. New York: Academic Press

Metals and Metalloids

ARSENIC I: INORGANIC, ALIPHATIC AND TRIVALENT ORGANIC ARSENICALS

For the most part, toxicoses caused by inorganic, aliphatic and trivalent organic arsenicals are manifested by an entirely different syndrome from that caused by the phenylarsonic feed additives. Thus, phenylarsonic feed additives will be discussed in the next section.

Arsenic appears to be second only to lead in importance as a toxicant in farm and household animals. Inorganic arsenic is found in nature and is synthesized in complex and varied forms, having many uses varying from medicinal to forensic (over 50,000 tons produced each year, world wide).

Source

Inorganic arsenical compounds are widely found in soils and ores, usually combined with other metals or elements such as sulfur. Much of the natural arsenic occurs in the form of pyrites ($FeS_2 \bullet FeAs_2$) and sulfides ($As_2S_{2,3}$). During the process of refining metal ores using heat, arsenic trioxide (As_2O_3) is produced and some is carried into the surrounding countryside in the dust or smoke. Much of the inorganic arsenic presently being produced is used in pesticide formulations. Arsenic trioxide (white arsenic) and sodium arsenite are frequently used as herbicides as are other alkali salts of arsenic such as sodium, potassium, calcium, and lead arsenates (fig. 1). These compounds are not only used as weed and brush killers but also defoliants, especially for cotton and fruit trees. Copper acetoarsenite (Paris green), arsenic trioxide, and lead arsenate all have good insecticidal qualities. Other sources of inorganic arsenic include pesticides for use against ants, snails, and rodents; insulation material such as vermiculite and Celotex® [1]; and wood building materials treated with arsenical preservatives. Arsenic is also found in certain paint pigments (emerald green), detergents, and medicaments such as Fowler's solution. It recently has been reported that ruminatorics such as Carmilax® [2] and Rumide® [3] had arsenic contamination which, although at levels not thought to be toxic, gave misleading results when rumen contents were tested for arsenic in connection with diagnostic cases. (Reagor, 1972)

In small animals, organic arsenical compounds such as Sodium Caparsolate® [4] and Filcide® [5] are used for the treatment of blood parasites such as *Dirofilaria immitis* (fig. 2). Although these are phenyl organic compounds they are never-the-less trivalent arsenicals and act similar to inorganic and aliphatic organic arsenical compounds rather than the phenylarsonic feed additives.

Since the synthesis of arsphenamine (salvarsan) in 1907 for the treatment of syphilis, many organic arsenical compounds have been developed for the treatment of various blood parasitic and infectious diseases in humans. Some of these compounds, for example, acctarsol (3-acetylamino-4-hydroxyphenylarsonate) and sodium cacodylate (sodium dimethylarsonate), have been used in veterinary medicine as general stimulants and for their antiblood parasitic properties. The results of their use probably have been more disappointing than beneficial.

Certain organic arsenicals are used as herbicides such as monosodium methanearsonate (MSMA) and disodium methanearsonate (DSMA). Poisoning by these compounds results in clinical signs and lesions identical to those produced by inorganic arsenicals. (Palmer, 1972)

Some of the more common sources of arsenic poisoning include grass clippings from lawns that have been previously treated with arsenical crabgrass control preparations; grass, weeds, shrubbery, and other foliage that have been sprayed with arsenical herbicides; dipping animals in vats that years before had been charged with arsenic trioxide; soils heavily contaminated with arsenic, either through the burning of arsenic formulations in rubbish piles or application of arsenic pesticides to orchards and truck gardens; and in the case of small animals, especially cats, ant and snail baits containing 1-2 percent arsenic.

1. Celotex Corporation, Tampa, Florida.
2. Norden Laboratories, Inc., Lincoln, Nebraska.
3 Pittman-Moore, Inc., Washington Crossing, New Jersey.
4. Diamond Laboratories, Des Moines, Iowa.
   Pittman-Moore, Inc., Washington Crossing, New Jersey.

As_2O_3
Arsenic Trioxide

As_2O_5
Arsenic Pentoxide

H_3AsO_3
Ortho Arsinious Acid*

H_3AsO_4
Ortho Arsenic Acid**

$HAsO_2$
Meta Arsinious Acid*

As_4S_4
Realgar

As_2S_3
Orpiment
(arsenic trisulfide)

As_2S_5
Arsenic Pentasulfide

$CH_3AsO(OH)_2$
Methylarsonic Acid

$(CH_3)_2AsO$
Cacodylic Acid
(dimethylarsinic acid)

$(CH_3)_3As$
Trimethylarsine

$CH_3As(OH)_2$
Methyldihydroxyarsine

$(CH_3)_2AsOH$
Dimethylhydroxyarsine

$(CH_3)_3AsO$
Trimethylarsine Oxide

*Salts of arsinious acids are called "arsenites."
**Salts of arsenic acids are called "arsenates."

Figure 1. Inorganic and aliphatic organic arsenicals commonly found in the environment.

Toxicity

Man and all lower animals are highly susceptible to inorganic arsenic, but poisoning is most frequently encountered in the bovine and feline species resulting from contamination of their food supply. Frequency of incidence of arsenical poisoning in these two species is closely followed in other forage-eating animals such as the sheep and horse. Poisoning by inorganic arsenicals is only occasionally seen in the dog and rarely seen in swine and poultry.

The toxicity of the various formulations of inorganic arsenicals varies with the species of animal exposed, the formulation of the arsenical (trivalent arsenicals more toxic than pentavalent), solubility of the formulation, route of exposure, rate of absorption from the gastrointestinal tract, and rate of metabolism and excretion by the exposed individual. (Clarke and Clarke, 1967; Radeleff, 1970) In practice, the most dangerous arsenical preparations are dips, herbicides, and defoliants in which the arsenical is in a highly soluble trivalent form,

usually trioxide or arsenite. Unfortunately, animals will frequently seek out and eat materials such as insulation, rodent baits, dirt, and foliage that have been contaminated with an inorganic arsenical.

Because of the many factors influencing the toxicity of arsenic, as noted above, there is little point in attempting to state its toxicity on a mg/kg body-weight basis. The lethal oral dose for most species of animals, however, appears to be from 1-25 mg/kg body weight as sodium arsenite with arsenic trioxide being three to ten times less toxic.

The fact that the toxicity of an arsenical is greatly influenced by its solubility and particle size and, thus, absorbability from the intestinal tract or skin is illustrated by an experiment we conducted with swine. Sodium arsenite was given in the feed at levels up to 500 ppm continuously for two weeks. The pigs readily ate the contaminated feed but manifested no signs of acute arsenic poisoning. When the level was increased to 1,000 ppm, the pigs refused to eat the feed. When an equivalent amount of sodium arsenite was added to their

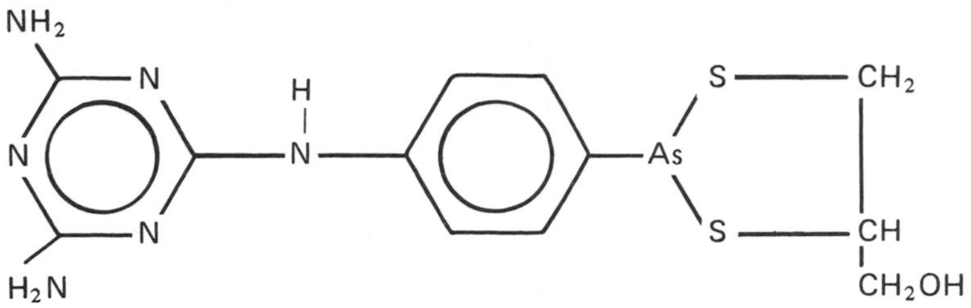

Melarsoprol

(2—[p—(4, 6— Diamino—*s*—triazin—2—ylamino) phenyl] —
4—hydroxymethyl—1, 3—dithia—2—arsacyclopentane)

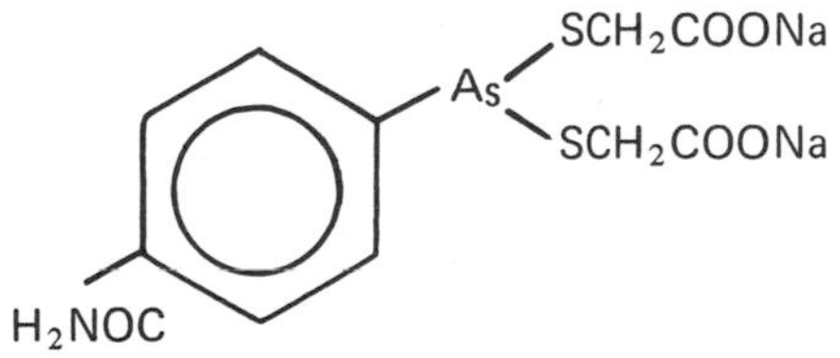

Caparsolate, Arsenamide

(Bis [carboxymethylmercapto] (p-carbamylphenyl) arsine disodium salt)

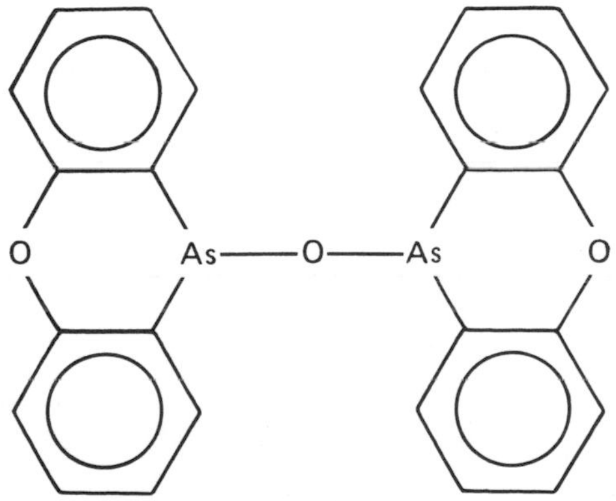

Vinyzene

(10, 10—Bis (phenoxarsine)

Figure 2. Some common trivalent phenyl organic arsenicals.

drinking water, severe poisoning and death occurred within a few hours. It was concluded that the lethal dose via drinking water of sodium arsenite was 100-200 mg/kg body weight.

Experience with field cases of arsenic poisoning indicates that animals which are weak, debilitated, and dehydrated are much more susceptible to arsenic poisoning than the normal animal. This probably is because of reduced excretion rate via the kidneys.

Arsenical poisoning in most animals is usually manifested by an acute or subacute syndrome. Chronic poisoning, although it has been reported, is seldom seen and has not been clearly documented. In humans,

chronic arsenical poisoning is manifested by symmetrical hyperkeratosis of the hands and feet, pigmentation of the exposed skin, conjunctivitis, tracheitis, acrocyanosis, and polyneuritis. The polyneuritis involves both sensory and motor functions. Other chronic effects include anorexia, cachexia, cirrhosis, and dementia. (Chisolm, 1970) Some animals appear to develop a tolerance to arsenic after prolonged oral exposure.

Caparsolate® is recommended for the treatment of adult heartworms in dogs at the rate of 1/10 ml of a 1 percent solution twice daily per pound of body weight for two days (1.6 mg/kg body weight total) or, in cases of heavily infested and poor-risk individuals, 1/10 ml of 1 percent solution daily for fifteen days (6 mg/kg total). The safety margin in the dog is quite low. Dogs have died of arsenic poisoning after five daily doses of 1.8 mg/kg body weight (a total of 5.4-9.0 mg/kg). However, dogs did not suffer ill effects from thirty daily doses of 0.9 mg/kg body weight (totaling 27 mg/kg). (Otto and Maren, 1950) Apparently, the most serious untoward reaction from the use of thiacetarsamide is the sudden death of the adult heartworm dislodging it into the pulmonary capillary bed causing embolism and fatal pulmonary embarrassment. Systemic arsenic poisoning is not uncommon, however, following the routine treatment of apparently healthy dogs.

In recent years, thiacetarsamide has been used in the treatment of *Hemabartonella felis* in cats. It is reasonable to assume, therefore, that poisoning will occur in a certain percentage of cats treated with this regimen.

Palmer (1972) has studied the toxicity of organic arsenical herbicides, monosodium methanearsonate (MSMA) and disodium methanearsonate (DSMA), in cattle, sheep, and chickens. Cattle were poisoned and died after receiving five daily doses of 10 mg/kg MSMA and six daily doses of 25 mg/kg DSMA. Ten daily doses of 5 mg/kg MSMA and 10 mg/kg DSMA produced no ill effects. Sheep were poisoned and died after receiving six daily doses of 50 mg/kg MSMA and six daily doses of 25 mg/kg DSMA. Animals receiving ten daily doses of 25 mg/kg MSMA and 10 mg/kg DSMA showed no ill effects. Chickens failed to exhibit ill effects after receiving ten daily doses up to 250 mg/kg of either compound. He also studied the toxicity of hydroxydimethylarsine oxide (cacodylic) acid in these three species. Cattle and sheep were poisoned after receiving eight and ten daily doses, respectively, at a rate of 25 mg/kg body weight. Chickens had reduced weight gains after ten daily doses of 100 mg/kg body wieght.

MSMA is recommended at 2 lbs per acre, DSMA at 3 lbs per acre, and cacodylic acid at 8 lbs per acre. It was concluded that if these arsenicals were applied at the recommended rate, MSMA would be hazardous for cattle but not sheep and chickens; and DSMA and cacodylic acid would be hazardous for cattle and sheep but not chickens. (Palmer, 1972)

Mechanism of Action

Soluble forms of arsenic, such as sodium arsenite, are readily absorbed from all body surfaces. Arsenic trioxide and other less soluble arsenicals are poorly absorbed from the digestive tract and are largely excreted unchanged in the feces. Once absorbed, pentavalent arsenic is readily excreted by the kidneys, whereas trivalent arsenic is more readily excreted into the intestine via the bile.

Is is generally considered that regardless of whether an arsenical is introduced into the body as trivalent or pentavalent arsenic, all the major actions can be attributed to the trivalent form. All arsenicals are believed ultimately to exert their effects by reacting with sulfhydryl groups in cells:

$$R-As=O + 2\ R'SH \longrightarrow R-As\begin{array}{c} SR' \\ \diagdown \\ SR' \end{array} + H_2O$$

As a result, sulfhydryl enzyme systems essential to cellular metabolism are inhibited. Thus, the net effect is the blocking of fat and carbohydrate metabolism and cellular respiration. The affinity of trivalent arsenic for the $-SH$ radical provides the rationale for the use of dimercaprol (BAL) as a specific antidote. The thioarsenite formed by the reaction between dimercaprol and arsenic provides for its rapid removal from tissue and excretion by the kidneys. The arsenate or pentavalent ion is capable of uncoupling phosphorylation. The importance of this phenomenon is not known, although it could account for some of the effects on peripheral nerves and spinal cord reported in humans. Arsine (AsH_3), a highly toxic industrial gas, combines with hemoglobin and is oxidized to a hemolytic compound that does not appear to act by sulfhydryl inhibition.

Arsenic affects those tissues rich in oxidative systems, primarily the alimentary tract, kidney, liver, lung, and epidermis. It is a potent capillary poison; and although injury involves all beds, the splanchnic area is the most commonly affected. Capillary damage and dilatation results in transudation of plasma into the intestinal tract and sharply reduced blood volume. Blood pressure usually falls to shock levels, and heart muscle becomes depressed contributing to circulatory failure. The capillary transudation of plasma results in vesicles and edema of the gastrointestinal mucosa, eventually leading to epithelial sloughing and discharge of the plasma into the gastrointestinal tract.

Toxic arsenic nephrosis is commonly seen in small animals and man. Capillaries in the glomeruli dilate, allowing the escape of plasma which results in swelling and varying degrees of tubular degeneration. The anhydremia resulting from the loss of fluid through other capillary beds and low blood pressure contribute to oliguria characteristic of arsenic poisoning. The urine usually contains protein, red blood cells, and casts.

Following percutaneous exposure, capillary dilatation and degeneration may result in blistering and edema, after which the skin may become dry and papery. At this latter stage, the skin may crack and bleed, providing a choice spot for secondary invaders.

While most textbooks report that arsenic is accumulated in the tissues and slowly excreted, this phenomenon appears to be true only in rats. Most species of livestock and pet animals apparently rapidly excrete arsenic. (Peoples, 1964) This phenomenon is very important when one considers arsenic levels in tissues as a means of confirming suspected poisoning. Experience with field cases in the Veterinary Diagnostic Laboratory, Iowa State University, indicates that if an animal lives several days after consuming a toxic level of arsenic, liver and kidney tissues may be below the level ordinarily considered diagnostic. Other laboratories have reported similar findings. (Moxham and Coup, 1968)

Many of the trivalent organic arsenicals such as thiacetarsamide and arsphenamine apparently act similarly to inorganic arsenicals in poisoning the intracellular sulfhydryl systems. Poisoning by these compounds results in a syndrome very similar to that produced by the inorganic arsenicals. The pentavalent arsenical herbicides DSMA and MSMA apparently also have actions similar to inorganic arsenicals.

Clinical Signs

Peracute and acute episodes of poisoning by inorganic arsenic are usually explosive with high morbidity and mortality over a two to three-day period. Symptoms are manifested by intense abdominal pain, staggering gait, extreme weakness, trembling, salivation, vomition (in dogs, cats, pigs, and perhaps even cattle), diarrhea, fast feeble pulse, prostration, rumen atony, normal to subnormal temperature, collapse, and death.

In subacute arsenic poisoning, animals may live for several days exhibiting depression, anorexia, watery diarrhea, increased urination at first followed by anuria, dehydration, thirst, partial paralysis of the rear limbs, trembling, stupor, cold extremities, subnormal temperature, and death. The watery diarrhea may contain shreds of intestinal mucosa and blood. Convulsive seizures have been reported but are not a usual manifestation. Poisoning resulting from arsenical dips usually results in some of the signs noted previously, in addition to blistering and edema of the skin followed by cracking and bleeding with associated secondary infection.

Chronic arsenical poisoning is rarely seen in most domestic animals but has been well documented in man. Reports of chronic arsenic poisoning indicate that a general wasting and unthriftiness with accompanied rough hair coat and brick red coloration of visible mucous membranes are the principle clinical signs seen.

In cases of poisoning by the toxic gas arsine, acute anemia and hemolysis occur in addition to other characteristic signs of arsenic poisoning. (Levinsky et al., 1970)

Small animals, especially dogs, suffering from thiacetarsamide poisoning exhibit vomiting and a diarrhea within twenty-four hours of intravenous administration. The diarrhea may be projectile and vary in color from reddish to black. The animals usually are listless, depressed, anoretic, and severely dehydrated. Renal damage resulting in oliguria is usually followed by death. Occasionally, a dog suffering from thiacetarsamide poisoning will exhibit gastric tympany, nonproductive retching, and terminal shock. (Hoskins, 1972)

In man, the trivalent organic arsenicals affect the circulatory system, gastrointestinal tract, kidneys, skin, and nervous system, much like the inorganic arsenicals. A polyneuritis has been described which may be similar to that seen in swine and poultry poisoned by the phenylarsonic acids. (Harvey, 1966)

Clinical signs of poisoning by the organic arsenical herbicides MSMA, DSMA, and cacodylic acid in cattle and sheep were anorexia, hematuria, diarrhea, and depression. Chickens exhibited only reduced weight gains.

Physiopathology

Characteristic gross lesions associated with inorganic arsenic poisoning include reddening of the gastric mucosa (abomasum in ruminants) which may be localized or general, reddening of the small intestinal mucosa (often limited to the first few feet of the duodenum), fluid gastrointestinal contents which are sometimes foul smelling, soft yellow liver, and red edematous lungs. In peracute cases of poisoning, occasionally no gross postmortem changes are noted. The inflammation is usually followed by edema, rupture of the blood vessels, and necrosis of the mucosa and submucosa. Sometimes the necrosis progresses to perforation of either the stomach or intestine. The fluid gastrointestinal contents may contain blood and shreds of mucosa. Hemorrhages on all surfaces of the heart and on the peritoneum may occasionally be observed.

Histopathologic changes include gastrointestinal edema of the mucosa and submucosa, necrosis and sloughing of mucosal epithelium, renal tubular degeneration, hepatic fatty change and necrosis, and capillary degeneration in vascular beds of the gastrointestinal tract, skin, and other organs. In cases involving cutaneous exposure, a dry, cracked, leathery, peeling skin may be a prominent feature.

The urine of poisoned animals will often contain

protein, red blood cells, and casts. The arsenic level in the urine varies with the form of arsenic, route of exposure, and species but usually ranges from 2-100 ppm.

In peracute, acute, and subacute poisoning, arsenic tends to be concentrated in the liver and kidneys. Normal animals usually have a background level of arsenic in these tissues of less than 0.5 ppm. Animals dying of acute or subacute arsenic poisoning may contain from 2-100 ppm arsenic on a wet-weight basis in these two organs with the kidney usually having a higher concentration than the liver. Certainly, levels above 10 ppm would be confirmatory of arsenic poisoning.

Postmortem lesions associated with poisoning by organic arsenical herbicides MSMA, DSMA, and cacodylic acid include inflammation, hemorrhages, and edema of the gastrointestinal mucosa in cattle and sheep. (Palmer, 1972) Organic arsenicals used as therapeutic agents in man such as arsphenamine and organic compounds such as thiacetarsamide used for the treatment of heartworms in dogs also produce lesions characteristic of those produced by inorganic arsenicals.

Diagnosis

Whenever an episode of illness occurs that is characterized by rapid onset and gastroenteritis, with only minor signs of central nervous system involvement, resulting in weakness, prostration, and rapid death, inorganic or aliphatic organic arsenical poisoning should be considered. The diagnosis is further substantiated by finding excessive fluid in the gastrointestinal tract together with varying degrees of inflammation and necrosis of the gastrointestinal mucosa. Liver, kidney, stomach and intestinal contents, and urine should be obtained for arsenic analysis. A modified Gutzeit method has worked well. (Buck, 1969) This method involves the dry ashing in a muffle furnace or digestion of wet tissue in nitric-perchloric-sulfuric acid, and utilizing an arsine generator and silver diethyl dithiocarbamate arsenic-sensitive color reagent.

Depending upon many factors as mentioned above, renal tissue and oftentimes hepatic tissue will contain greater than 8 ppm arsenic on a wet-weight basis in acute poisoning. If several days have elapsed since exposure, however, the liver and kidney tissue may contain only 2-4 ppm. Levels of arsenic in gastrointestinal contents and urine may range from 2-100 ppm and will also aid in determining the route and degree of arsenic exposure.

Diseases frequently confused with arsenic poisoning, especially in the ruminant, include hypomagnesemia (grass tetany); urea poisoning; organophosphorus insecticide poisoning; bovine virus diarrhea (mucosal disease complex); and poisoning from plants containing nitrates, cyanide, oxalates, selenium, or alkaloids. Sometimes lead poisoning in the bovine results in sudden death and could be confused with arsenic poisoning. However, in most instances central nervous system signs are more prominent in lead poisoning such as blindness, circling, depression, and convulsive seizures.

Conditions which may be easily confused with arsenic poisoning in dogs and cats include other heavy metal intoxications, such as thallium, mercury, and lead, and ethylene glycol poisoning. Arsenic poisoning is considerably more acute than the syndromes associated with other heavy metals. Enteric infections, which cause vomiting, diarrhea, and collapse, can also resemble arsenic poisoning.

Treatment

The key to successful treatment of inorganic and aliphatic organic arsenical poisoning is early diagnosis. Even so, the prognosis should be heavily guarded. In the ruminant and horse, which do not readily vomit, large doses of saline purgative in an attempt to remove the unabsorbed material from the GI tract may be indicated. Demulcents may be given to coat the irritated gastrointestinal mucous membrane. Sodium thiosulfate should be given orally and intravenously. Adult horses and cattle should be given 20-30 grams orally in approximately 300 ml of water and 8-10 grams in the form of a 10-20 percent solution intravenously. Sheep and goats should receive about one-fourth of this amount. British Anti-Lewisite (BAL) is a sulfhydryl containing specific antidote for trivalent arsenic. Its value as a therapeutic agent for arsenic poisoning in large animals is questionable. Disappointing therapeutic results with this compound in large animals may be because veterinarians have not repeated the treatment every four hours for the first two days, four times on the third day, and twice daily for the next ten days until recovery is complete, as has been recommended. BAL should be given in a 5 percent mixture in a 10 percent solution of benzyl benzoate in arachis oil at a rate of 3 mg/kg body weight I.M. (Clarke and Clarke, 1967) It is important to give supportive therapy such as electrolytes to replace body fluids and to provide plenty of drinking water.

In small animals, if there is an opportunity for treatment early in the course of the syndrome, the stomach should be emptied before the arsenic can pass into the intestine and be absorbed. Gastric lavage with warm water or a 1 percent solution of sodium bicarbonate is preferred, although emetics such as apomorphine may be used early in the treatment regimen. When signs of arsenic poisoning are already present, gastric lavages or emetics should not be used. BAL should be given intramuscularly at a dosage of 3 mg/kg body weight three times daily until recovery. Fluids should be administered parenterally to rehydrate animals which have been vomiting or had diarrhea. If uremia has developed, lactated Ringer's solution should be used; B-complex vitamins may be added to the Ringer's solution. Following rehydration, 20 ml/kg body weight of 10 percent dextrose solution should be administered, and this should result in diuresis. The urinary bladder should be catheterized to determine the rate of urine flow. If flow increases considerably following the administration of 10 percent dextrose and the urine contains considerable sugar, the uremia may be controlled by alternately administering lactated Ringer's solution and 5-10 percent dextrose. If acidosis is present, 50 percent sodium lactate may be added to the lactated Ringer's solution at the rate of 2.5-5.0 ml/1,000 ml.

Protein hydrolysates may be added to supply amino acids, but they must be given slowly to avoid inducing more vomiting. B-complex vitamin should be injected daily, and whole blood should be transfused when indicated by the occurrence of anemia or shock.

There should be no effort to administer drugs or food orally during the period that the animal is vomiting. When emesis has stopped, kaolin-pectin preparations can be given orally to aid in controlling diarrhea. Antibiotics are indicated to prevent secondary infections, and meperidine should be given as needed to lessen abdominal pain. As improvement occurs, a high protein, low residue diet should be fed and other supportive therapy discontinued.

Case History 1

A farmer had 75 head of heifers and steers which he had raised and to which he was feeding poor quality hay in a 25 acre lot. Very little other forage was available. In this lot there were various types of junk and rubbish, including old batteries, bags of fertilizer, antifreeze, paint cans, and wornout farm machinery. In addition, a bag of Johnson grass killer labelled ANVAR was accessible to the animals. Their source of water was a pond. Seven of the 75 animals died acutely; most were found dead. Clinical signs observed included depression, droopy ears, weakness, and recumbency. Some had a black diarrhea. After becoming recumbent, the animals were unable to rise and death ensued within twelve to twenty-four hours. Postmortem changes included severe inflammation of the mucosa of the rumen, reticulum, abomasum, and the cranial portion of the small intestine. The stomach and intestinal contents were very fluid. There was edema of the stomach walls and some straw-colored fluid in the abdominal cavity.

Since the clinical signs, postmortem changes, and course of events were compatible with inorganic arsenic

poisoning specimens from two animals were analyzed for arsenic:

| | Elemental Arsenic (PPM) | |
Specimen	Animal 1	Animal 2
Liver	12.8	18.2
Kidney	42.5	60.0
Spleen	not analyzed	9.6

A diagnosis of arsenic poisoning was made on the basis of clinical signs, postmortem findings, and chemical analyses of the liver and kidney. The source of arsenic in this case was not definitely established. However, AN-VAR grass killer contained sodium arsenite and was certainly a probable source of poisoning in this case.

Case History 2

The backyards of several homes in West Des Moines, Iowa, adjoined to form a small, one to two-acre pasture in which several of the families maintained pleasure horses. One of the backyard lawns was treated with a crabgrass control formulation containing, in addition to other ingredients, 47 percent arsenic trioxide and 3.5 percent arsenate of lead. Approximately three weeks later after several rains and after the lawn had been watered, the grass was clipped with a lawn mower and the clippings thrown over the fence to the horses. The horses readily ate the clippings and five died within a period of four days.

Clinical signs included weakness, depression, profuse diarrhea, icterus, extreme dehydration, prostration, and death. Postmortem changes included ecchymotic hemorrhages on the peritoneum, pleura, and epicardia. The mucous membranes in all horses had a muddy, brownish appearance. There was a severe hyperemia of the mucosa of the stomachs and small intestines. The large intestines were filled with fluid and were greatly distended. Finely chopped green grass was found in the stomachs of all the horses. In some horses, free blood was present in the small intestine, while in other horses there was only a severe hyperemia of the gastrointestinal mucosa. In one horse, the gastrointestinal mucosa was fibronecrotic.

Specimens obtained from two horses were analyzed for arsenic content. The results were as follows:

| | Elemental Arsenic (PPM) | |
Specimen	Horse 1	Horse 2
Liver	21.6	21.0
Kidney	21.6	24.0
Stomach Contents	>2,000	>2,000
Grass Clippings (composite of 3 piles)	>60,000	

Case History 3

An eight-year-old, 70-lb Doberman male dog was submitted to a veterinary hospital with a history of other dogs in the kennel having heartworms. Microfilaria were found in the peripheral blood. Other hematologic parameters were within the normal range.

It was decided that he should be treated for heartworms using thiacetarsamide at the rate of 1/10 ml of 1 percent solution per pound of body weight twice a day for two days (1.6 mg/kg total). He was given the recommended dosage intravenously in the morning and in the afternoon of the first day. The second injection was given about 4:30 p.m. By 7 p.m. the first day the dog was bloating severely and could be relieved by the passing of a stomach tube. He also began vomiting and continued with a nonproductive retching for several hours. The bloat continued as he continued to retch. His condition had worsened by 9 p.m. and appeared to be entering a state of shock. A laparotomy was performed revealing a stomach the size of a basketball. It was incised revealing a very friable stomach wall with hemorrhagic mucosal and serosal surfaces. The gas was removed from the stomach along with approximately two cups of food. The stomach was sutured to the abdominal wall and incision closed. Supportive therapy included intravenous fluids (lactated Ringer's), intravenous antibiotics, vitamin B-complex, and corticosteroids. The next morning the dog was improved, and recovery was uneventful within one week. The day following the arsenical treatment, the serum glutamic pyruvic transaminase activity was 4,500 Sigma-Frankel units. (Hoskins, 1972)

REFERENCES

Buck, W. B. 1969. Laboratory Toxicologic Tests and Their Interpretation. *JAVMA* 155: 1928-41.

Chisolm, J. J. 1970. Poisoning Due to Heavy Metals. *Pediat. Clin. N. A.* 17:591-615.

Clarke, E. G. C., and Clarke, M. L. 1967. *Garner's Veterinary Toxicology.* 3rd ed. Baltimore: The Williams & Wilkins Co. pp. 44-54.

Harvey, S. E. 1966. Heavy Metals. In *The Pharmacological Basis of Therapeutics.* 3rd ed. L. S. Goodman and A. Gilman, eds. New York: The Macmillan Co., pp. 944-51

Hoskins, J. 1972. Thiacetarsamide Poisoning in Dogs. Personal communication. Asst. Prof., Dept. of Vet. Clin. Sci., College of Vet. Med., I.S.U., Ames, Iowa.

Levinsky W. J.; Smalley, R. V.; Hillyer, P. N.; and Shindler, R. L. 1970. Arsine Hemolysis. *Arch. Environ. Health.* 20:436-40.

Moxham, J. W., and Coup, M. R. 1968. Arsenic Poisoning of Cattle and Other Domestic Animals. *N. Z. Vet. Jour.* 16:161-65.

Otto, G. F., and Marin, T. H. 1950. Studies on the Chemotherapy of Filariasis, Parts V-VIII. *Am. J. Hyg.* 51:353-95.

Palmer, J. S. 1972. Toxicity of 45 Organic Herbicides to Cattle, Sheep and Chickens. USDA-ARS Prod. Res. Rep. No. 137:22-23.

Peoples, S. A. 1964. Arsenic Toxicity in Cattle. *N. Y. Acad. Sci.* 111:644-49.

Reagor, J. C. 1972. Misleading Positive Arsenic Reactions. Personal Communication. Texas Veterinary Medical Diagnostic Laboratory, College Station, Texas.

Radeleff, R. D. 1970. *Veterinary Toxicology.* Philadelphia: Lea & Febiger pp158-61.

SUPPLEMENTAL REFERENCES

Buck, W. B. 1969. Pesticides and Economic Poisons in the Food Chain. Proc. 73rd Ann. Meet., U. S. Anim. Health Assoc. pp. 221-26.

———. 1970. Diagnosis of Feed-Related Toxicoses. *JAVMA* 156:1434-43.

Byron, W. R.; Bierbower, G. W.; Brouwer, J. B; and Hansen, W. H. 1965. Pathologic Changes in Rats and Dogs from Two-Year Feeding of Sodium Arsenite and Sodium Arsenate. *Tox. Appl. Pharm.* 10:132-47.

Done, A. K., and Peart, A. J. 1971. Acute Toxicities of Arsenical Herbicides. *Clin. Tox.* 4:343-55

Hatch, R. C. 1969. Inorganic Arsenic Levels in Tissues and Ingesta of Poisoned Cattle: An Eight-Year Study. *Canadian Vet. J.* 10:117-20.

Hood, R. D., and Bishop, S. L. 1972. Teratogenic Effects of Sodium Arsenate in Mice. *Arch. Environ. Health.* 24:62-65.

Moeschlin, S. 1965. *Poisoning Diagnosis and Treatment* 1st Amer. ed. New York: Grune & Stratton pp. 162-73.

Schroeder, H. A.; Kanisawa, M.; Frost, D. V.; and Mitchener, M. 1968. Germanium, Tin and Arsenic in Rats: Effects on Growth, Survival, Pathological Lesions and Life Span. *J. Nutr.* 96:37-45.

Teitelbaum, D. T., and Kier, L. C. 1969. Arsine Poisoning. *Arch. Environ. Health* 19:133-43.

Vallee, B. L.; Ulmer, D. D.; and Wacher, W. E. C. 1960. Arsenic Toxicology and Biochemistry. *A. M. A. Archs. Ind. Health* 121:132-51.

ARSENIC II:
PHENYLARSONIC COMPOUNDS

Poisoning by phenylarsonic compounds is usually manifested by a syndrome that is distinctly different from that produced by inorganic, aliphatic and trivalent organic arsenicals. In general, they are also less hazardous to mammals.

Source

Organic arsenical formulations have been used as animal feed additives for disease control and improvement of weight gain in swine and poultry since the mid-1940s. These compounds, of which there are four, are phenylarsonic acids and their salts. Their structural formulas are given in figure 1.

The most widely used compounds include arsanilic acid and its salt, sodium arsanilate, and 3-nitro-4-hydroxyphenylarsonic acid. Other organic arsenical feed additives include 4-nitro-phenylarsonic acid, and p-ureido-benzenearsonic acid. (Baron, 1969; Feed Additives Compendium, 1975) These compounds are all considered to improve weight gain, feed efficiency, and to aid in the prevention and control of certain enteric diseases of swine and poultry. (Frost, 1967; Morehouse and Mayfield, 1946; Morehouse, 1949; Bird et al., 1949; Buck, 1969b)

The registered uses of the phenylarsonic feed additives are given in table 1. (Feed Additive Compendium, 1975) Arsanilic acid and sodium arsanilate are recommended at 50-100 ppm (0.005-0.01%) in swine and poultry feeds for increased weight gains and improvement of feed efficiency. They are recommended at 250-400 ppm (0.025-0.04%) in swine feed for a duration of five to six days for the control of swine dysentery.

Toxicity

The margin of safety for arsanilic acid and its salt is quite wide in normal animals. However, the effective level and the chronically toxic level may impinge upon one another under certain conditions. The health status of the exposed animals and management practices, especially those involving availability of water, are important contributing factors for adverse reactions resulting from the addition of organic arsenicals to feed. Animals suffering with a diarrhea are usually dehydrated and, thus, are excreting very little urine. Since these arsenicals are excreted via the kidneys, their toxicity becomes greatly increased when given to animals with diarrhea. Usually the morbidity is high and mortality very low. Experimentally, clinical signs appear after three to ten days of exposure to high levels in the feed (1,000 ppm) and within three to six weeks on lower levels (250 ppm). (Buck et al., 1973)

The maximum safe dietary level of arsanilic acid for

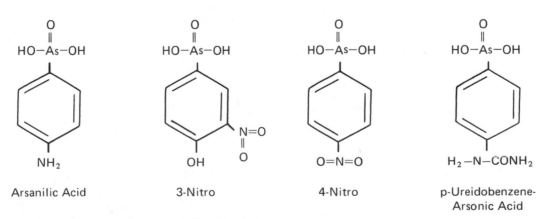

Figure 1. Structural formulas of phenylarsonic compounds.

TABLE 1
Arsenicals Used as Feed Additives

Arsenical	Level in Complete Feed, %	Species	Value
Arsanilic acid	0.005-0.01	Broilers	Increase rate of gain and feed efficiency
		Growing turkeys	Improve pigmentation
		Laying hens	Improve egg production
		Swine	Increase rate of gain and improve feed efficiency
			Prevent swine dysentery
	0.025-0.04	Chickens (up to 8 days)	Prevent coccidiosis
		Swine (5-6 days)	Control swine dysentery
3-nitro-4-hydroxy-phenylarsonic acid	0.0025-0.005	Chickens and turkeys	Growth promotion and improved feed efficiency
	0.0025-0.0075	Swine	Growth promotion and improved feed efficiency
	0.02	Swine	Control swine dysentery
4-nitrophenylarsonic acid	0.01875	Growing turkeys and chickens	Aid in prevention of blackhead
p-ureidobenzenearsonic acid	0.0375	Growing turkeys	Prevent blackhead and increase rate of gain

young turkeys to twenty-eight days of age was reported to be between 300-400 ppm (0.03-0.04%). (Al-Timimi and Sullivan, 1972)

Roxarsone or "3-nitro" is recommended at 25-50 ppm (0.0025-0.005%) for chickens and turkeys and at 25-75 ppm (0.0025-0.0075%) for swine for improving weight gains and feed efficiency. It is also recommended at a level of 200 ppm (0.02%) for five to six days for the control of swine dysentery. (Feed Additive Compendium, 1975) Swine may exhibit clinical signs after consuming 250 ppm in the feed for three to ten days, and have been chronically poisoned on 3-nitro at 100 ppm for two months. (Buck, 1969a,b)

The compound 4-nitrophenylarsonic acid ("4-nitro") has been recommended for chickens and turkeys at 188 ppm for the improvement of weight gains and feed efficiency. It has not been recommended for ducks or geese and, at the present time, has only limited use as a feed additive. Para-ureido-benzenearsonic acid is recommended for the prevention and control of blackhead in turkeys at 250-375 ppm in the feed.

Arsanilic acid and arsanilate are more commonly used as a swine feed additive. Toxicoses may occur, however, with any of the formulations in any of the species. The circumstances usually associated with tox-

icoses by the organic arsenicals used as a feed additive include:

1. Unwisely incorporating excessive levels in feed or water. (Ledet et al., 1973)
2. Mistaken feed formulation resulting in excessive levels.
3. Prolonged and excessive administration in combination with other drugs.
4. Treating animals with a severe diarrhea and debilitation, thus having increased susceptibility because of reduced renal excretion of the arsenical.
5. Limiting the water supply to animals being exposed to therapeutic levels of organic arsenic. (Buck et al., 1973) Vorhies et al., 1969)

Poisoning by organic arsenicals in swine is not uncommon and probably is second only to water deprivation-sodium ion toxicity in frequency of occurrence. (Ledet et al., 1973)

Mechanism of Action

The arsenic cation incorporated in the various organic formulations may be either in the trivalent or pentavalent form. Those in the trivalent form are usually referred to as arsenoso compounds, whereas those in the pentavalent form are termed arsonic acids.

There is still considerable discussion regarding the exact mode of action of the organic arsenicals. However, it seems certain that the phenylarsonic compounds have a different action to that of inorganic and aliphatic organic arsenicals. The arsenic incorporated in the various organic formulations is in the pentavalent form. It is likely that they have their primary action as pentavalent arsenicals, which may account for their characteristic rapid renal excretion.

There have been several postulations with regard to the possible therapeutic and nutritional effects of organic arsenical feed additives. We know that certain organisms cause a thickening of the intestinal wall and that the arsenicals inhibit these organisms by interfering with their enzyme systems. Another theory is that the arsenicals, by interfering with the development of the bacterial cell wall or by the inhibition of normal cellular production of proteins and nucleic acids, lower the harmful bacterial population. Yet another possibility is that this type of compound may have a sparing action on one or more of the essential nutrients required by the growing animal. (Baron, 1969)

Some workers have suggested that both the toxicity and efficacy of these compounds are due to their degradation and reduction to inorganic trivalent forms. (Harvey, 1966; Eagle and Doak, 1951; Voegtlin and Thompson, 1923) Eagle and Doak (1951) reported that arsenoso compounds have direct activity, while arsonic acid compounds became active by virtue of their conversion to arsenoso compounds in the animal body. More recent work, however, clearly established that arsanilic acid and acetylarsonic acid were excreted unchanged by chickens and that there is no evidence that these compounds are changed to any other compound or converted to inorganic arsenic. (Crawford and Levvy, 1947; Moody and Williams, 1964a; Overby and Fredrickson, 1963, 1965; Overby and Straube, 1965) Similar results were obtained in studies with "3-nitro" and "4-nitro" in chickens. Similar experiments by other workers with rats, rabbits, and swine indicate that the phenylarsonic acids for the most part are excreted unchanged by the kidneys, although some apparently undergo a limited amount of biotransformation. (Moody and Williams, 1964b and 1964c)

Since pentavalent arsenic compounds do not react with sulfhydryl groups and since the phenylarsonic acids are apparently excreted unchanged, then one must conclude that the mechanism of their action is by a method other than by interaction with sulfhydryl-containing enzymes and proteins. Since the predominant lesions produced by these compounds in swine and poultry are

peripheral nerve demyelination and gliosis, it has been postulated that the phenylarsonic acids may act to produce a vitamin B-complex deficiency, such as B_6 or B_1. (Buck *et al.,* 1973) This postulation has not been studied experimentally.

When the phenylarsonic compounds are injected parenterally, they are mostly excreted in the urine within twenty-four to forty-eight hours. When they are given orally, a considerable percentage is excreted in the feces, indicating that they are poorly absorbed by the intestinal tract. That proportion which is absorbed, however, apparently is excreted rapidly by the kidneys. (Overby and Fredrickson, 1965; Moody and Williams, 1964a,b,c; Baron, 1969)

Clinical Signs

Acute clinical signs may appear after three to five days of exposure to high levels of phenylarsonic compounds in the feed. Signs include incoordination, inability to control body and limb movements, and ataxia. After a few days, swine and poultry may become paralyzed but will continue to eat and drink (fig. 2). Arsanilic acid and its sodium salt may produce blindness, but this effect rarely is seen with "3-nitro." Erythema of the skin, especially in white animals, and sensitivity to sunlight may also be observed. The clinical signs are reversible up to a certain point. Removing the excess arsenical will result in recovery within a few days unless the clinical signs have progressed to partial or complete paralysis resulting from peripheral nerve degeneration. (Buck *et al.,* 1973; Oliver and Roe, 1957)

Chronic poisoning occurs in swine and poultry when excessive but lower levels of phenylarsonic compounds

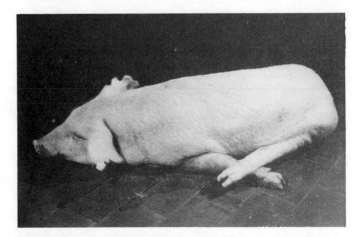

Figure 2. Pig with advanced quadriplegia manifested by nearly total lack of muscle control in the limbs. The pig has been fed arsanilic acid (1,000 ppm) for 15 days. (From Buck, 1969b).

are given in the feed or water for periods of three to six weeks or longer. Animals will continue to eat and drink and remain alert while progressively developing blindness and partial paralysis of the extremities. The onset of signs are usually insidious and therefore, not alarming to the herdsman. Goose-stepping, knuckling of the hock joints, and other manifestations of abnormal locomotion occur. Usually such animals have poor weight gain and food efficiency.

Poultry usually become incoordinated and ataxic after consuming excessive levels of "3-nitro" but more commonly exhibit ruffled feathers, anorexia, depression, coma, and death when exposed to excessive levels of arsanilic acid or sodium arsanilate. (Harding et al., 1968; Buck, 1969a, 1969b; Ledet, 1970; Menges, et al., 1970)

Calves dosed with toxic levels of arsanilic acid exhibit gastrointestinal signs similar to those produced by inorganic arsenic poisoning. They are more resistant, however, to organic arsenic in the feed. Levels up to 500 ppm and greater have been fed for several weeks without producing harmful effects. (Buck, 1969a)

Physiopathology

Postmortem findings in swine and poultry affected with organic arsenicals have no gross changes except for skin erythema in white pigs and muscle atrophy in chronic cases. (Buck, 1969a, 1969b) Harding et al., (1968) reported abnormal distension of the urinary bladders in pigs poisoned on arsanilic acid.

Detectable histopathologic changes in swine and poultry are confined to the optic tracts, optic nerves,

and peripheral nerves. Major lesions noted are necrosis of myelin-supporting cells, degeneration of myelin sheaths and axons, and gliosis of affected tracts (fig. 4). Damage is first seen after about six to ten days of feeding on excessive arsenical and is characterized by fragmentation of the myelin into granules and globules followed several days later by breaking up of the axons. There is an obvious increase in the severity of the lesions with the progression of the toxic syndrome. No microscopic changes are seen in the brain, cord, kidneys, liver, or other organ systems. (Harding et al., 1968; Ledet, 1970)

Excretion and Recommended Withdrawal Time

In general, the phenylarsonics are rapidly excreted by the urinary system in domestic animals and poultry. Once they are absorbed from the gastrointestinal tract, 50-75 percent are excreted within a 24-hour period. Excretion of the remaining 25 percent is greatly reduced and may take up to eight or ten days. (Moody and Williams, 1964a,b,c; Ledet, 1970) Although nervous tissue tends to accumulate relatively low levels of the phenylarsonic compounds, their excretion rate from this tissue appears to be relatively slow, less than 50 percent excretion after eleven days of withdrawal. (Ledet, 1970)

Ledet (1970) measured arsenic content of various organs from swine following their consumption of 1,000 ppm arsanilic acid in the diet (10 times the recommended level for continuous feeding for improving weight gains and feed efficiency) for nineteen days. The results are presented in table 2.

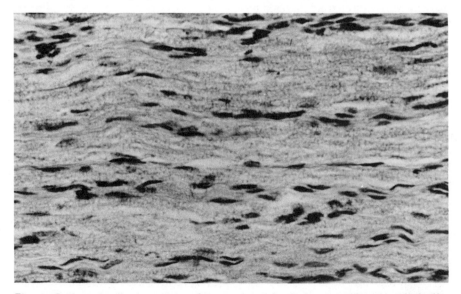

Figure 3. Longitudinal section of a portion of sciatic nerve from a clinically normal pig. Notice the feathery appearance of normal myelin. H & E stain x 250. (From Buck, 1969b).

TABLE 2

Specimen	Control	Days After Arsanilic Acid Withdrawal[a] (ppm Elemental Arsenic on Wet-Weight Basis)*			
		0	3	6	11
Kidney	< 0.02	8.33	2.90	2.24	1.90
Liver	< 0.02	9.67	3.10	1.65	1.75
Muscle	N[b]	0.92	0.29	0.29	0.31
Blood	< 0.02	1.94	0.25	0.19	0.45
Rib	N	0.46	0.18	0.24	0.08
Peripheral nerve	< 0.02	1.57	1.17	1.06	0.61
Spinal cord	< 0.02	0.74	0.76	0.80	0.25
Brain stem	< 0.02	1.04	0.90	0.91	0.62
Cerebellum	< 0.02	1.23	1.58	1.10	0.85
Cerebrum	N	0.82	1.09	0.84	0.51

*Adapted from Ledet et al., 1973.

[a]Control = mean of 3 animals; 0 = mean of 3 animals; and 3, 6, and 11 = mean of 2 animals each.

[b]Negative to test.

Evans and Bandemer (1954) measured the arsenic content of eggs from hens fed diets containing 100 and 200 ppm of arsanilic acid for ten weeks and found levels below the tolerance, established by the FDA, of 0.5 ppm.

Baron (1969) reported on the accumulation and depletion of arsenic in tissues of chickens fed a ration containing 50 parts per million (0.005%) 3-nitro-4-hydroxyphenylarsonic acid. Medication was started when the chickens were four weeks old and the birds were killed at 1, 2, 3, 4, 5, 7, 9, 11, 14, 28, 56, and 70 days of medication, and on day 1 through 14 after withdrawal of medication. Five birds of each sex from both the medicated and nonmedicated groups were killed on the days indicated. The arsenic levels found in kidney, liver, muscle, and skin are presented in table 3.

Federal Food and Drug Administration regulations require that all labels of feeds containing any of the four phenylarsonic compounds have a warning statement that such feed must be withdrawn from swine and poultry five days prior to slaughter. A tolerance of 2.0 ppm elemental arsenic has been set for uncooked swine liver and kidney tissues, and 0.5 ppm in uncooked pork muscle, edible chicken and turkey tissue and eggs.

Diagnosis

Diagnosis of organic arsenical poisoning in swine and poultry can be made tentatively on the basis of the characteristic signs of wobbly, incoordinated gait and ataxia. Animals and birds evidencing paralysis of the extremities without central nervous system involvement, high morbidity with low mortality, continuing to eat and drink if food and water are made available, especially swine, and upon postmortem examination evidencing little or no gross changes should be suspected of having been exposed to excessive levels of organic arsenical.

Levels of arsenic in tissue are rarely diagnostic since the organic arsenicals are excreted unmetabolized by the kidneys. If the animal has not been eating for three to five days, the arsenical will have been excreted from the

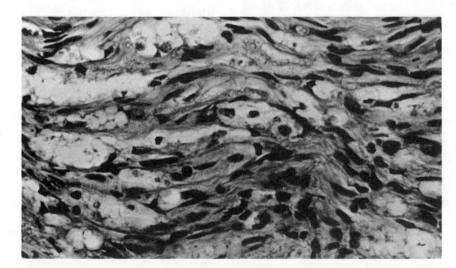

Figure 4. Longitudinal section of a portion of sciatic nerve from a paralyzed pig that was poisoned on excessive arsanilic acid in the feed. Extensive myelin degeneration is evident. Notice interruption of nerve fibers by vacuolated areas where myelin breakdown is taking place. H & E stain x 250. (From Buck, 1969b).

TABLE 3
Summation of Arsenic Levels in ppm Found in Chicken Tissues

Days									
On test	1	7	56	70	71	75	80	84	
On medication	1	7	56	70	—	—	—	—	
Off medication	—	—	—	—	1	5	10	14	Nonmedicated
Kidney	.93	.76	.52	.64	.22	.10	.09	.08	.05
Liver	1.31	2.43	1.26	1.26	.69	.43	.32	.19	.08
Muscle	.03	.07	.05	.04	.03	.01	.02	.02	.02
Skin	.05	.11	.06	.05	.08	.02	.03	.03	.02

body tissue for the most part and will not be of diagnostic significance. If liver and kidney specimens are obtained from animals which have been on feed containing excessive levels of organic arsenical, 3-10 ppm arsenic on a wet-weight basis would have diagnostic significance. Blood levels of 1-2 ppm would also be diagnostically significant. A more important diagnostic procedure is determining the level of organic arsenical or arsenic in the feed. (Buck, 1969a) Levels of 250 and 100 ppm arsanilic acid and 3-nitro, respectively, should be viewed with significance if other factors such as diarrhea or limited water intake are evident in swine and poultry.

Microscopic examination of longitudinal sections of peripheral and cranial nerves is an important procedure in confirming a diagnosis of organic arsenical toxicosis in swine and poultry. It should be kept in mind, however, that demyelination and gliosis will not be evident in the optic tract prior to ten days after beginning exposure nor will these lesions be evident in sciatic and brachial nerves prior to two weeks after beginning of exposure. (Harding *et al.,* 1968; Ledet, 1970)

There are several disease and nutritional conditions that somewhat mimic organic arsenical poisoning in swine and poultry. Those that must be differentiated from organic arsenical poisoning include:

1. Vitamin B-complex deficiency, especially B_1 and B_6. These vitamin B-complex deficiencies reportedly produce peripheral and central nervous system demyelination which may be indistinguishable from that produced by the organic arsenicals.
2. Organic mercurial poisoning—Clinical signs are very similar to those produced by the organic arsenicals including incoordination and ataxia. However, central nervous system depression and derangement are usually characteristic. In mercurial poisoning the death rate is very high, and fibrinoid degeneration of the small vessels and cyton degeneration in the brain are characteristic lesions.
3. Calcium-phosphorous imbalance resulting in skeletal fractures, rickets, and other problems resulting in incoordination and ataxia.
4. Husbandry practices—especially in pigs in which there is excessive erosion of their feet on rough concrete or injury on slatted floors.
5. Water deprivation—sodium ion toxicity. This is a very common, noninfectious problem in pigs but can be differentiated from organic arsenical poisoning because of the convulsive seizures which invariably occur, high levels of cerebrospinal fluid and plasma sodium, and characteristic eosinophilic meningoencephalitis.

Treatment

The best treatment for swine and poultry being fed excessive organic arsenicals in water or feed is complete and immediate withdrawal of the arsenical. It is important to make sure that adequate drinking water is available and that the animals or birds are consuming it. A diuretic may increase the rate of renal excretion.

Case History

A farmer owned 125 feeder pigs for which he mixed home-grown grain with a commercial concentrate containing the recommended level of arsanilic acid. However, besides mixing the concentrate at the recommended level, he purchased additional arsanilic acid from the local feed store and mixed it with the feed at a rate of an estimated 0.5 lb/ton of feed. The farmer was not sure how much arsanilic acid was actually mixed with the feed.

Approximately one week after the commencement of feeding the pigs on the above mixture, the pigs became ataxic. The farmer removed the feed containing the arsanilic acid, and all but one pig recovered shortly thereafter. This pig became blind, gained poorly, developed torticollis, and at six months of age weighed about 60 lbs.

Approximately two weeks later the farmer diluted the mixture 1:1 with home-grown grain and began feeding another group of 175 pigs. Within two weeks several pigs in the second group began to show a gradual weakness of the limbs manifested by incoordination, knuckling of the pasterns, exaggerated stepping movements, and reluctance to rise. Many pigs became progressively paralyzed and unable to rise and walk. Six weeks after he began feeding the diluted mixture to the second group of pigs, approximately one-fourth of them were showing some type of incoordination and paralysis. Some were completely paralyzed, others were weak in their pelvic limbs and knuckling the pastern joints. Many pigs were blind.

Despite signs of toxicosis in his pigs, the farmer continued to feed the mixture in the belief that the problem was a mineral or vitamin deficiency. However, he supplemented the contaminated feed with another ration containing a grain mixture with no (added) arsanilic acid. The pigs, although incoordinated, continued to eat and drink normally. They gained poorly; and at six months of age, only a few had reached market size. At this time the farmer sold several for slaughter.

Four of the affected pigs were euthanatized, and postmortem examinations were performed. No gross lesions were observed except for muscle atrophy in those pigs which had been paralyzed for a considerable period of time. Histopathologic examination of the sciatic nerve, optic tracts, and brachial plexus revealed demyelination and gliosis. No changes were observed in the brain, spinal cord, or other tissues.

Samples of the feed in question contained 450 ppm of arsanilic acid, whereas the feed that was presumed to have no arsanilic acid contained 180 ppm. Thus, it can be extrapolated that the feed containing high levels of arsanilic acid and diluted 1:1 with home-grown grain originally contained at least 900 ppm. Analysis of tissues from the four pigs which were necropsied revealed less than 1 ppm arsenic in their liver, kidney, skeletal muscle, spleen, brain, bone, fat, and blood. Their stomach contents ranged from 0-5.2 ppm arsanilic acid, and their feces ranged from 1.4-149 ppm.

REFERENCES

Al-Timimi, A. A., and Sullivan, T. W. 1972. Safety and Toxicity of Dietary Organic Arsenicals Relative to Performance of Young Turkeys. *Poultry Sci.* 51:111-16.

Animal Health Institute. 1976. *Feed Additive Compendium.* Minneapolis: Miller Publishing Co.

Baron, R. R. 1969. The Use of Arsenicals in Feeding Stuffs. Proceedings of a Seminar held at the Criterion, Lower Regent Street, London, S. W. 1, March 20. London: Salsbury Laboratories.

Bird, H. R.; Groschke, A. C.; and Rubin, M. 1949. Effect of Arsonic Acid Derivatives in Stimulating Growth of Chickens. *J. Nutr.* 37:215-26.

Buck, W. B. 1969. Laboratory Toxicologic Tests and Their Interpretation. *J. Amer. Vet. Med. Assoc.* 155:1928-41.

Buck, W. B. 1969. Untoward Reactions Encountered with Medicated Feeds. *Use of Drugs in Animal Feeds, Publication 1679.* Washington, D.C.: National Academy of Sciences.

Buck, W. B; Osweiler, G. D.; and Van Gelder, G. A. 1973. *Clinical and Diagnostic Veterinary Toxicology.* Dubuque, Iowa: Kendall-Hunt Publishing Co.

Crawford, T. B. B., and Levvy, G. A. 1947. Changes Undergone by Phenylarsenious Acid and Phenylarsonic Acid in the Animal Body. *Biochem. J.* 41:333-36.

Eagle, H., and Doak, G. O. 1951. The Biological Activity of Arsenosobenzenes in Relation to Their Structure. *Pharmacol. Rev.* 3:107-43.

Evans, R. J., and Gandemer, S. 1954. Determination of Arsenic in Biologic Materials. *Anal. Chem.* 26:595-98

Frost, D. V. 1967. Arsenicals in Biology—Retrospect and Prospect. *Fed Proc.* 26:194-208.

Harvey, S. E. 1966. Heavy Metals, pp. 944-51. L. S. Goodman and A. Gilman, eds. in *The Pharmacologic Basis of Therapeutics* 3rd ed. New York: The Macmillan Company.

Harding, J. D. J.; Lewis, G.; and Done, J. T. 1968. Experimental Arsanilic Acid Poisoning in Pigs. *Vet. Rec.* 83:560-64.

Ledet, A. E. 1970. Clinical, Toxicological and Pathological Aspects of Arsanilic Acid Poisoning in Swine. Ph.D. Thesis. Ames: Iowa State University.

Menges, R. W.; Kintner, L. D.; Selby, L. A.; Stewart, R. W.; and Marionfeld, C. J. 1970. Arsanilic Acid Blindness in Pigs. *Vet. Med. Small Anim. Clin.* 65:565-68.

Morehouse, N. W. 1949. Accelerated Growth of Chickens and Turkeys Produced by 3-nitro-4-hydroxyphenylarsonic Acid. *Poultry Sci.* 28:375-84.

Moorehouse, N. W., and Mayfield, O. J. 1964. The Effect of Some Aryl Arsonic Acids on Experimental Coccidiosis. Infection of Chickens. *Parasitol.* 32:20-24.

Moody, J. P., and Williams, R. T. 1964. The Fate of Arsanilic Acid and Acetylarsanilic Acid in Hens. *Food Cosmet. Toxicol.* 2:687-93.

———. 1964. The Fate of 4-nitrophenylarsonic Acid in Hens. *Food Cosmet. Toxicol.* 2:695-706.

————. 1964. The Metabolism of 4-hydroxy-3-nitrophenylarsonic Acid in Hens. *Food Cosmet. Toxicol.* 2:707-15.

Oliver, W. T., and Roe, C. K. 1957. Arsanalic Acid Poisoning in Swine. *J. Amer. Vet. Med. Assoc.* 130:177-78.

Overby, L. R., and Fredrickson, R. L. 1965. Metabolism of Arsanilic Acid. II. Localization and Type of Arsenic Excreted and Retained by Chickens. *Tox. Appl. Pharm.* 7:855-67.

Overby, L. R., and Fredrickson, R. L. 1963. Metabolic Stability of Radioactive Arsanilic Acid in Chickens. *J. Agric. Food Chem.* 11:378-81.

Overby, L. R., and Straube, L. 1965. Metabolism of Arsanilic Acid. I. Metabolic Stability of Double-Labelled Arsanilic Acid in Chickens. *Toxicol. Appl. Pharmacol.* 7:850-54.

Voegtlin, C., and Thompson, J. W. 1923. Rate of Excretion of Arsenicals, a Factor Governing Toxicity and Parasitical Action. *J. Pharm. Exp. Therp.* 20:85-105.

Vorhies, M. W.; Sleight, S. D.; and Whitehair, C. K. 1969. Toxicity of Arsanilic Acid in Swine as Influenced by Water Intake. *Cornell Vet.* 59:3-9.

COPPER-MOLYBDENUM

Copper and molybdenum are essential elements for plants and animals, although under naturally occurring conditions uncomplicated molybdenum deficiency has never been reported in man or farm animals.

The metabolism of copper, molybdenum, and inorganic sulfate is extremely complex and interrelated. Other elements also affect this interaction; namely, manganese, zinc, and iron. (Underwood, 1971) Several excellent reviews concerning this essentiality, metabolic interrelationships and toxicity of copper have been published. (Underwood, 1971; Ammerman, 1970; Prasad et al., 1970; Dowdy, 1969; Anon. 1967; Todd, 1962; Scheinberg and Sternlieb, 1960; Marston, 1952; and Boughton and Hardy. 1934)

In mammals, a copper deficiency results in anemia and reduced hematopoiesis, cardiovascular lesions, defects in pigmentation, keratinization, bone formation, reproduction, myelination of the spinal cord, connective tissue formation and reduced growth. Chronic excess copper intake results in sudden release of copper from hepatic storage sites into the bloodstream causing hemolysis, icterus and anemia with accompanying hepatic and renal necrosis.

Since the copper-molybdenum-sulfate interaction is more prominent in ruminants than nonruminants, this discussion is separated accordingly.

RUMINANT ANIMALS

The first evidence of the relation between copper and molybdenum metabolism was obtained when it was learned that the drastic scouring disease of cattle, known as "teart," was shown to be a manifestation of chronic molybdenum poisoning and could be controlled by treating the cattle with large amounts of copper. (Ferguson et al., 1938; Underwood, 1971) Additional evidence of copper-molybdenum interaction was reported by Dick and Bull (1945) when molybdenum was found to be effective treatment for copper poisoning in sheep. From these investigations came the realization of the profound interrelationship of molybdenum and cop-

per and the dependence of this interaction upon inorganic sulfate in the diet. Subsequent investigations have quantified these interactions in ruminants. (Dick, 1953a,b; Dick, 1954; Pierson and Aanes, 1958; Cunningham et al., 1959; Kowalczyk et al., 1962; Todd, 1962; Kowalczyk et al., 1964; Goodrich and Tillman, 1966; Dowdy and Matrone, 1968a,b; Adamson and Valks, 1969; Marcilese et al., 1969; Todd, 1969; Ross, 1970; Huber et al., 1971; Underwood, 1971) These interactions are more fully discussed under the section Mechanism of Action.

Excess Copper-Deficient Molybdenum

Source

Copper toxicity and interactions of copper with other trace elements present complex and significant consequences for animal husbandry in the United States. Dietary imbalances of copper and molybdenum may result from either ad libitum consumption of mineral mixtures, or of conventional feeds that have been fortified with inappropriate mineral mixtures. (Boughton and Hardy, 1934; Kowalczyk et al., 1962, 1964; Buck and Sharma, 1969. Buck, 1970; Suveges et al., 1971) Copper is generally recognized as safe (GRAS) as a livestock feed ingredient by the Food and Drug Administration (FDA), whereas molybdenum is not. Therefore, copper is routinely and ubiquitously added to commercial trace element mixtures used in livestock feeds. Since FDA regulations do not recognize molybdenum as being an essential and safe element, its addition to such mixtures is prohibited. Unfortunately, these regulations do not recognize species differences between cattle and sheep in their requirements for a balance between copper and molybdenum. Cattle can tolerate mineral mixtures and feeds with added copper and without molybdenum, even when their natural grain and forages contain adequate levels of copper. But they are more susceptible to copper deficiency than sheep. In contrast, sheep are susceptible to the toxic effects of added copper, especially when the natural forage contains adequate levels of copper and low levels of molybdenum. Since the cattle-feeding industry is of major economic importance, and the sheep-feeding industry is not, it has not been economically feasible for manufacturers of livestock mineral mixtures to provide special formulations for sheep with the proper balance between copper and molybdenum (6-10 parts copper/1 part molybdenum).

Further complications arise because in certain areas of the United States—such as Florida and states west of the Rocky Mountains—it is not uncommon to find molybdenum-induced copper deficiencies in plants, cattle, and occasionally sheep. (Berger, 1962; Cordy, 1971; Clawson, 1972) Copper deficiences in plants and animals are unusual in most areas east of the Rocky Mountains.

Copper toxicoses in sheep are not rare in the Midwest and Great Plains states. They extend northward well into Canada. Since the levels of copper found in plants vary greatly and depend upon many factors, no general geographical distribution of copper and molybdenum levels in plants have been mapped. However, it appears that grains and forages grown in the upper Midwest and Great Plains states contain sufficient copper and are low enough in molybdenum content to make the addition of the GRAS 15 ppm copper to the total diet of sheep cause excessive accumulations of copper in the liver. In these areas, 1-5 percent of sheep consuming such feed develop hemolytic crises. Sheep may develop copper toxicosis on a diet containing a normal concentration of copper (8-10 ppm) if the molybdenum levels are below 0.5 ppm. (Hogan *et al.,* 1968) When a vitamin-mineral preparation containing copper but not molybdenum is added to a ration, the copper concentration of the ration may be elevated to 25-30 ppm or more. Since the natural molybdenum concentration in most feedstuffs is usually below 2 ppm, the copper: molybdenum ratio in the resulting diet is greater than 10:1. Over 20 episodes of chronic toxicosis in sheep were found in Iowa from June 1968—June 1970, especially in feeder lambs, show lambs, and ram lambs being tested for weight gain and feed efficiency. (Buck, unpublished data; Buck, 1970)

Causes of copper toxicosis in ruminants, in addition to dietary trace element imbalances as discussed above, include:

1. consumption of plants contaminated by copper-containing pesticides used to spray orchards, such as Bordeaux mixture with 1-3 percent copper sulfate;
2. use of copper sulfate to control helminthiasis and infectious pododermatitis in cattle and sheep;
3. contamination of soils and vegetation in the vicinity of mining and refining operations;
4. use of calcium-copper ethylenediaminetetraacetic acid as an injectable source of copper in countries where sheep frequently are subject to copper deficiency problems; (Ishmael and Gopinath, 1971, 1972)
5. confining sheep (Bracewell, 1958; Todd, 1962; Adamson and Valks, 1969) with no access to green forage containing sufficient molybdenum to prevent excessive accumulation of copper in the liver, (Todd, 1972) and
6. feeding sheep certain forage plants containing an imbalance of copper and molybdenum, or forage plants that produce hepatic necrosis, thus imparing copper metabolism.

The latter example illustrates the problems which may arise from an imbalance of copper and molybdenum in forage plants. In Australia *Trifolium subterraneum* is used extensively to raise the nitrogen level of soils, and this clover may grow abundantly because of the climatic conditions associated with an early autumn break. Since the plants contain little or no molybdenum, (Bull *et al.,* 1956; Beck and Bennetts, 1963) sheep grazing on the plants store high levels of copper in their livers and become predisposed to the hemolytic crisis of chronic copper poisoning.

In western Australia, sheep grazing on pastures containing various species of *Lupinus,* develop hepatic toxicosis from lupine alkaloids more readily in the presence of excess copper. (Gardiner, 1966, 1967) Susceptibility to copper poisoning in sheep may be enhanced by the forage. Thus, in Australia and New Zealand, plants of the *Heliotropium, Echium,* and *Senecio* genera contain pyrrolizidine alkaloids that cause hepatic necrosis; animals grazing on these plants will be unable to metabolize and excrete normal dietary levels of copper. (St. George-Grambauer and Rac, 1962; Underwood, 1971)

Toxicity

When discussing the deficiency or toxicity of copper or molybdenum, it should be understood that the interaction of these elements in the presence of inorganic sulfate makes it impossible to delineate between the toxicity of one and a deficiency of the other. Thus, copper deficiency is manifested by the same syndrome as chronic molybdenum poisoning; and chronic copper poisoning is identical to molybdenum deficiency.

If sheep, for instance, are fed a diet containing a normal concentration of copper (8-11 ppm) but with no molybdenum, copper toxicity may result. Therefore, when a vitamin-mineral preparation containing copper but no molybdenum is added to the ration, the copper concentration of the ration may be elevated to 25-30 ppm or greater; and since the natural molybdenum concentration in feed is usually low (1-2 ppm), copper poisoning may occur. Usually from 1-5 percent of a flock is affected, and over 75 percent of those clinically affected die.

Sheep are more susceptible than cattle to excess copper and deficient molybdenum in their diet. This has been shown by numerous accounts in the literature. Young calves are susceptible; but as they mature, their tolerance increases. (Todd, 1962)

In acute copper poisoning, copper chloride ($CuCl_2$) is more toxic than $CuSO_4$. Cattle are poisoned by 200-800 mg $CuSO_4$/kg body weight, and sheep are poisoned by 20-100 mg/kg single dose.

Mechanism of Action

There is evidence that copper and molybdenum form an *in vivo* complex with a molar ratio of 4:3, (Dowdy and Matrone, 1968a,1968b; Huisingh and Matrone, 1972) and that copper bound in a copper-molybdenum complex is biologically unavailable. Although this complex may not prevent intestinal absorption of copper, the copper-molybdenum complex inhibits copper accumulation in the liver. Copper may not accumulate because liver cells which take up copper become impaired, or because of a primary intracellular metabolic disturbance in the synthesis of copper proteins, including ceruloplasmin. (Marcilese *et al.*, 1969)

Moreover, copper and molybdenum, especially in ruminants, appear to interact with inorganic sulfate in the diet. (Cunningham *et al.*, 1959; Hogan *et al.*, 1968; Marcilese, *et al.*, 1969; Todd, 1969) This copper-molybdenum-sulfate interaction affects biliary and urinary excretion of copper and molybdenum. Dick (1953a) reported that increased urinary excretion of molybdenum occurs with an increased diet of inorganic sulfate, and Marcilese *et al.*, (1969, 1970) found that increased dietary levels of molybdenum and sulfate result in more urinary and biliary excretion of copper.

Huisingh and Matrone (1972) investigated the interaction of molybdate with the sulfate-reducing system in the rumen contents of sheep fed purified diets; the effect of copper on the system in the presence of molybdate was also observed. They found that molybdate inhibited the reduction of sulfate to sulfite, and that copper reduced this inhibition greatly. Molybdate inhibition of sulfate reduction increased as the concentration of sulfate decreased.

It has been suggested (Buck, 1970) that copper

added to sheep diets in the form of the sulfate is less toxic than copper added as the acetate, oxide, carbonate, gluconate, iodide, chloride, orthophosphate or pyrophosphate. Todd *et al.*, (1962) demonstrated that the acetate salt of copper was more toxic to sheep than was its sulfate salt. If it is true that copper sulfate is less toxic to sheep than other copper salts, much of the copper toxicity data in the literature should be reevaluated because copper sulfate has been the most commonly studied copper salt.

The liver metabolizes considerable copper without ill effects, providing molybdenum and sulfate are present. The sheep liver stores copper more readily than that of other species of animals, and a copper concentration of 10-50 ppm on a wet-weight basis is normally present. When it reaches about 150 ppm or more, the animal is predisposed to the characteristic hemolytic crisis of copper poisoning. Poisoning is brought about by the sudden release into the bloodstream of copper which has been stored in the liver. This sudden release of copper by the liver may be spontaneous or may be associated with stress such as reduced food intake, unaccustomed handling, or strenuous exercise. (Todd, 1962) The hepatic storage of copper may occur as a result of: (1) intake of copper-contaminated feed; (2) the consumption of diets containing improper levels of copper, molybdenum, and sulfate; (3) liver damage affecting the copper metabolism of the hepatocyte.

When acute poisoning occurs from consuming a high dose of a soluble copper salt, coagulation necrosis of the gastrointestinal mucosa may be the primary effect.

Clinical Signs

When an animal consumes small but excessive amounts of copper over a period of weeks to months, particularly when the copper to molybdenum ratio is greater than 10:1, no toxic signs are manifested until a critical level of copper is reached in the liver. The clinical signs are sudden, and the course is usually twenty-four to forty-eight hours. The animal becomes weak, trembles, and is anoretic. Hemoglobinuria, hemoglobinemia, and icterus are usually present. Occasionally an animal will show only pale mucous membranes without icterus and hemoglobinuria. Although the morbidity is usually less than 5 percent, the mortality is usually over 75 percent.

In acute poisoning by large oral doses of copper formulation, vomition, excessive salivation, abdominal pain, and diarrhea (greenish tinged fluid feces) are usual signs. Collapse and death follow within twenty-four to forty-eight hours.

Physiopathology

A sudden hemolytic crisis accounts for nearly all of the signs of chronic copper poisoning, although not all animals that die of chronic copper poisoning have a hemolytic crisis and jaundice. (Sutter *et al.,* 1958) Reduced hemoglobin and PCV with increased WBC and unchanged platelet counts are characteristic hematologic findings. Concomitant with the release of copper from the liver into the plasma, there is an elevation of plasma bilirubin and decreased liver function. (McCosker, 1968)

One of the important features of chronic copper poisoning in sheep and cattle is that blood copper concentrations may remain within normal range during the period of accumulation of copper yet increases very markedly and abruptly twenty-four to twenty-eight hours before clinical signs appear. (Albiston *et al.,* 1940; Barden and Robertson, 1962; Todd and Thompson, 1963, 1965) McCosker (1968) describes an intermediate stage, however, when blood copper levels are slightly increased before the stage of acute hemolytic crisis.

Normal levels of copper in the blood range from 75 to 135 $\mu g/100$ ml (0.75-1.35 ppm); but at the onset of the hemolytic crisis, concentrations may be much higher. (Beck, 1955)

Postmortem changes are usually characteristic and include generalized icterus (occasionally absent, however); greatly enlarged gunmetal-colored kidneys that sometimes have hemorrhagic mottling; slightly enlarged, friable, yellowish liver (may also be small, firm, and pale); gallbladder distended with thick, greenish bile; and enlarged spleen with a brown to black parenchyma of blackberry jam consistency.

The hepatocytes may exhibit cytoplasmic vacuolation and necrosis. All lobules may contain clusters of dead cells with fragmented nuclei and acidophilic cytoplasm. Fibrosis begins early and is distributed portally. (Jubb and Kennedy, 1970) The kidney tubules are clogged with hemoglobin accompanying degeneration and necrosis of the tubular and glomerular cells occurs. The spleen is crowded with fragmented erythrocytes, and status spongiosus in the white matter of the central nervous system has been reported.

Morphological and histochemical changes occur in sheep when copper accumulates in their livers. (Ishmael *et al.,* 1971) In biopsies taken six months before the hemolytic crisis, swelling and necrosis of isolated hepatic parenchymal cells have been noted, together with swollen Kupffer's cells rich in acid phosphatase and containing PAS-positive, diastase-resistant material and copper. Various increases in liver-related serum enzyme activities have been recorded six to eight weeks before the hemolytic crisis. These enzymes include serum glutamic oxaloacetic transaminase, lactic dehydrogenase, sorbitol dehydrogenase, arginase, and glutamic dehydrogenase. (Todd and Thompson, 1963, 1965; Van Adrichem, 1965; Ross, 1966; MacPherson and Hemingway, 1969; Ishmael *et al.,* 1971, 1972) The increased serum activities of these enzymes often subside to nearly normal levels one to two weeks before the hemolytic crisis, but very high levels of activity occur shortly before or during the crisis. It is important to note that these elevations are not correlated with increases of copper levels in the blood. They only occur shortly before and during the hemolytic crisis and therefore are of little diagnostic value.

During the hemolytic crisis, the activities of hydrolytic adenosine triphosphatase, nonspecific esterase, and succinic dehydrogenase are reduced. (Ishmael *et al.,* 1971, 1972; Peters *et al.,* 1965)

Todd and Thompson (1963, 1964) reported a marked reduction in blood glutathione concentration and an accumulation of methemoglobin associated with the hemolytic crisis of copper toxicosis. They postulated that the effect of high blood copper levels is to initiate a chain of events which results in the premature death of the red cell. Death may result from blockage of the kidneys by hemoglobin and resulting kidney failure.

Copper is absorbed from the small intestine of most species. Generally, less than 30 percent of the copper consumed is absorbed in any species, and its absorption and retention is greatly affected by the chemical forms in which the metal is ingested, by the dietary levels of other minerals and organic substances, and by the acidity of the intestinal contents in the absorptive area. (Underwood, 1971) Little is known, however, about the mechanism of copper absorption, although it is generally believed that a copper-protein binding or a copper-metal or organic complex may be formed.

Copper entering the blood plasma from the intestine and from body tissues becomes loosely bound to serum albumin and is distributed widely to the tissues and the erythrocytes. Copper in ceruloplasmin does not appear to be so readily available for exchange or for transfer. (Underwood, 1971)

When copper reaches the liver, the primary organ of its metabolism, it is incorporated into the mitochrondia, microsomes, nuclei and soluble fraction of the parenchymal cells. (Gregoriadis and Sourkes, 1967; Milne and Weswig, 1968) The copper is either stored in these sites or released for incorporation into erythrocuprein, ceruloplasmin or the various copper-containing enzymes. Hepatic copper is also secreted into the bile and excreted into the intestine. Smaller amounts of plasma copper is also excreted into the urine. (Cartwright and Wintrobe, 1964; Underwood, 1971)

Diagnosis

Diagnosis of chronic copper poisoning may be confirmed using chemical analysis of the tissues and blood of affected animals correlated with copper and molybdenum concentration in the ration, clinical signs, and necropsy findings. Normal copper concentration in whole blood ranges from 0.7-1.3 ppm. Concentrations above this level are often associated with copper poisoning. (McCosker, 1968) Liver concentrations associated with copper poisoning are usually greater than 150 ppm on a wet-weight basis, whereas kidney concentrations are usually greater than 15.0 ppm. (Buck, 1969) Complete sheep feed containing 25.0 ppm or greater copper with no added molybdenum (2 ppm or less) may produce copper poisoning. (Todd, 1962; Adamson and Valks, 1969) Because cattle are less susceptible to excess copper-deficient molybdenum than are sheep, somewhat greater dietary concentrations of copper may be necessary to produce poisoning in this species.

Other disease conditions which must be differentiated from copper poisoning-molybdenum deficiency include leptospirosis, postparturient hemoglobinemia, bacillary hemoglobinemia, rape (*Brassica napus*) poisoning, hepatitis, phenothiazine poisoning, onion poisoning, babesiosis, and anaplasmosis. Poisoning by other metals such as arsenic, mercury, lead, and thallium may mimic the gastrointestinal effect of acute massive copper poisoning.

Treatment

Administration of small amounts of molybdenum, 50-500 mg of ammonium molybdate per day, and 0.3-1 gram of thiosulfate daily for three weeks is recommended for the prevention of copper toxicity. Molybdenumized superphosphate (4 oz molybdenum/acre) is valuable to increase the molybdenum content of pasture and reduce the retention of copper. Molybdenumized licks or mineral mixture (190 lbs salt, 140 lbs finely ground gypsum, and 1 lb sodium molybdate) can be used alternately. (Ross, 1966, 1970; Pierson, 1958)

According to the "Food and Drug Administration Code of Federal Regulations," Section 121.101, Subpart B, p. 8, copper is officially recognized as a suitable mineral ingredient in animal feeds. Molybdenum is not recognized as a safe and necessary additive to the diet of animals. This means that animal feeds may contain added copper but no molybdenum. Complete feeds fed to sheep and cattle may, therefore, contain mineral mixtures which in effect increase the copper content without providing the molybdenum necessary for metabolism of the excessive copper. Our investigations of field cases of

copper poisoning in sheep revealed that losses have occurred because no molybdenum was incorporated into the complete feed to which copper had been added. Because the sulfate ion facilitates molybdenum enhanced excretion of copper, copper in combination with sulfate is less toxic than other combinations of copper such as oxide, carbonate, orthophosphate, pyrophosphate, chloride, gluconate, and hydroxide.

Buck (1970) has proposed three alternative solutions to this problem:

1. Change the regulations allowing molybdenum to be added along with copper to ruminant feeds (especially sheep) at a ratio of 1 part molybdenum:10 parts copper.
2. Provide for copper to be added to sheep feeds only in the form of copper sulfate at concentrations no greater than 15 ppm in the complete feed.
3. Discontinue the practice of adding copper to sheep feeds.

Case History

An Iowa lamb testing station had approximately 80 six-month-old animals on feed tests. They were being fed a complete pelleted ration. Six animals became suddenly affected: weakness, dark-colored urine, anorexia, yellowing of the lighter areas of the skin, and collapse and death of four within 72 hours. Postmortem changes included icterus of all tissues; hemoglobinemia; bladder filled with dark, coffee-colored urine; and dark, swollen, pulpy spleen and kidneys.

Chemical analysis and clinical pathologic results are presented:

	Affected Lambs		Unaffected Lambs	
	#656	#363	#255	#299
Copper (ppm whole blood)	2.64	1.50	0.95	1.0
Hemoglobin	8.3%	7.9%	11.4%	10.7%
PCV	22.5	19.0	34.0	32.5
WBC (corrected)	21,535	34,683	9,500	6,650
Platelets	Adequate	Adequate	Adequate	Adequate
Comments	Many nucleated RBC; severe anisocytosis; moderate poikilocytosis; basophilic stippling; plasma hemolyzed		Plasma clear; no RBC changes	

The complete feed was found to contain 35 ppm copper. The label indicated that a mineral mixture containing copper carbonate and copper oxide had been added to the feed. The molybdenum concentration in the feed was less than 1.0 ppm.

Excess Molybdenum-Deficient Copper

Source

Cattle apparently are more susceptible than sheep to excess molybdenum-deficient copper in their diet. (Britton and Goss, 1946; Fleming *et al.,* 1961; Underwood, 1971)) When the ratio of copper to molybdenum in feed drops below 2:1, molybdenum poisoning can be expected in cattle. (Miltimore and Mason, 1971) This syndrome is manifested by emaciation, liquid diarrhea full of gas bubbles, swollen genitalia, anemia, and achromotrichia. Poor weight gains and death from prolonged purgation may occur. The average morbidity is about 80 percent. (Britton and Goss, 1946) Osteoporosis and bone fractures have been reported in prolonged cases of molybdenosis. (Underwood, 1971)

Some conditions under which excess molybdenum-copper deficiency occur are as follows:

1. Contamination of soils and forages in the vicinity of certain mining operations where molybdenum-containing ores are heated at high temperatures.
2. Industrial contamination of farmland near metal alloy production plants.
3. Contamination of soil with molybdenum fertilizers.
4. Feeding of forages and grains grown on soils naturally high in molybdenum and/or low in copper. In the United States, such soils have been found in California, Oregon, Nevada, and Florida. (Britton and Goss, 1946; Fleming *et al.,* 1961; Underwood, 1971) Cattle grazing pastures on muck or shale soils in England, Ireland, New Zealand, and Holland have suffered severe molybdenosis. (Underwood, 1971)

Miltimore and Mason (1971) apparently have made the first extensive report of molybdenum and copper concentrations and copper:molybdenum ratios in ruminant feeds. The overall mean copper:molybdenum ratio of all feeds in the area of Canada studied (legume hay, grass hay, sedge hay, oat forage, corn silage, and grains) was 5.7:1. The copper:molybdenum ratio in sedge hays was 2.1·1, near the critical ratio of 2:1. The mean ratio of other hays was 4.4:1, and the ratio for other feeds was 5:1 or higher. They reported that 19 percent of all samples had ratios below 2:1; the lowest copper:molybdenum ratio was 0.1:1 and the highest was 52.7:1. Molybdenum levels were generally low, 35 percent of all samples being below 1 ppm. Only 1 percent was above 8.0 ppm, and the highest molybdenum concentration was 9.9 ppm. Copper concentrations were generally low, 95 percent being below 10 ppm with legumes having 7.5 ppm and grass hays 3.3 ppm.

Disorders that have been associated with a *relative* copper deficiency in various animal species include anemia, depressed growth, bone disorders, depigmentation of hair and wool, abnormal wool growth, neonatal ataxia, impaired reproductive performance, heart failure, cardiovascular defects and gastrointestinal disturbances. (Underwood, 1971) Many factors influence the severity of these dysfunctions, especially species, age, dietary interrelationships, environment, sex, and even breed or strain characteristics.

Anemia associated with copper deficiency occurs in most species and is characteristic of the anemia associated with iron deficiency (see section Copper-Iron-Zinc Interrelationships under Nonruminant Animals).

Bone abnormalities associated with copper deficiency have been reported in rabbits, mice, chicks, dogs, pigs, foals, sheep and cattle. (Underwood, 1971) In ruminants, osteoporosis and spontaneous bone fractures are usually associated with excess dietary molybdenum and thus a relative copper deficiency. Suttle *et al.,* (1972) have presented evidence, however, of the development of osteoporosis in the offspring of ewes given copper-deficient diets.

Sheep suffering from simple copper deficiency and/or excess molybdenum also develop depigmentation of dark wool together with loss of crimp and quality of their fine wool. (Underwood, 1971; Dick, 1954) In Australia a syndrome called "enzootic ataxia" and in the United Kingdom a condition termed "swayback" are thought to be due to copper deficiency. Ewes become anemic with stringy wool, which corresponds with neurological signs in their lambs in enzootic ataxia; whereas the typical case of swayback is more acute in lambs with the ewes' wool being normal. These diseases are noted in lambs under one month of age. Lambs are severely incoordinated, ataxic, and usually blind. Death is the result of starvation, exposure, or pneumonia. (Jubb and Kennedy, 1970; Underwood, 1971) Cordy (1971) has also reported that this condition occurs in the United States.

Toxicity

When the copper levels of feed or forages are in the normal range of 8-11 ppm, cattle can be poisoned on levels of molybdenum above 5-6 ppm and sheep on levels above 10-12 ppm. When the dietary copper level falls much below 8-11 ppm or the sulfate ion level is high, even 1-2 ppm molybdenum may be toxic to cattle.

Increasing the copper level in the diet even 5 ppm

above normal (13-16 ppm) will protect cattle against 150 ppm dietary molybdenum.

Calves may be poisoned by milk from cows on high molybdenum.

Mechanism of Action

The mechanism(s) responsible for the interaction of copper-molybdenum-sulfate is not entirely understood. There is good evidence that copper and molybdenum form an *in vivo* complex having a molar ratio of 4:3 (Dowdy and Matrone, 1968a,b) but that this complex may not prevent the intestinal absorption of copper. It is more likely that the copper-molybdenum complex inhibits copper and perhaps molybdenum utilization. As a tentative explanation of the mechanism of this interference, either an impairment of copper uptake by liver cells or a primary intracellular metabolic disturbance in the synthesis of copper-protein compounds, including ceruloplasmin or both, are postulated by Marcilese *et al.*, (1969). Regardless of the mechanism(s), this phenomenon is dependent upon the presence of inorganic sulfate. The copper-molybdenum-sulfate interactions also strongly affect urinary excretion of these elements. Dick (1953a) reported that increased urinary molybdenum excretion was associated with increased dietary inorganic sulfate, and Marcilese *et al.*, (1970) reported that increased dietary levels of molybdenum and sulfate resulted in increased urinary excretion of copper. The modes of action of copper at the cellular level have been the subject of many basic researches. Many copper-protein compounds have been isolated from living tissues, many of which are enzymes with oxidative functions. Probably no metal ion is more versatile than copper as a catalyst of enzymic reactions. Tyrosinase, lactase, ascorbic acid oxidase, uricase, monoamine oxidase, delta aminolevulinic acid dehydrase, dopamine-B-Hydroxylase and cytochrome oxidase have all been identified as copper enzymes. (Underwood, 1971) The diminished activity of cytochrome oxidase is a sensitive indicator of copper deficiency. (Jubb and Kennedy, 1970)

The first evidence of cardiovascular disorders in copper deficiency emerged from studies by Bennetts and coworkers (1939, 1942, 1948) studying a disorder in cattle known as "falling disease." The primary lesion is progressive atrophy of the myocardium with replacement fibrosis. Sudden deaths characteristic of the disease were attributed to heart failure, usually after exercise or excitement. The disease can be prevented by copper supplementation. This condition has not been reported in sheep or horses but has occurred in pigs and chickens. (Shields *et al.*, 1961; Odell *et al.*, 1961) There

is a derangement of the elastic tissue in major blood vessels resulting in spontaneous ruptures. The tensile strength of the aorta becomes markedly reduced and the myocardium becomes friable. The primary biochemical lesion has been described by Hill *et al.*, (1967) as a reduction in the aorta of amine oxidase activity, a copper containing enzyme. This reduction in enzymic activity results in reduced capacity for deaminating lysine in elastin, which, in turn, results in less lysine being converted to desmosine, a cross-linkage group of elastin, and therefore lessened elasticity of the aorta and other major vessels. Rucker *et al.*, (1969) reported that reduced bone cytochrome oxidase activity was also associated with copper deficiency in chicks.

Clinical Signs

In cattle with molybdenosis, there is a persistent severe scouring with many gas bubbles in the liquid feces, which usually begins eight to ten days after animals are placed on a high-molybdenum diet. Depigmentation (achromotrichia) of the hair coat gradually develops, beginning around the eyes. Animals become emaciated and anemic with a rough coat and general unthriftiness. Milk production decreases; there is often loss of libido and reduced fertility. Animals exhibit evidence of pain in the joints and develop anemia.

If the condition becomes chronic, osteoporosis, bone fractures, beaded ribs, and overgrowth of the ends of long bones are common. Animals suffering from molybdenosis often develop pica.

Sheep suffering from simple copper deficiency and/or excess molybdenum also develop depigmentation of dark wool together with loss of crimp and quality of their fine wool. In Australia a syndrome called "enzootic ataxia" and in the United Kingdom a condition termed "swayback" are thought to be due to copper deficiency. Ewes become anemic with stringy wool, which corresponds with neurological signs in their lambs in enzootic ataxia; whereas the typical case of swayback is more acute in lambs with the ewes' wool being normal. These diseases are noted in lambs under one month of age. Lambs are severely incoordinated, ataxic, and usually blind. Death is the result of starvation, exposure, or pneumonia. (Jubb and Kennedy, 1970)

Physiopathology

Cytochrome oxidase is a copper-dependent enzyme, and diminished activity of this enzyme is a sensitive indicator of copper deficiency which apparently limits the synthesis of heme, the prosthetic group of cytochrome oxidase. (Jubb and Kennedy, 1970) Copper undoubtedly is involved in many other biochemical functions, but many of the signs of deficiency apparently result from insufficient cytochrome oxidase. Copper is important to the formation and maintenance of myelin.

Postmortem changes associated with excess molybdenum-deficient copper include harsh, stringy wool and hair; achromotrichia; microcytic, hypochromic anemia; emaciation; osteoporosis; bone rarification and fractures; and hemosiderosis. Lesions associated with enzootic ataxia and swayback in lambs are characterized by lysis of the white matter of the cerebrum and degeneration of the motor tracts of the spinal cord. The destruction of the white matter varies from microscopic foci to massive subcortical destruction. There is often neuronal degeneration as well as demyelination (Jubb and Kennedy, 1970; Cordy, 1971)

Diagnosis

The clinical appearance of animals together with their response to copper therapy are good diagnostic criteria of molybdenosis-copper deficiency. Copper and molybdenum levels in tissues and forages can be confirmatory. Liver levels of copper less than 10-30 ppm on a wet-weight basis and molybdenum levels greater than 5 ppm are significant. Whole blood copper levels less than 0.6 ppm and molybdenum levels greater than 0.1 ppm are usually present in copper deficiency-molybdenosis syndromes. Normal blood copper levels range from 0.7-1.3 ppm, while a normal molybdenum level is around 0.05 ppm. Normal liver copper levels range from 30-140 ppm on a wet-weight basis, and liver molybdenum is normally below 3-4 ppm.

Milk from animals consuming a diet having an optimum concentration of molybdenum usually contains 30-50 ppb molybdenum. One would likely find up to 300 ppb or greater molybdenum in milk from animals consuming excessive dietary molybdenum.

It should be kept in mind that molybdenum concentrations in blood and milk reflect the level of molybdenum consumption within the past 24-36 hours. Both blood and milk concentrations decrease rapidly when the molybdenum is removed from the diet.

Forage levels of copper and molybdenum are important in establishing the source of the problem. For cattle, the safe ratio of copper:molybdenum is greater than 2:1. Copper should be 8-11 ppm to protect cattle against 5-6 ppm molybdenum and sheep against 10-12 ppm molybdenum. Copper levels below 7 ppm in forages may result in a copper deficiency.

Several disease conditions must be differentiated from molybdenosis-copper deficiency. Imbalance of calcium-phosphorus-vitamin D metabolism, massive parasitism, Johne's disease, and demyelinating diseases of the brain and cord should be included in the list.

Treatment

Providing copper parenterally or orally is the best treatment for molybdenosis-copper deficiency. Copper sulfate may be added to a salt-mineral mixture at 1-5 percent, depending upon molybdenum levels in the feed. Various other formulations have been recommended to provide approximately 1 gram of copper sulfate to an adult cow; e.g., (1) 1 oz $CuSO_4$ to 250 gal of water; (2) 1/2-1 lb of $CuSO_4$ to 100 lbs of salt; (3) 100 lbs of protein concentrate (soybean oilmeal or cottonseed meal), 100 lbs of fine salt, and 2 1/2 lbs of $CuSO_4$ (given at a rate of 1/6 lb/day/cow).

Copper glycinate can be given subcutaneously at 60 mg for calves and 120 mg for mature cattle. Treatment may need to be repeated during a season. Response to copper therapy is usually good.

Case History

During the start-up of a major refinery unit in 1960, some 40 tons of molybdenum-containing catalysts were emitted due to equipment malfunction; and downwind of the plant the catalyst (containing 8.2 percent molybdenum trioxide) settled out. Five to eleven days later the older cattle in this area began to have an acute diarrhea (bloody dysentery in at least one case) accompanied by loss of condition and fall in milk yield. A degree of diarrhea was also present in younger animals (3 months to 2 1/2 years of age), but in these younger cases the most prominent symptom was a marked stiffness of the legs and back which caused difficulty in rising and great reluctance to move. The gait was stilted, but it was not possible to detect any painful areas or to produce pain by manipulation of muscles or joints. Appetite remained good and temperatures were normal, but the affected animals appeared more placid and were handled more easily than usual; they were somewhat unresponsive to stimuli. Knowledge of the catalyst emission suggested a diagnosis of molybdenosis, and this was supported by high molybdenum levels found on herbage samples and blood analysis. Blood molybdenum levels ranged from 0.005-0.047 mg/100 ml (0.05-0.47 ppm) and blood copper levels ranged from 0.05-0.180 mg/100 ml (0.15-1.8 ppm) in 24 animals tested. Forage levels ranged from 34-16.7 ppm molybdenum and 11.5-6.9 ppm copper on a dry-matter basis. Treatment with copper sulfate (1 gm/100 lbs body weight as a single oral dose, repeated in a few instances in 48 hours) was immediately initiated, and scouring was controlled almost at once. Subsequent treatments were by means of copper glycinate injections. All animals improved after copper treatment, and no illness occurred in any animal that received copper glycinate before the onset of symptoms. (Gardner and Hall-Patch, 1962)

NONRUMINANT ANIMALS

Copper-Molybdenum-Sulfate Interrelationships

The combined effects of copper, molybdenum, and sulfate are much less marked in the nonruminant. Gip *et al.,* (1967) and Hays and Kline (1969) were unable to demonstrate any effect of molybdenum and sulfate on the liver storage of pigs fed varying levels of copper. Dale (1971) observed similar results but also observed a depression of ceruloplasmin levels when sulfate was added to swine diets containing about 10 ppm of copper. Cromwell (1971) reported that a combination of molybdenum and *sulfate* were ineffective in preventing the depressive effects upon weight gains, hematological changes, and the buildup of liver copper stores in swine associated with feeding a high (500 ppm) level of dietary copper; however, a combination of molybdenum and *sulfide* appeared to be quite effective in preventing excessive copper accumulation in the liver of pigs fed a diet containing a high level of copper. In rats fed copper-deficient diets, Gray and Daniel (1964) observed greater growth reduction when sulfate was added to high levels of molybdenum. In diets with adequate copper, no effects were noted.

Copper-Zinc-Iron Interrelationships

Zinc and iron have a profound effect upon copper metabolism in nonruminant animals, especially swine. Both zinc and iron have been shown to protect swine from the adverse effects of high levels (250-750 ppm) of dietary copper. (Hanrahan and O'Grady, 1968; Ritchie *et al.,* 1963; Suttle and Mills, 1966 a,b) Similarly, zinc and iron deficiency tended to accentuate copper toxicity in swine. (Suttle and Mills, 1966 b)

In rats, copper was shown to prevent the occurrence of anemia and reduced liver catalase and cytochrome oxidase associated with zinc toxicosis, but did not prevent the growth inhibition produced by zinc. (Van Reen, 1953; Smith and Larson, 1946) Subsequent studies have revealed an influence of zinc on copper metabolism in rats. (Whanger and Weswig, 1971)

Severe anemia is a prominent manifestation of cop-

per deficiency in swine and other animals. (Lahey *et al.,* 1952; Cartwright *et al.,* 1956; Underwood, 1971) Copper deficiency is first manifested by a slow depletion of body copper stores, including blood plasma. The type of anemia associated with copper deficiency is identical to that caused by iron deficiency and appears to be a defect in hemoglobin synthesis. Lee *et al.,* (1968a,b) however, showed that copper deficient pigs did not have abnormalities in the heme biosynthetic pathway. On the contrary, as the anemia developed, the activity of heme biosynthetic enzymes increased. Copper, it was concluded, is not a part of heme biosynthesis. For many years it was accepted that iron absorption was unaffected by copper deficiency but that copper was necessary for iron utilization by the blood-forming tissues. Chase *et al.,* (1952a,b) showed that copper deficiency in rats reduced their ability to absorb iron, to mobilize iron from the tissues and to utilize iron in the hemoglobin synthesis. Subsequently, Lee *et al.,* (1968a,b) confirmed that copper deficient pigs failed to absorb iron at a normal rate and observed increased amounts of iron in the duodenal mucosa. When radioiron was administered orally, the mucosa of copper-deficient animals extracted iron from the duodenal lumen at a normal rate but transfer to the plasma was impaired. These and other experiments provided evidence that copper deficiency causes an impaired ability of duodenal mucosa, the reticuloendothelial system, and the hepatic parenchymal cells to release iron into the plasma. This hypothesis is compatible with the suggestion that the transfer of iron from tissues to plasma requires the enzymic oxidation of ferrous iron and that ceruloplasmin is the enzyme (ferroxidase) that catalyzes the reaction. The authors (Lee *et al.,* 1968a,b) proposed an additional defect in iron metabolism in copper deficiency, residing within the normoblast itself. The excessive levels of iron in normoblasts suggested that a defect in these cells plays a major role in the development of anemia. As a result of this defect, iron cannot be incorporated into hemoglobin and, instead, accumulates as nonhemoglobic iron.

Copper and Other Interactions

There is some indication that the source or quality of dietary protein may also be a factor in these interrelationships. (Hanrahan and O'Grady, 1968) Suttle and Mills (1966 b) observed severe copper toxicosis in swine receiving white-fish meal but not in those receiving soybean-oil meal with both diets containing up to 425 ppm copper. Other workers did not obtain such decisive results. (MacPherson and Hemingway, 1965; Paris and McDonald, 1969) At any rate, there appears to be a regional difference in susceptibility of swine to dietary copper. (Anon., Nutrition Reviews, 1966) Significantly, Gregoriadis and Sourkes (1968) demonstrated that protein synthesis is required for the removal of copper from the liver of the rat. It is also possible that the effects of dietary protein source upon copper toxicity are related to their concentration of elements such as zinc and iron.

In 1969, Moore suggested an inverse relationship between vitamin A and copper metabolism. He suggested that in the latter stages of human gestation there is a decrease in maternal blood vitamin A but an increase in copper, and that the fetal livers of animals usually have low levels of vitamin A while concentrating high levels of copper. He further suggested that studies of vitamin A and copper metabolism might give interesting results. Underwood (1971) reviewed the role of copper in keratinization of wool, although vitamin A was not mentioned. Subsequently, Moore et al., (1972) reported that experimental chronic copper poisoning in sheep was accompanied by much-reduced plasma concentrations of retinol.

Copper Deficiency

Copper is not only essential to life in mammals but also to plants and lower forms of organisms. It has varied and numerous biologic effects as an essential element. Gallagher and Reeve (1971) have suggested that an uncomplicated copper deficiency in the rat causes two major biochemical dysfunctions and that one is directly caused by the other. One, the loss of cytochrome oxidase activity, leads to the other, depressed synthesis of phospholipids by liver mitochrondria, by interfering with the provision of endogenous ATP to maintain an optimal rate of synthesis. Copper undoubtedly is involved in many other biochemical functions, but many of the signs of deficiency apparently result from insufficient cytochrome oxidase. Copper is important to the formation and maintenance of myelin.

Copper deficiency in the nonruminant results in anemia, bone deformation and reduced calcification, cerebral edema and cortical necrosis, achromotrichia, fetal absorption, and aortic rupture. (Underwood, 1971) The levels of ceruloplasmin and copper in serum and the levels of cytochrome oxidase and copper in tissues decrease in animals fed a copper-deficient diet. (Owen and Hazelrig, 1968; Dowdy et al., 1969; Ragen et al., 1969; Hunt et al., 1970)

Nonruminants are more tolerant of excess levels of molybdenum than ruminants. Pigs appear to be the most tolerant of the nonruminants since Davis (1950) reported that a diet containing 1,000 ppm molybdenum for a period of three months had no ill effects on pigs. In pigs, the storage of copper in the liver does not appear to be influenced by the level of molybdenum in the diet. (Hays and Kline, 1969; Kline et al., 1970; Kline et al., 1971)

Molybdenum excess in rats can result in symptoms that are similar to copper deficiency. The level of molybdenum that is required to produce toxicity depends upon the copper status of the rat. Nielands et al., (1948) and Gray and Daniel (1964) have demonstrated that growth and hemoglobin levels of rats can be reduced by feeding 100 ppm of molybdenum when a diet low in copper is fed. When the diet contains adequate amounts of copper, 500-1,000 ppm of molybdenum are required to cause such effects. In rats, the blood and liver copper level tends to increase when the dietary level of molybdenum is increased. (Compere et al., 1965)

Supplemental ascorbic acid has been demonstrated to accentuate copper deficiency in chicks, swine, and rabbits. Hunt et al., (1970) found that 0.5 percent dietary ascorbic acid reduced liver copper levels and increased mortality associated with the rupture of the aorta. Voelker and Carlton (1969) have reported that 2.5 percent ascorbic acid in the diet of swine resulted in intensification of copper deficiency symptoms. Ascorbic acid is thought to interfere with the absorption of copper.

Copper Toxicity

There is a marked difference between species in their ability to tolerate high levels of copper. Levels that are toxic to ruminants (30-50 ppm) are well tolerated by nonruminants. Dietary levels in excess of 250 ppm are required to produce toxicity in swine and rats. (Boyden et al., 1938; Wallace et al., 1960; Suttle and Mills, (1966a,b) Milne and Weswig (1968) have shown that sheep accumulate copper in the liver in proportion to the dietary intake, while rats maintain normal liver copper levels until a high dietary level is reached (1,000 ppm). This may partially explain the difference in the effects of high levels of copper between the ruminants and nonruminants.

Swine

Copper levels of 125-250 ppm have been noted to increase the rate of gain and feed efficiency of swine. (Bowler et al., 1955; Barber et al., 1957; Bunch et al., 1965; DeGoey, 1971) Such dietary levels also increase the unsaturation of depot fat resulting in soft fat. (Taylor and Thomke, 1964; Elliot and Bowland, 1970; De Goey et al., 1971)

The levels of zinc and iron are important when high levels of copper are fed since low levels of these minerals accentuate the toxic properties of copper. (Bunch *et al.*, 1963; Suttle and Mills, 1966a,b; De Goey *et al.*, 1971)

A recent report (NCR-42 Committee on Swine Nutrition, 1974) indicated that swine fed diets high in copper (up to 250 ppm) during the eight weeks of the early postweaning period increased their daily weight gains. However, continuous feeding at these levels did not affect overall rate of gain; or feed-gain ratios. Copper stores in the liver increased linearly with increasing dietary copper but removal of the added dietary copper reduced hepatic copper content. Significant differences were discovered from location to location, suggesting that genetic, managemental, housing, and environmental factors may contribute to the differences observed in swine. Also, there is no indication that the dietary levels of iron or zinc were considered by the various investigations.

The diverse effects of feeding swine high levels of copper are well illustrated by the accompanying table from the Committee Report 1974. Feeding 125-250 ppm of copper for up to eight weeks after weaning did cause an average increase in daily gain over no added copper, but there were wide variations. Ohio stations reported better than 20 percent increased daily gain when the higher levels of copper were supplied; Illinois and Iowa showed mixed gains and losses in rate of gain. When results are examined for a complete feeding period, the rate of gain and feed efficiency are less significant than for gains made during the first eight weeks, the variations among stations was considerable.

Poultry

Poultry may be more resistant to copper toxicosis than most mammals, except rats. Smith (1969) fed copper sulfate to day-old chicks for 25 days at 0, 100, 200, or 350 ppm copper in a basal ration containing 10 ppm copper. Those chicks on the 100 ppm copper diet had a slight increase in daily gain while those on 350 ppm had

TABLE 0
Effects of Levels of Supplementary Copper on Rate of Gain and Feed/Gain (Total Period)[a]

| Cu, ppm (0 to 8 weeks) | 0 | 125 | 125 | 187.5 | 187.5 | 250 | 250 | 0 | 125 | 125 | 187.5 | 187.5 | 250 | 250 |
| Cu, ppm (8 weeks to final) | 0 | 0 | 125 | 0 | 187.5 | 0 | 250 | 0 | 0 | 125 | 0 | 187.5 | 0 | 250 |
Station	Daily gain (g) by replicate							Feed/gain by replicate						
Illinois	730	694	653	699	721	—	640	3.85	3.58	3.70	3.77	3.58	—	3.65
	630	590	594	694	540	—	635	3.51	3.41	3.75	3.50	4.10	—	3.56
Indiana	780	771	789	767	721	780	780	3.24	3.42	3.29	3.26	3.10	3.31	3.43
	748	762	807	785	744	794	803	3.27	3.27	3.14	3.02	3.36	3.03	2.89
Iowa	750	810	730	760	—	690	770	3.72	3.72	3.86	3.72	—	4.02	3.65
	710	750	740	780	—	740	740	3.90	3.86	3.75	3.87	—	4.01	4.10
	690	740	680	690	—	650	730	3.83	3.67	4.02	3.91	—	4.12	3.71
	810	670	740	740	—	700	680	3.37	3.80	3.48	3.83	—	3.61	3.93
Kansas	640	700	730	670	730	710	700	3.06	3.15	3.12	2.91	2.96	3.00	2.90
	690	720	770	780	750	740	780	3.08	2.91	3.09	2.84	2.83	2.86	2.88
Kentucky	692	690	709	744	713	716	700	3.49	3.34	3.33	3.25	3.41	3.37	3.17
	621	658	668	671	655	681	704	3.53	3.41	3.34	3.41	3.64	3.30	3.20
Michigan	604	599	627	627	613	622	636	3.23	3.03	3.12	3.23	3.33	3.12	3.23
Missouri	830	810	830	790	820	—	—	2.83	2.91	3.02	3.03	3.17	—	—
	810	790	820	790	820	—	—	3.01	3.10	2.94	3.20	2.97	—	—
Nebraska	760	820	730	780	820	—	740	3.50	3.13	3.70	3.52	3.36	—	3.52
	710	780	730	670	700	—	740	3.33	3.23	3.21	3.36	3.32	—	3.31
Ohio	708	735	—	789	—	730	—	3.05	2.97	—	2.87	—	2.92	—
	717	—	780	—	762	—	785	2.90	—	2.78	—	2.86	—	2.76
South Dakota	735	735	789	730	753	776	767	3.30	3.47	3.03	3.49	3.39	3.54	3.57
	757	739	680	780	757	803	717	3.18	3.45	3.65	3.16	3.20	3.47	3.58
	689	671	699	726	748	798	771	3.32	3.50	3.43	3.50	3.12	3.40	3.36
Treatment means (x)[b]	710	724	725	730	726	727	735	3.30	3.26	3.29	3.29	3.31	3.27	3.25

[a]Taken from NCR-42 Committee on Swine Nutrition (1974).

[b]Station sig. (P $<$ .01) for rate of gain and feed/gain.

a slight but statistically significant reduced weight gain. These differences were attributed only to feed consumption. Goldberg *et al.,* (1965) gave copper acetate to adult chickens (weighing 1.8 ± 0.25 kg) via capsule at a rate of 50 mg copper per chicken/day for one week, 75 mg/day for a second week and 100 mg/day until anemia or toxicosis appeared or death occurred. After two to six weeks of copper administration the birds became weak, anorexic and lethargic. Eight of 23 chickens developed anemia concomitant with toxicosis. They suggested that erythrocytes are destroyed in the liver as a consequence of copper exposure. McGhee *et al.,* (1965) reported iron and copper interacted in the diet of chicks. They found that copper at 80 ppm or above depressed growth in young chicks when iron was fed at the level of 40 ppm or above for a duration of 4 weeks. No signs of toxicosis were observed, however, even in levels up to 160 ppm copper and 1,600 ppm iron. Turkey poults have been reported to tolerate up to 676 ppm dietary copper (as copper sulfate) for 21 days, but growth depression occurred when fed 910 or 1,000 ppm copper. Signs of toxicosis occurred at 1,620 ppm. (Vohra and Kratzer, 1968) Wiederanders (1968) tried to produce copper toxicosis in turkeys by injecting copper sulfate subcutaneously. He injected 0.5 mg per bird for 84 days followed by 5 mg per bird for an additional 17 days without producing copper toxicosis. He concluded that turkeys and perhaps other fowl have metabolic and excretory pathways for copper different from those of mammals because there was no increase in ceruloplasmin in the copper-loaded turkeys.

Extensive acute and chronic copper toxicity studies in chickens, pigeons and ducks were conducted by Pullar (1940 a,b). He found the MLD of copper sulfate for chickens on a mg/kg body weight basis to be as follows: single crystal, 900; powdered, 300-500; 4% solution, 1,000-1,500; mixed with twice its weight with sodium chloride, 300-500. The MLD of copper carbonate to chickens was found to be 900 mg/kg single dose. The MLD of copper carbonate to chickens was found to be 900 mg/kg single dose. The MLD of copper fed to pigeons on a mg/kg basis were as follows: single copper sulfate crystal, 1,000-1,500; copper carbonate, 1,000-1,500. The single MLD's of a single copper sulfate crystal to domestic mallards and muscovy ducks were 400 and 600 mg/kg body weight, respectively. The maximum daily intake of copper carbonate tolerated by chickens was 60 mg/kg body weight and by mallards was 29 mg/kg. It was not possible to produce poisoning in chickens given copper sulfate in drinking water at a level of 250 ppm (1:4,000 dilution of copper sulfate in drinking water) and no obvious signs of copper poisoning were observed in mallards consuming 250 ppm copper sulfate in their feed.

Rats and Mice

Numerous studies in rats and mice have been conducted in an effort to learn more about hepatolenticular degeneration (Wilson's disease) in humans. (Vogel, 1960; Wolff, 1960; Lal and Sourkes, 1971a,b, Barka *et al.,* 1964; McNatt *et al.,* 1971; Verity *et al.,* 1967; Lindquist, 1967, 1968) As with other animals, copper seems to have a propensity for the liver. Prolonged daily intraperitoneal injections of as little as 0.3 mg Cu/kg will result in elevated hepatic levels. (Lal and Sourkes, 1971a) There is indication that an increase in hepatic copper occurs without saturation of the excretory capacity of the rat. Copper levels in the kidney also increase with copper exposure, but this seems to be unrelated to liver storage. (Lal and Sourkes, 1971a) Both hepatic and renal necrosis is observed in rats and mice associated with increased copper levels. (Vogel, 1960; Wolff, 1960) However, there is no apparent deposition of copper in the brain, skeletal and cardiac muscle or skin, and only transient elevations of copper in bone following copper exposure. (Lal and Sourkes, 1971a)

Studies with rats and mice injected with copper compounds have shown that copper accumulates in liver lysosomes.(Barka *et al.,* 1955; Goldfischer, 1967; Lal and Sourkes 1971b) Some researchers have postulated that acid hydrolases capable of producing cellular injury are released from lysosomes, once copper is accumulated, thus causing hepatic damage. (Lindquist 1967, 1968; Verity *et al.,* 1967) Conversely, it has been demonstrated that high concentrations of copper in the toad, *Bufo marinus,* are localized to liver lysosomes and are made innocuous because of this localization. (Goldfischer *et al.,* 1970)

Dogs

Very recently, Hardy *et al.,* (1975) have described a form of hepatic cirrhosis in Bedlington terriers that has striking similarities to Wilson's disease. The disorder appears to be hereditary and autosomal, and the histologic and functional abnormalities of the liver are extraordinarily like those seen in man. The concentrations of hepatic copper found in these terriers exceed 10 mg/g (10,000 ppm) dry liver, to be compared to 0.25-3.0 mg/g in patients with Wilson's disease and normal levels of less than 0.1 mg/g in humans and dogs. Although this disorder is fatal to the dogs, Kayser- Fleischer rings and neurologic dysfunction have not been observed so far.

Aquatic Organisms

Copper is poisonous to many aquatic organisms. It may reach toxic levels either from mining or industrial operations, influxes of copper-containing fertilizers, use of copper salts to control aquatic vegetation or mollusks. Desalinization plants may cause local excessive concentrations of copper in the ambient salt water because their effluent is hot, hypersaline and of low pH—all are conditions that will dissolve the metal in the copper pipes or vessels through which the waste flows. Toxic concentrations are also functions of the species, the age of the individual organism, the concentrations of mineral and organic material, temperature of the water, and whether the copper is ionic or not.

In fresh water, acute toxicity to fish is unusual if the concentration is below 0.025 ppm. (The accepted standard for drinking water is 1.0 ppm.) (Doudroff and Katz, 1953) In soft fresh water, however, 0.01-0.02 ppm has been found to be toxic. (Powers, 1917; Jones, 1938; and Pickering and Henderson, 1966) Slightly higher concentrations of copper can be lethal in regions where the surface water is very soft. (Sprague, 1968)

As exposure time is lengthened, the minimal toxic concentration diminishes. The 48-hour LC_{50} (lethal concentration for 50 percent of the animals) in rainbow trout (*Salmo gairdnerii*) has been found to be 0.67-0.84 ppm. (Brown and Dalton, 1970) The 96 hour TL_m (median threshold limit, killing 50% of test animals in 96 hrs) of copper for blue gills (*Lepomis macrochirus*) is reported as 0.24 ppm, (O'Hara, 1971) although levels over 0.01 ppm alter oxygen consumption. The 10-day lethal concentration of copper for brook trout (*Salvelinus fontinalis*) is about 0.05 ppm. (Sprague, 1968) Chinook salmon eggs can withstand 0.08 ppm, (Hazol and Meith, 1970) but the fry exhibit acute toxicity at 0.04 ppm, and even 0.02 ppm copper inhibited their growth and increased mortality.

Relatively few data are available on more chronic exposures of fish to copper. Mount (1968) found that fathead minnows (*Pimiphales promelas, rafinesque*) exposed to copper for 11 months did not show impaired growth or reproduction at 3-7 percent of the 96-hour TI_m of 0.43 ppm. That, is, they were unaffected by 0.02 ppm. Minnows are unaffected by 3 times this concentration of copper if the water has an ethylenediamenetetraacetic acid hardness of 30 mg/liter as calcium carbonate ($CaCO_3$). (Mount and Stepan, 1969) In surprising contrast, Arthur and Leonard found that 8-14.8 ppm copper had no effect on fish after 6 weeks in soft water.

Copper pollution of waters has significant effect on marine invertebrates. Copper concentrations of 0.1 ppm are acutely toxic to nereis. (Raymond and Shields, 1963)

Certain metal chelating agents, nitrilotriacetic acid (NTA) and ethylenediaminetetraacetic acid (EDTA) have been shown to protect fish from poisoning by copper and zinc. (Sprague, 1968) The ratio of NTA to copper must be at least 3:1 for protection of most fish and is

effective against concentrations up to 300-400 times the toxic level. About 6 times as much EDTA as metal is required for protection, and this chemical is more expensive than NTA. These chelating agents are not cure-alls, however, since they are biodegradable in natural waters in a few days. It has been suggested that they are effective as temporary treatment for metal pollution or to carry a slug of pollution harmlessly past a critical section of river.

Molybdenum Essentiality

The only suggestion of the essential nature of molybdenum is the presence of the metal in the enzyme, xanthine oxidase. In rats, molybdenum depletion results in decreased xanthine oxidase activity but does not affect growth or purine metabolism. (de Renzo *et al.,* 1953; Richert and Westerfeld, 1953) In chicks, an antagonist to molybdenum, tungstate, can cause a reduction in growth and a reduction in the ability of the birds to oxidize xanthine to uric acid. (Higgins *et al.,* 1956; Leach and Norris, 1957)

REFERENCES

Adamson, A. H., and Valks, D. A. 1969. Copper Toxicity in Housed Lambs. *Vet. Rec.* 85:368-69.

Albiston, H. D.; Bull, L. B.; Dick, A. T; and Keast, J. C. 1940. A Preliminary Note on the Aetiology of Enzootic Jaundice, Toxaemic Jaundice, or "Yellows," of Sheep in Australia. *Aust. Vet. J.* 16:233-43.

Anmerman, C. B. 1970. Symposium: Trace Minerals. Recent Developments in Cobalt and Copper in Ruminant Nutritian: A Review. *J. Dairy Sci.* 53(8):1097-1107.

Anon. 1966. Copper Toxicity. *Nutrition Reviews* 24:305-8.

———. 1967. Site of Copper Toxicity: Microsomal Membranes Adenosinetriphosphatase. *Nutrition Reviews* 25(7):213-15.

Barber, R. S.; Braude, R.; Mitchell, K. G.; Rook, J. A. F.; and Rowell, J. G. 1957. Further Studies on Antibiotic and Copper Supplements for Fattening Pigs. *Brit. J. Nutr.* 11:70-79.

Barden, P. J., and Robertson, A. 1962. Experimental Copper Poisoning in Sheep. *Vet. Rec.* 74:252-56.

Barka, T.; Scheuer, P. J.; Schaffner, F.; and Popper, H. 1964. Structural Changes of Liver Cells in Copper Intoxication. *Arch. of Path.* 78:331-49.

Beck, A. B. 1956. The Copper Content of the Liver and Blood of Some Vertebrates. *Aust. J. Zool.* 4:1-18.

Beck, A. B., and Bennetts, H. W. 1963. Copper Poisoning in Sheep in Western Australia. *J. Roy. Soc. West. Aust.* 46:5-10.

Bennetts, H. W., and Hall, H. T. B. 1939. "Falling Disease" of Cattle in the South-West of Western Australia. *Aust. Vet. J.* 15:152-59.

Bennetts, H. W.; Harley, R.; and Evans, S. T. 1942. Studies on Copper Deficiency of Cattle: The Fatal Termination ("Falling Disease"). *Aust. Vet. J.* 18:50-63.

Bennetts, H. W.; Beck, A. B.; and Harley, R. 1948. The Pathogenesis of Falling Disease." *Aust. Vet. J.* 24:237-44.

Berger, K. C. 1962. Micronutrient Deficiencies in the United States. *Agric. Food Chem.* 10:178-81.

Boughton, I. B., and Hardy, W. T. 1934. Chronic Copper Poisoning in Sheep. Tex. Agric. Expt. Sta. Bull. No. 499, 32 pages.

Bowler, R. J.; Braude, R.; Campbell, R. C.; Craddock-Turnbull, J. N.; Fieldsend, H. F.; Grifiths, E. K.; Lucas, I. W. M.; Mitchell, K. G.; Nickalls, N. J. D.; and Taylor, J. H. 1955. High Copper-Mineral Mixtures for Fattening Pigs. *Brit. J. Nutr.* 9:358-62.

Boyden, R.; Potter, V. R.; and Elvehjem, C. A. 1938. Effect of Feeding High Levels of Copper to Albino Rats. *J. Nutr.* 15:397-402.

Bracewell, C. D. 1958. A Note on Jaundice in Housed Sheep. *Vet. Rec.* 70:342-44.

Britton, J. W., and Goss, H. 1946. Chronic Molybdenum Poisoning in Cattle. *JAVMA* 108:176-78.

Brown, V. M., and Dalton, R. A. 1970. The Acute Lethal Toxicity to Rainbow Trout of Mixtures of Copper, Phenol, Zinc, and Nickel. *J. Fish Biol.* 2:211-16.

Buck, W. B. 1969. Laboratory Toxicologic Tests and Their Interpretation. *JAVMA* 155:1928-41.

———. 1970. Diagnosis of Feed-Related Toxicoses. *JAVMA* 156:1434-43.

Buck, and Sharma, R. M. 1969. Copper Toxicity in Sheep. *I.S.U. Vet.* 31:4-8.

Bull, L. B.; Albiston, H. E.; Edgar, G.; and Dick, A. T. 1956. Toxaemic Jaundice of Sheep: Phytogenous Chronic Copper Poisoning, Heliotrope Poisoning, and Hepatogenous Chronic Copper Poisoning. *Aust. Vet. J.* 32:220-36.

Bunch, R. G.; Speer, V. C.; Hays, V. W.; and McCall, J. T. 1963. Effects of High Levels of Copper and Chlorotetracycline on Performance of Pigs. *J. Anim. Sci.* 22:56-60.

Bunch, R. G.; McCall, J. T.; Speer, V. C.; and Hays, V. W. 1965. Copper Supplementation for Weanling Pigs. *J. Anim. Sci.* 24:995-1000.

Carnes, W. H.; Shields, G. S.; Cartwright, G. E.; and Wintrobe, M. M. 1961. Vascular Lesions in Copper-Deficient Swine. *Fed. Proc., Fed. Amer. Soc. Expr. Biol.* 20:118. (abstract)

Cartwright, G. E.; Gubler, C. J.; Bush, J. A.; and Wintrobe, M. M. 1956. Studies on Copper Metabolism. XVII. Further Observations on the Anemia of Copper Deficiency in Swine. *Blood* 11:143-53.

Cartwright, G. E., and Wintrobe, M. M. 1964. Copper Metabolism in Normal Subjects. *Amer. J. Clin. Nutr.* 14:224-32.

Chase, M. S; Gubler, C. J.; Cartwright, G. E.; and Wintrobe, M. M. 1952. Studies on Copper Metabolism. IV. The Influence of Copper on the Absorption of Iron. *J. Biol. Chem.* 199:757-63

———. 1952. Studies on Copper Metabolism. V. Storage of Iron in Liver of Copper-Deficient Rats. *Proc. Soc. Expr. Biol. Med.* 80:749-50.

Clawson, W. J. 1972. Copper, Molybdenum, and Selenium in the West. *Animal Nutr. Health.* April, p. 14-15.

Compere, R.; Burny, A.; Riga, A.; Francois, E.; and Vanuytrecht, S. 1965. Copper in the Treatment of Molybdenosis in the Rat: Determination of the Toxicity of the Antidote. *J. Nutr.* 87:412-18.

Cordy, D. R. 1971. Enzootic Ataxia in California Lambs. *JAVMA* 158:1940-42.

Cromwell, G. L. 1971. Copper, Molybdenum, Sulfate and Sulfide Interrelationships in Swine. *An. Nutr. and Health* 26(12):5-7.

Cunningham, I. J.; Hogan, K. G.; and Lawson, B. M. 1959. The Effect of Sulfate and Molybdenum on Copper Metabolism in Cattle. *New Z. J. Agric. Res.* 2:145-52.

Dale, S. E. 1971. Effect of Molybdenum and Sulfate on Copper Metabolism in Young Growing Pigs. M. S. Thesis, Iowa State University, Ames, Iowa.

Davis, G. K. 1950 *Symposium on Copper Metabolism.* W. D. McElroy and B. Glass, eds. Baltimore: Johns Hopkins Press.

De Goey, L. W.; Wahlstrom, R. C.; and Emerick, R. J. 1971. Studies of High Level Copper Supplementation to Rations for Growing Swine. *J. Anim. Sci.* 33:52-57.

de Renzo, E. C.; Kaleita, E.; Heyther, P.; Oleson, J. J.; Hutchings, B. L.; and Williams, J. H. 1953. Identification of the Xanthine Oxidase Factor as Molybdenum. *Arch. Biochem. Biophys.* 45:247-53.

Dick, A. T. 1953a. The Effect of Inorganic Sulfate on the Excretion of Molybdenuin Sheep. *Aust. Vet. J.* 29:18-26.

———. 1953b. The Control of Copper Storage in the Liver of Sheep by Inorganic Sulfate and Molybdenum. *Aust. Vet. J.* 29:233-39.

———. 1954. Preliminary Observations on the Effect of High Intakes of Molybdenum and of Inorganic Sulfate on

Blood Copper and on Fleece Character in Crossbred Sheep. *Aust. Vet. J.* 30:196-202.

Dick, A. T., and Bull, L. B. 1945. Some Preliminary Observations on the Effect of Molybdenum on Copper Metabolism in Herbivorous Animals. *Aust. Vet. J.* 21:70-72.

Doudoroff, P., and Katz, M. 1953. Critical Review of Literature on the Toxicity of Industrial Wastes and Their Components to Fish. II. The Metals, as Salts. *Sewage Ind. Wastes* 25:802-39.

Dowdy, R. P. 1969. Copper Metabolism. *Amer. J. Clin. Nutr.* 22(7):887-92.

Dowdy, R. P.; Kunz, G. A.; and Sauberlich, H. E. 1969. Effect of a Copper-Molybdenum Compound Upon Copper Metabolism in the Rat. *J. Nutr.* 99:491-96.

Dowdy, R. P., and Matrone, G. 1968a. Copper Molybdenum Interactions in Sheep and Chicks. *J. Nutr.* 95:191-96.

———. 1968b. A Copper-Molybdenum Complex: Its Effects and Movements in the Piglet and Sheep. *J. Nutr.* 95:197-201.

Elliot, J. I., and Bowland, J. P. 1970. Effects of Dietary Copper Sulfate and Protein on the Fatty Acid Composition of Porcine Fat. *J. Anim. Sci.* 30:923-30.

Ferguson, W. S.; Lewis, A. H.; and Watson, S. J. 1938. Action of Molybdenum in Nutrition of Milking Cattle. *Nature (London)* 141:553.

Fleming, C. E.; McCormick, J. A.; and Dye, W. B. 1961. The Effects of Molybdenosis on a Breeding Experiment. Nevada Agric. Expr. Sta. Bull. No. 220. 15 pages.

Gallagher, C. H., and Reeve, V. E. 1971. Copper Deficiency in the Rat. Effect of Synthesis of Phospholipids. *Aust. J. Expr. Biol. Med. Sci.* 49:21-31.

Gardiner, M. R. 1966. Mineral Metabolism in Sheep Lupinosis. II. Copper. *J. Comp. Path.* 76:107-20.

———. 1967. The Role of Copper in the Pathogenesis of Subacute and Chronic Lupinosis of Sheep. *Aust. Vet. J.* 43:243-48.

Gardner, A. W., and Hall-Patch, P. K. 1962. An Outbreak of Industrial Molybdenosis. *Vet. Rec.* 74:113-15.

Gipp, W. F.; Pond, W. G.; and Smith, S. E. 1967. Effects of Level of Dietary Copper, Molybdenum, Sulfate, and Zinc on Body Weight Gain, Hemoglobin, and Liver Storage of Growing Pigs. *J. Anim. Sci.* 26:727-30.

Goldberg, A.; Williams, C. B.; Jones, R. S.; Yamagita, M.; Cartwright, G. E.; and Wintrobe, M. 1956. Studies on Copper Metabolism. XXII. Hemolytic Anemia in Chickens Induced by the Administration of Copper. *J. Lab. Clin. Med.* 48:442-53.

Goldfischer, S. 1967. Demonstration of Copper and Acid Phosphatase Activity in Hepatocyte Lysosomes in Experimental Copper Toxicity. *Nature* 215:74-75.

Goldfischer, S.; Schiller, B.; and Sternlieb, I. 1970. Copper in Hepatocyte Lysosomes of the Toad, *Bufo marinus L. Nature* 228:172-73.

Goodrich, R. D., and Tillman, A. D. 1966. Copper, Sulfate, and Molybdenum Interrelationships in Sheep. *J. Nutr.* 90:76-80.

Gray, L. F., and Daniel, L. J. 1964. Effect of the Copper Status of the Rat on the Copper-Molybdenum-Sulfate Interaction. *J. Nutr.* 84:31-37.

Gregoriadis, G., and Sourkes, T. L. 1967. Interacellular Distribution of Copper in the Liver of the Rat. *Can. J. Biochem.* 45:1841-51.

———. 1968. Role of Protein in Removal of Copper from the Liver. *Nature* 218:290-91.

Hanrahan, T. J., and O'Grady, J. F. 1968. Copper Supplementation of Pig Diets. The Effect of Protein Level and Zinc Supplementation on the Response to Added Copper. *Anim. Prod.* 10:423-32.

Hardy, R. M.; Stevens, J. B.; and Stowe, C. M. 1975. Chronic Progressive Hepatitis in Bedlington Terriers Associated with Elevated Liver Copper Concentrations. *Minn. Vet.* 15:13-24.

Hays, V. W., and Kline, R. D. 1969. Copper-Molybdenum-Sulfate Interrelationships in Growing Pigs. *Feedstuffs* 41(44):18.

Hazel, C. R., and Meith, S. J. 1970. Bioassay of King Salmon Eggs and Sac Fry in Copper Solutions. *Calif. Fish. Game.* 56:121-24.

Higgins, E. S.; Richert, D. A.; and Westerfield, W. W. 1956. Molybdenum Deficiency and Tungstate Inhibition Studies. *J. Nutr.* 59:539-59.

Hill, C. H.; Strarcher, B.; and Kim, C. 1967. Role of Copper in the Formation of Elastin. *Fed. Proc., Fed. Amer. Soc. Expr. Biol.* 26:129-33.

Hogan, K. G.; Money, D. F. L.; and Blayney, A. 1968. The Effect of Molybdate and Sulfate Supplement on the Accumulation of Copper in the Livers of Penned Sheep. *New Z. J. Agric. Res.* 11:435-44.

Huber, J. T.; Price, N. O.; and Engel, R. W. 1971. Response of Lactating Dairy Cows to High Levels of Dietary Molybdenum. *J. Anim. Sci.* 32:364-67.

Huisingh, J., and Matrone, G. 1972. Copper-Molybdenum Interactions with the Sulfate-Reducing System in Rumen Microorganisms. *P.S.E.B.M.* 139:518-21.

Hunt, C. E.; Landesman, J.; and Newberne, P. M. 1970. Copper Deficiency in Chicks: Effects of Ascorbic Acid on Iron, Copper, Cytochrome Oxidase Activity, and Aortic Mucopolysaccharides. *Brit. J. Nutr.* 24:607-14.

Ishmael, J., and Gopinath, C. 1971. Blood Copper and Serum Enzyme Changes Following Copper Calcium E.D.T.A. Administration to Hill Sheep of Low Copper Status. *J. Comp. Path.* 81:455-61.

Ishmael, J., and Gopinath, C. 1972. Effect of a Single Small Dose of Inorganic Copper on the Liver of Sheep. *J. Comp. Path.* 82:47-57.

Ishmael, J.; Gopinath, C.; and Howell, J. M. 1971. Studies with Copper Calcium E.D.T.A. *J. Comp. Path.* 81: 279-91.

———. 1972. Experimental Chronic Copper Toxicity in Sheep. Biochemical and Hematological Studies During the Development of Lesions in the Liver. *Res. Vet. Sci.* 13:22-29.

———. 1971. Experimental Chronic Copper Toxicity in Sheep. Histological and Histochemical Changes During the Development of the Lesions in the Liver. *Res. Vet. Sci.* 12:358-66.

Jones, J. R. E. 1938. The Relative Toxicity of Salts of Lead, Zinc, and Copper to the Stickleback *(Gasterosteus aculeatus L.)* and the Effect of Calcium on the Toxicity of Lead and Zinc Salts. *J. Exp. Biol.* 15:394-407.

———. 1939. The Relation Between Electrolytic Solution Pressures of the Metals and Their Toxicity to the Stickleback *(Gasterosteus aculeatus L.).* *J. Exp. Biol.* 16:425-37.

Jubb, K. V. F., and Kennedy, P. C. 1970. *Pathology of Domestic Animals.* Vol. I. New York: Academic Press. pp. 304-8.

Kline, R. D.; Hays, V. W.; and Cromwell, G. L. 1971. Effects of Copper, Molybdenum and Sulfate on Performance, Hematology and Copper Stores of Pigs and Lambs. *J. Anim. Sci.* 33(4):771-79.

———. 1970. Effects of Molybdenum, Sulfate, and Sulfide on Copper Store of Pigs. *J. Anim. Sci.* 31:205.

Kowalczyk, T.; Pope, A. L.; Berger, K. C.; and Muggenburg, B. A. 1964. Chronic Copper Toxicosis in Sheep Fed Dry Feed. *JAVMA* 145:352-57.

Kowalczyk, T.; Pope, A. L.; and Sorensen, D. K. 1962. Chronic Copper Poisoning in Sheep Resulting from Free-Choice Trace Mineral-Salt Ingestion. *JAVMA* 141: 362-66.

Lahey, M. E.; Gubler, C. J.; Chase, M. S.; Cartwright, G. E.; and Wintrobe, M. M. 1952. Studies on Copper Metabolism. II. Hematologic Manifestations of Copper Deficiency in Swine. *Blood* 7:1053-74.

Lal, S., and Sourkes, T. L. 1971. Deposition of Copper in Rat Tissues—the Effect of Dose and Duration of Administration of Copper Sulfate. *Toxicol. Appl. Pharmacol.* 20:269-83.

———. 1971. Intracellular Distribution of Copper in the Liver During Chronic Administration of Copper Sulfate to the Rat. *Toxicol. Appl. Pharmacol.* 18:562-72.

Leach, R. M., Jr., and Norris, L. C. 1957. Studies on Factors Affecting the Response of Chicks to Molybdenum. *Poultry Sci.* 36:1136. (abstract)

Lee, G. R.; Cartwright, G. E.; and Wintrobe, M. M. 1968. Heme Biosynthesis in Copper-Deficient Swine. *Proc. Soc. Exper. Biol. Med.* 127(4):977-81.

Lee, G. R.; Nacht, S.; Lukens, J. M.; and Cartwright, G. E. 1968. Iron Metabolism in Copper-Deficient Swine. *J. Clin. Invest.* 47:2058-69.

Lindquist, R. R. 1967. Studies on the Pathogenesis of Hepatolenticular Degeneration. I. Acid Phosphatase Activity in Copper-Loaded Rat Livers. *Amer. J. Path.* 51:471-81.

Lindquist, R. R. 1968. Studies on the Pathogenesis of Hepatolenticular Degeneration. III. The Effect of Copper on Rat Liver Lysosomes. *Amer. J. Path.* 53:903-27.

MacPherson, A., and Hemingway, R. G. 1965. Effects of Protein Intake on the Storage of Copper in the Liver of Sheep. *J. Sci. Food Agric.* 16:220-27.

———. 1969. The Relative Merit of Various Blood Analyses and Liver Function Tests in Giving an Early Diagnosis of Chronic Copper Poisoning in Sheep. *Brit. Vet. J.* 125:213-20.

Marcilese, N. A.; Ammerman, C. B.; Valsecchi, R. M.; Dunavant, B. G.; and Davis, G. K. 1969. Effect of Dietary Molybdenum and Sulfate Upon Copper Metabolism in Sheep. *J. Nutr.* 99:177-83.

———. 1970. Effect of Dietary Molybdenum and Sulfate Upon Urinary Excretion of Copper in Sheep. *J. Nutr.* 100:1399-1406.

Marston, H. R. 1952. Cobalt, Copper and Molybdenum in the Nutrition of Animals and Plants. *Physiol. Rev.* 32:66-121.

McCosker, P. J. 1968. Observations on Blood Copper in the Sheep. II. Chronic Copper Poisoning. *Res. Vet. Sci.* 9:103-16.

McGhee, F.; Creger, C. R.; and Couch, J. R. 1965. Copper and Iron Toxicity. *Poultry Sci.* 44:310-12.

McNatt, E. N.; Campbell, W. G. Jr.; and Callahan, B. C. 1971. Effects of Dietary Copper Loading on Livers of Rats. I. Changes in Subcellular Acid Phosphatases and Detection of an Additional Acid p- nitrophenylphosphatase in the Cellular Supernatant During Copper Loading. *Amer. J. Path.* 64:123-44.

Milne, P. B., and Weswig, P. H. 1968. Effect of Supplementary Copper on Blood and Liver Copper-Containing Fractions in Rats. *J. Nutr.* 95:429-33.

Miltmore, J. E., and Mason, J. L. 1971. Copper to Molybdenum Ratio and Molybdenum and Copper Concentrations in Ruminant Feeds. *Can. J. Anim. Sci.* 51:193-200.

Moore, T. 1969. Vitamin A and Copper. *Amer. J. Clin. Nutr.* 22(8):1017-18.

Moore, T.; Sharman, I. M.; Todd, J. R.; and Thompson, R. H. 1972. Copper and Vitamin A Concentrations in the Blood of Normal and Copper-Poisoned Sheep. *Br. J. Nutr.* 28:23-29.

Mount, D. I. 1968. Chronic Toxicity of Copper to Fathead Minnows (*Pimephales promelas, Rafinesque*). *Water Research* 2:215-23.

Mount, D. I., and Stephan, C. E. 1969. Chronic Toxicity of Copper to the Fat Head Minnow *(Pimephales promelas)* in Soft Water. *J. Fish. Res. Bd. Can.* 26:2449-57.

NCR-42 Committee on Swine Nutrition. 1974. Cooperative Regional Studies with Growing Swine: Effects of Vitamin E Levels of Supplementary Copper During the Growing-Finishing. Period on Gain, Feed Conversion and Tissue Copper Storage in Swine. *J. Anim. Sci.* 39:512-20.

Nielands, J. B.; Strong, F. M.; and Elvehjem, C. A. 1948. Molybdenum in the Nutrition of the Rat. *J. Bio. Chem.* 172:431-39.

O'Dell, B. L.; Hardwich, B. C.; Reynolds, G.; and Savage, J. E. 1961. Connective Tissue Defect in the Chick Resulting from Copper Deficiency. *Proc. Soc. Expr. Biol. Med.* 108:402-5.

O'Hara, J. 1971. Alterations in Oxygen Consumption by Bluegills Exposed to Sublethal Treatment with Copper. *Water Research* 5:321-27.

Owen, C. A., and Hazelrig, J. B. 1968. Copper Deficiency and Copper Toxicity in the Rat. *Amer. J. Phys.* 215:334-38.

Parris, E. C. C., and McDonald, B. E. 1968. Effect of Dietary Protein Source on Copper Toxicity in Early-Weaned Pigs. *Can. J. Anim. Sci.* 49:215-22.

Peters, R. A.; Shorthouse, M.; and Walshe, J. M. 1965. The Effect of Cu^{++} on the Membrane ATPase and its Relation to the Initiation of Convulsions. *J. Physiol.* 181:27P-28P.

Pickering, Q. H., and Henderson, C. 1966. The Acute Toxicity of Some Heavy Metals to Different Species of Warm Water Fishes. *Air Water Pollut.* 10:453-63.

Pierson, R. E., and Aanes, W. A. 1958. Treatment of Chronic Copper Poisoning in Sheep. *JAVMA* 133:307-11.

Powers, E. B. 1917. The Goldfish *(Carassius carassius)* as a Test Animal in the Study of Toxicity. *Illinois Biol. Monographs.* 4:127-93.

Prasad, A. S.; Oberleas, D.; and Rajasekaran, G. 1970. Essential Micronutrient Elements., *Amer. J. Clin. Nutr.* 23(5):581-91.

Pullar, E. M. 1940. The Toxicity of Various Copper Compounds and Mixtures for Domesticated Birds. *Aust. Vet. J.* 16:147-62.

————. 1940. The Toxicity of Various Copper Compounds and Mixtures for Domesticated Birds. *Aust. Vet. J.* 16:203-13.

Ragen, H. A.; Nacht, S.; Lee, G. R.; Bishop, C. R.; and

Cartwright, G. E. 1969. Effect of Ceruloplasmin on Plasma Iron in Copper-Deficient Swine. *Amer. J. Phys.* 217:1320-23.

Raymount, J. E. G., and Shields, J. 1963. Toxicity of Copper and Chromium in the Marine Environment. *Air Water Pollut.* 7:435-43.

Richert, D. A., and Westerfield, W. W. 1953. Isolation and Identification of the Xathine Oxidase Factor as Molybdenum. *J. Biol. Chem.* 203:915.

Ritchie, H. D.; Luecke, R. W.; Baltzer, B. V.; Miller, E. R.; Ulrey, O. E.; and Hoefer, J. A. 1963. Copper and Zinc Interrelationships and Parakeratosis. *J. Nutr.* 79(2):117-23.

Ross, D. B. 1966. The Diagnosis, Prevention and Treatment of Chronic Copper Poisoning in Housed Lambs. *Br. Vet. J.* 122:279-84.

Ross, D. B. 1970. The Effect of Oral Ammonium Molybdate and Sodium Sulfate Given to Lambs with High Liver Copper Concentrations. *Res. Vet. Sci.* 2:295-97.

Rucker, R. B.; Parker, H. E.; and Rogler, J. C. 1969. Effect of Copper Deficiency on Chick Bone Collagen and Selected Bone Enzymes. *J. Nutr.* 98:57-63.

St. George-Grambauer, T. D., and Rac, R. 1962. Hepatogenous Chronic Copper Poisoning in Sheep in South Australia Due to the Consumption of *Echium plantagineum* (Salvation Jane). *Aust. Vet. J.* 38:288-93.

Scheinberg, I. H., and Sternlieb, I. 1960. Copper Metabolism. *Pharmacol. Rev.* 12:355-81.

Smith, M. S. 1969. Responses of Chicks to Dietary Supplements of Copper Sulphate. *Br. Poult. Sci.* 10:97-108.

Smith, S. E., and Larson, E. J. 1946. Zinc Toxicity in Rats; Antagonistic Effects of Copper and Liver. *J. Biol. Chem.* 163:29-38.

Sprague, J. B. 1968 Promising Anti-Pollutant: Chelating Agent NTA Protects Fish from Copper and Zinc. *Nature* 220:1345-46.

Sutter, M. D.; Rawson, D. C.; McKeown, J. A.; and Hashell, A. R. 1958. Chronic Copper Toxicosis in Sheep. *Amer. J. Vet. Res.* 19:890-92.

Suttle, N. F.; Angus, K. W.; Nisbet, D. E.; and Field, A. C. 1972. Osteoporosis in Copper-Depleted Lambs. *J. Comp. Path.* 82:93-97.

Suttle, N. F., and Mills, C. F. 1966a. Studies of the Toxicity of Copper to Pigs. I. Effects of Oral Supplements of Zinc and Iron Salts on the Development of Copper Toxicosis. *Brit. J. Nutr.* 20:135-47.

————. 1966b. Studies of the Toxicity of Copper to Pigs. 2. Effect of Protein Source and Other dietary Components on the Response to High and Moderate Intakes of Copper. *Brit. J. Nutr.* 20:149-61.

Suveges, T.; Ratz, F.; and Salyi, G. 1971. Pathogenesis of

Chronic Copper Poisoning in Lambs. *Acta Vet. Hung.* 21(4):383-91.

Taylor M., and Thomke, S. 1964. Effect of High-Level Copper on the Depot Fat of Bacon Pigs. *Nature:* 201:1246.

Todd, J. R. 1962. Chronic Copper Poisoning in Farm Animals. *Vet. Bull.* 32:573-80.

Todd, J. R. 1969. Chronic Copper Toxicity of Ruminants. Symposium on Nutritional Disorders of Ruminants 28:189-97.

———. 1972. Copper, Molybdenum and Sulphur Contents of Oats and Barley in Relation to Chronic Copper Poisoning in Housed Sheep. *J. Sci. Comb.* 79:191-95.

Todd, J. R.; Gracey, J. F.; and Thompson, R. H. 1962. Studies on Chronic Copper Poisoning. I. Toxicity of Copper Sulphate and Copper Acetate in Sheep. *Brit. Vet. J.* 118:482-91.

Todd, J. R., and Thompson, R. H. 1963. Studies on Chronic Copper Poisoning. II. Biochemical Studies on the Blood of Sheep During the Hemolytic Crisis. *Brit. Vet. J.* 119:161-73.

———. 1964. Studies on Chronic Copper Poisoning. III. Effect of Copper Acetate Injected into the Blood Stream of Sheep. *J. Comp. Path.* 74(4):542-51.

———. 1965. Studies on Chronic Copper Poisoning IV. Biochemistry of the Toxic Syndrome in the Calf. *Brit. Vet. J.* 121:90-97.

Underwood, E. J. 1971. *Trace Elements in Human and Animal Nutrition.* New York: Academic Press, pp.57-106.

Van Adrichem, P. W. 1965. Changes in the Activity of Serum-Enzymes and in the LDH Isoenzymes Pattern in Chronic Copper Intoxication in Sheep. *Tydschr. Diergeneesk* 90(20):1371-81.

Van Reen, R. 1953. Effects of Excessive Dietary Zinc in the Rat and the Interrelationship of Copper. *Arch. Biochem. Biophys.* 46:337-44.

Verity, M. A.; Gambell, J. K.; Reith, A. R.; and Brown, W. Jann. 1967. Subcellular Distribution and Enzyme Changes Following Subacute Copper Intoxication. *Lab. Invest.* 16(4):580-90.

Voelker, R. W., and Carlton, W. W. 1969. Effects of Ascorbic Acid on Copper Deficiency in Miniature Swine. *Amer. J. Vet. Res.* 30:1825-30.

Vogel, F. S. 1960. Nephrotoxic Properties of Copper Under Experimental Conditions in Mice With Special Reference to the Pathogenesis of the Renal Alterations in Wilson's Disease. *Amer. J. Path.* 36:699-11.

Vohra, P., and Kratzer, F. H. 1968. Zinc, Copper and Manganese Toxicities in Turkey Poults and Their Alleviation by E.D.T.A. *Poult. Sci.* 47:699-704.

Wallace, H. D.; McCall, J. T.; Bass, B.; and Combs, G. E. 1960. High Level Copper for Growing-Finishing Swine. *J. Anim. Sci.* 19:1153-63.

Wiederanders, R. E. 1968. Copper Loading in the Turkey. *Proc. Soc. Exptl. Biol. Med.* 128:627-29.

Whanger, P. D., and Weswig, P. H. 1971. Effect of Supplementary Zinc on the Intracellular Distribution of Hepatic Copper in Rats. *J. Nutr.* 101:1093-98.

Wolff, Sh. M. 1960. Copper Deposition in the Rat. *A.M.A. Arch. Path.* 69:217-23.

IRON

Young animals born to mothers that have been raised in confinement or on soils deficient in iron may have a deficiency of this element at birth. Young piglets are born with approximately 50 mg of iron in their bodies. It has been estimated that they will utilize approximately 7 mg/day. Therefore, if they receive no supplemental iron their tissues will be depleted after one week. It is necessary that they receive iron either by the parenteral or oral route during the first week after birth. This can be accomplished by natural means, that is giving pigs access to soil, or by supplementing their milk diet orally with an iron preparation, or by injecting 100-200 mg of iron which will meet the pig's needs for the next several weeks when he will be receiving iron in his feed.

Iron toxicosis usually results when too much iron is either injected or given orally to the neonatal animal. In general two types of problems may result: (1) an anaphylactoidlike reaction following the use of injectable iron preparations and (2) iron toxicosis per se.

Source

Several injectable preparations of iron are used for the prevention of anemia, especially in baby pigs. The injectable preparations include iron dextran, iron dextrin, iron polysaccharide, iron sorbital and ferric ammonium citrate. Oral iron preparations include iron sulfate and ferrous sulfate.

Toxicity

Problems following iron therapy are most usually seen in baby pigs one to three days of age. Cattle and sheep have been killed by excessive dosing with ferric ammonium citrate and other iron preparations. All animals are potentially susceptible including humans.

Apparently two syndromes are involved. (1) A peracute syndrome characterized by sudden death within a few minutes to hours after iron injection. This resembles an anaphylactic reaction, however the triggering mechanism is unknown. (2) A subacute syndrome characterized by death accompanied by severe depression and coma. This syndrome is related to direct toxic effects of the iron resulting from an overdosage.

It should be remembered that most animals and humans do not have a mechanism for excretion of iron; therefore, the toxicity of iron depends upon the amount of iron already present in the body. This is why some animals may die from an iron injection while others receiving the same dosage from the same vial may show no signs of toxicosis. Pigs born from vitamin E and selenium deficient sows are reported more susceptible to iron toxicosis. (Tollerz, 1965)

Toxicity of iron is greatest by the intravenous route followed by intramuscular injection with the oral route being the least toxic.

Oral dosages greater than 150 mg/kg are considered excessive and may lead to iron toxicosis. Levels of iron in the diet of baby pigs (5,000 ppm) may cause reduced growth and rickets because of the precipitation of phosphate by iron.

Mechanism of Action

Excessive levels of iron cause a cardiovascular collapse. There is increased capillary permeability, decreased plasma volume and sudden vascular collapse. Liver injury may result from direct toxic effects of the iron. Witzleben and Chaffey (1966) demonstrated acute liver damage in rabbits following intravenous injection of ferrous sulfate. Initially there was an increase in activity of oxidative enzymes followed by loss of activity.

Large doses of ferrous sulfate given orally may break down the mechanism controlling absorption of iron from the intestine resulting in increased absorption, development of a ferritin complex and cardiovascular shock and liver damage.

Absorbed iron is carried in the serum by transferrin. When the dose is excessive then the binding capacity of the transferrin is exceeded and serum iron concentration

315

rises rapidly. When the serum iron passes through the liver, the liver sequesters large amounts as does the spleen. At the cellular level, excessive iron is a protoplasmic poison capable of inactivating metabolic oxidative enzymes. A severe metabolic acidosis occurs and the clinical picture is one of profound shock. Elevated serum iron also interferes with the clotting mechanism augmenting any hemorrhagic process.

Some endogenous chemical, possibly ferritin from mucosal cells, serves as a vasodepressor.

Clinical Signs

In the peracute shock syndrome animals develop a vascular collapse, and die rapidly within a few hours. In the subacute syndrome animals become drowsy and vomit followed by a period of apparent improvement. This is followed by cardiovascular collapse and death. There is often swelling and edema of the limb in which an iron injection has been made.

Physiopathology

The physiology of iron absorption has been reviewed by Bothwell et al., (1970). Najean et al., (1967), developed a model describing the storage and transport of iron in mammalian systems.

Iron is distributed in the body as follows: 70 percent in hemoglobin; 25 percent stored as ferritin and hemosiderin; 5 percent as muscle myoglobin and less than 0.5 percent as tissue enzymes and plasma transferrin. Excess iron absorbed over a period of years finds its way mainly to harmless stores. Large amounts of iron taken as a single dose can be extremely toxic.

Experimentally, about 5-10 percent of an oral dose is absorbed by the intestinal mucosa. In iron deficient states up to 60 percent is absorbed. The divalent forms (ferrous) are absorbed to a greater extent than the ferric forms, probably due to lower solubilities of ferric salts. Both ferric and ferrous iron can be absorbed as long as they are in ionized form. A high sugar diet increases the absorption of iron. Phosphates reduce the absorption of iron.

The duodenum and jejunum have the highest absorptive activity for iron. There is a rate limited mucosal transfer system.

There is often a yellowish-brown discoloration of all tissues, especially those near the site of injection. The lymph nodes, liver and kidneys may be very dark. There is usually severe edema near injection sites and in the subcutaneous connective tissue. There may be liver damage, especially periportal necrosis. Gastric ulceration and edema may be associated with oral toxicosis.

Diagnosis

There is usually a history of iron injection or oral exposure. Clinical signs indicating a rapid cardiovascular collapse and shock and postmortem lesions including dark and edematous kidneys, lymph nodes, liver and musculature at the site of injection are all compatible with a diagnosis of iron toxicosis.

In children serum iron levels of 500 micrograms per 100 ml are likely to be associated with severe poisoning. Serum levels have exceeded 2,500 micrograms in some cases.

In dogs normal serum iron levels were 100-900 micrograms/100 ml. After oral dosing with 225 mg iron/kg serum iron levels rose to 1,000-32,000 micrograms/100ml.

There appears to be a profound lack of information on serum iron levels associated with iron toxicosis in most domestic animals.

Treatment

Treatment of peracute iron toxicosis is usually futile. Supportive therapy with glucose and norepinephrine have given beneficial effects. When the iron exposure has been oral, magnesium oxide can be given to form an insoluble iron hydroxide.

Chelating agents have been used in an attempt to reduce mortality in children. EDTA (ethylenediaminetetraacetic acid) and DTPA (diethylenetriamine pentaacetic acid) have not reduced mortality in acute iron poisoning in experimental animals. Deferoxamine (Desferal®, Ciba) a new chelating agent with a stronger and more selective affinity for iron than EDTA or DTPA has been used in children with iron poisoning. Experimental work in dogs suggests that an intravenous dose of 0.75 mg desferrioxamine/kg/min is sufficient to complex all of the circulating iron. The use of corticosteroids in conjunction with desferrioxamine did not alter the survival rate. Levarterenol restored arterial blood pressure and maintained cardiac output but also increased mortality.

Plasma extenders and other intravenous fluids may be of some value in countering the cardiovascular shock. Deferoxamine given intravenously can cause a marked drop in blood pressure. For this reason the drug should be given slowly in an IV drip.

REFERENCES

Anonymous. 1959. Parenteral Iron Therapy May Induce Iron Toxicosis. *Bordon Review of Nutrition.* 20:71.

Apri, T., and Tollerz, G. 1965. Iron Poisoning in Piglets—Autopsy Findings and Experimental and Spontaneous Cases. *Acta. Vet. Scand.* 6:360-73.

Bothwell, T. H., and Charlton, R. W. 1970. Absorption of Iron. *Ann. Rev. Med.* 21:145-56.

Clarke, E. G. C., and Clarke, M. L. 1967. *Garner's Veterinary Toxicology.* Baltimore: Williams & Wilkins Co., pp. 90-91.

Forth, W., and Rummel, W. 1973. Iron Absorption. *Physiological Reviews.* 53:724-92.

Harrison, P. M. 1971. Biochemistry of Iron. *Clinical Toxicology* 4:529-44.

James. J. A. 1970. Acute Iron Poisoning: Assessment of Severity and Prognosis. *J. of Ped.* 77:117-19.

Miller, E. R.; Ullrey, D. E.; Brent, B. E.; Merkel, R. A.; Laidlaw, V. A.; and Hoefer, J. A. 1965. Iron Retention and Ham Discoloration: A Comparison of Five Injectable Iron Preparations. *JAVMA.* 146:331-36.

Najean, Y.; Dresch, C.; Ardaillou, N.; and Bernard, J. 1967. Iron Metabolism—Study of Different Kinetic Models in Normal Conditions. *Am. J. Physiol.* 213:533-46.

Robertson, W. O. 1967. Treatment of Acute Iron Poisoning. *Mod. Treatm.* 4:671-78.

Tollerz, G. 1965. Studies on the Tolerance to Iron in Piglets. Dept. Med. I, Royal Vet. Coll., Stockholm.

Witzleben, D. L, and Chaffey, N. J. 1966. Acute Ferrous Sulfate Poisoning. *Arch. Path.* 82:454-61.

LEAD

Lead poisoning has been a part of history since 4,000 years before Christ. Yet, even today with an increased awareness of the toxicity associated with lead, it is one of the most common toxicants in large and small animals. Zook *et al.,* (1969) reported lead as the most common cause of poisoning in dogs. Buck (1969) reported that lead is a common toxicant of cattle, and Perlstein and Attala (1966) reported that in the Chicago area lead accounted for 80 percent of all deaths in children due to accidental poisoning. When one considers that about 600,000 tons of lead are mined each year in the United States and another 600,000 tons are reclaimed the opportunity for exposure of animals and man is not surprising. The uses of lead in the United States for 1972 are given in table 1.

Oral consumption is the major route of exposure for animals. Almost everyone is aware that some paints contain lead. In fact, some paints may contain nearly 50 percent lead. The lead in paint may be in the form of red lead (Pb_3O_4), white lead ($2PbCO_3 \bullet Pb[OH]_2$), lead sulfate ($PbSO_4$), or lead chromate ($PbCrO_4$). Equally important, of course, the veterinarian must recognize that not all paint contains lead and, therefore, paint eating by young calves, dogs, or other animals is not conclusive evidence for a diagnosis of lead poisoning. The practitioner should be aware that buckets of old, unused lead-based paint may be discarded in junk piles, groves, or gullies where cattle are allowed to graze. Other sources of lead associated with the barn area include window putty and plumbing caulk.

Two sources of lead associated with farm machinery are grease, containing up to 50 percent lead in some cases, and used crankcase oil. As gasoline is burned in the engine, the tetraethyl lead is burned with approximately 30 percent of the lead ending up in the lubricating oil, 50 percent being exhausted, and 20 percent deposited in the engine.

Motto *et al.,* (1970) found levels as high as 255 mg lead/kg dry weight grass immediately adjacent to roadways. The levels decreased to 165 mg/kg at 7.6 m, 99 mg/kg at 22.8 m, and 67 mg/kg at 68.6 m from the road. Since a cow can be expected to eat 22.5 gm dry matter/kg/day, the lead exposure would range from 5.7 to 1.0 mg/kg from eating the contaminated forage. Potential exposure in horses would be equivalent since a horse averages eating 21 gm dry matter/kg/day. Consumption of only the most heavily contaminated forage would be likely to cause any overt adverse health effects. Grass growing near heavy trafficked roads is generally not available to grazing animals so the hazard is low. To date, no instances of poisoning from motor vehicle pollution of forage have been reported. However, the lead intake from contaminated pasture or hay

TABLE 1
Uses of 1,445,600 Tons of Lead
in United States for 1972[a]

Use	Tons	% of Total[b]
Storage batteries	695,000	48.0
Antiknock additives	278,300	19.3
Ammunition	85,567	5.9
Red lead and litharge	69,000	4.7
Solder	71,400	4.9
Cable covering	48,700	3.4
Caulking	23,000	1.6
Sheet lead	23,000	1.6
Brass and bronze	18,600	1.3
Pipe	18,500	1.3
Weights	18,300	1.3
Type metal	18,000	1.2
Pigment colors	16,300	1.1
Bearing metals	15,000	1.0
Casting metals	6,500	0.4
Foil	4,500	0.3
Terne metal	4,500	0.3
Annealing	4,100	0.3
Collapsible tubes	3,800	0.3
White lead	2,900	0.2
Galvanizing	1,300	0.1
Other	18,900	1.3

[a]Source: Adapted from Annual Review 1972, US Lead Industry, Lead Industries Assn. Inc., 292 Madison Ave., New York 10017.

[b]Rounded to nearest 0.1%.

319

would be expected to contribute to the total body burden of lead.

Surprisingly cattle will drink crankcase oil or will lick machinery grease if allowed access to these materials. Discarded lead-acid batteries and plumbing lead should be considered as potential sources. Many times these items are available in rural trash piles within the confines of a pasture. Such articles may also be found around barns where calves may be able to gnaw at them.

In a survey of lead poisoning in livestock conducted at Iowa State University, lead poisoning was diagnosed in a total of 63 separate cases from 1965 through 1970. Paint and petroleum products accounted for 60 percent of all lead poisoning diagnosed in the six-year period of study. Unknown or general sources such as trash piles involved 35 percent of the cases.

Another Iowa State University survey involved 58 additional cases of lead poisoning. Results were similar to the six-year study with paint and used motor oil as the leading sources. The higher yearly incidence of poisoning in 1971 and 1972 most likely represents increased awareness of potential toxicosis and improved and refined diagnostic methods. (Buck, 1975)

In horses most episodes have involved contaminated pastures near smelters. Airborne particulate lead settles upon forage and vegetation around smelters and is ingested with the natural herbage intake of the animals. In a relatively old report, Haring (1915) investigated 32 farms located near a smelter. Twelve cases of laryngeal paralysis were identified in horses grazing contaminated pastures. The estimated lead dose was 250 mg/horse/day. Cattle and hogs raised in the area were not affected.

Linoleum, lead toys, drapery weights, or ornaments are sources of lead for household pets, especially young pups which are predisposed to chewing on everything and anything.

Industrial contamination can cause isolated problems where fumes or residue runoffs from lead reclaiming or processing plants are located in the immediate vicinity. In the United States, England, and Australia lead mine tailings have been a problem.

The impact of lead mining and ore processing activities on lead contamination in an area in southeast Missouri that produces 75% of the current United States supply has been reported by Dorn et al., (1972). Test cows placed in the area were estimated to have their lead exposures increased from a background of 0.18 mg/kg up to 8.6 mg/kg in the test site. As in other similar situations, the horse seemed to be either more sensitive or somehow achieved a higher total exposure.

Waterfowl can be poisoned on as few as eight No. 6 lead shot. The gizzard retains the shot as grit which increases the chances for absorption of toxic amounts of lead.

Water from lead pipes or pipes with soldered joints is a potential source. The veterinarian should also be alert for the use of lead-lined drinking or feeding utensils.

Lead arsenate pesticides are a cause of poisoning in cattle, although it is usually due to the more acute toxicity of the arsenic.

In captive primates the major sources have been the paint used on the cages.

Canned cat and dog pet food was reported to contain about 3 ppm lead with a range of 0.9-7 ppm. To what extent the lead comes from organ meats used in pet food and what portion comes from the solder in the can is not known. (Hankin et al., 1975) These levels are not sufficient to cause any clinical illness. This data is cited to call attention to two aspects. First, it is an example of the probable cycling of toxic substances from one animal to another. Second, this is an example of the background exposure to lead experienced by most animals. Therefore, it is to be expected that randomly collected blood samples will contain trace amounts of lead.

Toxicity

Lead accumulates in the body so that chronic exposure to small amounts may lead to toxicosis. Silage containing 140 ppm lead has poisoned cattle. Herbage grown on lead-contaminated soil has contained 260-914 ppm and caused death in calves. Normal herbage should contain 3 to 7 ppm or less. Forage with levels less than 45-60 ppm did not cause problems in lambs.

Acute lethal single exposures are usually considered to be 400-600 mg/kg in calves and 600-800 mg/kg in adult cattle. However, a case has been reported in dairy cattle where an estimated single exposure to 4.8 mg/kg red oxide of lead in paint killed 18 of 20 animals. The daily intake of approximately 6-7 mg/kg body weight appears to be the minimum dose which will eventually result in toxicosis in horses and cattle.

Reports of horses affected while cattle grazing in the same area remain unaffected suggest that horses are more susceptible to lead toxicosis. However, since horses tend to eat grass closer to the ground and occasionally pull plants up by the roots they may receive additional exposure from contaminated soil.

Sheep were fed metallic lead daily during gestation at levels ranging from 0.5-16.0 mg/kg to maintain blood lead levels of 0.4-0.6 ppm. Severe nonfatal poisoning occurred, manifested by anorexia, emaciation, and abortion. (Sharma, 1971)

Lead toxicosis is rarely reported in swine, and pigs were found experimentally to be relatively resistant to lead. (Link and Pensinger, 1966) In addition the eating and foraging habits of swine do not suggest their consumption of foreign objects.

The approximate toxic dose for wildfowl such as mallard ducks is 1 gm, based on feeding trials where birds were fed eight No. 6 shotgun pellets. The nonlethal dose is approximately 380 mg (three No. 8 pellets). Birds have a remarkable capacity for retaining lead shot in the gizzard; frequently six of eight shot are retained. (Bates *et al.,* 1968) In some cases birds die while others develop nonlethal poisoning. Ducks have been shown experimentally to be susceptible to poisoning from consumption of marsh soil containing disintegrated lead shot.

All species of animals are susceptible; but due to eating habits or greater sensitivity, lead poisoning is more frequently observed in cattle, horses, waterfowl, and dogs. Young animals are more susceptible than mature animals. Goats, chickens, and pigs are more tolerant. Vengris (1972) fed six-week-old chickens lead as the acetate at 160 mg/kg daily for 30 days without producing signs of toxicosis. Levels of 320 and 640 mg/kg daily caused toxicosis at 25 and 7 days, respectively.

Mechanism of Action

Lead is relatively insoluble, and even soluble forms such as lead acetate form insoluble compounds such as lead sulfate in the gastrointestinal tract.

Only 1-2 percent of orally administered lead acetate (soluble form), lead carbonate (insoluble form), or metallic lead is absorbed from the digestive tract. However, a large portion of the absorbed lead is retained in the soft tissues initially and later in the bone. Organic compounds such as tetraethyl lead can rapidly penetrate the skin. Inorganic lead cannot, except through wounds. Lead may be absorbed from subcutaneous and intramuscular sites (shot) and through the respiratory tract. (Goodman and Gilman, 1966)

Although lead is poorly absorbed from the digestive tract, blood lead levels may rise to 2.5-4.0 ppm within 12 hours of ingestion and decline to 1-1.5 ppm in 48-72 hours. However, the blood level will be elevated for one to two months. (Allcroft, 1951) This slow decline in blood lead emphasizes the slow excretion of lead in untreated animals and the role of lead as a chronic cumulative toxicant.

Lead appears to affect all major organs. Circulating lead combines with erythrocytes and, unless in very high concentrations, is not found in plasma. Anemia may result from first an increased fragility of red cells which leads to premature destruction and, secondly, by depression of bone marrow so that fewer cells are produced. The nervous system is affected by a decreased blood supply due to damage to capillaries which results in either edema or a collapse of the small arteries. Peripheral nerves are affected by a segmental demyelination which interferes with nerve conduction. The roaring that is observed in horses, the pharyngeal or buccal paralysis in cattle, and the paralysis of the masseter muscles in dogs are evidence of neurological damage of either cranial nerves or brain stem nuclei.

In the kidney, lead causes degeneration and necrosis of renal tubule cells. In acute exposures, lead may cause necrosis of gastrointestinal mucosa. Liver degeneration and necrosis can follow both acute and chronic exposures. In young animals, lead will affect metabolically active growth centers of long bones and result in increased densities on radiographs. Experimentally, lead will suppress growth in young animals. Lead crosses the placental barrier, and the fetal liver can accumulate toxic levels. Lead can be a cause of abortion, fetal resorption, and sterility.

Lead is removed slowly from the body, primarily by the kidneys. For instance, sheep can excrete a maximum of 0.8 mg lead per day in the urine. Four to six months may be required to reduce the blood lead levels to control levels following acute nonfatal exposure. The magnitude of biliary excretion of lead is poorly understood. Lead is also excreted in the milk which is a potential source for nursing animals.

The subcellular effects of lead have not been fully investigated. However, lead will cause rupture of lysosomes and release acid phosphatase which is required for energy production and protein synthesis. Lead interferes with several enzymes involved in heme synthesis. One important effect is in blocking the metabolism of aminolevulinic acid (ALA), causing abnormally large amounts of deltaminolevulinic acid (Δ- ALA)to appear in the plasma and urine. The detection of abnormal levels of Δ-ALA in urine has been used as a diagnostic tool in human and veterinary medicine. Lead also blocks the incorporation of iron into the heme molecule. In general, it is thought that lead will interfere with thiol-containing enzymes (—SH).

Lead has recently been shown to reduce the resistance of mice to bacterial infection by inhibiting antibody production or tying up antibodies already produced (Hemphill *et al.,* 1971), even at exposure levels insufficient to cause other signs of poisoning. This finding could have profound influence upon our attitude toward environmental contamination by lead, if similar effects of lead are found in other species of animals.

Studies at the Behavioral Toxicology Laboratory, College of Veterinary Medicine, Iowa State University, have recently shown that lambs produced by ewes being exposed to subclinical levels of lead during their entire gestation period (4.5 mg lead/kg/day) showed no learning or behavioral deficit until they were about one year old. At this time, the lambs from exposed ewes required nearly twice the time and number of trials to learn a two-choice visual discrimination operant task. (Carson *et al.,* 1972)

Clinical Signs

The first evidence of lead intoxication is often depression and anorexia. It is important to remember that anorexia is almost a constant occurrence in lead poisoning. A transient constipation may occur early followed by diarrhea, which is not frequently seen. In cattle, rumen motility is decreased or abolished. The animals will show abdominal distress, and the abdomen may appear tucked. Cattle may grind their teeth and appear to be chewing, although they may not actually be swallowing. This can give the impression of excessive salivation.

Animals may circle, push against objects, and be ataxic. A slow, rhythmic twitching of the ears and bobbing of the head is frequently seen in cattle. The eyelids may blink in a violent manner, and fine muscle tremors may be seen. The occurrence of marked excitement and convulsive seizures indicates an unfavorable prognosis since these animals frequently die shortly thereafter. Some animals will show very little evidence of intoxication prior to the onset of a sudden convulsive seizure and rapid death.

Signs of clinical toxicity may develop in a few days, especially from drinking used motor oil, or may take two weeks to develop even after fairly large exposures.

There are two syndromes in animals associated with lead poisoning; namely, abdominal and neurological.

In a survey conducted by the authors 90 percent of affected cattle exhibited signs of central nervous system (CNS) involvement, and 60 percent exhibited signs of gastrointestinal involvement. This information is summarized in table 2. Body temperatures were recorded in only 15 cases and were normal in 8, but increased (up to 111 °F) in the other 7. Acute death (less than 24 hours after onset of clinical signs) was reported in about one-third of the episodes. Many animals, however, survived for a longer period of time, ranging from a few hours to about 10 days. Table 3 shows the seasonal occurrence of these cases.

The horse shows more peripheral nerve involvement with muscular weakness and "roaring" which results from paralysis of the recurrent laryngeal nerve. There is also loss of weight, stiffness of joints, progressive arching of the back and cachexia. Young foals are more severely affected than older horses. Lead will cause colic and diarrhea in the horse.

The clinical picture of lead toxicosis in dogs usually

TABLE 2
Clinical Signs Observed in Lead-Poisoned Cattle
(Iowa Veterinary Diagnostic Laboratory)

System	Clinical Sign	No. of Episodes	Percent of Total Episodes
CNS	Blindness	32	51
	Muscle twitching	25	40
	Hyperirritability	21	33
	Depression	20	32
	Convulsions	20	32
	Grinding teeth	15	24
	Ataxia	11	18
	Circling	10	16
	Pushing against objects	7	11
	(One or more of these signs were reported in 90% of the episodes)		
Gastrointestinal	Excessive salivation	26	45
	Anorexia	16	21
	Tucked abdomen	6	10
	Diarrhea	6	10
	(One or more of these signs were reported in 60% of the episodes)		
Other	Acute death	22	35
	Bellowing	8	13

begins with anorexia, vomiting, colic, diarrhea or constipation. The pet owner's attention is usually not attracted until signs of neurologic disorders occur, such as CNS depression, hyperexcitability, hysterical barking, champing fits, convulsions, opisthotonos, paraplegia, muscular spasms, hyperesthesia or blindness. Clarke (1973) cites evidence that gastrointestinal signs are more common in older dogs.

Gastrointestinal symptoms occurred in 87 percent of 60 clinical cases reviewed, while nervous system disorders occurred in 76 percent of the same cases. Although a lead gum line has been reported twice it appears that this is a rare finding and may have resulted from confusion with natural gingival pigments.

Because of some similarities between the clinical signs of lead poisoning and infectious canine distemper of dogs, it has been suggested that the incidence of lead poisoning in dogs may be even higher than presently recognized. It is difficult to establish a firm diagnosis of canine distemper and many clinicians may not suspect lead poisoning. The basis for differentiating the two diseases has been reported. (Zook *et al.,* 1972a) The main features include reticular stippling of red blood cells and the presence of 5-40 nucleated red blood cells (metarubricytes or rubricytes) per 100 white blood cells.

Clinical signs in young rhesus monkeys include short convulsive seizures, eye blinking, decreased activity and visual impairment. There is no apparent effect on hemoglobin or packed cell volume. Intranuclear inclusions are found in the kidney. After six months there was no gross evidence of permanent neurologic damage. (Houser and Frank, 1970)

The clinical signs in waterfowl include weakness, anorexia, weight loss, anemia, and paralysis of wings and legs.

Physiopathology

It is important to recognize that deaths may occur in the absence of any visible lesions. In the authors' experience, most cases of bovine lead poisoning result in acute onset of clinical symptoms and rapid deaths; consequently few cellular lesions have been observed.

Depending on the nature of the exposure pieces of lead may be found in the digestive tract. If the source was used crankcase oil, the digestive contents will be blackened and oily.

Lesions seen following acute or subacute lead poisoning usually include a mild gastritis. The liver in acute exposures is pale with centrilobular degeneration. Acidophilic and acid-fast intranuclear inclusions may be present in hepatocytes. The muscle may appear pale and cooked.

TABLE 3

Seasonal Occurrence of Bovine Lead Poisoning
(Iowa Veterinary Diagnostic Laboratory)

Period	No. of Cases	Percent of Total
January-March	33	27
April-June	48	40
July-September	28	23
October-December	12	9

The kidneys are hyperemic with some hemorrhages in acute deaths; and in chronic cases, the kidneys are degenerated with some fibrosis. Histologically, the glomerular capsule is increased in thickness and hyalinized. Degeneration and necrosis of proximal convoluted and descending tubular epithelium is a prominent lesion along with acid-fast intranuclear inclusion bodies.

Some observe one or more of the following brain changes, ranging from mild to severe, in acute lead poisoning in the bovine: moderate brain edema, swelling, severe congestion of cerebral cortical tissue, prominence of capillaries and endothelial swelling, petechial hemorrhage and laminar neuronal necrosis. (Little and Sorensen, 1969) Christian and Tryphonas (1970) recently reviewed the brain histopathology of lead poisoning in cattle. The more severe changes are limited to protracted cases where animals linger with marked signs for one to two weeks. The histopathology of prolonged cases may include laminar cortical necrosis, endothelial and astrocytic proliferation, microglial accumulation and eosinophilic infiltration of leptomeninges. A study of 55 confirmed cases of lead poisoning revealed that 63 percent of the animals had intranuclear acid fast inclusions characteristic of lead poisoning.

Necropsies were done in 37 of the 63 episodes in the authors' survey. Of these, no gross lesions were observed in ten. In the remaining cases, the following lesions were observed: oil in the gastrointestinal tract (30%); gastritis and/or enteritis (24%); petechiation of epicardium and/or myocardium (21%); pulmonary congestion (16%) and kidney degeneration (16%).

Other lesions observed (in less than 10% of the episodes) were: fatty liver; pale and watery muscle; petechiation of subcutaneous tissues, thymus and trachea; cystitis; cloudy cornea; ocular hemorrhage; brain edema and hyperemia; metal or paint materials in rumen and reticulum and swollen mesenteric lymph nodes.

Zook (1972) described gross and microscopic lesions in dogs affected with lead poisoning. Gross lesions, while generally nondiagnostic included abnormal red bone marrow, brain congestion, petechial hemorrhages, esophageal dialatation and reduction in thickness of adrenal cortex. All lead poisoned dogs had histologic lesions of renal tubular damage and a majority of affected dogs had intranuclear inclusion bodies in proximal renal tubular epithelium. In the bone, metaphyseal sclerosis was observed in young dogs poisoned by lead. The most obvious and consistent lesions in the brain included vascular endothelial swelling and degenerative to necrotic vascular changes. The reader is referred to the specific paper cited for a detailed account of histopathologic lesions.

Electroencephalographic (EEG) changes consisting of high amplitude (200 microvolts) delta waves (1-2 Hertz) have been observed in lead-poisoned dogs. The EEG changes were reversed after EDTA treatment. Analysis of cerebrospinal fluid did not reveal consistent changes in pressure or protein and cellular content. (Zook *et al.,* 1972a)

No definitive brain lesions have been reported for lead-poisoned waterfowl. Vacuolation of liver cord cells and acid-fast intranuclear inclusions in proximal convoluted kidney tubules have been reported. Evidence has been reported for lead-induced anemia in wildlife.

The presence of intranuclear inclusion bodies is frequently observed. Richter *et al.,* (1968) demonstrated that the inclusions were distinct from the nucleoli and that some were surrounded by Feulgen positive material but did not contain DNA. The core of the inclusion was compact and amorphous, probably containing proteins other than histones. The inclusion was surrounded by a fringe of microfibrils.

Diagnosis

As with other toxicoses, consideration must be given to obtaining a good history, noting clinical signs, determining the likelihood of exposure and interpreting chemical analyses. The clinical signs, important histopathologic factors, and hematologic findings, especially in dogs, have been discussed previously.

The major analyses presently used to assist in establishing a diagnosis of lead toxicosis are blood, liver, kidney and stomach content lead levels.

Because of the variability in urinary lead levels and the difficulty of routinely obtaining 24-hour urine specimens in domestic animals, urine lead levels are of little use in establishing a diagnosis. The best use of urine specimens is in comparing pretreatment and posttreatment levels after EDTA chelation therapy. A large increase in lead levels should be observed.

One investigator has found that tissues stored in formalin can still be used for lead analysis to obtain

retrospective information of lead poisoning. (Zook, *et al.,* 1970)

The analysis of hair specimens for lead and other metals is of use in human studies but of more limited value in animals because of seasonal growth changes and shedding.

Before the diagnostic toxicologist can interpret the significance of tissue lead levels, the normal background levels should be known. Background tissue lead levels (table 4) were obtained from animals submitted to the Iowa Veterinary Diagnostic Laboratory for which a diagnosis other than lead poisoning was made.

Dorn, *et al.,* (1972) found milk lead levels of 0.034-0.25 ppm in cows placed in a lead-contaminated test site. Blood levels were 0.28-0.58 ppm. Background levels were 0.06-0.13 ppm in milk and 0.06-0.18 ppm in blood.

The background blood lead level in 89 clinically normal dogs from a suburban Illinois area was .078 ppm. In 50 dogs from the pound the average level was 0.26

TABLE 4
Background Tissue (Wet Weight) Lead Levels for Domestic Animals Submitted to Iowa Veterinary Diagnostic Laboratory

Species and Tissue	No. of Samples	Lead — PPM Mean ± S.D.
Equine		
Blood	2	0.18, 0.05
Liver	9	0.82 ± 0.58
Kidney	7	0.93 ± 0.59
Bovine		
Blood	92	0.103 ± 0.044
Liver	197	1.12 ± 1.36
Kidney	181	1.21 ± 1.69
Rumen contents	52	1.07 ± 1.44
Canine		
Blood	20	0.093 ± 0.031
Liver	31	1.00 ± 0.98
Kidney	27	0.81 ± 0.82
Stomach contents	7	0.91 ± 1.36
Porcine		
Blood	2	0.12, 0.09
Liver	27	0.93 ± 0.73
Kidney	24	0.95 ± 0.97
Stomach contents	8	0.95 ± 0.88
Ovine		
Blood	2	0.09, 0.05
Liver	13	0.72 ± 0.58
Kidney	13	0.72 ± 0.58
Rumen contents	4	0.55 ± 0.30

ppm and for 98 dogs from low-income families in the city the level was 0.17 ppm. Eleven of the pound and 15 of the low-income dogs had blood levels greater than 0.35 ppm. None of the regular hospital patients had elevated blood levels. Four dogs from the pound and low-income groups had blood levels greater than 0.6 ppm. (Thomas *et al.*, 1975) Zook *et al.*, (1969) reported blood leads of 0.19 ± 0.18 ppm (mean ± standard deviation) in clinically normal dogs, while the average blood lead in poisoned dogs was 1.2 ppm. Diagnostic levels were considered to be 0.6 ppm or greater, although occasionally levels of 0.35 ppm when coupled with appropriate clinical signs were considered diagnostic. (Zook *et al.*, 1972b)

The tissue lead levels associated with clinical bovine lead poisoning based on cases submitted to the Iowa Veterinary Diagnostic Laboratory are shown in table 5.

Previously reported tissue lead levels associated with toxicosis are summarized in table 6.

It is considered diagnostically significant when liver or kidney tissues contain at least 10 ppm lead on a wet-weight basis. Whole blood lead levels of at least 0.35 ppm are considered significant in cattle and probably other ruminants. Furthermore, for a clinician to render a positive diagnosis of lead poisoning it is imperative that symptomatology, history or circumstantial evidence be compatible with the lead poisoning. In some cases diagnoses may be confirmed at less than 10 ppm liver lead if clinical signs, exposure, or other tissue levels are known.

Generally those animals with blood lead concentrations in excess of 1.0 ppm should be given a guarded prognosis. However, recovering animals may maintain blood levels well in excess of the clinically significant level of 0.35 ppm and still continue to improve. In the authors' experience, blood lead levels may range from 0.4 to 0.8 ppm for one to three weeks. Thus any one blood level at one point in time may not be sufficient as a prognostic tool. Knowledge of concomitant chelation therapy, peak blood lead concentration, time since clinical disease first occurred, and continued exposure to lead should all enter into evaluation of the animal.

The possibility exists that liver and kidney levels from 1 to 10 ppm and bovine blood levels from 0.10 to 0.35 ppm are significant either as a primary etiological agent or as a predisposing or contributory factor. Dodd and Staples (1965) found that young dogs with lead poisoning sometimes had liver lead levels less than 10 ppm.

Chickens may have blood lead levels of 8.0 ppm without manifesting clinical signs and 13.0 ppm before death. (Vengris, 1972)

In the cow, approximately 0.1 percent of the red cells will have basophilic stippling in chronic lead poisoning. The hematologists must study the smears carefully and eliminate other causes of stippling. Zook *et*

TABLE 5

Levels of Lead in Tissues and Rumen Contents Associated with Clinical Lead Toxicosis in Cattle (Iowa Veterinary Diagnostic Laboratory)

Tissue	No. of Cases	Mean	Range
Liver	100	26.40	1.0 -83.0 ppm
Kidney	105	50.30	3.0 -200 ppm
Blood	50	0.81	0.19-3.80 ppm
Rumen contents	52	400.80	0.0 -11,875 ppm

al., (1969) considered the appearance of large numbers of immature (especially nucleated) RBC and basophilic stippling of RBC in the presence of a normal or slightly lowered PCV (PCV of 28-34%) as almost pathognomonic for lead poisoning in dogs. Whether this is diagnostic in itself is open to debate; however, this should serve as a clue to consider lead poisoning in a diagnosis. This is also an important diagnostic aid since this represents two easily conducted tests (blood smear and PCV).

Although not well established as diagnostic criteria for lead poisoning in animals, tests for aminolevulinic acid (ALA) dehydrase inhibition by lead (in the heme synthesis reaction) have been employed in human medicine. It is probable that the test for serum aminolevulinic acid dehydrase has more diagnostic value than does the test for urinary ALA. (Blumenthal *et al.*, 1972; National Academy of Sciences, 1972) The urinary ALA test has been shown to correlate with clinical signs of poisoning in the cow, dog, and cat. (McSherry *et al.*, 1971)

Background urinary ALA (delta-aminolevulinic acid) levels in normal cows averaged 139.2 ± 75 ug/100 ml and elevated ALA levels above 500 micrograms were associated with bovine lead toxicosis. (McSherry *et al.*, 1971) Sharma (1971) reported background urinary ALA levels in sheep to be less than 50 ug/100ml. Blood lead and urinary ALA levels were directly correlated. Clinical signs of lead poisoning were accompanied by ALA levels of 300-1,400 ug/100 ml of urine.

Both the urinary ALA and the serum ALA dehydrase tests are relatively easily performed and could be done as a routine clinical procedure.

At necropsy, samples of liver, kidney, and digestive tract contents should be obtained. The kidney should be divided into cortex and medulla. If an animal is necropsied on a lead-covered postmortem table, extreme care should be exercised to prevent contamination of the specimens.

Lead levels in brain, lung, and spleen will be a few parts per million in animals dying from lead toxicosis.

TABLE 6
Tissue Lead Levels in Animals Associated with Lead Toxicoses

Animal	Tissue	No. of Samples	Lead Level (Average)
Horses	Blood	6	.39 ppm
	Liver	6	18 ppm
	Kidney	6	16 ppm
Horses	Liver	2	50, 98 ppm
Calves	Liver	10	38 ppm
	Kidney cortex	10	173 ppm
	Kidney medulla	8	10.3 ppm
Calves	Blood	5	1 ppm
Cow	Liver	2	16.1, 11.1 ppm
	Kidney	2	39.0, 61.4 ppm
Cattle	Kidney	158	137 ppm
	Liver	170	43 ppm
	Rumen contents	133	3,427 ppm
Dog	Blood	209	.94 ppm
	Liver	30	24 ppm
Barbary ape	Liver	1	110 ppm
	Kidney	1	120 ppm
Red-faced macaque	Liver	1	65 ppm
	Kidney	1	90 ppm
Spot-nosed guenon	Liver	1	10 ppm
Rhesus	Blood	9	1.56 ppm
Baboons	Blood	2	4-45 ppm
Dove	Liver	1	72 ppm
Geese	Liver	7	5-32 ppm
	Blood	10	.81-16.8 ppm
Mallard duck	Liver	10	33 ppm
	Brain	10	5 ppm
Andean condor	Liver	1	34 ppm
23 avian species	Liver	1-37/species	0.5-3.7 ppm

A fecal lead determination gives the diagnostician some clue as to the time and duration of the exposure. The control fecal level is approximately 12 ppm, while fecal levels greater than 35 ppm are suspect. A high-blood level with a low fecal level indicates that exposure occurred one to three weeks prior to sample collection. Note the wide variation in rumen content lead levels shown in table 5, which emphasizes the point that fecal levels may have time to reach low levels before the animal is severely affected by the ingested lead. Very acute exposures result in high-kidney levels and lower bone and liver levels, while chronic exposures result in low-liver and kidney levels but bone levels of 100 ppm or greater.

In waterfowl, a simple diagnostic test involving microscopic examination of red blood cells for red fluorescence has been shown to be of value. (Barrett and Karstad, 1971)

One must differentiate lead poisoning from rabies, distemper, hepatitis, and other heavy metal toxicoses in dogs. In cattle, hypovitaminosis A (which can result in blindness), rabies, nervous acetonemia (lead-poisoned cattle may have ketone bodies in the urine), other heavy metals (abdominal signs), organic pesticides (salivation and convulsions), and infectious encephalitis, polioencephalomalacia, or thromboembolic meningoencephalomyelitis should be differentiated from lead poisoning. (Buck, 1970) Certain forms of coccidiosis in cattle cause intermittent seizures that may be confused with lead poisoning. Brain abscesses, hemorrhages, and edema may be confused with lead toxicosis. In horses, chronic lead poisoning must be differentiated from heaves.

Treatment

The treatment recommended by Hammond and Sorensen (1957) for cattle consists of the intraperitoneal or subcutaneous administration of a 1-2 percent (weight/volume) solution of CaEDTA in 5 percent dextrose at the rate of 110 mg/kg. This should be given twice daily for two days, the treatment withheld for two days, followed by two more days of therapy. Success is best achieved when the blood lead is less than 1 ppm. Cattle require 10 to 14 days to recover and may require several series of treatment in severe cases.

Supportive therapy of forced feeding and oral fluids is very important since these animals are frequently anoretic, emaciated, and dehydrated. In the presence of neurologic involvement, fluids should not be given since water loading will compound the brain edema. Oral magnesium sulfate may be of some value in limiting further absorption of lead in animals as well as serving as a purge.

Zook et al., (1969) also used CaEDTA (10 mg/ml in 5 percent dextrose) to treat dogs. EDTA should be given subcutaneously for five days at the rate of 110 mg/kg in 4 divided doses daily. The daily dosage should not exceed 2 gm/day. A second treatment is given if clinical signs persist. Supportive therapy may include barbiturates or tranquilizers to control convulsions, mannitol for cerebral edema, fluids for dehydration, and cortisones as indicated. Enemas and lavages can be used to clear the digestive tract of unabsorbed lead particles.

Animals with neurologic involvements are accorded a poor prognosis.

Case History 1

An Iowa farmer lost 3 of 125 six-week-old beef calves. The clinical signs were of short duration, the calves dying within 24 hours after initial signs of illness. They included listlessness, central nervous system depression, groaning, frothy salivation, and twitching of the eyelids and facial muscles. One calf was submitted for postmortem examination revealing congestion and excessive mucus in the intestinal tract. There was an oily smell and consistency to the rumen contents. Microscopic examination of the tissues failed to reveal significant lesions.

Samples of rumen contents, liver, and kidney were submitted for lead analysis. The following levels of lead were found: liver, 70 ppm; kidney, 103 ppm; rumen contents, 180 ppm.

It was apparent from the postmortem findings that these calves had consumed used motor oil containing lead precipitated from the burning of gasoline in a tractor engine.

Case History 2

Seven cattle being fattened for slaughter in a small pasture exhibited convulsive seizures, blindness, and severe central nervous system depression. Only 1 of 100 head in the herd died, the other 6 recovering slowly over a period of several days. The one that died was submitted for postmortem examination revealing hemorrhages on the epicardium and endocardium. No other lesions were noted. Many of the animals were anoretic. An investigation of the premises revealed a junk and trash pile in a small pasture where the cattle were located. There was evidence that these animals had been browsing through the trash, which contained paint buckets, oil and grease buckets, and lead storage batteries.

Appropriate specimens were submitted for lead analysis from the animal that died as well as whole blood from one affected animal. The following levels of lead were obtained: liver, 25.7 ppm; kidney, 68.1 ppm; rumen contents, 110.0 ppm; whole blood (affected animal), 0.84 ppm.

Discussion

The following is intended to provide additional information for the interested student by discussing some basic work and examining selected aspects of lead toxicosis in humans.

Allcroft (1951) showed that lead would cross the placental barrier. Fetal lambs accumulated 37 ppm lead in the liver from ewes receiving 50 mg lead acetate daily during gestation. Blood levels may rise to high levels in a few hours following acute exposures but will require weeks to months to return to normal. For example, Allcroft (1951) showed blood levels rising to 2.5-4.0 ppm in less than 12 hours and falling to 1.0-1.5 ppm in a day or two. However, the blood levels remained at 1.0 ppm for four to eight weeks.

In children, recurrent seizures (20 percent) and mental retardation (22 percent) are common sequelae. (Perlstein and Attala, 1966)

Smith (1964) reported that lead-induced encephalopathy in children resulted in a 25 percent fatality rate,

40 percent recurrent convulsive seizures, and 29 percent with paralysis or significant neurologic defects. Ninety percent of the cases were in children 15 to 36 months of age.

The average daily intake from food for man is 0.12-0.35 mg. (Kehoe, 1964a) (Kehoe, 1964b) reported the safety threshold for humans at 0.15 mg lead/liter urine and 0.8 ppm in blood. This blood level is significantly higher than that of animals. He estimated that daily exposures of 3.27 mg, 2.35 mg, and 1.27 mg would result in critical body levels at eight months, four years, and eight years, respectively. The brain levels in fatal cases of lead poisoning range from 2-6 ppm.

Goyer (1968) reported intranuclear inclusions and swelling of mitochondria in proximal convoluted tubules in rats. In his opinion, the aminoaciduria was due to failure of reabsorption in the renal tubules. Yodaiken (1966) found that radioactive lead was incorporated into mitochondria and nuclei of renal tubule cells.

Effect on Nervous System

Gombault (1880) first described segmental demyelination in peripheral nerves following lead poisoning. Segmental demylination consists of degeneration of one or more internodes with internodes on either side unaffected. Recovery occurs by formation of several short segments along a length of nerve which previously consisted of a single internode segment. Fullerton (1966) confirmed these observations in guinea pigs. Axonal degeneration was also described. Motor nerve conduction velocity was decreased 30 percent, and there was a loss of large nerve fibers. Not all motor axons were equally affected. The loss of fast, unified motor nerve conduction would decrease unity of muscle action and could lead to ataxia and slower, uncoordinated muscle movements.

Lead was shown to increase acid phosphatase in neurons, presumably by causing rupture of lysosomes which liberated the enzyme into the cytoplasm. Acid phosphatase is involved in the production of energy, in protein synthesis, and intracellular metabolism. Acid phosphatase activity was decreased in capillaries, which may account for at least part of the toxic effects of lead on the vascular structures. (Brun and Brunk, 1967) Rosenblum and Johnson (1968) studied young nursing mice receiving lead via postparturient feeding of 0.5 or 1 percent lead carbonate to the maternal mice. This lead to a large number of deaths by three weeks of age. The eyes remained closed for up to 23 days, the young had an abnormal gait, and had difficulty in righting themselves.

Histologic examination of the brain revealed fibrous intravascular strands which were thought to represent thinning and occlusion of cerebral capillaries, with the greatest number occurring in the hippocampus and basal ganglia.

Schlaepfer (1969) found a poor correlation between the amounts of axonal and segmental damage. Either can occur independently and, therefore, axonal degeneration may reflect additional cellular lesions. There was increased nodal acid phosphatase in peripheral nerves which preceded the morphologic evidence of myelin sheath disruption and breakdown. The capsule cells surrounding the dorsal root ganglia cells were increased in number and contained numerous dense bodies in the vicinity of the nucleus. These dense bodies were electron dense comparable to lead.

The axonal degeneration or damage was of two types. First, there was a replacement of neurofilaments and neurotubules with amorphous granular material; and second, membrane-bound glycogen granules were observed in both myelinated axons with normal neurotubular and neurofilament components. Segmental but not axonal degeneration was seen in dorsal and ventral spinal nerve roots.

Metabolism

Figure 2 shows the effect of lead on heme synthesis. Lead inhibits this process in several places. Lead (A on diagram) will cause increased excretion of ALA in the urine. This is due to a depression of ALA dehydrase activity. ALA dehydrase is a copper-containing enzyme. CaEDTA in addition to increasing the excretion of lead will also chelate copper and may inhibit ALA dehydrase by limiting its formation due to decreased availability of copper. Lead (B on diagram) inhibits the conversion of coproporphyrinogen III to protoporphyrin, but the effect is only 1/25 to 1/50 of that on ALA metabolism.

Heme synthetase is a thiol-containing enzyme (—SH) which is needed to incorporate iron into the molecule. This enzyme appears to be inhibited by lead. Of interest here is the report by Bessis and Brenton-Gorius (1959) where ferratin granules were observed to accumulate around mitochondria of erythroblasts.

Diagnosis

Hair has a chemical affinity for heavy metals such as arsenic, lead, thallium, selenium, bismuth, and mercury. These metals react with sulfhydryl groups, particularly cysteine, in the follicular proteins and are incorporated into the keratin molecule. (Flesch, 1965) Since hair is metabolically inactive after its formation, it can be used as a record of the past exposure to heavy

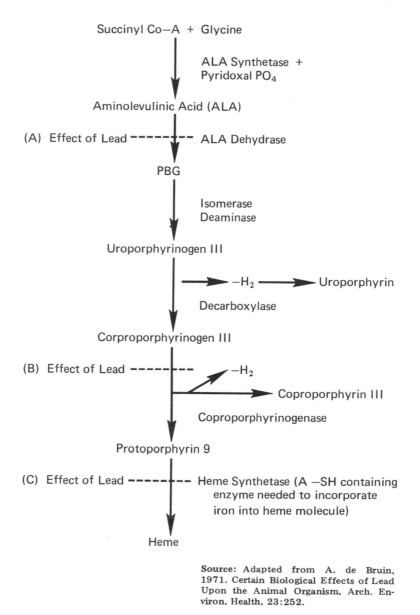

Source: Adapted from A. de Bruin, 1971. Certain Biological Effects of Lead Upon the Animal Organism. Arch. Environ. Health. 23:252.

Figure 2.

metals. In normal children, hair contains 31 ppm lead while lead poisoning results in levels of 200-300 ppm. Considering the relative ease of getting hair samples, this could be used in field surveys to determine the chronic lead exposure in animals.

Treatment

Three drugs are predominately used in treating lead; namely, BAL (2,3-dimercapto-1-propanol); d-penicillamine (β,β- dimethylcystein, a monothiol degradation product of penicillins F, G, K, and X); and CaEDTA (ethylenediaminetetraacetic acid).

All of these drugs act by combining with lead to

presumably form a soluble complex that can be eliminated from the body (see fig. 3).

In biologic systems, N, O, S, and P serve as the chief donors and are tied up by heavy metals. Calcium, barium, and strontium form the most stable complexes with N and O_2, while mercury, silver, and gold complex with S and P. Lead forms complexes equally with all four atoms. The d-isomer of penicillamine should be used rather than the l- or dl-isomers to avoid the antipyridoxine effects of the l-isomer. The d-isomer of penicillamine is a better metal-binding agent than other monothiols such as glutathione and cystein because the thiol (—SH) group is more resistant to oxidation. The chief advantage of penicillamine is that it is effective orally and will increase lead loss in urine four to five

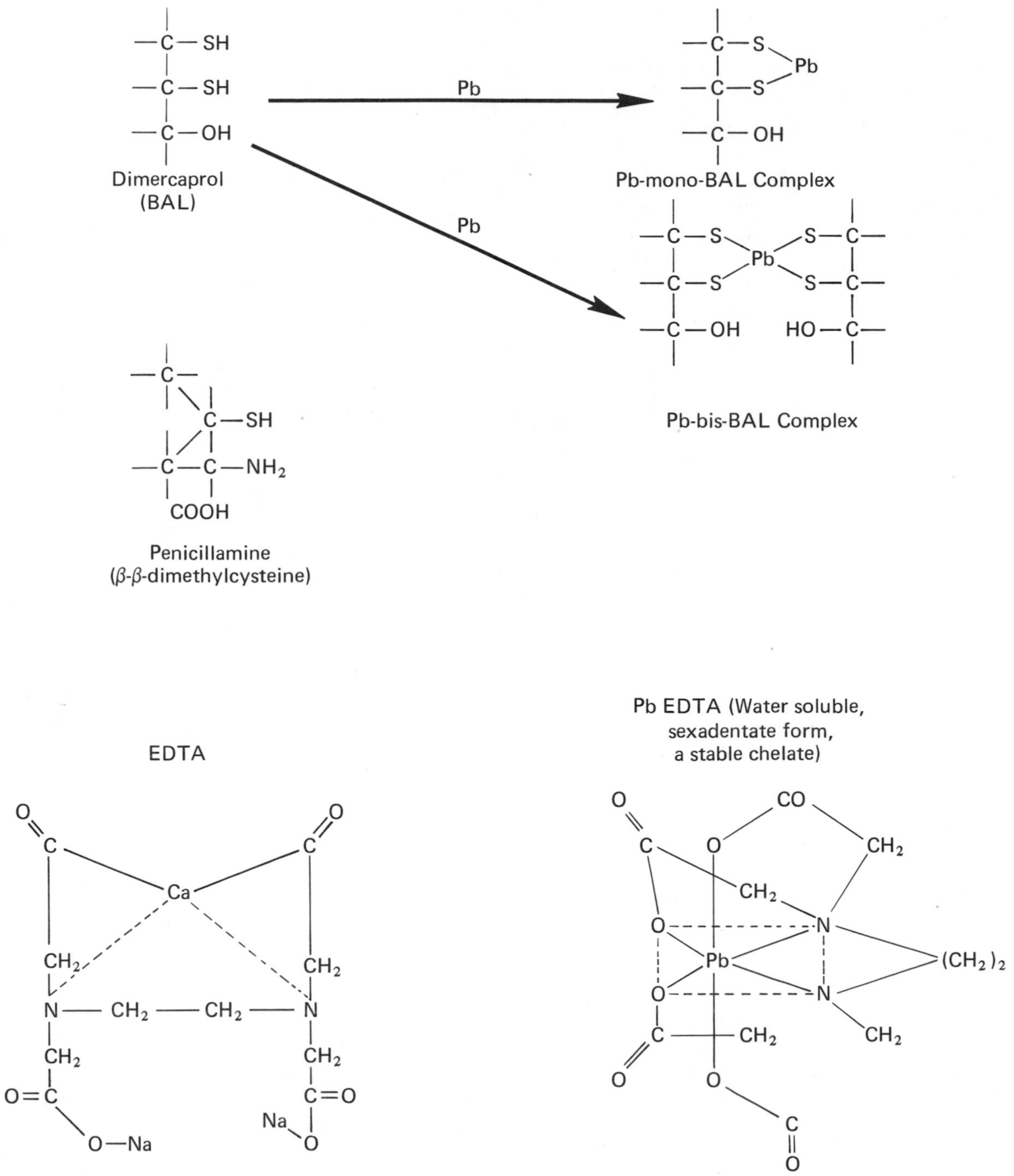
Pb
Pb
Dimercaprol
(BAL)
Pb-mono-BAL Complex
Pb-bis-BAL Complex
Penicillamine
(β-β-dimethylcysteine)
EDTA
Pb EDTA (Water soluble,
sexadentate form,
a stable chelate)

Figure 3.

times. A disadvantage is that it does not remove lead from red cells. Penicillamine will chelate copper, mercury, gold, and lead.

BAL is the drug of choice for stimulating excretion of arsenic and gold. This drug is only active for 4-6 hours and, therefore, repeated doses are required. BAL increases the urinary and fecal excretions of lead. Some BAL reaches the brain. BAL is also effective in restoring the —SH groups on thiol enzymes and cofactors. BAL removes lead from red cells, which may be an important consideration.

EDTA is not metabolized in the body and does not penetrate red cells and only slowly diffuses into cerebrospinal fluid. Oral EDTA promotes the absorption of lead by the intestine and is, therefore, contraindicated. Parenteral EDTA enhances lead excretion twenty to fifty-fold and is probably the most effective drug currently used. A problem that has been encountered with the use of EDTA is the occasional precipitation of severe clinical signs following the start of treatment. This is most likely to occur in severe exposures which are likely to involve neurologic damage, exactly the cases in which this is the most undesirable. For this reason, Chisolm (1968) advocated the simultaneous use of EDTA and BAL and was able to reduce the mortality in children with encephalopathy. His recommendation was to give one dose of BAL first and then start with a combination of BAL and EDTA.

BAL-EDTA together reduced the blood lead by 50 percent in 15 hours while EDTA alone required 68 hours for a 50 percent reduction. Since a major portion of the lead is carried by the red cells, the use of BAL is significant in helping to excrete this portion.

Once chelation therapy is started, it is important to keep it up because stored lead is being mobilized. It is also important to maintain a proper chelant to metal molar ratio.

REFERENCES

Allcroft, R. 1951. Lead Poisoning in Cattle and Sheep. *Vet. Rec.* 63:583-90.

Barrett, M. W., and Karstad, L. H. 1971. A Fluorescent Erythrocyte Test for Lead Poisoning in Waterfowl. *J. Wild. Mgt.* 35:109-18.

Bates, F. Y.; Barnes, D. M.; and Higbee, J. M. 1968. Lead Toxicosis in Mallard Ducks. *Bull. Wildl. Dis. Assoc.* 4:116.

Bessis, M., and Breton-Gorius, J. 1959. Ferritin and Ferruginous Micelles in Normal Erythroblasts and Hypochromic Hypersideremic Anemias. *Blood.* 14:423.

Blanksma, L. A.; Sachs, H. K.; Murray, E. F.; and O'Connell, M. J. 1969. Failure of Urinary Δ -Aminolevulinic Acid (ALA) Test to Detect Pediatric Lead Poisoning.*Am. J. Clin. Pediat.* 52:96.

Blumenthal, S.; Davidow, B.; Harris, D.; and Oliver-Smith, F. 1972. A Comparison Between Two Diagnostic Tests for Lead Poisoning. *Am. J. Pub. Health.* 62:1060-64.

Brun, A., and Brunk, U. 1967. Histochemical Studies on Brain Phosphatases in Experimental Lead Poisoning. *Acta. Path. Microbiol. Scandinavia.* 70:531-36.

Buck, W. B. 1969. Laboratory Toxicologic Tests and Their Interpretation. *JAVMA* 155:1928-41.

———. 1970. Lead and Organic Pesticide Poisonings in Cattle. *JAVMA* 156:1468-72.

———. 1975. Toxic Materials and Neurologic Disease in Cattle. *J. American Veterinary Medical Association* 166:222-26.

Carson, T. L.; Van Gelder, G. A; Buck, W. B.; Hoffman, L. J.; Mick, D. L.; and Long, K. R. 1973. Effects of Low Level Lead Ingestion in Sheep. *Clin. Toxicol.* 6:389-403.

Carson, T. L.; Van Gelder, G. A.; Karas, G. G.; and Buck, W. B. 1974. Slowed Learning In Lambs Prenatally Exposed to Lead. *Archieves of Environmental Health* 29:154-56.

Chisolm, J. J. 1968. The Use of Chelating Agents in the Treatment of Acute and Chronic Lead Intoxication in Childhood. *J. Pediat.* 73:1-38.

Christian, R. G., and Tryphonas, L. 1971. Lead Poisoning in Cattle: Brain Lesions and Hematologic Changes. *Am. J. Vet. Res.* 32:203-16.

Clarke, E. G. C. 1973. Lead Poisoning in Small Animals. *Journal Small Animal Practice* 14:183-93.

Clegg, F. G., and Rylands, J. M. 1966. Osteoporosis and Hydronephrosis of Young Lambs Following the Ingestion of Lead. *J. Comp. Path.* 76:15-26.

Dodd, D. C., and Staples, E. L. J. 1965. Clinical Lead Poisoning in the Dog. *N.Z. Vet. J.* 4(1):1-7

Dorn, R. C., *et al.,* 1972. Study of Lead, Copper, Zinc and Cadmiun Contamination of Food Chains of Man. Report of Environmental Protection Agency Contract 68-2-0092. University of Missouri, Columbia, Missouri.

Flesch, P. 1965. *Hair Growth: Physiology and Biochemistry of the Skin.* 4th ed. Chicago: University of Chicago Press, pp. 641-741.

Fullerton, P. M. 1966. Chronic Peripheral Neuropathy Produced by Lead Poisoning in Guinea Pigs. *J. Neuropath. Exper. Neurol.* 25:214-36.

Garner, R. J. 1961. *Veterinary Toxicology.* 2nd ed. Baltimore: The Williams & Wilkins Co.

Goldberg, A.; Smith, J. A.; and Lochhead, A. C. 1963.

Treatment of Lead Poisoning with Oral Penicillamine. *British Med. J.* 1:1270-75.

Gombault, M. 1880. Contribution a L'etude Anatomique de la Nevite Parenchymateuse Subaique et Chronique-Nevite Segmentaire Peri-axile. *Arch. Neurol.* (Paris). 1:11.

Goodman, L. S., and Gilman, A. 1966. *The Pharmacological Basis of Therapeutics.* 3rd ed. New York: The Macmillan Company, pp. 966-71.

Goyer, R. A. 1968. The Renal Tubule in Lead Poisoning. I. Mitochondrial Swelling and Aminoaciduria. *Lab. Invest.* 19:71-77.

Goyer, R. A.; Krall, A.; and Kimball, J. P. 1968. The Renal Tubule in Lead Poisoning. *Lab. Invest.* 19:78-83.

Hammond, P. B., and Aronson, A. L. 1960. The Mobilization and Excretion of Lead in Cattle: A Comparative Study of Various Chelating Agents. *Ann. N.Y. Acad. Sci.* 88:498-511.

———. 1964. Lead Poisoning in Cattle and Horses in the Vicinity of a Smelter. *Ann. N.Y. Acad. Sci.* 111: 595-611.

Hammond, P. B., and Sorensen, D. K. 1957. Recent Observations on the Course and Treatment of Bovine Lead Poisoning. *JAVMA* 130:23-25.

Hankin, L.; Heichal, G. H.; and Botsford, R. A. 1975. Lead in Pet Foods and Processed Organ Meats. *J. American Medical Association* 231:484-85.

Haring, C. M., and Meyer, K. F. 1915. Investigation of Livestock Conditions and Losses in the Selby Smoke Zone. US Bureau of Mines Bulletin No. 98:474.

Hatch, R. C., and Funnell, H. S. 1969. Lead Levels in Tissues and Stomach Contents of Poisoned Cattle: A Fifteen-Year Survey. *Can. Vet. J.* 10:258-62.

Hemphill, F. E.; Kaeberle, M. L.; and Buck, W. B. 1971. Lead Suppression of Mouse Resistance to *Salmonella typhimurium. Science.* 172:1031-32.

Hirschler, D. A., and Gilbert, L. F. 1964. Nature of Lead in Automobile Exhaust Gas. *Arch. Environ. Health.* 8:297-313.

Houser, W. D., and Frank, N. 1970. Accidental Lead Poisoning in a Rhesus Monkey *(Macaca mulatta). J. Am. Vet. Med. Assoc.* 157:1919.

Kehoe, R. A. 1964a. Normal Metabolism of Lead. *Arch. Environ. Health.* 8:232-35.

———. 1964b. Metabolism of Lead Under Abnormal Conditions. *Arch. Environ. Health.* 8:235-43.

Kopito, L.; Briley, A. M.; and Shwachman, H. 1969. Chronic Plumbism in Children. *JAMA* 209:243-48.

Kradel, D. C.; Adams, W. M.; and Guss, S. B. 1965. Lead Poisoning and Eosinophilic Meningoencephalitis in Cattle. *Vet. Med. Small Anim. Clin.* 60:1045-50.

Leary, S. L; Buck, W. B.; Lloyd, W. E.; and Osweiler, G. D. 1970. Epidemiology of Lead Poisoning in Cattle, *I.S.U. Vet.* 3:112-17.

Link, R. P., and Pensinger, R. R. 1966. Lead Toxicosis in Swine. *American Journal Veterinary Research* 27:759-63.

Little, P. B., and Sorensen, D. K. 1969. Bovine Polioencephalomalacia, Infectious Embolic Meningoencephalitis, and Acute Lead Poisoning in Feedlot Cattle. *JAVMA* 155:1892-1903.

Macadam, R. F. 1969. The Early Glomerular Lesion in Human and Rabbit Lead Poisoning. *British J. Exper. Path.* 50:239.

McSherry, B. J.; Willoughby, R. A.; and Thomson, R. G. 1971. Urinary Delta Aminolevulinic Acid (ALA) in the Cow, Dog, and Cat. *Can. J. Comp. Med.* 35:136-40.

Motto, H. L., *et al.,* 1970. Lead in Soils and Plants: Its Relationship to Traffic Volume and Proximity to Highways. *Environ. Sci. Technol.* 4:231.

National Academy of Sciences. 1972. *Lead: Airborne Lead in Perspective.* Conmittee on Biologic Effects of Atmospheric Pollutants. Washington, D.C.

Osweiler, G. D. 1969. Incidence and Diagnostic Considerations of Major Small Animal Toxicoses. *J. Am. Vet. Med. Assoc.* 155:2011-15.

Pentschew, A., and Garro, F. 1966. Lead Encephalomyelopathy of the Suckling Rat and Its Implications on the Porphyrinopathic Nervous Diseases. *Acta Neuropath.* 6:266-78.

Perlstein, M. A., and Attala, R. 1966. Neurologic Sequelae of Plumbism in Children. *Clin. Pediat.* 5:292-98.

Radeleff, R. D. 1964. *Veterinary Toxicology.* Lea & Febiger.

Richter, G. W.; Kress, Y.; and Cornwall, C. C. 1968. Another look at Lead Inclusion Bodies. *Am. J. Pathol.* 53:189.

Sharma, R. M. 1971. *Effects of Lead Exposure on Pregnant Sheep and Their Progeny.* M.S. Thesis. Iowa State University, Ames, Iowa. p. 134.

Smith, H. D. 1964. Pediatric Lead Poisoning. Arch. Environ. Health. 8:256-261.

Vengris, V. E. 1972. Personal communication. Dept. of Vet. Microbiology, College of Vet. Med., Iowa State University, Ames, Iowa.

Wilson, M. R., and Lewis, G. 1963. Lead Poisoning in Dogs. Vet. Rec. 75:787-791.

Yodaiken, R. E. 1966. The Use of Lead as a Tracer in Ultrastructural Research. Lab. Invest. 15:403.

Zook, B. C.; Carpenter, J. L.; and Leeds, E. B. 1969. Lead Poisoning in Dogs. JAVMA. 155:1329-1342.

Zook, B. C.; Carpenter, J. L.; and Roberts, R. M. 1972a. Lead Poisoning in Dogs: Occurrence, Source, Clinical Pathology, and Electroencephalography. Am. J. Vet. Res. 33:891-902.

Zook, B. C.; Kopito, L.; Carpenter, J. L.; Cramer, D. V.; and Shwachman, H. 1972b. Lead Poisoning in Dogs: Analysis of Blood, Urine, Hair, and Liver for Lead. Am. J. Vet. Res. 33:903-909.

ORGANIC AND INORGANIC MERCURY

Problems encountered with mercury in veterinary medicine during the past years have primarily involved the feeding of seed grain treated with an organic mercury fungicide. Recently the environmental aspect of mercury pollution, especially affecting birds and fish, has been much discussed in the scientific and lay media.

As early as 1705, mercuric chloride was used as a wood preservative. In the late 1700s, mercuric chloride was used as a fungicide for control of wheat smut. Other uses included bedbug control (1822), earthworm control (1860), pesticide for cabbage maggot (1864), and potato seed scab (1891). In 1907 the organic mercury compounds were first used in Europe. By 1924 organic mercury fungicides similar to Semesan (hydroxymercurinitrophenol and hydroxymercurichlorophenol) were being used. In the late 1950s, the use of liquid methyl (alkyl) mercury compounds was started.

The major uses of mercury and consumption figures for the United States in 1969 are given below.

Use	Pounds
Electrolytic chlorine (chlorine-alkali plants)	1,572,000
Electrical apparatus (batteries, switches, fluorescent lights)	1,382,000
Paint (anti-fouling formulations)	739,000
Instruments	391,000
Catalysts	221,000
Dental preparations	209,000
Agriculture (fungicides)	204,000
General laboratory	126,000
Pharmaceuticals	52,000
Pulp and paper (slimicides)	42,000
Amalgamation	15,000
Other	1,082,000
TOTAL	6,035,000

In 1968 a total of 5,732,072 pounds of mercury was used. Of this amount, 17 percent (947,000 pounds) was used for pesticide manufacture for (percent given for each use):

1. Mildew-proof paints (66%).
2. Agricultural chemicals (28%).
3. Paper and pulp (3%).
4. Antifouling paints (3%).

Seed treatment use totaled 76,500 pounds of mercury in 1969. It is estimated that contamination of plants from mercury-treated seed would be at the most 1-3 ppb, which is less than the 5 ppb allowed for potable waters.

Pulp and paper mills are reported to have substituted NaOH for phenylmercuric acetate in 1969 as a slimicide.

The U.S. Department of Interior reported that during the summer of 1970, mercury discharges were reduced 86 percent. Fifty factories that had been discharging a total of 287 pounds of mercury a day reduced losses to 40 pounds/day by September, 1970.

Most of the mercury present in food products is in the form of methylmercury. Studies have demonstrated that regardless of the nature of the mercury pollutant, essentially only methylmercury is present in fish tissue. This has led to studies demonstrating the transformation reactions of various mercury compounds. The biotransformation reactions are given at the top of the following page. Note especially the conversion of inorganic to organic mercury.

The following generalizations can be made about the environmental impact of mercury:

1. Mercury, in whatever form, is potentially exchangeable among air, land, and other phases.
2. Mercury, in whatever form, is potentially capable of being taken up by aquatic animals in the form of methylmercury or ethylmercury.
3. In an aquatic system, methylmercury can be formed directly from inorganic mercury (Hg^{+2}) under anaerobic conditions; except that under *permanently* anaerobic conditions, mercury will tend to accumulate in bottom sediments as either HgS or $Hg°$.

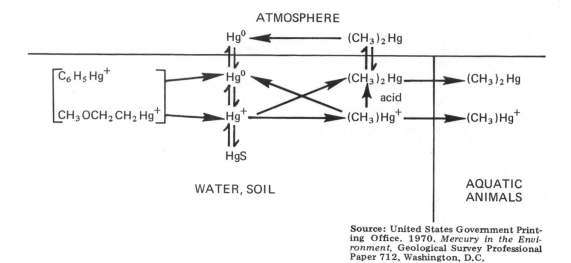

Source: United States Government Printing Office. 1970. *Mercury in the Environment*, Geological Survey Professional Paper 712, Washington, D.C.

Figure 4.

4. Methylmercury and dimethylmercury can be formed from either HgS or Hg° in the presence of oxygen or under oxidizing conditions.
5. Alkaline conditions will tend to promote the release of mercury from aquatic systems via dimethylmercury.

Source

The mercury levels of rocks and soils is estimated to average 50 ppb, however, some soils may contain levels of 15 ppm (England and North Ireland where the residues are thought to be of geological origin). Levels in water are estimated to be 0.2 ppb for ocean and rain and less than 0.1 ppb for inland waters except in cases near natural or manmade sources of contamination.

Mercury is also found in fossil fuels with upper limits of 20 ppm for petroleum oils, 300 ppm for anthracite coal, and 500 ppm for tars.

Mercury in soil will volatize into the atmosphere with a turnover time of two years. Ground air at mercury ore sites has been found to contain 16-20 ppb peak values at midday. Air levels decrease with elevation and lower ambient temperatures. Rain will return the mercury to the soil and estimates have been made that this results in 500 mg of mercury per acre per year.

Average background mercury levels are given below for air, water, plants and animals.

I. Environmental.
  A. Air.
    1. In nonmineralized areas—0.003-0.009 microgram/m³.
    2. Mineral areas—20 microgram/m³.
    3. In urban areas—.01-0.17 microgram/m³.
    4. In industries using mercury—100 microgram/m³.
    5. In mines—20,000 microgram/m³.
  B. Water.
    1. Ocean—0.03 to 2.0 ppb varying with area and depth.
    2. Minamata Bay, Japan—1.6-3.6 ppb.
    3. Normal ground water—0.02-0.07 ppb.
    4. Surface water—most less than 0.1 ppb, some 1-5 ppb.
    5. Sludge from sewage—0.8-120 ppm.
II. Biological.
  A. Plants—natural (levels vary with plant and locality—upper limits reported).
    1. Pome fruit—0.04 ppm or less.
    2. Tomatoes—0.02 ppm.
    3. Potatoes—0.01 ppm.
    4. Wheat, barley—0.08 ppm—occasional sample reported at 0.15-0.40 ppm.
    5. Rice—0.015 ppm.
    6. Marine algae—0.023-0.037 ppm.
  B. Plants treated with fungicide.
    1. Apples—0.1 ppm.
    2. Tomatoes—0.1 ppm.
    3. Potatoes—0.05 ppm.
    4. Seeds treated with fungicide—23-34 ppm, washing seed removed 10-40%.
  C. Animals—levels in eggs, birds, and mammals generally below 0.1 ppm.
    1. Brain—0.1ppm.
    2. Kidney—2.75 ppm.
    3. Liver—0.30 ppm.
    4. Large intestine—0.05 ppm.
    5. Muscle—0.15 ppm.

The most frequent source of mercury for domestic animals is the consumption of seed grains treated with organic mercury fungicides. This source will disappear as the very toxic methyl- and ethylmercury fungicides are no longer used to treat seed grain.

Toxicity

Mercury exists in a variety of both organic and inorganic forms. In table 1, particularly note the high toxicity of the methyl and ethyl organic mercury compounds.

The alkyl (noncyclic saturated hydrocarbon radical) forms such as methyl- and ethylmercury are the most toxic. These mercury forms also show delayed and cummulative effects. Symptoms and lesions may occur 7-21 days after a single exposure. The aryl (aromatic or benzene ring derived radical) forms are less toxic than the alkyl forms but more toxic than the elemental salts. This appears to be due to greater absorption of the aryl form. The aryl mercurial forms, such as phenylmercury, are catabolized in the liver within 24 hours and the mercuric ion is excreted via the kidneys and large intestine.

Mercury vapor is almost completely absorbed from inhaled air and represents a very serious problem in certain situations. It is unlikely that animals would be exposed to mercury vapors since this is an industrial and laboratory problem.

Mechanism of Action

Inorganic mercury compounds are absorbed from the lungs and GI tract, but only poorly through the skin. After ingestion of inorganic mercury, the highest residues are found in the kidney and liver. *Organic* mercury is absorbed from the lung, GI tract, and also through the skin. Phenylmercury and methoxyethylmercury are degraded in the body to inorganic mercury and disappear fairly rapidly from the blood and accumulate in the kidney prior to excretion. All of the forms of mercury may be converted to methylmercury. Hens fed inorganic methoxyethylmercury or phenylmercury laid eggs containing methylmercury in the egg white. Methyl and ethyl (alkymercury) mercury compounds are more stable in the body and circulate attached to the RBC rather than plasma as with the inorganic forms. Attachment to the RBC reduces the portion available for excretion by the liver.

Methylmercury accumulates in the brain to a much greater extent than other forms of mercury. Methylmercury in the CNS appears, at least in man, dog, and primates, to concentrate in the cerebrum and cerebellum. Approximately 10-20 percent of the body burden is located in the head. Alkylmercury is excreted by the liver, but up to 90 percent can be reabsorbed from the gut and recirculated (enterohepatic circulation). The half-life of methylmercury for man is 70-74 days.

Inhaled mercury vapors also show an affinity for nervous tissue.

The affinity of methylmercury for various parts of the dog brain is given in table 2. (Yoshikazu *et al.,* 1966)

In fractionation studies of brain tissue from methylmercury treated animals, the mercury was found in the protein fraction with little in the lipid and nucleic acid fractions. Initially, mercury was highest in the mitochondrial fraction but after 24 hours the amounts in the mitochondrial, microsomal, and supernatant were about equal. Peak brain levels were found 1-2 days after administration.

The hen will excrete methylmercury in the egg, with the level in the albumin four to six times the level in the yolk. (table 3; Smart and Lloyd, 1963)

Clinical Signs

In cattle the clinical signs of inorganic, aryl and methoxyethyl forms of mercury poisoning are similar. Cattle fed methylmercury also develop the CNS form of toxicosis associated with methylmercury in other species.

Symptoms include stomatitis, salivation, loosening of teeth, gastroenteritis, cough, nasal discharge, dyspnea, bronchopneumonia, eczema, skin pustules and ulcers, depilation (starting at the root of the tail), skin keratinization, weakness, anorexia, CNS depression, emaciation, nephritis, hemorrhage (especially of mucous membranes), epistaxis, hematuria, and bloody feces. Convulsive CNS involvement was rarely reported. The percentages of these symptoms in 29 animals studied by Sonoda *et al.,* (1956) are given in table 4.

Herigstad *et al.,* (1972) fed six, four-week-old calves varying levels of methylmercury. Dosages of 0.2 or 0.4 mg/kg produced ataxic after 75-90 days in two calves. The onset of clinical signs was sudden and rapidly progressed from ataxia to stumbling, hyperesthesia, convulsions and prostration.

The average time from onset of symptons till death occurred was 20 days and ranged from 1-43 days. Some animals recovered over a 3-6 month period. Animals with a high fever, severe skin damage, and hemorrhagic symptoms all died.

Clinical pathologic tests showed evidence of a nonregenerating anemia and elevated blood sugar. Serum protein and globulin were slightly depressed, while albumin, phosphorous, calcium, iron and ketone

TABLE 1
Toxicity Data of Mercury Compounds

Species	Compound	Toxicity
Cattle	Ceresan M (1.5% Hg) (ethyl mercury p-toluene sulfonanilide)	1 mg Hg/kg/day leads to anorexia and CNS depression (8 days), lachrymation and depilation (day 17), fever, diarrhea (day 18-22), staggering (28 days).
Cattle	Mercuric chloride-($HgCl_2$) (corrosive sublimate)	4-8 gm (Toxic Dose)
Cattle	Calomel (mercurous chloride-Hg_2Cl_2)	8-10 gm (Toxic Dose)
Cattle	Methylmercury dicyandiamide	0.23 mg Hg/kg for 56 days—mild clinical signs, ataxia.
Horse	Calomel (mercurous chloride-Hg_2Cl_2)	12-16 gm (Toxic Dose)
Horse	Mercuric chloride-($HgCl_2$) (corrosive sublimate)	5-10 gm (Toxic Dose)
Swine	Phenylmercuric chloride	90 day exposure to 0.38 mg Hg/kg resulted in no detectable changes.
Swine	Phenylmercuric chloride	90 days of exposure to 0.76 mg Hg/kg caused reduced growth, but no clinical signs.
Swine	Phenylmercuric chloride	15 days at 2.28 gm Hg/kg resulted in diarrhea followed by tissue lesions. 10 days at 4.56 mg Hg/kg resulted in diarrhea followed by tissue lesions.
Swine	Methylmercury dicyandiamide	Estimated single dose LD_{50} = 13.4 mg Hg/kg.
Swine	Methylmercury dicyandiamide	Single dose 1.7 mg Hg/kg—no clinical toxicity
Swine	Methylmercury dicyandiamide	Single dose 3.4 mg Hg/kg—mild symptoms 3 weeks post-exposure.
Swine	Methylmercury dicyandiamide	Single dose 6.7 mg Hg/kg—clinical sings 6-7 days post-exposure similar, but more severe than 3.4 mg group.
Swine	Methylmercury dicyandiamide	Single dose 10 mg Hg/kg—CNS depression early, followed in 3 weeks by onset of usual signs (i.e., anorexia, staggering, etc.).
Swine	Methylmercury dicyandiamide	Single dose 13 mg Hg/kg—vomiting and diarrhea during first few days. Neurological involvement in 10-20 days. Some deaths after 3-4 weeks.
Swine	Methylmercury dicyandiamide	Single dose 27 mg Hg/kg—severe signs and deaths in 7 days.
Swine	Methylmercury dicyandiamide	Single dose 50-100 mg Hg/kg death in 24 hours.
Swine	Methylmercuric	0.38 mg/kg for 60 days, no clinical signs.
Swine	Methylmercury dicyandiamide	0.76 mg/kg for 44 days, progressive cerebral deficiency. (see text)
Swine	Ethylmercuric chloride	0.38 mg/kg for 64-90 days, 2 of 5 showed progressive cerebral deficiency (see text).
Swine	Ethylmercuric chloride	0.76 mg/kg for 22-30 days, progressive cerebral deficiency (see text).

TABLE 1 (Cont.)

Species	Compound	Toxicity
Sheep	Mercuric chloride-($HgCl_2$) (corrosive sublimate)	4 gm (Toxic Dose)
Sheep	Calomel (mercurous chloride Hg_2Cl_2)	1-2 gm (Toxic Dose)
Sheep	Methylmercury dicyandiamide	0.23 mg Hg/kg for 42 days—mild clinical signs, ataxia.
Sheep	Ethyl mercury p-toluene sulfonalide, Ceresan M, 3.2% Hg	13-38 mg Ceresan/kg for 12-33 days resulted in death.
Cat	Bisethylmercuric sulfide, ethylmercuric chloride, or S-ethylmercurithiouria hydrobromide	2 or 3 mg compound/kg body weight/day in food. No change in 1 week, cerebellar ataxia in 2-3 weeks, moribund 2 weeks later.
Cat	Diethyl mercury	Daily doses of 2-3 mg/kg, via stomach tube, symptoms same as above.
Cat	Mercuric ethyl mercaptide	2-3 mg/kg for 52 days. No effect.
Cat	Phenylmercuric acetate	2-3 mg/kg for up to 52 days. No effect.
Chicken	Methylmercury dicyandiamide	0.42-0.46 mg/kg/day for 40-44 days resulted in no clinical signs. This equaled a total dose of 27-28 mg Hg/chicken. Tissue residues were 10 ppm for muscle and 40 ppm for liver.
Chicken	Ceresan M	5 mg Ceresan/kg for 26-30 days—lethal.
Chicken	Ceresan M	10-20 Ceresan/kg for 10-12 days—lethal.
Chickens	Methylmercury dicyandiamide	0.15 mg Hg/kg for 84 days—no clinical signs.
Rat	Methylmercury	Multiple dose over 10-90 days, a cumulative dose of 100 mg/kg leads to neurological symptoms.
Mouse	4.2% Methoxyethlen mercuric chloride (USPULN) 2.5% Hg	Oral LD_{50} = 47 mg/kg Subcut. LD_{50} = 60 mg/kg
Mouse	5% Phenylmercuric acetate (SANMICRON)	Oral LD_{50} = 25 mg/kg Subcut. LD_{50} = 36 mg/kg
Mouse	4.7% Phenylmercuric acetate plus 0.5% tolyl mercury p-toluene sulfonanilide (MERAN)	Oral LD_{50} = 35 mg/kg Subcut. LD_{50} = 51 mg/kg
Mouse	Phenylmercuric acetate plus phenylmercury triethanol ammonium acetate (SINMEL)	Oral LD_{50} = 24 mg/kg Subcut. LD_{50} = 32 mg/kg
Mouse	1.75% Ethyl mercuric phosphate (RUBERON)	Oral LD_{50} = 61 mg/kg
Dog	Calomel (mercurous chloride-Hg_2Cl_2)	1-2 gm (Toxic Dose)
Dog and Cat	Mercuric chloride-($HgCl_2$) (corrosive sublimate)	0.1-0.3 gm (Toxic Dose)
Rat and Mouse	Alkylmercury	LD_{50} = 20-30 mg/kg
Rabbits, Dogs, Cats	Methylmercury	Multiple feeding 10-90 days, 0.4-1 mg Hg/kg per day will result in neurological symptoms, this equals a cumulative dosage of 10-20 mg/kg.

TABLE 2
Average Level (ppm) for 3 Dogs Given
60 mg Hg/kg

Area	
Calcarine grey	44
Calcarine white	42
Frontal cortex	27
Temporal cortex	33
Parietal cortex	17
Occipital cortex	17
Cerebellar grey	25
Cerebellar white	30
Caudate nucleus	17

TABLE 3
Comparative Egg and Kidney Residues for
2 Hens Fed 6 ppm Methylmercury
Dicyandiamide for 8 Weeks

Sample	Level—ppm
Yolks	4.1
Albumin	18.2
Kidney	7.5

TABLE 4
Distribution of Symptoms of 29 Cattle Fed Ceresan
(1.5% Mercury in the Form of Chlorophenyl-Mercuric
Chloride, Phenyl-Di-Mercuric Chloride and
Methoxyethyl-Mercuric Chloride)

Sympton	Percent Occurence in 29 Animals
Fever	65%
Depression and anorexia	76%
Lachrymation	48%
Decline of milk	79%
Cramp	7%
Depilation	79%
Eczema	41%
Itchiness	27%
Salivation	65%
Diarrhea	17%
Bronchial catarrh	58% (especially in severe cases)
Anemia of mucosa	34% (especially in severe cases)
Petechia (mucosa)	27% (especially in severe cases)
Swelling of lymph nodes	55% (especially in severe cases)
Cardiac disturbance	31% (especially in severe cases)

bodies were within normal ranges. Urine samples from severely affected animals contained protein.

Tissue residue levels were 2.26-70 ppm in kidney and 0-1.40 ppm in liver.

Most of the reported field episodes of mercury poisoning in domestic animals have involved swine. The recent report by Piper *et al.*, (1971) provides data on the responses of pigs to single acute exposures of varying amounts of methylmercury dicyandiamide (alkylmercury). The following summarizes their findings in relationship to single dose exposures. Exposure to 1.7 mg Hg/kg resulted in no apparent damage. Pigs given 3.4-6.7 mg Hg/kg became sick and then recovered. Initially anorexia, loss of weight, CNS depression, weakness, gagging and vomiting were seen 6-21 days postexposure. A few days later, postural abnormalities, slight staggering and stiffness were reported. Other signs noted were cyanosis, constipation, and thickened, scaly skin. Depending on the dose, the pigs either recovered or the symptoms become gradually more severe. The higher doses resulted in a more rapid onset of clinical signs.

Pigs given 10-26 mg Hg/kg vomited following the acute exposure. CNS depression and anorexia were apparent in a few days followed by loss of weight, weakness, fever, abnormal posturing and incoordination. Some pigs had a diarrhea and experienced a CNS

excitatory phase. Some animals were severely affected (*in extremis*) in 6-7 days.

Massive exposure (50-100 mg Hg/kg) resulted in diarrhea, vomiting, tachycardia, CNS depression, cyanosis, subnormal temperature, labored respiration, coma, and death within 12-24 hours.

A summary of the residue levels in various tissues is given in table 5. Be careful to note that the duration between exposure and postmortem varied with dosage. In terms of diagnostic utility, samples of kidney and liver would be most useful.

Tryphonas and Nielsen (1973) extended the acute studies of Piper *et al.*, to include chronic exposures of 20-90 days by feeding low levels of methylmercuric dicyandiamide (MMD) or ethylmercuric chloride (EMC) to swine. Pigs fed 0.76 mg/kg of MMD or 0.38 to 0.76 mg/kg of EMC developed a progressive cerebral deficiency after 20-90 days. The clinical signs included anorexia, retarded growth rate, incoordination, aimless walking, blindness, chewing without prehension of food, flaccid abdominal musculature, paresis, raucous voice, tremor, paddling movements, coma, and death. The duration of the disease averaged 8 days at the high dose.

Exposure of swine to 0.76 mg Hg/kg (as phenylmercuric chloride, an arylmercury) resulted in depression of growth rates without other signs of toxicosis. Exposure to higher levels consistently resulted in diarrhea and progressive weight loss. Diarrhea appeared after 15 days

TABLE 5
Tissue Residues (PPM—Wet-Weight Basis) in Pigs Exposed to a Single Oral Dose of Methylmercury Dicyandiamide*

Dose (mg Hg/kg)	0	1.7	6.7	26.9	107.4
Days post-exposure	28-33	32	29-34	7	0.5
No. of animals	4	2	4	2	2
Muscle	.29	.67	3.95	36.8	4.9
Brain stem	.25	.65	3.5	22.6	2.6
Cerebrum	.23	.75	3.93	25.7	9.2
Kidney medulla	.25	1.05	4.63	24.2	23.6
Kidney cortex	.35	2.1	13.4	83.7	32.5
Liver	.38	1.95	7.83	82.6	54
Duodenum	.30	.3	1.95	21	293.5
Colon	.23	.23	1.1	18.7	43.8

*Adapted from Piper et al., 1971.

TABLE 6
Mercury Residue Levels in Pigs Fed Phenylmercuric Chloride*

	Residue Level—ppm				
Dose (mg Hg/kg)	0.19	0.38	0.76	2.28	4.56
No. of days	64	74	66	33	13
No. of pigs	5	5	5	5	5
Tissue					
Kidney	40	140	200	220	220
Liver	5	5	11	66	72
Muscle	0	0	0	1	1
Intestine	4	4	14	34	34
Brain	1	1	1	3	2

*Adapted from Tryphonas and Nielsen, 1971.

of 2.28 mg Hg/kg and after 10 days of 4.56 mg Hg/kg exposure. As the disease progressed the pigs became weak and were reluctant to move. This was followed by lethargy, prostration, and terminal coma. Elevated BUN levels were reported for the higher exposed pigs. Residue levels are given in table 6.

Wright et al., (1973) produced mild poisoning in sheep after 42-60 days of feeding 0.33 mg methylmercury dicyandiamide/kg body weight. In cattle and sheep residue levels were highest in the kidney, reaching 100-150 ppm after 6-8 weeks. Liver levels were 40-50 ppm, muscle 14-23 ppm and brain 12-13 ppm after 8-9 weeks.

Chickens were fed 0.11 and 0.22 mg MMD/kg for 12 weeks without producing toxicosis. Residue levels were highest in the liver (12 ppm) followed by kidney (10 ppm) and muscle (4-5 ppm) after 12 weeks.

Physiopathology

In cattle postmortem changes include subacute interstitial nephritis, subacute catarrhel bronchitis, enlargement and edema of lymph nodes, enlargement of splenic follicles, subendocardial and subepicardial hemorrhages, multiple petechiae in general subserosa and submucosa, catarrh and hemorrhages in digestive tract, and hepatic focal necrosis. CNS involvement is primarily due to circulatory disturbances (hyperemia and hemorrhages).

In calves fed methylmercury there was a reduction of the number of cells in the granular layer of the cerebellum. There was swelling and necrosis of proximal convoluted renal tubular cells. Brain mercury levels in two calves were 9 and 20 ppm.

Howe et al., (1972) feed three lactating goats low levels of HgCl₂ (doses less than 1 mg/goat). About 90 percent of the dose was recovered in the feces, 3-4 percent in the urine and only .01-0.04 percent in the mild over a 9-18 day period. Peak blood and mild levels occurred on day 3.

Only a small amount (0.03-0.17%) of ingested mercury is excreted in cow's milk. (Neathery and Miller, 1975)

Postmortem tissue changes in swine primarily involved the kidney, liver and large intestine. The lesions in the large intestine reflect the fact that mercuric ions are excreted by the large intestine. The tissue changes reflect a degenerative and necrotic reaction in the large intestine. In the kidney the tubular epithelial cells are affected.

In pigs fed phenylmercuric chloride (PMC) at dosages of 2.28 and 4.56 mg/kg one of 24 pigs had a mild pharyngeal hyperemia. In all 24 pigs, the mouth, esophagus, stomach and small intestine were unaffected. In pigs fed 2.28 and 4.56 mg PMC/kg which had diarrhea the large intestine was affected by a diffuse necrotic process extending caudally from the ileocecal valve. The wall of the cecum and portions of the spiral colon were thickened and contracted. The proximal portion of the large intestine was more severely involved. The livers were tawny and slightly reduced in size but not friable. The kidneys of clinically affected pigs were swollen and pale yellow. Gross lesions were not found in the CNS.

Histologically the mucosa of the cecum, ileocecal valve and proximal colon was affected by a necrotizing process. The surface was covered with fibrin and the epithelium was degenerating or necrotic. In regions with coagulation necrosis of the mucosa and exposure of the lamina propria, the surface of the intestine was covered by a structureless and finely granular eosinophilic exudate.

The liver showed diffuse hydropic degeneration. Histologic renal lesions consisted of a small number of necrotic tubular cells. The lesions were more intense with longer exposures. Mitotic figures (regeneration) were seen in proximal convoluted tubular epithelium. Tubular casts were observed. The renal blood vessels and glomeruli were free of visible injury. The distal part of the nephrons were not primarily affected. (Tryphonas and Nielsen, 1970)

Pigs fed toxic levels of MMD or EMC had mottled livers. In some pigs there was necrotizing inflammatory pharyngitis. Pronounced gross atrophy of the cerebral hemispheres was seen in pigs fed EMC for about two months. Pigs fed higher levels but for shorter periods did not show this atrophy. Pigs fed EMC but not those fed MMD had severe focal erosive and ulcerative hemorrhagic gastritis. Edema and focal hyperemia occurred in the colon and cecum.

Histologic lesions consisted of mild to moderate hydropic degeneration of hepatocytes and renal proximal tubular epithelium. Lesions in the CNS included pronounced laminar neuronal loss of the third, fourth and fifth cerebrocortical laminae. Severe loss of myelin and degeneration and necrosis of axons occurred in the affected areas. In more severely affected brains the laminar neuronal stratification was destroyed. There was a marked reduction in number of cerebral neurons. Severe astrogliosis and microgliosis were seen. Mineralization was found in many neurons. The blood vessels were affected with proliferation of the tunica intima and moderate narrowing of the lumen. The precapillary arterioles had an advanced stage of fibrinoid degeneration.

Focal malacia was found in the basal ganglia and thalamus of clinically affected pigs. Lesions were less severe in the brainstem and cerebellum. The spinal cord was not affected. (Tryphonas and Nielsen, 1973)

Brain levels of 14 ppm or more were associated with clinical signs and severe lesions. A brain level less than 7 ppm was difficult to correlate with lesions. (Tryphonas and Nielsen, 1973)

The response of the pig to alkylmercurials appears to be different from that of man and other animals. In pigs the cerebellar granular cells are not as vulnerable while the cerebral cortex is more severely affected. The degenerative vascular lesions appear to be more pronounced in swine and cattle than in other species.

The changes seen in the cat brain following alkylmercury poisoning have been described as a granular type of cerebellar atrophy and atrophy of the calcarine and central cortices.

It has been demonstrated in two cats fed 2-3 mg/kg of biethylmercuric sulfide that transplacental transfer occurred with delayed neurotoxicity evident in the offspring. All kittens died within 3 months. Lesions included atrophy of the cerebellum and cerebellar cortex.

Hollins et al., (1975) found the whole body half-life of methylmercury chloride in the cat to be 117 days if storage in hair was considered. Ignoring mercury in hair resulted in a half-life of 76 days.

The IV administration of 30-60 mg/kg of methylmercury thioacetamide to dogs results in marked degeneration and loss of nerve cells in all layers near the calcarine fissure and temporal cortex, while the frontal, parietal, and occipital areas other than calcarine are only mildly affected.

In a study with low exposures (1 mg/rat/day) of diethylmercury sulfide it has been reported that peripheral sensory nerves were affected. Changes reported included swelling and degeneration of Schwann cells and noticeable changes in myelin sheaths and axons.

There is some concern that methylmercury may possess a genetic effect. It has been known since 1930 that organic mercury compounds have a c-mitotic effect. [Note: A c-mitotic effect means that the compound causes inactivation of the spindle mechanism in the same way as colchicine, an alkaloid ($C_{22}H_{25}NO_6$) obtained from colchicum. In the extreme form, c-mitosis implies that the chromosomes divide without the cells dividing. The result is a cell with twice the normal number of chromosomes.] Methyl- and phenylmercury compounds are c-mitotic active at levels of less than 0.1 ppm, while methoxyethyl mercury is active at a level of 0.6 ppm.

Recent observations of Minamata disease in Japan suggest that there are significant delayed neurotoxic effects that may not be manifested until several years after exposure. These observations are supported by recently published work in experimental animals. In some regards the delayed effects appear similar to an increase in the aging process.

Diagnosis

The practitioner should be able to demonstrate that a source of mercury exposure was present. The incidence of mercury poisoning in the past has been closely tied to the use of organic mercurial fungicides on wheat, barley and other small grains. This has resulted in a geographical distribution of mercury poisoning cases in livestock.

Kidney, and especially kidney cortex, is the best postmortem tissue for residue analysis. In acute cases kidney mercury residues will exceed 10-15 ppm. However, with lower exposures the delayed onset of clinical signs may provide enough time for the kidney residues to decrease to only a few ppm.

Mercury poisoning has been mistaken in the past for acute infectious diseases. The febrile response and skin color changes have resulted in mercury poisoning being confused with hog cholera and erysipelas. In the early part of the clinical syndrome mercury poisoning in pigs also resembles the early skin reddening and abnormal gait seen in organic arsenic poisoning. However, as the toxicosis progresses, mercury poisoned pigs are anoretic while organic arsenic poisoned pigs continue to eat.

Treatment

There is no specific treatment for mercury poisoning. In many cases, by the time the toxicosis is recognized extensive tissue changes including neurologic damage will have occurred.

Treatment consists of removing the source and giving supportive therapy such as fluids and dietary changes appropriate for the amount of renal damage.

In individual animals of significant economic or sentimental value sodium thiosulfate and BAL may be used. But this will require repeated administrations and close supervision.

With acute exposures the oral administration of protein, such as egg, may help to tie up mercury in the gastrointestinal tract.

The meat from a herd of animals poisoned with mercury and showing clinical signs is not fit for human consumption, and may very well result in illness or death in individuals consuming the contaminated meat. If a mercury poisoning case is encountered, the appropriate state officials should be notified immediately. If sufficient time is allowed the animals will eliminate the mercury and may be suitable for marketing. Individual circumstances and local laws will dictate the disposition of a contaminated herd or flock.

Episodes of Mercury Poisoning

Minamata, Japan

The first cases were originally thought to have occurred in 1953, but recent evidence traces the problem back to 1947. (Kurland, et al., 1960) A factory manufacturing nitrogenous fertilizer, vinyl chloride, sulfuric acid, and acetic acid was located on the sac-shaped Minamata Bay. The bay is relatively isolated by a small island at its mouth from the outer sea.

The initial cases primarily involved fishermen along the bay. Fishing was banned in 1956. In 1957 the effluent from the factory was channeled from the bay to the Minamata River. In 1959 and 1960 cases occurred in

people living at the mouth of the river some 5-10 km from the factory. In 1960 and 1966, improvements in waste water treatment were made and the mercury content of fish in the discharge area decreased. From 1953 to April, 1971, 134 persons were poisoned with 78 adult cases, 31 infantile cases and 25 fetal cases.

Shellfish caught in 1958 had mercury levels of 27-102 ppm (dry weight). The estimated dose was 2 mg Hg/day or less for those with symptoms. A total of 48 persons died, with deaths related to secondary infection and inanition.

The predominant symptoms included constriction of the visual field, sensory disturbance (numbness), ataxia, speech impairment, hearing deficits, tremor, and slight mental disturbance.

Cats in the area were also affected.

Sweden—1955-1958

A decrease in population of some seed-eating and predatory birds was noticed in 1955. (Lofroth, 1970) In 1958, mercury residues of 4-200 ppm in kidneys and liver were reported for dead birds. Birds captured and analyzed had levels of 1-53 ppm with 50 percent of the birds having levels greater than 2 ppm in liver.

Seed-eating rodents and predatory animals had levels of 2.0 ppm while levels in herbivorous animals were 0.006 to 0.055 ppm.

Levels in some fish were 9.8 ppm. Neutron activation analysis of museum feathers indicated stable background mercury levels from 1840 to 1940. Levels after 1940, when methyl- and ethylmercury fungicides were used, were 10-20 times higher.

Sweden switched to methoxyethylmercury compounds after 1965 and also reduced the amount of dressed seed. Levels in predatory birds dropped in 1966 and 1967. Levels in fish remained elevated.

Alamagordo, New Mexico—1969-1970

In this much publicized episode (Curley, et al., 1971; Snyder, 1971; Pierce, et al., 1972) waste seed grain treated with Panogen or Ceresan was fed to a number of pigs on six farms. The feeding started in late August. After two or three weeks, one pig, which received more mercury than the others, was slaughtered for home use. The family (father, mother, one son and two daughters) ate the pork during the next 3.5 months. The remaining pigs were fed smaller quantities of the contaminated feed and by mid-October, 14 pigs were blind, incoordinated, and had posterior paralysis. During the next three weeks, twelve of the fourteen pigs died. In early December, one child (an 8 year-old girl) became ill. Symptoms included ataxia, decreased vision, and depression of consciousness progressing to coma over a three-week period. Two weeks after the first child became ill, her 13 year-old brother developed the same signs and became comatose over a 2-3 week period. The 20 year-old daughter became ill in late December and proceeded to a semicomatose condition. The mother was six months pregnant at this time. The pork eaten by the family was reported to contain 27-29 ppm mercury.

The mother stopped eating the contaminated pork at six months of pregnancy. Urine levels during the last trimester were 0.06-0.18 ppm. A 3 kg male infant was delivered at term. The infant displayed intermittent gross tremulous movements of the extremities during the first few days of life. Urine mercury levels were 2-2.7 ppm.

Electroencephaograms of the infant were within normal variation during the first three months. At six months of age, myoclonic jerks developed and the electroencephalograms were markedly abnormal with paroxysmal high-voltage spikes, poly-spike and spike and slow wave patterns. At eight months the infant was hypotonic, irritable, and had nystagmoid eye movements. With the exception of the spike activity, the findings were similar to those reported in children with mercury poisoning (Minamata Disease).

Iraq (1972)

A large epidemic of methylmercury poisoning in farmers and their families occurred in Iraq. This epidemic is the most catastrophic ever recorded in terms of extent, morbidity and mortality. A total of 6,530 cases with 459 hospital deaths were recorded through February, 1972.

Treated wheat and barley seed grain was distributed to farmers in September, 1971. The treated seed was used by individual families for food.

Epidemologic studies were done through a joint effort of the University of Baghdad and the University of Rochester, U.S.A. Blood levels were as high as 5,000 nanograms/ml. Deaths occurred with blood levels exceeding 3,000 ng/ml. Blood levels of 500 ng/ml or higher were associated with paresthesia, ataxia, visual changes and dysarthria. The blood samples were taken after ingestion was stopped so caution must be exercised in extrapolating the data.

The estimated half-life in the blood was 65 days. Levels in human milk were 3 percent of whole blood levels. The number of days of ingestion ranged from 43-68 and the latent period ranged from 16-38 days. It was estimated that the flour contained 9 ppm mercury with each loaf of bread containing 1.4 mg mercury. (Bakir *et al.*, 1973)

Impact of Mercury Pollution on Wild Fowl

During the past several years, mercury contamination of wild fowl (especially pheasants) has caught the attention of the lay press. For this reason a few reports are included to provide some background for those who might need to respond to questions in this area.

In the United States Benson *et al.*, (An analysis of mercury residues in Idaho pheasants. *The Journal of the Idaho Academy of Science*, Research Issue No. 2, 1971) has published data on the seasonal variation in mercury residues in leg muscle of Idaho pheasants. A summary of their results is given in table 7.

The highest levels were found during the June-July sampling period with the highest level being 7.60 ppm. The residues also varied by area with eleven of twelve

TABLE 7
Mercury Residues in Leg Muscle of Wild Pheasants*

Period	No. of Birds	%>0.5 ppm	x̄Hg ppm
Oct.-Nov., 1969	27	0	0.025
June-July, 1970	90	43	1.120
Oct. 1-7, 1970	16	0	<.003
Oct. 10, 1970	12	0	<.004
Oct. 24, 1970	72	2.7	0.024
January, 1971	29	0	0.065

*Adapted from *The Journal of the Idaho Academy of Science*, Research Issue No. 2, 1971.

TABLE 8
Liver Mercury Residues in Pheasants Fed Methylmercury Dicyandiamide*

| Cumulative dose (mg/hen) | Liver Hg—ppm | |
	Mean	Range
Fed 2 weeks, off 8 weeks		
1.71	0.68	0-1.55
3.38	0.59	0.34-1.11
6.25	0.98	0.37-2.28
Fed 4 weeks, off 6 weeks		
3.05	1.15	0.39-3.26
6.29	1.87	0.93-2.97
12.38	4.44	2.20-6.80
Fed 10 weeks		
9.69	1.86	0.59-5.08
18.91	4.47	3.36-7.62
33.66	7.83	4.03-13.70

*Adapted from Fimreite, 1971.

birds having residues greater than 0.5 ppm and an average of 2.55 ppm in one area.

Fimreite (1971), who has published a number of papers on the effects of mercury on wildlife, reported on the effects of feeding methylmercury dicyandiamide to ring-necked pheasants. Levels which did not adversely affect hens resulted in reductions in hatchability, reduced egg production and an increased number of shell-less eggs. Tissue levels (table 8) were reported for various levels and periods of feeding.

REFERENCES

Bakir, F. *et al.* 1973. Methylmercury Poisoning in Iraq. *Science* 181:230-41.

Butler, G. M. 1965. A Case of Overeating of Grain Which Had Been Dressed with Mercurial Dressing. *Irish Vet. J.* 19:94.

Curley, A. *et al.* 1971. Organic Mercury Identified as the Cause of Poisoning in Humans and Hogs. *Science.* 172:65.

Fimreite, N. 1971. Effects of Methylmercury on Ring- Necked Pheasants. *Can. Wldlf. Ser.* 9.

Fujimoto, Y. *et al.* 1956. Pathological Studies on Mercury Poisoning in Cattle. *Jap. J. Vet. Res.* 4:18.

Herigstad, R. R.; Whitehair, C. K.; Beyer, N.; Mickelsen, O.; and Zabik, M. J. Chronic Methylmercury Toxicosis in Calves. *Journal American Veterinary Medical Assn.* 160:173-82.

Hollins, J. G.; Willes, R. F.; Bryce, R. A.; Charbonneau, S. M.; and Munro, I. C. 1975. The Whole Body Retention and Tissue Distribution of 203 Hg- Methylmercury in Adult Cats. *Toxicology and Applied Pharmacology* 33:438-49.

Howe, M.; McGee, J.; and Lengemann, F. W. 1972. Transfer of Inorganic Mercury to Milk in Goats. *Nature* 237: 516-18.

Kahrs, R. F. 1968. Chronic Mercurial Poisoning in Swine: A Case Report of an Outbreak with Some Epidemiological Characteristics of Hog Cholera. *Cornell Vet.* 58:67.

Kurland, L. T.; Faro, S. N.; and Siedler, H. 1960. Minamata Disease. *World Neurology* 1:370-95.

Lofroth, G. 1970. Methyl Mercury: A Review of Health Hazards and Side Effects Associated with the Emission of Mercury Compounds into Natural Systems. Editorial Service, Swedish Natural Resource Council, Box 23-136, S-104-35, Stockholm.

McEntee, Kenneth. 1950. Mercurial Poisoning in Swine. *Cornell Vet.* 40:143.

Morikawa, N. 1961. Pathological Studies on Organic Mercury Poisoning, Part II. *Kumamoto Med. J.* 14:87.

Palmer, J. G. 1963. Mercurial Fungicidal Seed Protectant Toxic for Sheep and Chickens. *JAVMA* 142:1385.

Neathery, M. W., and Miller, W. J. 1975. Metabolism and Toxicity of Cadmium, Mercury and Lead in Animals: A Review. *Journal Dairy Science.* 58:1767-81.

Pierce, P. E.; Thompson, J. F.; Likosky, W. H.; Nickey, L. N.; Barthel, W. F.; and Hinman, A. R. 1972. Alkyl Mercury Poisoning in Humans. *JAMA* 220:1439-42.

Piper, R. *et al.* 1971. Toxicity and Distribution of Mercury in Pigs with Acute Methylmercurialism. *AJVR* 32(2):263.

Platonow, N. S., and Funnell, H. S. 1971. The Accumulation of Mercury in Chickens Following the Prolonged Administration of Low Levels of an Inorganic Mercurial. *Vet. Rec.* 188:503.

Smart, N. A., and Lloyd, M. K. 1963. Mercury Residues in Eggs, Flesh and Livers of Hens Fed on Wheat Treated with Methylmercury Dicyandiamide. *J. Sci. Food. Agr.* 14:734.

Snyder, R. D. 1971. Congenital Mercury Poisoning. *New England J. Med.* 284:1014-16.

Sonada, M., *et al.* 1956. Clinical Studies of Mercury Poisoning in Cattle. *Jap. J. Vet. Res.* 4:1.

Swensen, A. *et al.* 1968. Distribution and Excretion of Various Mercury Compounds After Single Injections in Poultry. *Acta Pharm. et Tox.* 26:259.

Taylor, E. L. 1947. Mercury Poisoning in Swine. *JAVMA.* 111:46.

Tryphonas, L., and Nielsen, N. 1970. The Pathology of Aryl-Mercury Poisoning in Swine. *Can. J. Comp. Med.* 34:181.

Tryphonas, L., and Nielsen, N. O. 1973. Pathology of Chronic Alkylmercurial Poisoning in Swine. *American Journal of Veterinary Research* 34:379-92.

United States Government Printing Office. 1970. *Mercury in the Environment.* Geological Survey Professional Paper 713, Washington, D.C.

Wright, F. C.; Palmer, J. S.; and Riner, J. C. 1973. Accumulation of Mercury in Tissues of Cattle, Sheep and Chickens Given the Mercurial Fungicide, Panogen 15, Orally. *Journal Agricultural Food Chemistry.* 21:414-16.

Yoshikazu, Y.; Mozai, T.; and Nakao, K. 1966. Distribution of Mercury in the Brain and Its Subcellular Units in Experimental Organic Mercury Poisonings. *J. Neurochem.* 13:397-406.

SELENIUM

Selenium is a metalloid discovered in the 18th century. A chemical relationship exists between sulfur and selenium, although both differ in their action. Only during the last three decades has selenium been recognized as a toxic material present in indicator plants grown on seleniferous soils. It has been recognized that small amounts of selenium are essential as a trace mineral, and it has been used in conjunction with vitamin E for prevention of muscular dystrophies and other selenium-responsive diseases in livestock and poultry.

Selenium toxicosis is a worldwide problem and has been reported from the United States, Canada, Germany, France, South Africa, and other countries. Forage crops grown on seleniferous soils contain sufficient amounts of selenium to cause poisoning in domestic animals. Selenium may be present in soil as selenates, elemental selenium, and organic selenium. Plants utilize either the organic or selenate forms.

Selenium may cause acute or chronic poisoning in all animals, especially sheep, cattle, horses, swine, poultry, and dogs. Selenium is distributed to all organs of the body by the blood vascular system and causes severe damage to the vital organs. Acute selenium poisoning (blind staggers) is associated with single or multiple feeding of high amounts of seleniferous plants and is usually fatal. A severe gastroenteritis, anorexia, depression, incoordination, coma, and death are the usual clinical signs.

Alkali disease is a form of selenium poisoning resulting from the consumption of moderate amounts of seleniferous plants over a long period of time and is manifested by ataxia, incoordination, partial blindness, and paralysis. A loss of hair or wool, and deformation and sloughing of the hoof is seen in cattle, sheep, and horses with chronic selenium poisoning.

Selenium poisoning in animals increases the prothrombin time resulting from hepatic injury and decreases the synthesis of adenosine triphosphate (ATP). Selenium also interferes with vitamin A and ascorbic acid metabolism. Synthesis of sulfur containing amino acids is reduced in the liver. Selenium can pass the placental barrier and interfere with the cellular oxidative processes during embryonic development and may cause congenital malformations.

A high protein diet gives protection against selenium poisoning. Inorganic and organic compounds of arsenic have been used in the treatment and prevention of selenium poisoning. Arsenic aids in the excretion of selenium through the bile duct.

Source

Selenium was discovered in 1817 by Berzelius, a Swedish chemist. In addition to its numerous industrial uses, it has medicinal and insecticidal properties. It was only 30 years ago that selenium was recognized as a toxic material in plants which caused huge losses sustained by the livestock industry in South Dakota, Wyoming, and some of the adjacent states in the U.S.A. Since then, many investigators have worked on the different aspects of selenium poisoning and deficiencies, and it is now known to occur in many countries of the world.

Selenium is a metalloid and classed in Group VI of the Periodic Table. It resembles sulfur and tellurium. Sulfur and selenium are somewhat related chemically but differ in their physiologic actions. Sulfur is present in certain amino acids and is useful, while selenium is toxic in low levels; but also it has been recognized as an essential trace element for animals and birds.

Selenium toxicosis has been recognized in many arid and semiarid regions of the world, including much of the western third of the United States. In problem areas an appreciable amount of selenium is present in the soil, which is taken up by *obligate* indicator plants, ones which require selenium for growth. *Faculative* indicator plants may absorb selenium if it is present in the soil but do not require it for growth. Many factors, including plant species, stage of maturity, chemical form of selenium, and climate affect the uptake of selenium by plants.

Species of *Xylorrhiza* (woody aster), *Oonopsis* (goldenweed), *Stanleya,* and *Astragalus* are obligate indicators and may accumulate several hundred ppm sele-

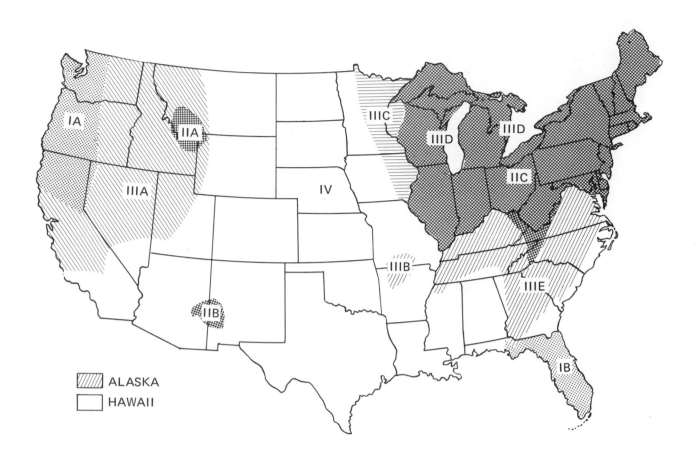

Area Group	Mean Concentration of Selenium in Forages (ppm)
IA	0.03
IB	0.02
IIA	0.05
IIB	0.05
IIC	0.05
IIIA	0.09
IIIB	0.05
IIIC	0.09
IIID	0.10
IIIE	0.06
IV*	0.26

*Approximately 30% of specimens of wheat and feed grains contained between 1-5 ppm selenium.

Figure 1. Selenium in crops in different regions of U.S. (Adapted from Kubota *et al.,* 1967)

nium. Fortunately, most of the plant species that have the ability to accumulate large quantities of selenium are not palatable and are only eaten by animals when there is nothing else to eat. Faculative indicator plants *(Asters, Atriplex, Sideranthus,* and *Machaeranthera)* are commonly grazed by livestock and often cause poisoning.

Geological Distribution of Selenium

Selenium has been found in toxic amounts in wheat and other plants in North and South America, Australia, New Zealand, South Africa, France, and Germany. It has also been found in soil and vegetation in many regions of the western part of the United States from North Dakota to Texas and west to the Pacific Ocean. Seleniferous soils have also been found in Mexico and Alberta, Canada. Figure 1 gives selenium levels in crops in the United States. Table 1 summarizes selenium levels in corn grain in the midwestern states.

High concentrations of selenium in rocks are found in two types of situations. The most widely studied occurrences are those in sedimentary rocks that have resulted from volcanic ejection of selenium and the deposition of this selenium in seas followed by the uplift of sea floor sediments.

The other major occurrence of selenium is in deposits of sulfide ores of heavy metals, including copper, silver, bismuth, and mercury. Most of the large selenium-bearing geologic formations in the United

States have been located. This has been done by realizing the close association between the occurrence of seleniferous rocks and the presence of selenium indicator plants.

On the other hand, the recognition of areas where selenium levels are too low to support optimum biologic performance is probably not complete at this time. During the past fifteen years, selenium deficiencies in livestock have been reported in the United States, Canada, New Zealand, Australia, and most of the countries of Europe. In the U.S. selenium deficient areas are in the Northwest, Northeast, Southwest, and areas in Ohio, Indiana, Minnesota, Wisconsin, and eastern Iowa, anywhere there is a sandy, acid-leached soil.

Selenium in the soil may be present as selenates, elemental selenium, pyritic selenium, ferric selenium, and organic selenium compounds. The most available forms for plant absorption are organic selenium compounds and selenates. Slow oxidation or elemental selenium in the soil can take place and, thereby, become available for absorption by crop plants. Certain bacteria in the soil may also be capable of converting elemental selenium to selenite.

Selenium as an Animal Feed Additive

In 1973 the Commissioner of Food and Drugs, U.S. Department of Health, Education, and Welfare, amended the food additive regulations to provide for the safe use of selenium as a nutrient in the feed for chickens, turkeys, and swine. The amendment provides for the addition of sodium selenite or sodium selenate up to 0.1 ppm in the complete diet for growing chickens and swine and 0.2 ppm in the complete diet for turkeys. The selenium must be added in a premix formulated in such a way that at least 1 lb but no more than 2 lbs of premix are added per ton of complete feed. Feeds containing added selenium may not be administered to laying hens, cattle or sheep.

Toxicity

All animals and humans are susceptible to selenium toxicosis. Poisoning is most common, however, in forage-eating animals such as cattle, sheep and horses which may graze selenium-containing plants. Poisoning may occur in swine and poultry consuming grain raised on seleniferous soils. Laboratory animals such as rats and mice are equally susceptible to poisoning if fed grain containing excessive selenium.

Horses and other livestock may discriminate against selenium-containing indicator plants because of their offensive odor. This is especially true of horses who are

TABLE 1
Selenium Content of Corn in Midwestern States*

State	Number of Samples	Low ppm	High ppm	Average ppm	Median ppm
North Dakota	6	0.09	0.26	0.19	0.22
South Dakota	10	0.11	2.03	0.40	0.24
Nebraska	6	0.04	0.81	0.35	0.28
Kansas	1	—	0.99	—	—
Minnesota	22	0.02	0.29	0.09	0.06
Iowa	25	0.02	0.16	0.05	0.05
Missouri	4	0.02	0.09	0.05	0.05
Wisconsin	5	0.02	0.13	0.05	0.02
Illinois	31	0.02	0.15	0.05	0.04
Michigan	5	0.03	0.04	0.03	0.03
Indiana	20	0.01	0.15	0.04	0.04
Total	135	0.01	2.03	0.11	0.05

*From George Patrias, *Feedstuffs,* 41:33, 1969. Used by permission.

more selective in their grazing habits than cattle or sheep. Forages and grains which are moderately seleniferous or which have withered may lack the highly offensive odor and, therefore, be more dangerous than the selenium indicator plants.

Selenium poisoning in humans is uncommon because animal tissues do not store excessive levels of selenium, even in those cases where toxicosis has occurred. About the only opportunity for selenium poisoning in humans is associated with industrial contamination or mining operations and perhaps the use of selenium-containing shampoos and other medicinal agents.

Organically bound selenium as found in forages and grains may be more toxic than inorganic selenium salts and metallic selenium. A complicating factor, however, is the concomitant presence of phytotoxins, which may be present along with selenium in plant material.

The toxicity of selenium to the various species of animals varies with the diet being consumed. For instance, a high protein diet may protect an animal from selenium poisoning. While many factors enter into selenium toxicosis, the following appear to be the most important: (1) size and frequency of the doses; (2) characteristics of the compound; (3) presence of combining, reducing, diluting, or synergistic substances; (4) inherent susceptibility of the animal; and (5) efficiency of elimination after absorption. It is not yet possible to state with any degree of accuracy what constitutes the minimum toxic dose of selenium in each of its forms for the different kinds of livestock.

It may be stated in general, however, that the single acute oral minimum lethal dose of selenium for most animals is in the range of from 1-5 mg/kg body weight. Levels in the total diet of 25 ppm and greater may be sufficient to produce acute poisoning in most animals.

Table 2 summarizes the selenium requirements, tolerance levels, and toxic levels in livestock and poultry feeds.

Selenium Deficiency Syndrome

Selenium responsive diseases have been reported, especially in swine and poultry, during the last fifteen years in various areas of the United States. Borderline deficiency problems are difficult to diagnose because of other factors which apparently are involved such as vitamin E, iron, and moldy feeds. Selenium is necessary for normal function of the muscle, heart, liver, kidneys, pancreas, and perhaps other organs. White muscle disease in ruminants is thought to be related to a selenium-vitamin E deficiency. Hepatosis dietetica, Hertzod, and porcine stress syndrome are diseases of swine which may be related to selenium deficiency. Exudative diathesis is

a disease of chickens and turkeys which only selenium will prevent or correct.

There is some indication that mold-damaged grain may contain lower levels of selenium than grain of good quality.

Since arsenic has been shown to facilitate the biliary excretion of selenium, it has been postulated that perhaps arsenic-containing feeds may contribute to the problems of selenium deficiency in these species. The recognition of diseases such as hepatosis dietetica, porcine stress syndrome, and exudative diathesis have coincided with the increased use of arsenicals in animal feeds.

Mechanism of Action

Biochemical mechanisms of selenium in animals remain obscure. Selenium apparently exerts its toxic effect by enzymatically inhibiting oxidation-reduction systems of the body. Selenium requirements are less in animal diets containing antioxidants such as vitamin E. It seems likely that physiologic levels of selenium perform some antioxidant function, but it cannot be stated that this is its only biochemical role. Selenium has not been found to be an essential component of an enzyme system.

Selenium is usually bound to proteins in animal tissues. Although it is easy to speculate that certain biochemical mechanisms such as replacement of sulfur by selenium may be involved in selenium toxicity, it is difficult to prove that these mechanisms are the primary cause of the clinical signs observed.

There is some indication that selenium and sulfate antagonism exists in both plants and animals. Certain enzyme systems such as succinic dehydrogenase are apparently inhibited by selenite.

The biliary excretion of selenium in rats has been shown to be stimulated several fold by the administration of arsenic but not by mercury, thallium, or lead.

TABLE 2
Selenium Requirements and Toxicity in Livestock and Poultry Feeds (levels expressed as ppm of ration)*

Type of Livestock	Requirement Level	Non-Toxic Level	Toxic Level
Cattle	0.10	2.0	8.0
Sheep	0.10	?	10.0
Swine	0.10	2.5	7.0
Poultry	0.15	5.0	15.0
Turkey	0.20	?	?

*Adapted from Patrias, George: *Feedstuffs,* March 1969, Vol. 41, p. 24.

Many workers have reported that selenosis is associated with decreased tissue ascorbic acid and glutathione and that the decrease of ascorbic acid may be a contributing factor to vascular damage observed. Other workers have noted that formation of ATP, as measured by P_{32} uptake in rat liver, indicated that ATP formation was depressed in chronic selenosis. (Rosenfeld, *et al.*, 1953, 1964) There also appears to be a significant reduction of methionine in the liver supposedly due to the oxidation of sulfhydryl groups.

Reproductive and Teratogenic Effects

It is generally accepted that selenium passes the placental barrier and may interfere with embryonic development. Selenium apparently interferes with cellular oxidative processes during embryonic formation. Since such tissues have very critical oxygen requirements, fertility and reproduction may be reduced even in low-grade chronic selenium poisoning. Congenital alkali disease was reported by Smith, *et al.*, (1936) in a 14-day old colt of a mare that developed symptoms of disease during gestation. Malformation in lambs that were the progeny of ewes which grazed seleniferous plants was reported by Beath, *et al.*, (1939). The joints of the extremities were thickened and nodular in appearance. Most of the young lambs were unable to stand and died soon after birth. It has been reported in the literature that the developmental arrest occurred rather early in gestation. It is interesting to note in this case, however, that more recent reports by Binns and co-workers and the USDA Laboratory at Logan, Utah, indicate that species of the genus *Astragalus* produce similar effects in the absence of excessive levels of selenium.

Clinical Signs

Acute Poisoning

The onset of acute poisoning is characterized by changes in movement and posture of the animal. The animal may walk a short distance with an uncertain gait and then stop and assume a characteristic stance, with the head lowered and ears drooped. Dark, watery diarrhea usually develops. The temperature may be elevated to 103-105° F. The pulse may be rapid and weak, 90-300. Respiration may be labored with mucous rales and there may be bloody froth from air passages. Bloating and abdominal pain is usually pronounced. Urine excretion is greatly increased. The mucous membranes become pale or bluish in color. The pupils become dilated. The animal usually becomes completely prostrate before death. Death is due to respiratory failure. The course of the illness is from a few hours to several days, depending upon the amount and toxicity of selenium ingested. In the pig, emesis, diarrhea, lethargy, and paresis develop upon consumption of a toxic dose of selenium.

Subacute and Chronic Poisoning

The discussion of subacute and chronic selenosis in livestock will be divided into three groups: (1) blind staggers, caused by organic selenium compounds with or without small amounts of selenate which are readily extractable with water from native selenium indicator plants; (2) alkali disease, produced in livestock having consumed the plants or grain in which selenium is bound in proteins and is relatively insoluble in water; and (3) chronic selenosis produced experimentally by the administration of selenate or selenite to livestock.

Some of the characteristic manifestations of selenosis in the above three forms are given in table 3.

A type of subacute or chronic selenosis, commonly referred to as blind staggers appears in cattle and sheep when they consume moderately toxic amounts of seleniferous weeds over a considerable period of time. Clinical manifestations are often suddenly followed by acute death. The term "blind staggers" is a misnomer commonly used by stockmen. Affected animals may be neither blind nor do they necessarily stagger. In the early stage of illness, the poisoned animal wanders, frequently circles, disregards objects in its path, and stumbles over or walks through them. The body temperature and respiration may be normal. The animal usually shows little desire to eat or drink and may give some evidence of impaired vision. In the second stage, the earlier manifestations become more pronounced; and in addition, the front legs seem to become weak and unable to support the animal. Anorexia becomes complete. A third stage prior to death is manifested primarily by paralysis. The tongue and the mechanism of swallowing become partially or totally paralyzed. The animal may be nearly blind. Respiration is labored and accelerated. There is evidence of great abdominal pain manifested by constant grating of the teeth and salivation. The body temperature may be subnormal, the eyelids are swollen and inflamed, and the cornea distinctly cloudy. In most cases the third stage appears suddenly and is fatal within a few hours. The immediate cause of death is respiratory failure. A gradual loss of weight always accompanies the disease; and, in the final stage, the animal appears emaciated.

Recovery may occur in the first and second stages; but if the third stage is reached, it is usually fatal.

TABLE 3

Manifestations of Chronic Selenosis and Associated Syndromes
Produced by Different Chemical Forms of Selenium*

	Alkali Disease	Blind Staggers	Experimental Selenosis
Sources of selenium	Seleniferous grains and grasses	Selenium indicator plants: *Astragalus, Machaeranthera, Haplopapus,* and *Stanleya*	Salts of selenate and selenite
Effects of selenium on food intake	Rarely affected	Decreased—followed by anorexia	Decreased—followed by anorexia
Visible signs of the disease	Lameness, loss of vitality, elongated hoofs, loss of hair from mane and tail	Emaciation. Neuromuscular involvement in 3 stages in cattle. Sheep, neuromuscular involvement not well defined	Emaciation. Some neuromuscular involvement not well defined (cattle)
Reproduction	Rarely affected	Cattle: impaired Sheep: malformations	Not studied
Selenium accumulation	Cattle: hoofs 5-8 ppm; hair 5-10 ppm Horses: hoofs 11.0 ppm; hair 11-45 ppm Other tissues: 4-25 ppm	Cattle: hair variable Sheep: wool undetermined Other tissues: 10-25 ppm	Cattle: hair 2.7-9.5 ppm; horn 0.25 ppm. Other tissues: 10-25 ppm
Characteristic gross pathology	Liver: atrophy and cirrhosis; kidney: chronic nephritis; gall bladder: rarely enlarged; heart: soft and flabby; intestinal tract: rarely involved	Liver: necrosis with cirrhosis; kidney: subacute and chronic nephritis; gall bladder: generally enlarged; heart: soft and flabby; intestinal tract: impacted with irritation	Liver: necrosis with occasional cirrhosis; kidney: acute nephritis; intestinal tract: ulceration and gangrene

*Adapted from Rosenfeld, Irene and Beath, Orville: *Selenium.* Academic Press. 1964. p. 146.

Mature animals that recover do not become vigorous and young animals remain stunted.

Animals may show a delayed effect of selenium exposure for several weeks or months. Cattle may show no outward signs of poisoning, but suddenly symptoms may develop and death occur within a few days. This has been known to occur after cattle have been shipped to a feedlot and are being fattened for market.

Subacute-chronic selenium poisoning in sheep is not as readily diagnosed as in cattle. The three stages are not clearly differentiated.

Chronic Poisoning of the Alkali-Disease Type

Chronic selenium poisoning, commonly known as alkali disease, is characterized by loss of hair and deformation and sloughing of the hoofs in cattle, hogs, and horses that have consumed moderately seleniferous grains and forage grasses over a period of several weeks or months. Clinical manifestations of this syndrome differ from blind staggers in that animals affected only occasionally show the emaciation characteristic of blind staggers. The term "alkali disease" is a misnomer and is not related to problems associated with the consump-

tion of alkaline salts in water. The general clinical signs include lack of vitality, anemia, stiffness of joints, lameness, roughened coat, loss of long hair, and hoof lesions and deformities. The first sign may be loss of long hair from the mane and tail. For this reason the disease has been called "bob-tailed disease." This is followed by soreness of the feet. A circular break appears on the wall of the hoof below the coronary band. As new growth of the hoof continues in the region of the coronary band, the break in the wall of the hoof moves downward. In severe cases, the crack is so deep that the upper part of the old wall becomes separated from the new growth. As the new hoof develops, the old hoof is gradually pushed down and is finally sloughed. During this time the animal is in severe pain and may die of thirst or starvation. Cattle may be seen to be grazing on their knees. Such hoof lesions have been mistaken for frostbite.

Selenium Deficiency Signs

Clinical signs of selenium deficiency are more difficult to describe, primarily because of other factors which are involved such as vitamin E deficiency, moldy feeds, and perhaps other toxins that produce similar clinical signs. It is difficult to estimate whether the disease is due primarily from borderline selenium deficiency or a combination of factors. If the grain ration or forage is low in selenium (less than 0.1 ppm) and damaged by mold and weather, it will usually be deficient in vitamin E. Animals then fed such rations which are stressed by other diseases, bad weather, handling, parasites, etc., may not grow normally.

Selenium is necessary for normal function of most of the organ systems especially the muscle, heart, liver, and kidney. Nutritional muscular degeneration (NMD) or white muscle disease is commonly associated with selenium and vitamin E deficiency. In ruminants and pigs the skeletal muscles are severely affected, and the animals become unable to walk or stand. Young animals are more severely affected than older animals. A nursing lamb or calf may die of starvation. Heart failure and pulmonary edema are usually associated with advanced stages. Appetite usually remains good.

In pigs NMD is often observed in association with the feeding of poor grains low in vitamin E and selenium. In such cases young pigs injected with iron often develop the muscular degeneration syndrome. Hepatosis dietetica (liver degeneration) is also a common deficiency syndrome attributed to selenium. Pigs become dull, often vomit, and have diarrhea. The liver is often swollen and has a mottled appearance due to focal necrosis.

Exudative diathesis is a disease of chickens and turkeys commonly associated with selenium deficiency. It is characterized by a gelatinous subcutaneous edema, poor growth, and hemorrhages throughout the muscles. Birds are listless and anemic, and fluid which collects under the skin is often a blue green color. Degeneration of the smooth muscle of the gizzard, skeletal muscles, and heart are seen in this condition.

Physiopathology

Pathologic changes attributed to selenium toxicosis vary with the species of animal affected and the duration of the disease. The lesions involve most of the organs and systems of the body. Major changes described in the literature are: (a) swelling and congestion of the liver with varying degrees of degeneration progressing to focal necrosis and fibrosis in some animals; (b) congestion, degeneration, and necrosis of tubular epithelium and fibrosis of the kidneys; (c) congestion of the spleen with hyperplasia of splenic nodules; (d) hemorrhagic enteritis ranging from mild to severe; (e) ulceration of the abomasum; (f) subserous and subendocardial hemorrhages in the heart with myocardial congestion, necrosis, cellular infiltra-

tion, and fibrosis; (g) edema and congestion of the brain with neuronal degeneration in the cerebral and cerebellar cortices; (h) articular erosions and deformed hoofs; and (i) various developmental anomalies of the embryo.

It is interesting that the organs affected by excessive levels of selenium are also those affected by selenium deficiency. Skeletal and heart muscle degeneration is commonly associated with selenium deficiency and the liver and other organs may exhibit degenerative changes and necrosis.

Diagnosis

When selenium toxicosis is suspected, it is important that a source of selenium be located and the level of exposure established. Because of the various stages of clinical signs varying from acute through chronic, it may be difficult to diagnose selenium toxicosis on the basis of clinical signs. If the clinical signs, postmortem changes, and course of events are compatible with selenium toxicosis, one should establish the level of selenium in the ration or other avenues of exposure as well as establish levels of selenium in tissue and body fluids. Thus, selenium levels in the diet which are greater than 5 ppm may produce signs of toxicosis after extended exposure. Levels of 10-25 ppm could be expected to produce more severe poisoning.

Selenium tends to be distributed throughout the body in both acute and chronic cases of poisoning. The concentration in the blood, however, would be much greater in acute than in chronic poisoning. Blood levels may reach 25 ppm in acute cases whereas they are more likely to be from 1-4 ppm in chronic cases of poisoning. The kidney and liver usually contain the largest amounts of selenium, and the brain the least amount. The concentration in these tissues depends not only upon the length of time during which selenium was ingested but also the quantity ingested. Organic selenium also accumulates in higher quantities in these tissues than does inorganic selenium. Levels of from 4-25 ppm may be seen in liver and kidney in both chronic and acute cases of poisoning.

As pointed out above, the level of selenium in the tissues is directly related to the duration of illness. If death occurs soon after clinical signs develop, the concentrations will be at the level of 20 ppm whereas if the animal lingers for several days prior to death, the tissue levels may be between 1 and 5 ppm. In chronic cases, the hoof tissue usually contains from 8-20 ppm. Tissues of animals not exposed to excessive selenium will be free of selenium residue.

The urine from animals suffering from selenium toxicosis may contain from 0.1 to 8.0 ppm selenium. Other chemical changes associated with selenium toxicosis include decreased vitamin A, ascorbic acid, and serum protein levels and an increase in nonprotein nitrogen levels.

Differentiation

Differentiation between acute selenium toxicosis and other diseases such as pneumonia, anthrax, infectious necrotic hepatitis, enterotoxemia, pasteurellosis, and many other types of poisonings must be made. Chronic diseases that may be confused with chronic selenosis include freezing of the extremities, ergotism, molybdenum toxicosis, fluoride poisoning, and laminitis due to founder. In some species, loss of hair from thallium toxicosis may be confused with chronic selenosis.

Treatment

Acute selenium poisoning is not amenable to treatment. The various forms of chronic selenosis may be treated by feeding a salt preparation containing about 40 ppm arsenic. Feeding a ration containing 50-100 ppm arsanilic acid has also provided benefit for calves and pigs. Mature cattle and horses have been treated successfully by the oral administration of 4-5 grams of naphthalene daily for 5 days, resting for 5 days, then repeating the dosage.

Of course, removal of the animals from the selenium-containing forage or grain or supplementing nonselenium grain so that a dilution effect is obtained is always indicated.

In the case of selenium deficiency problems, the addition of selenium-bearing grains to rations would be indicated to bring the overall selenium level up to 0.1 ppm of the total ration. Federal regulations permit the adding of selenium as sodium selenite or selenate to growing swine and chicken diets at a level up to 0.1 ppm and to growing turkey diets up to 0.2 ppm.

Case History*

This case involved a flock of 56 grade ewes and 63 lambs in which 5-10 percent of the lamb crop was lost in previous years from nutritional muscular dystrophy. Following the death of 2 lambs due to this condition, 12 lambs between 1 and 3 weeks of age were treated with 2 mg of sodium selenite orally. These remained unaffected. Twenty lambs from 4-14 days of age were treated with 10 mg of sodium selenite orally at 1 p.m. on March 27. The treated lambs were observed to be normal by the owner at 8 p.m. of that day. On March 28 at 6 a.m. there were 7 dead lambs. They had loose yellow fecal material around the anus; 8 others had diarrhea.

Other signs included depression and ataxia, which was followed by progressive dyspnea. The temperature in some of the lambs was as high as 104.5° F and pulse was 170/min. Urination was frequent and bloating was noted terminally. Pupils were dialated and the mucous membranes were cyanotic just prior to death.

The 8 lambs exhibiting diarrhea were treated symptomatically twice daily for two days with a preparation containing 300 mg of neomycin sulfate and 3 mg of methscopolamine bromide. The time from treatment with selenium to death was 10-16 hours.

The 8 lambs with diarrhea were normal 48 hours after treatment with neomycin-methscopolamine preparation. The remaining 5 selenium-treated lambs showed no signs of illness.

Postmortem findings in the dead lambs included serumlike fluid in the thoracic cavity (approximately 50 cc). The heart had moderate bilateral dilation. The pericardium contained clear, yellow transudate. The lungs were severely hyperemic and edematous with the bronchi and distal half of the trachea filled with frothy fluid. There was a moderate number of small submucosal hemorrhages in the trachea and bronchi. The bronchial and mediastinal lymph nodes were hyperemic and edematous. There were localized hemorrhagic areas in the wall of the small intestine. The kidneys were hyperemic, especially in the medulla. There was subcapsular petechiation and a hemorrhagic infarct in the cortex of one kidney. The bladders were distended with urine and contained petechial hemorrhages. Other organs, including the thymus gland, were moderately hyperemic with minute hemorrhages.

Microscopic examination of the tissues revealed pulmonary edema, hyperemia, and hemorrhages. The alveoli were lined with red blood cells. There was severe acute necrotizing nephrosis which primarily affected the proximal convoluted tubules. Hemorrhages were frequent and extensive in the renal cortex. The medulla had severe hyperemia but no inflamation. The only important changes in the brain and other organs was moderate hyperemia.

Chemical analysis of the liver revealed 20 ppm selenium, and the kidneys revealed 8 ppm on a dry-weight basis (approximately 4 and 1.7 ppm respectively on a wet-weight basis).

BIBLIOGRAPHY

Allaway, W. H. 1968. Control of the Environmental Levels of Selenium. Proc., 2nd Annual Conf. on Trace Substances in Environmental Health. University of Missouri, Columbia, Missouri. 181-206.

*Adapted from Morrow, 1968.

————. 1969. Selenium Concentrations in Crops from Different Parts of the U.S. Proc., Georgia Nutrition Conf., University of Georgia. 61-66.

Allaway, W. H.; Kubota, J.; Losee,F.; and Roth, M. 1968. Selenium Molybdenum, and Vanadium in Human Blood. *Arch. Environ. Health.* 16:342-48.

Beath, O. A.; Eppson, H. F.; and Gilbert, C. S. 1935. Selenium and Other Toxic Minerals in Soils and Vegetation. University of Wyoming. Agricultural Experiment Station Bulletin 206.

Bieri, J. G.; Pollard, C. J.; and Cardenas, R. R. 1951. Utilization of Vitamin A and Carotene by Selenium Poisoned Rats. *Proc. Soc. Exptl. Biol. Med.* 94:140-43.

Byers, H. G.; Miller, J. T.; Williams, K. T.; and Lankin, H. W. 1938. Selenium Occurrences in Certain Soils in the United States with a Discussion of Related Topics. USDA Tech. Bul., 601.

Clarke, E. G. C., and Clarke, M. L. 1967. *Garner's Veterinary Toxicology.* Baltimore: The Williams & Wilkins Co., pp. . 114-19.

Draize, J. H., and Beath, O. A. 1935. Observations on the Pathology of "Blind Staggers and Alkali Disease." *JAVMA* 86:753-63.

Fimiani, R. 1949. Ascorbic Acid in Blood and Urine in Chronic Experimental Selenium Poisoning. *Folia Med.* 32:452-58.

————. 1951. Prothrombin Time in Experimental Chronic Selenium Poisoning.*Folia Med.*34:140-43.

Glenn, M. W.; Jensen, R.; and Griner, L. A. 1964. Sodium Selenate Toxicosis: The Distribution of Selenium Within the Body After Prolonged Feeding of Toxic Quantities of Sodium Selenate to Sheep. *Amer. J. Vet. Res.* 25:1495-99.

————. 1964. Sodium Selenate Toxicosis; The Effects of Extended Oral Administration of Sodium Selenate on Mortality, Clinical Signs, Fertility, and Early Embryonic Development in Sheep.*Amer. J. Vet. Res.* 25:1479-85.

————. 1964. Sodium Selenate Toxicosis: Pathology and Pathogenesis of Sodium Selenate Toxicosis in Sheep. *Amer. J. Vet. Res.* 25:1486-94.

Hamdy, A. H Pounden, W. D.; Trapp, A. L.; Bell, D. S.; and Lagace, A. 1963. Effect on Lambs of Selenium Administered to Pregnant Ewes. *JAVMA* 143:749-51.

Hendrick, C. M., and Olson, O. E. 1953. The Effect of Sodium Methyl Arsonate and Calcium Methyl Arsonate on Chronic Selenium Toxicity in the Rat. Proc. South Dakota Acad. Sci 321:68-71.

Kingsbury, J. M. 1964. *Poisonous Plants of the United States and Canada.* Englewood Cliffs, N.J.: Prentice-Hall, pp. 44-50.

Klug, H. L.; Moxon, A. L.; Petersen, D. F.; and Potter, V. R. 1950. The *In Vitro* Inhibition of Succinic Dehydrogenase by Selenium and Its Release by Arsenic. *Arch. Biochem.* 28:253-59.

Knott, S. G.; McCray, C. W. R.; and Hall, W. T. K. 1958. Selenium Poisoning in Horses in North Queensland. *Queensland. J. Agr. Sci.* 15:43-58.

Kubota, J.; Allaway, W. H.; Carter, D. L.; Cary, E. E.; and Lazar, V. A. 1967. Selenium in Crops in the United States in Relation to Selenium-Responsive Diseases of Animals. *Ag. and Food Chem.* 15:448-53.

Levander, O. A., and Argrett, L. C. Effects of Arsenic, Mercury, Thallium, and Lead on Selenium Metabolism in Rats. *Tox. and Appl. Pharmacol.* 14:308-14.

Maag, D. D.; Osborn, J. S.; and Clopton, J. R. 1960. Effect of Sodium Selenite on Cattle. *Amer. J. Vet. Res.* 21:1049-53.

Miller, W. T., and Schoening, H. W. 1938. Toxicity of Selenium Fed to Swine in the Form of Sodium Selenite. *J. Ag. Res.* 56:831-42.

Morrow, D. A. Acute Selenite Toxicosis in Lambs. 1968. *JAVMA* 152:1625-29.

Moxon, A. L. 1937. Alkali Disease or Selenium Poisoning. South Dakota State College. Agricultural Experiment Station Bulletin 311.

————. 1941. Influence of Arsenic on Selenium Poisoning in Hogs. Proc. South Dakota Acad. Sci. 21:34-36.

Munsell, H. E.; DeVaney, G. M.; and Kennedy, M. H. 1936. Toxicity of Food Containing Selenium as Shown by Its Effects on the Rat. USDA Tech. Bull. 534.

Muth, O. H., and Binns, W. 1964. Selenium Toxicity in Domestic Animals. *Veterinary Toxicology. Ann. N.Y. Acad. Sci.* 111:583-90.

National Academy of Sciences, NRC, Committee on Medical and Biologic Effects of Environmental Pollutants, Assembly of Life Sciences. Selenium, Report of Subcommittee. 1975.

Orstadius, K. 1960. Toxicity of a Single Subcutaneous Dose of Sodium Selenite in Pigs. *Nature.* 188:1117.

Patrias, G. 1969. Selenium—A Missing Link in Animal Nutrition. *Feedstuffs.* 41:24-25.

Potter, R. L.; DuBois, K. P.; and Moxon, A. L. 1939. A Comparative Study of Liver Glycogen Values of Control Selenium and Selenium-Arsenic Rats. Proc. South Dakota Acad. Sci. 19:99-106.

Radeleff, R. D. 1970. *Veterinary Toxicology.* Philadelphia: Lea & Febiger, pp. 180-183.

Rigdon, R. H.; Grass, G.; and McConnell, K. P. 1953. Inhibition of Maturation of Duck Erythrocytes by Sodium Selenite. *AMA Arch. Pathol.* 56:374-85.

Rosenfeld, I. 1964. Metabolic Effects and Metabolism of Selenium in Animals. Wyoming Agricultural Experiment Station Bulletin 414, pp. 1-64.

Rosenfeld, I., and Beath, O. A. 1964. The Influence of Protein Diets on Selenium Poisoning. II. The Chemical

Changes in the Tissues Following Selenium Administration. *Amer. J. Vet. Res.* 7:57-61.

———. 1964. *Selenium. Geobotany, Biochemistry, Toxicity, and Nutrition.* New York: Academic Press, 411 pages.

Smith, M. I.; Franke, K. W.; and Westfall, B. B. 1936. The Selenium Problem in Relation to Public Health. A Preliminary Survey to Determine the Possibility of Selenium Intoxication in the Rural Population Living on Seleniferous Soil. U.S. Public Health Report 51:1496-1505.

Toxic Gases

TOXIC GASES

Under unique circumstances there are a large number of gases that could adversely affect the health of domestic animals. Such situations might involve leakage in storage areas, industrial accidents or animals located adjacent to industrial plants. However, there are several toxic gases which are more frequently and more commonly involved in animal poisonings with which the veterinarian should be familiar. These include carbon monoxide (CO), carbon dioxide (CO_2), hydrogen sulfide (H_2S), sulfur oxides (SO_2,SO_3), ammonia (NH_3) and nitrogen dioxide (NO_2). Much of the information in this section was obtained from the review of Lillie, 1970.

One newer source of toxic gases is the slurry tanks used to hold animal wastes in some confinement feeding operations. The four major gases released are carbon dioxide, methane, ammonia and hydrogen sulfide.

Ammonia

Ammonia is liberated from the decomposition of animal wastes and other nitrogenous materials. Ammonia (NH_3), ammonium hydroxide (NH_4OH) and other ammonium salts are also used as fertilizers. Compressed anhydrous ammonia gas (NH_3) is used in large quantities. Exposure to the rapidly released gas from a hose or vent results in freezing of exposed surfaces plus a severe caustic reaction.

Ammonia has been more of a problem with confined poultry than with other animals.

Source

Levels in chicken houses have been reported to be 9-60 mg/m^3 without any apparent harmful effects on broilers. At levels of 40-50 mg/m^3 (60-75 ppm) there is eye irritation that may result in erosion of the cornea. Prolonged exposure to levels of 35 mg/m^3 (50ppm) seems to increase susceptibility to respiratory diseases. Egg production is decreased with levels of 14 mg/m^3 (20 ppm). For comparison, man can detect NH_3 at 15 ppm

(10 mg/m^3) and the eyes burn at 25-35 ppm (17-24 mg/m^3).

Mechanism of Action

NH_3 acts as a mucous membrane irritant. Ammonia in the blood also upsets the acid-base balance which is discussed under urea.

Clinical Signs

The major visible effect in birds is the keratoconjunctivitis. There may be pulmonary edema leading to respiratory distress.

Physiopathology

Inhalation exposure leads to pulmonary edema and congestion, dilation of veins and capillaries and hemorrhage. Prolonged high exposures may cause a purulent tracheitis and bronchopneumonia.

Diagnosis

The diagnosis will be primarily based on the history and field observation. Laboratory analysis will be of limited value in cases of inhalation exposures.

Treatment

The maintenance of adequate ventilation and good sanitary procedures will alleviate the problem. Good ventilation for adult chickens is 1 c.f.m./bird.

Carbon Dioxide

Carbon dioxide (CO_2) results from the *complete* combustion of hydrocarbon fuels. CO_2 is heavier than air and will settle to low spots in a room. The use of unvented space heaters in tightly closed spaces can result in the buildup of CO_2 at the lower spaces of the room. Dry ice can be used as a source of CO_2 for euthanizing small animals.

Toxicity

The relationship between atmospheric CO_2 and effect is given in table 1.

Mechanism of Action

The body normally produces CO_2 which is released from the lungs. A high alveolar CO_2 level prevents the release of CO_2 resulting in CO_2 retention and acidosis. The body tries to compensate by increasing alveolar ventilation to maximal values. But, if atmospheric CO_2 is sufficiently high there is incomplete compensation. This results in tissue pH changes and if severe enough cessation of CNS function and death.

Clinical Signs

Animals may appear anxious and struggle with mild exposures. High exposure results in staggering, incoordination, anesthesia, coma and death. The blood and tissues will be dark.

Diagnosis

Diagnosis will usually be based on the clinical history, clinical signs and lack of other obvious causes. Blood pCO_2 could be measured if suitable equipment is available. Samples would have to be protected from exposure to the air for even brief periods of time.

TABLE 1
Effect of Increasing Levels of Carbon Dioxide

Level	Effect
5%	Tolerated by organism, increase in respiratory rate.
9-10%	Organism is distressed, there is maximal increase in respiration.
15%	Respiratory rate has decreased from peak reached at 9-10%, but is elevated above normal. Considerable distress.
25%	Respiratory rate is near normal and animal goes into coma.
35%	Slow respiratory rate, animal is anesthetized.
40-50%	Death occurs.

Treatment

Treatment is simply to provide fresh air. If the respiratory mechanisms are still intact, the body is able to rapidly eliminate the excess CO_2. Chronic damage may result depending on the severity and duration of apnea.

Carbon Monoxide

Source

Carbon monoxide results from the *incomplete* combustion of hydrocarbon fuels. Poisoning occurs when space heaters or furnaces are operated in tight buildings, such as farrowing houses or lambing sheds, and the heaters are either not vented or are improperly vented. The increased cost of hydrocarbon heating fuels is expected to result in more carbon monoxide toxicoses. As individuals become more energy cost conscious there will be a greater effort to reduce ventilation in buildings during the heating season to reduce heat loss. Sometimes fresh air vents are covered or flue pipes or chimneys become blocked and what was previously a safe operation becomes unsafe. Carbon monoxide is also present in the exhaust fumes of internal combustion engines. Animals have been poisoned when transported in the trunk of a car with a faulty exhaust system. CO is lighter than air and tends to rise to the ceiling in closed rooms.

There is a small amount of endogenously produced CO in mammals which arises from catabolized heme. One mole of CO is formed for each mole of heme degraded. (Landaw, 1970) The hemophagous organ of the placenta of multiparous mamalian species also produces CO as it degrades hemoglobin and glycoglobulin hemochromogens, probably as part of a physiologic mechanism to increase the supply of iron for the fetus. This endogenous CO production results in COHb levels of 0.5-3 percent. When COHb levels reach 12 percent the oxidase systems involved in hemoglobin degradation to CO are inhibited.

Ambient background levels of CO are 0.02 ppm in fresh air, 13 ppm in metropolitan city streets and 40 ppm in areas with high vehicular traffic.

Toxicity

The toxicity of CO to some domestic animals is shown in table 2. The decreasing order of CO toxicity is canary, mouse, chicken, small dog, pigeon, guinea pig and rabbit. The dog is more sensitive than man.

Based on COHb levels the following effects can be expected to occur with various levels of CO exposure.

TABLE 2
Toxicity of Carbon Monoxide

Species	Dose	Effect
Dog	0.05-1% (570-11,000 mg/m^3) for one hour	Decreased heart excitability
Dog	0.37% (4200 mg/m^3) for 1-2 hours	70% carboxyhemoglobin and apnea
Dog	0.01% (115 mg/m^3) for 5 hrs/day for 11 weeks	20% carboxyhemoglobin, disturbance of gait and position reflexes. Changes in ECG, brain lesions.
Chicken	160 ppm (183 mg/m^3) for 7 days	No effect
Chicken	600 ppm (687 mg/m^3) for 30 minutes	Distress
Chicken	2000-3600 ppm (2200-4120 mg/m^3)	Death in 1.5-2 hours

At 1-3 percent COHb no effects are observed or changes that have been reported are either mild or have not been replicated. At 6-8 percent COHb there is a decreased ability to maintain attention. At 20 percent COHb there is definite psychomotor disturbance. At 20-40 percent COHb there is lethargy, disturbance in gait and changes in EEG from an arousal to a slow wave plus spindle pattern. Death occurs with 60-70 percent COHb.

The amount of COHb formed depends on the length of exposure and the CO level. Considering levels of COHb associated with recognizable clinical illness (30% COHb) the time and CO level interactions are: one hour at 1,200 ppm (0.12%), two hours at 600 ppm (.06%), four hours at 400 ppm (.04%) and infinite time at 200 ppm (.02%). The higher the level the shorter the exposure time necessary to result in formation of 30 percent COHb.

Mechanism of Action

CO competes with O_2 for binding of such proteins as hemoglobins, myoglobins, cytochrome-c oxidase and cytochrome P450. The relative affinities vary ranging from 200 times as much binding of CO as O_2 in hemoglobin, to 30-50 times for myoglobins to less CO than O_2 affinity for cytochromes. CO binds in a competitive fashion at the oxygen site on hemoglobin.

CO combines with hemoglobin with 200 times the affinity of O_2. This blocks the transfer of O_2 from the lungs to the tissues and results in hypoxia. In addition, the oxygen dissociation curve is shifted to the left meaning that the release of O_2 from hemoglobin to tissues is impaired.

The O_2 carrying capacity of the remaining unreacted Fe(II) sites on a hemoglobin molecule is reduced if CO is present at one of the heme sites. Additionally, if O_2 is already present then the addition of CO results in a tighter bond of the already existing O_2 associated with the heme molecule.

Most of the body CO load is found in blood and is chemically bound to hemoglobin. Anywhere from 10-25 percent is located in extravascular tissues involving myoglobin, cytochromes, catalase and peroxidases. Very little CO is dissolved in body fluids. Mitochondrial respiration is not impaired if carboxyhemoglobin levels are 30 percent or less.

The CO binding to myoglobin is three times higher for myocardial muscle than skeletal muscle. The relationship between %CO saturation of hemoglobin and myoglobin is about 1:1 for skeletal muscle and 1:3 for cardiac muscle. Thus, if the COHb level is 10 percent then about 10 percent of skeletal myoglobin and 30 percent of cardiac myoglobin is saturated. Under conditions of reduced arterial PO$_2$ there is a shift of CO from Hb to myoglobin.

Fetal Hemoglobin and CO

Fetal hemoglobins have been identified for the following (The time that the fetal type disappears is given after each animal): calf (8-10 weeks postnatal), lamb (40-50 days postnatal), goat (after 60 days postnatal), and deer (8-12 weeks postnatal). Fetal and adult hemoglobins are the same for the pig, dog and cat. (Kitchen and Brett, 1974)

Most adult mammals have a high level of 2, 3-diphosphoglycerate (DPG) except for the cat, sheep, cow and goat which contain barely measurable levels. In the cat and the above ruminants hemoglobin has an intrinsically low oxygen affinity that does not interact with DPG. In the other species with high red cell DPG levels the hemoglobin has an intrinsically high oxygen affinity, which is markedly lowered by addition of DPG.

Fetal hemoglobin (Hb-F) is different than adult hemoglobin (Hb-A). Fetal hemoglobin is replaced by Hb-A after birth over a period of several months. The oxygen affinity of fetal blood is significantly greater than that of adult blood. In the sheep and goat the fetal hemoglobins have an intrinsically greater oxygen affinity than do adult hemoglobins, whereas in the horse, pig and dog fetal erythrocytes simply contain less DPG than their adult counterparts. (Bunn and Kitchen, 1973) DPG is produced by the catabolism of D-glucose and represents approximately 15 percent of the anionic content of the erythrocyte. The DPG interacellular concentration is nearly equimolar with hemoglobin. The DPG bonds with deoxyhemoglobin. DPG bonding with hemoglobin has the overall effect of lowering the affinity of Hb for O_2. At high PO_2, such as 100 mm Hg as in the alveoli, the Hb is nearly 100 percent O_2 saturated. At the tissues as the PO_2 falls to 40 mm Hg, the DPG binds with the deoxyhemoglobin thus reducing the affinity of hemoglobin for the reduced amount of available O_2. The net effect is to facilitate the movement of O_2 from the blood to the tissues.

The presence of 10 percent COHb shifts the O_2-hemoglobin dissociation curve to the left. This means that the O_2 tension in the tissue must be lower than normal before a given amount of O_2 will unload from hemoglobin. The usual comparative value is the P_{50} that is, the PO_2 associated with 50 percent saturation of hemoglobin. In maternal blood the P_{50} falls from 26.5 to 21 mm Hg and in the fetus the P_{50} falls from 20 to 15.5 mm Hg when there is 10 percent COHb. All of this interacts to reduce O_2 delivery to the fetus up to 40 percent.

Not only are there direct effects on the fetus but the metabolic function of the placenta may also be adversely affected.

Chronic exposure to CO may result in small litters based on experimental work with rats. However, exposure to 50 ppm during gestation did not effect reproduction in mice. The effects of CO on the development of the fetus and postnatal development have not been adequately studied.

The ratio of COHb-fetus to COHb-maternal varies from 0.6-2.2. Sheep, dogs and rabbits have higher ratios (2.2) because of the high O_2 affinity of fetal blood in these species. There is a delay in the placental transfer of CO. Following acute exposure maternal COHb levels peak in 5-10 minutes. Fetal COHb peaks after 2-4 hours. At four hours postexposure the fetal level is twice the maternal level and may be higher than the initial peak maternal level. The disappearance of COHb follows a first-order rate reaction with a half-time of two hours. Fetal COHb levels of 20-50 percent have resulted in stillbirths in humans. Liveborn offspring may subsequently develop neurologic sequelae, brain damage and die.

Clinical Signs

With high exposures death may occur rapidly. Lower exposures result in drowsiness, disorientation, incoordination, dyspenea and coma.

The tissues are pink and the blood becomes cherry red, which should serve as an immediate clue to aid in identifying the problem.

Physiopathology

The physiologic and pathologic changes observed are thought to be the direct results of hypoxia.

Changes in the ECG are thought to reflect necrosis of single heart muscle fibers.

Histological changes in the brain appear as necrosis in the cortex and white matter of the cerebral hemispheres, the globus pallidus and the brain stem. Also reported are edema and hemorrhage in the brain and necrosis in Ammon's horn of the hippocampus. Demyelination has also been reported.

Respiratory alkalosis occurs from hyperventilation caused by a metabolic acidosis. There is no evidence of CO_2 retention.

At postmortem the bronchi are dilated and major blood vessels may be distended.

The brain lesions may result in permanent damage manifested as deafness in dogs and cats.

Diagnosis

The bright cherry red color of the blood, lungs and general body tissues should cause one to suspect CO poisoning. This should be differentiated, usually by the species and history, from HCN toxicosis.

The presence of CO can be confirmed by measuring COHb. In lethal exposures the hemoglobin will be 60-70 percent saturated as COHb.

Treatment

The objective in treating CO poisoning is to restore an adequate O_2 supply to the brain and heart. A mixture of CO_2 plus O_2 is more effective than O_2 alone. The mixture commonly used is called carbogen and consists of 5-7 percent CO_2 plus 95-93 percent O_2.

Dogs have been shown to survive high acute CO exposure without brain damage resulting if they are kept under deep amobarbital anesthesia. (Rosenthal *et al.*, 1945)

Hydrogen Sulfide

Source

Hydrogen sulfide (H_2S) is a toxic gas released from the decomposition of organic matter containing sulfur. In veterinary medicine the major source is from slurry tanks, especially following agitation of the tank. Of the four toxic gases released from slurry pits H_2S is thought to be the major cause of deaths in exposed animals.

Toxicity

Fatalities occur following sudden exposure to 400 ppm (556 mg/m^3) or more. There do not appear to be overt chronic effects. However, changes in lung tissue enzyme levels have been reported following exposure at 100 mg/m^3 without apparent gross effects.

Mechanism of Action

Death occurs rapidly following exposure to high levels. Death may follow after only a few breaths. Respiration ceases rapidly and artificial respiration does not prevent death in H_2S intoxicated animals.

Clinical Signs

Prior to rapid death there may be a period of tetanic spasms and unconsciousness.

Physiopathology

Histologic examination of lung tissue reveals deterioration. The tissues are cyanotic and the lungs may be gray and edematous.

Diagnosis

The circumstantial evidence, history of rapid deaths and elimination of other causes of rapid death will help in making a diagnosis.

Treatment

As with most toxic gases treatment consists of adequate ventilation. In addition it may be necessary to install gas traps which prevent slurry gases from entering the animal quarters. The design of the physical facilities will dictate the changes required to prevent recurrence.

Nitrogen Dioxide

Source

On occasion a yellow or yellow brown gas has been observed seeping from silos. This gas has been identified as NO_2. Cattle, pigs, and chickens have been reported to die rapidly from exposure to this gas. Because of similarities between "silo fillers" disease in man and bovine pulmonary adenomatosis it has been postulated that NO_2 is the causative agent in both diseases.

It is postulated that high rates of nitrate fertilization increase the nitrate contents of plants. When the forage is placed in the silo and fermented, the nitrates are converted to nitric acid which then breaks down to release NO and NO_2.

Toxicity

Levels in silo gas have reached 100-150 ppm NO_2. The safety limit value for continuous exposure is only 1 ppm. Animals have survived exposures of 25 ppm.

A 12-week exposure to 8-12 ppm was lethal in about 50 percent of exposed rabbits.

Some evidence suggests that exposure to a few ppm is sufficient to lower resistance to respiratory diseases.

Mechanism of Action

The mechanism of action is poorly understood. There are pulmonary lesions, peroxidative changes in pulmonary lipids and changes in mechanical pulmonary resistance.

Clinical Signs

Acute exposure is followed by coughing and panting. Exposure to fresh air may not prevent deaths from occurring several hours later. Affected cows show elevated temperature, hypersalivation and severe dyspnea. In experimental exposures deaths occurred 3-25 days after exposure.

Physiopathology

In the bovine, experimental NO_2 exposures resulted in apnea, progressive dyspnea, lacrimation, excessive salivation, grunting, reduced feed and water consumption, emaciation and dehydration. The hematologic response was an increase in lymphocytes and a decrease in neutrophils.

The pathologic changes included methemoglobinemia, dark red kidneys and necrosis of skeletal muscles. Pulmonary lesions were hyperemia, edema, hemorrhage, fibrin deposition, hyperplasia, bronchiolitis, infarction and emphysema. The investigator concluded that NO_2 was not the cause of bovine pulmonary adenomatosis. (Cutlip, 1966)

One of the confounding facets of "silo fillers" disease has been the reports where cattle maintained outside in fresh air but which have been fed the silage have developed the disease just as if they stood by the silo and breathed the NO_2 gas.

Diagnosis

Inhalation of NO_2 results in severe lung damage which coupled with a history of exposure will serve as the basis for a diagnosis.

Additionally, KI-starch paper can be used to detect the presence of NO_2. The paper turns dark when exposed to NO_2. The KI-starch paper is available commercially and could be used by farmers before entering a silo.

Treatment

There is no reported treatment. Even animals given fresh air immediately after exposure may die in a few hours to several days.

Sulfur Oxides

Sulfur dioxide (SO_2) and sulfur trioxide (SO_3) are the two sulfur oxides of greatest concern in air pollution.

Sulfur oxides plus H_2SO_4 mist are thought to be major factors in deaths associated with major air pollution episodes. Both man and animals have died in these killer smogs.

Toxicity

The feeding of SO_2 damaged forage did not adversely affect the performance of dairy cattle. Forage containing 1,700-2,500 ppm H_2SO_4, formed from SO_2 emissions, was toxic to grazing livestock.

A single exposure to 5 ppm SO_2 results in eye irritation and salivation. Hemorrhage and emphysema occurs within 24 hours after an eight hour exposure to 40 ppm SO_2.

H_2SO_4 is more toxic than SO_2. The guinea pig is most sensitive, as it is killed by a three hour exposure to 22 ppm H_2SO_4/m^3.

Clinical Signs

At low concentrations there is eye and nasal irritation. Higher levels produce severe respiratory distress and deaths.

Physiopathology

In addition to the mucous membrane irritation of the eye and nose, hemorrhage and emphysema occur in the lung.

Chronic effects also occur. Two pigs exposed for a single eight hour exposure to 40 ppm SO_2 developed pulmonary fibrosis within 160 days postexposure.

In laboratory animals chronic exposures to SO_2 leads to decreases in cholinesterase, spleen dehydrase and carbohydrase and decreases in vitamin C content of several organs.

H_2SO_4 causes laryngeal spasm and deep lung damage. Lung damage includes degeneration of respiratory tract epithelium, hyperemia, edema, emphysema, atelectasis and occasionally hemorrhage.

Diagnosis

The diagnosis will be based on a history of exposure and the presence of pulmonary changes.

Treatment

There is no specific treatment.

REFERENCES

Biological Effects of Carbon Monoxide. 1970. R. F. Coburn, ed. *Annals New York Academy Sciences,* 174.

Bunn, H. F., and Kitchen, H. 1973. Hemoglobin Function in the Horse. The Role of 2, 3-diphosphoglycerate in Modifying the Oxygen Affinity of Maternal and Fetal Blood. *Blood* 42:471.

Cutlip, R. C. 1966. Experimental Nitrogen Dioxide Poisoning in Cattle. *Path. Vet.* 3:474.

George, M. E.; Murphy, J. P. F.; and Back, K. C. 1970. Effects of Carbon Monoxide on Brain Cellular Metabolism in Monkeys. AMRL-TR-70-88. Wright-Patterson Air Force Base, Ohio.

Hemoglobin: Comparative Molecular Biology Models for the

Study of Disease. 1974. H. Kitchen and S. Boyer eds., *New York Academy of Sciences*

Kitchen, H., and Brett, I. 1974. Embryonic and Fetal Hemoglobin in Animals. *Annals New York Academy Sciences* 241:653-71.

Landaw, S. A. 1970. Kinetic Aspects of Endogenous Carbon Monoxide Production in Experimental Animals. *Annals New York Academy Sciences* 174:32-48.

Lillie, R. J. 1970. Air Pollutants Affecting the Performance of Domestic Animals. A Literature Review. *Agriculture Handbook No. 380.* USDA.

Longo, L. D. 1970. Carbon Monoxide in the Pregnant Mother and Fetus and its Exchange Across the Placenta. *Annals New York Academy Sciences* 174:313-41.

Montgomery, R., *et al.,* 1974. *Biochemistry.* St. Louis, Missouri: C. V. Mosby Co.

Rosenthal, O.; Shenkin, H.; and Drabkin, D. L. 1945. Oxidation of Pyruvate and Glucose in Brain Suspensions from Animals Subjected to Irreversible Hemorrhagic Shock, Carbon Monoxide Poisoning on Temporary Arrest of the Circulation. A Study of the Effect of Anoxia. *Amer. J. Physiol.* 144:334-47.

Miscellaneous Chemicals

CORROSIVES
(ACIDS, ALKALIS, AND PHENOLS)

Occasionally, dogs ingest or are accidentally medicated with products containing strong bases, or phenols. Phenolic compounds are frequently present in ointments that may be used by uninformed individuals. At times, coal tar products become harmful when used for bathing animals to control external parasites or in the treatment of skin problems.

Strong acids, bases, and phenols have a primary corrosive action in the gastrointestinal mucosa or the skin. The immediate effect of ingestion is vomition resulting from the necrotizing effect on the mucosa. Less concentrated phenolic compounds cause little local irritation; however, they are general cellular poisons and may profoundly affect the liver and kidneys.

Signs following ingestion of corrosive materials include severe abdominal pain and stomatitis. There is a grayish-white or red color of the tongue, pharynx, and esophageal mucosa. Sometimes the lesions turn black and become wrinkled. Vomiting is stimulated by the corrosive action, and a severe thirst develops; there is circulatory collapse and death from asphyxia because of swelling of the glottis or larynx. If there is skin exposure, the lesions may vary from mild dermatitis to severe corrosion of the skin and systemic intoxication.

Ingestion of noncorrosive concentrations of phenols may result in loss of appetite, depression, weakness, icterus, and anemia. Convulsive seizures, coma, and death may be seen, especially in cats.

Lesions produced by acids, alkalis, and phenols depend upon the route of exposure. Corrosive compounds severely corrode the oral cavity, pharynx, larynx, esophagus, and stomach. These tissues may be edematous and hemorrhagic. The phenolic compounds cause severe centrilobular hyperemia, fatty degeneration, and necrosis of the liver. Nephritis is also often seen. Treatment should be directed toward removal of the offending agent. If the material has been ingested, milk or egg whites should be given immediately to inactivate the corrosive material. Following this, efforts should be made to remove the inactivated material from the stomach, either by gastric lavage or the use of emetics. If the corrosive material is on the skin, dilute the toxicant with warm, soapy water. Ethyl alcohol applied to the skin will neutralize the toxic effects of phenol but should not be given internally because then phenol and alcohol are rapidly absorbed. Symptomatic treatment should include CNS stimulants, parenteral injection of electrolytes if dehydration is present, administration of B vitamins, and placing of the patient in warm, comfortable surroundings.

Strong bases may be neutralized by vinegar or 5 percent acetic acid. If the toxic agent is acid, 5 percent sodium bicarbonate can be used to neutralize dermal exposure.

The damaged skin or gastrointestinal mucosa should be protected as much as possible. Antibiotic ointments should be applied to the skin. Emollients containing antibotics should be used to treat the damaged mucosa.

REFERENCE

Clarke, E G. C., and Clarke, M. L. 1967. *Garner's Veterinary Toxicology*. 3rd ed. Baltimore: The Williams & Wilkins Co.

COAL-TAR, PHENOL

Coal-tar poisoning is an acute and often fatal disease. Its clinical course usually progresses without noticeable physical symptoms, death often being the first sign of illness. Lesions of the liver are perhaps the most important indication of the disease. Clay pigeon poisoning and pitch poisoning are other names used to designate this disease.

Source and Toxicity

Poisonous substances in coal-tar pitch are the primary etiological factors. Coal-tar is a mixture of condensable volatile products formed during the destructive distillation of bituminous coal. The composition is variable but generally it consists of: 2-8 percent light oils, chiefly phenols, cresols, and naphthalene; 8-10 percent heavy oils (naphthalene and derivatives); 16-20 percent anthracene oils (mostly anthracene); and about 50 percent pitch. Phenols and their congeners have the highest acute toxicity.

Quinn and Shoeman (1933) described a disease of the liver in swine as an idiopathic hemorrhagic hepatitis for which a cause had not been found; although subsequently, they implicated clay pigeons. Graham, et al., (1940) were the first to discover that this degenerative liver disease resulted from the ingestion of expended clay pigeons.

After correlating the ingestion of clay fragments with the occurrence of the disease, Graham, et al., undertook to prove the toxicity of some of the suspected material that was obtained from a farm where pigs had died from coal-tar pitch poisoning. A group of five nine-week-old pigs were fed a diet composed of corn, oats, wheat middlings, tankage, minerals, and cod liver oil to which was added a measured quantity of powdered clay pigeons. The test substance was fed at the rate of 15 grams per pig per day. On the fourth day of the trial the pigs refused the feed mixture. Each was then given 6 grams of the powdered clay pigeons in a gelatin capsule for another two days. All five pigs died 8-20 days later. At necropsy, four showed evidence of liver injury, but no noticeable lesions were observed in

the remaining pig. This placed the burden of cause on the clay pigeons. Since they were prepared from a mixture of finely powdered limestone and coal-tar pitch, the next move was to study the pitch.

A liquid coal-tar preparation was put in gelatin capsules and administered to young pigs. Three grams were given to each of three pigs for five successive days, and all died within 10-18 days. Pronounced diffuse degenerative changes in the liver were found at necropsy. The researchers concluded that coal-tar pitch in clay pigeons caused toxicosis in swine if consumed for a period of several days in daily amounts of approximately 15 grams.

Since that time, Giffee (1945), Fenstermacher, et al., (1945), Schopen, et al., (1955), Beer (1956), and Fleischer and Schulte (1956) have reported losses in swine from coal-tar pitch poisoning. Thamm (1956) reported that floor slabs containing as little as 1/3 lignite tar pitch caused a 20-28 percent reduction in growth rate of pigs kept in sties floored with the slabs; pigs developed liver dystrophy and nephritis. Reuss (1956) mentioned that the clinical and postmortem findings in pigs kept on floors constructed from tar-containing slabs and cement were similar to those seen in natural cases. The condition was less marked in pigs kept on tar-containing slabs set in concrete. Control pigs confined to a floor consisting entirely of concrete remained healthy. Coal-tar pitch poisoning has been reported from the USA, Canada, Northern Ireland, Germany, and Poland.

Other sources of coal-tar pitch considered to be responsible for fatal cases of this liver disease have been reported. Giffee (1945) described cases that appeared to have been due to the consumption of tar that was used for sealing and surfacing a pipeline for the transportation of gas. The history of a case examined by the author suggests a similar source. In this instance the affected pigs had "chewed off" and consumed the tar substance on lumber dismantled from a tank that had been used for storing water. The pigs had access to the tar from this source for two or three weeks prior to their sudden death. In another of our cases the cause of death was traced to a tarry sludge contaminating a small area of pasture lot occupied by the affected pigs. The sludge or residue came from an establishment engaged in cleaning and restoring steel drum containers which had been collected from many different sources and which had been used for various purposes. A spillover from a drainage ditch carrying wastes from this establishment had flooded the area of the pasture and left shallow pools of oily water that slowly seeped away leaving a tarry sludge or residue on the surface of the soil. The source was not detected until the pasture had been carefully inspected. None of the adjoining, uncontaminated lots contained affected pigs.

Another interesting case, reported by Fenstermacher, et al., (1945), showed the necessity of continuing the search for a likely source of coal-tar pitch poisoning. The history disclosed that the pigs had developed a habit of eating tarred paper which had been placed around the base of several farm buildings as a protection against low temperatures and frost. Schipper and Anders (1959) mentioned a case where sows due to farrow in a few days were placed in crates with wooden floors freshly treated with preservatives containing pentachlorophenol or creosote. Many stillbirths occurred. The piglets were unthrifty and many died. Burns and necrosis of the udder of the sows and of the face of the piglets were seen. No toxicosis was seen when straw bedding was provided. Schiffer (1961) mentioned that such wood preservatives might prove extremely toxic to young pigs. The degree of toxicity lessened as the pigs grew older.

Flooring prepared from lignite pitch and bitumen was harmful because of the high phenol content (highest measured was 438 mg%); mineral-oil bitumen flooring materials were not toxic. Amounts of phenolic constituents of over 6 mg% were toxic, particularly for pigs up to 4 kg body weight. On floors with phenol content of 4.5 mg% piglets remained healthy. (Rummler, 1962) Libke, et al., (1967) fed 21 pigs, aged 8-9 weeks, on finely ground "clay pigeon" material until death or the end of a 14-day period, when the survivors were killed. All the pigs, on postmortem examination, showed centrilobular necrosis with subsequent intralobular hemorrhage. Our own experience and the experience of others with whom we have communicated indicate that clay pigeons are the source of the toxic compound in most outbreaks.

Cats are especially susceptible to the toxic effects of phenolic compounds, because of their inability to detoxify and excrete phenol from the blood. (Oehme, 1971)

Clinical Signs

The sudden death and rapid clinical course of this disease often occurs without the appearance of symptoms of diagnostic significance. Under these circumstances, death is the only physical sign indicative of the existence of a morbid process. However, some animals live for several hours or even days after the clinical onset, in which case the affected animals usually show signs of physical weakness and depression. They are recumbent much of the time and generally lie in the sternal position. Respiration rate is increased and a tenderness over the abdomen can be detected by digital palpitation. The disease is afebrile. A secondary anemia usually develops and the visible mucous membranes are icteric. The mucous membranes of the mouth and eyes are discolored by the bile pigments in the circulating blood. The respiratory rate may be increased and a "thumpy" type of breathing may be apparent. A high portion of the pigs that manifest these symptoms die.

Physiopathology

The outstanding lesion observed at necropsy in pigs poisoned with coal-tar pitch is the altered appearance of the liver. When the abdominal cavity of a pig with a typical and fully developed case of a coal-tar pitch poisoning is opened, the greatly enlarged liver with a varigated mottling makes a striking pathological picture. It is engorged and quite friable. The lobular architecture of the liver is very distinct. Some of the lobules are dark red in color and others are yellow with a shading toward a copper-colored tint. The intensity of the color varies between these extremes in other affected lobules. This accounts for the characteristic varigated mottling that stands out so sharply. When the liver is sliced, the mottling shows up distinctly on the cut surfaces. An excess of fluid in the peritoneal cavity is not uncommon. The lymph nodes of the abdominal cavity are swollen and hemorrhagic. As a rule, the kidneys are enlarged and turgid and somewhat pale in color. No other significant lesions have been found in the other organs or tissues. The subcutaneous tissue and mucous membranes are frequently yellowish or orange, indicative of a jaundiced condition. The necrosis of the liver cells and vascular tissues of the lobules allows bile to enter the circulation. Its subsequent distribution throughout the body produces jaundice.

From the standpoint of microscopic changes, the lobules are either partially or almost completely filled with blood. Generally the hemorrhage begins at the center of the lobule and extends towards the periphery, but sometimes it occurs only in the midzonal portion. The red cells in some lobules show evidence of destruction and lysis with the presence of hemosiderin. Other lobules show the changes characteristic of a central necrosis in which the cells of the liver cords are swollen and have a very granular cytoplasm with small and densely stained nuclei. Some cells may have undergone autolysis and appear as an amorphous substance.

Diagnosis

Diagnosis is based on history of access to coal-tar derivatives, clinical symptoms, severe hepatic centrilobular necrosis with subsequent intralobular hemorrhage and other postmortem lesions, and chemical identification of phenol or pitch derivatives.

Treatment

There is no specific treatment known for this disease. The use of demulcents and gastric lavage is helpful. When its presence in a herd is recognized, it is advisable to determine the source of the offending compound and take necessary steps to prevent the pigs from coming in contact with it. In the case of animals affected with it, the skin should be washed with soap and water to remove phenol. Local application of petrolatum base ointments may prove useful. Other symptomatic treatment may be carried out as deemed necessary.

It is important to know that a pasture can be contaminated with coal-tar pitch for long periods of time. The history on one of our cases revealed that approximately 35 years prior to the occurrence of coal-tar pitch poisoning an area of the pasture where the losses were occurring had been used as a target range for shooting clay pigeons. More often, however, the history indicates that it is a period of a year or two since the contamination occurred.

BIBLIOGRAPHY

Aitken, W. A. 1956. Coal-Tar Poisoning in Pigs. *JAVMA* 128:262.

Beer, J. 1956. Schwere Gesundheitschadigung bei Schweinen dwich Fussbodenbelag aus Branknohlenterrhartpech. *Arch. Exp. Vet. Med.* 10:321.

Buck, W. B., and Kernkamp, H. C. H. 1970. Coal-Tar Poisoning and Mercury Poisoning, in *Diseases of Swine*. H. W. Dunne, ed. 3rd ed. Ames, Iowa: Iowa State University Press.

Fleischer, R., and Schulte, F. 1956. Weiterer Beitrag uber die Gesundheitsschadliche Wirkung Teerhaltiger Stallfussbodenplatten auf Jungschweine. *Tiererztl. Umsch.* 11:250.

Giffee, J. W. 1945. Clay Pigeon (Coal-Tar) Poisoning in Swine. *JAVMA.* 96:135.

Libke, K. G., and Davis, J. W. 1967. Hepatic Necrosis in Swine Caused by Feeding Clay Pigeon Targets. *JAVMA* 151:426.

Quinn, A. H., and Shoeman, J. D. 1933. Idiopathic Hemorrhagic Hepatitis. *JAVMA* 82:707.

Reuss, U. 1956. Tierhygienische Erfahrungen mit Neuzeitlichen Stallfussbodenplatten in Schweinestall. *Berl. Munch Tierarztl. Wschr.* 69:343.

Rummler, H. J. 1962. Uber Terrpech-und Bitumenhalatige Fubbodenbelage in Schweinestallumgens. *Mh. Vet. Med.* 17:482.

Schipper, I. A. 1961. Toxicity of Wood Preservatives for Swine. *Am. J. Vet. Res.* 22:401.

Schipper, I. A., and Anders, R. 1959. Toxicity of Wood Preservatives to Swine. *Bi. M. Bull. N. Dak. Fm. Res.* 21:8.

Thamm, H. 1956. Versuche uber die Einwirkungen Teerhaltiger Stallbodenplatten auf die Gesundheit der Schweine. *Arch. Exp. Vet. Med.* 10:321.

Oehme, F. W. 1971. New Information on the Toxicity of Phenolic Compounds in Small Animals. *Gaines Newer Knowledge about Dogs.* 21:8-15.

INDEX